T0200197

THE WASHINGTON MANUAL®

Endocrinology

FOURTH EDITION

THE WASHINGTON MANUAL®

Endocrinology

FOURTH EDITION

Editors

Thomas J. Baranski, MD, PhD

*Associate Professor of Medicine
and Developmental Biology*
Division of Endocrinology, Metabolism,
and Lipid Research
Washington University School of Medicine
St. Louis, Missouri

Janet B. McGill, MD, MA, FACE

Professor of Medicine
Division of Endocrinology, Metabolism,
and Lipid Research
Washington University School of Medicine
St. Louis, Missouri

Julie M. Silverstein, MD

*Associate Professor of Medicine
and Neurological Surgery*
Division of Endocrinology, Metabolism,
and Lipid Research
Washington University School of Medicine
St. Louis, Missouri

Series Editors

Thomas M. De Fer, MD, FACP

Executive Editor
Professor of Medicine
Associate Dean for Medical Student
Education
Department of Medicine
Division of Medical Education
Washington University School of Medicine
St. Louis, Missouri

Thomas M. Ciesielski, MD

Assistant Professor of Medicine
Associate Program Director
Department of Medicine
Division of Medical Education
Washington University School of Medicine
St. Louis, Missouri

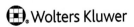 Wolters Kluwer

Philadelphia • Baltimore • New York • London
Buenos Aires • Hong Kong • Sydney • Tokyo

Acquisitions Editor: Rebecca Gaertner
Product Development Editor: Liz Schaeffer
Editorial Coordinators: Tim Rinehart, Katie Sharp
Marketing Manager: Rachel Mante Leung
Production Project Manager: Kim Cox
Design Coordinator: Joan Wendt
Manufacturing Coordinator: Beth Welsh
Prepress Vendor: Aptara, Inc.

4th edition

10 9 8 7

Printed in the United States of America

Library of Congress Cataloging-in-Publication Data

Names: Baranski, Thomas J., editor. | McGill, Janet B., editor. |
  Silverstein, Julie M., editor. | Washington University (Saint Louis, Mo.).
  School of Medicine, issuing body.
Title: Washington manual endocrinology subspecialty consult / editors,
Thomas
  J. Baranski, Janet B. McGill, Julie M. Silverstein.
Other titles: Endocrinology subspecialty consult | Washington manual
  subspecialty consult series.
Description: Fourth edition. | Philadelphia : Wolters Kluwer, [2020] |
  Series: Washington manual subspecialty consult series | Includes
  bibliographical references and index.
Identifiers: LCCN 2018060345 | ISBN 9781975113339 (paperback)
Subjects: | MESH: Endocrine System Diseases | Metabolic Diseases | Handbook
Classification: LCC RC648 | NLM WK 39 | DDC 616.4/8–dc23 LC record
available at https://lccn.loc.gov/2018060345

shop.lww.com

Contributing Authors

Ana Maria Arbelaez, MD
Associate Professor of Pediatrics
Division of Pediatric Endocrinology and
    Diabetes
Washington University School of Medicine
St. Louis, Missouri

Thomas J. Baranski, MD, PhD
*Associate Professor of Medicine and
    Developmental Biology*
Division of Endocrinology, Metabolism,
    and Lipid Research
Washington University School of Medicine
St. Louis, Missouri

Kevin T. Bauerle, MD, PhD
Clinical Fellow
Division of Endocrinology, Metabolism,
    and Lipid Research
Washington University School of Medicine
St. Louis, Missouri

Carlos Bernal-Mizrachi, MD
*Chief of Endocrinology, John Cochran
    Division, VA Medical Center*
Philip E. and Carolyn E. Cryer Professor in
    Medicine, Cell Biology, and Physiology
Division of Endocrinology, Metabolism, and
    Lipid Research
Washington University School of Medicine
St. Louis, Missouri

Conor J. Best, MD
Assistant Professor of Medicine
Department of Endocrine Neoplasia
    and Hormonal Disorders
University of Texas MD Anderson Cancer Center
Houston, Texas

Paulina Cruz Bravo, MD
Assistant Professor of Medicine
Division of Endocrinology, Metabolism,
    and Lipid Research
Washington University School of Medicine
St. Louis, Missouri

Kim Carmichael, MD, FACP
Professor of Medicine
Division of Endocrinology, Metabolism,
    and Lipid Research
Washington University School of Medicine
St. Louis, Missouri

Jacqueline L. Cartier, MD
Clinical Fellow
Division of Endocrinology, Metabolism,
    and Lipid Research
Washington University School of Medicine
St. Louis, Missouri

Roberto Civitelli, MD
*Sydney M. and Stella H. Schoenberg
    Professor of Medicine*
Professor of Orthopaedic Surgery and of
    Cell Biology and Physiology
Chief, Division of Bone and Mineral Diseases
Department of Medicine
Musculoskeletal Research Center
Washington University School of Medicine
St. Louis, Missouri

William E. Clutter, MD
Associate Professor of Medicine
Department of Medicine
Division of Medical Education
Washington University School of Medicine
St. Louis, Missouri

Philip E. Cryer, MD
Professor, Emeritus of Medicine
Division of Endocrinology, Metabolism,
    and Lipid Research
Washington University School of Medicine
St. Louis, Missouri

Cecilia A. Davis, MD
Clinical Fellow
Division of Endocrinology, Metabolism,
    and Lipid Research
Washington University School of Medicine
St. Louis, Missouri

Laura T. Dickens, MD
Clinical Instructor, Endocrinology Fellow
Section of Pediatric and Adult
    Endocrinology, Diabetes, and Metabolism
Kovler Diabetes Center
The University of Chicago Medicine
Chicago, Illinois

Kathryn Diemer, MD
Professor of Medicine
Division of Bone and Mineral Diseases
Washington University School of Medicine
St. Louis, Missouri

Julia P. Dunn, MD
Assistant Professor of Medicine
Division of Endocrinology, Metabolism,
    and Lipid Research
Washington University School of Medicine
Staff Physician
Division of Medicine, Endocrine Section
VA St. Louis Health Care System
St. Louis, Missouri

Anne C. Goldberg, MD, FACP, FAHA
Professor of Medicine
Division of Endocrinology, Metabolism, and
    Lipid Research
Washington University School of Medicine
St. Louis, Missouri

Andrea Granados, MD
Instructor in Pediatrics
Division of Pediatric Endocrinology and
    Diabetes
Washington University School of Medicine
St. Louis, Missouri

Charles A. Harris, MD, PhD
Assistant Professor of Medicine
Division of Endocrinology, Metabolism,
    and Lipid Research
Washington University School of Medicine
St. Louis, Missouri

Cynthia J. Herrick, MD, MPHS
Assistant Professor of Medicine
Division of Endocrinology, Metabolism, and
    Lipid Research
Assistant Professor of Surgery
Division of Public Health Sciences
Washington University School of Medicine
St. Louis, Missouri

Karin Hickey, MD
Instructor in Medicine
Division of Endocrinology, Metabolism,
    and Lipid Research
Division of Medical Oncology
Washington University School of Medicine
St. Louis, Missouri

Laura N. Hollar, MD
Clinical Fellow
Division of Endocrinology, Metabolism,
    and Lipid Research
Washington University School of Medicine
St. Louis, Missouri

Jing W. Hughes, MD, PhD
Instructor in Medicine
Division of Endocrinology, Metabolism,
    and Lipid Research
Washington University School of Medicine
St. Louis, Missouri

Sina Jasim, MD, MPH
Assistant Professor of Medicine
Division of Endocrinology, Metabolism,
    and Lipid Research
Washington University School of Medicine
St. Louis, Missouri

Emily S. Jungheim, MD
*Associate Professor of Obstetrics and
    Gynecology*
Division of Reproductive Endocrinology
    and Infertility
Washington University School of Medicine
St. Louis, Missouri

Christopher Lewis, MD
Instructor in Pediatrics
Medical Director of Differences of Sexual
    Development Clinic
Co-Director of Pediatric Transgender Health
Division of Pediatric Endocrinology and
    Diabetes
Washington University School of Medicine
St. Louis, Missouri

Marina Litvin, MD
Assistant Professor of Medicine
Division of Endocrinology, Metabolism,
    and Lipid Research
Washington University School of Medicine
St. Louis, Missouri

Ningning Ma, MD
Instructor in Medicine
Division of Hospital Medicine
Washington University School of Medicine
St. Louis, Missouri

Marjorie Ann Malbas, MD
Clinical Fellow
Division of Endocrinology, Metabolism,
    and Lipid Research
Washington University School of Medicine
St. Louis, Missouri

Janet B. McGill, MD, MA, FACE
Professor of Medicine
Division of Endocrinology, Metabolism,
    and Lipid Research
Washington University School of Medicine
St. Louis, Missouri

Brian D. Muegge, MD, PhD
Clinical Fellow
Division of Endocrinology, Metabolism,
    and Lipid Research
Washington University School of Medicine
St. Louis, Missouri

Johnathon S. Parham, MD
Clinical Fellow
Division of Endocrinology, Metabolism,
    and Lipid Research
Washington University School of Medicine
St. Louis, Missouri

Louis H. Philipson, MD, PhD, FACP
James C. Tyree Professor
Departments of Medicine and Pediatrics
Section of Endocrinology, Diabetes, and
    Metabolism
Director, Kovler Diabetes Center
The University of Chicago Medicine
Chicago, Illinois

Ritika Puri, MD
Clinical Fellow
Division of Endocrinology, Metabolism,
    and Lipid Research
Washington University School of Medicine
St. Louis, Missouri

Susan R. Reeds, MD, FACP
Assistant Professor of Medicine
Division of Geriatrics and Nutritional Science
Medical Director, Washington University
    Weight Management Program
Washington University School of Medicine
St. Louis, Missouri

Lauren D. Reschke, MD
Chief Resident
Department of Obstetrics and Gynecology
Washington University School of Medicine
St. Louis, Missouri

Amy E. Riek, MD, MSCI
Assistant Professor of Medicine
Division of Endocrinology, Metabolism,
    and Lipid Research
Washington University School of Medicine
St. Louis, Missouri

Sobia Sadiq, MD
Clinical Fellow
Division of Endocrinology, Metabolism,
and Lipid Research
Washington University School of Medicine
St. Louis, Missouri

Maamoun Salam, MD
Assistant Professor of Medicine
Division of Endocrinology, Metabolism,
   and Lipid Research
Washington University School of Medicine
St. Louis, Missouri

Julie M. Silverstein, MD
*Associate Professor of Medicine and
   Neurological Surgery*
Division of Endocrinology, Metabolism,
   and Lipid Research
Washington University School of Medicine
St. Louis, Missouri

Sudhir Singh, MD
Clinical Fellow
Division of Endocrinology, Metabolism, and
   Lipid Research
Washington University School of Medicine
St. Louis, Missouri

Richard I. Stein, PhD
Research Assistant Professor
Center for Human Nutrition
Behavioral Director, Weight Management
   Program
Washington University School of Medicine
St. Louis, Missouri

Garry S. Tobin, MD
Professor of Medicine
Division of Endocrinology, Metabolism, and
   Lipid Research
Washington University School of Medicine
St. Louis, Missouri

Michael P. Whyte, MD
*Professor of Medicine, Pediatrics, and
   Genetics*
Division of Bone and Mineral Diseases
Washington University School of Medicine
Medical-Scientific Director, Center for
   Metabolic Bone Disease and Molecular
   Research
Shriners Hospitals for Children
St. Louis, Missouri

Naga Yalla, MD
Assistant Professor of Medicine
Division of Endocrinology, Metabolism, and
   Lipid Research
Washington University School of Medicine
St. Louis, Missouri

Rong Mei Zhang, MD
Clinical Fellow
Division of Endocrinology, Metabolism, and
   Lipid Research
Washington University School of Medicine
St. Louis, Missouri

Chairman's Note

It is a pleasure to present the new edition of *The Washington Manual® Endocrinology Subspecialty Consult*. This pocket-size book continues to be a primary reference for medical students, interns, residents, and other practitioners who need ready access to practical clinical information to diagnose and treat patients with a wide variety of disorders. Medical knowledge continues to increase at an astounding rate, which creates a challenge for physicians to keep up with the biomedical discoveries, genetic and genomic information, and novel therapeutics that can positively impact patient outcomes. The *Washington Manual* Subspecialty Series addresses this challenge by concisely and practically providing current scientific information for clinicians to aid them in the diagnosis, investigation, and treatment of common medical conditions.

I want to personally thank the authors, which include house officers, fellows, and attendings at Washington University School of Medicine and Barnes Jewish Hospital. Their commitment to patient care and education is unsurpassed, and their efforts and skill in compiling this manual are evident in the quality of the final product. In particular, I would like to acknowledge our editors, Drs. Thomas J. Baranski, Janet B. McGill, and Julie Silverstein and the series editors, Drs. Tom De Fer and Thomas Ciesielski, who have worked tirelessly to produce another outstanding edition of this manual. I would also like to thank Dr. Melvin Blanchard, Chief of the Division of Medical Education in the Department of Medicine at Washington University School of Medicine, for his advice and guidance. I believe this subspecialty manual will meet its desired goal of providing practical knowledge that can be directly applied at the bedside and in outpatient settings to improve patient care.

Victoria J. Fraser, MD
Adolphus Busch Professor of Medicine
Chairman, Department of Medicine
Washington University School of Medicine
St. Louis, Missouri

Preface

This fourth edition of *The Washington Manual® Endocrinology Subspecialty Consult* was written largely by Washington University house staff, fellows, and endocrine faculty. The manual is designed to serve as a guide for students, house staff, and fellows involved in inpatient and outpatient endocrinology consults. It is not meant to serve as a comprehensive review of the field of endocrinology. Rather, it focuses on practical approaches to endocrine disorders commonly seen in consultation, with emphasis on key components of evaluation and treatment.

Several changes in content were made with the fourth edition. All chapters have been updated to provide the latest information on the pathophysiology and treatment of endocrine disorders. New chapters covering monogenic diabetes and transgender care have been added. Drug dosing information was also reviewed and updated in each chapter. Bulleted key points highlight the salient features of each chapter. Clinical pearls are highlighted in boldface text within the chapters.

We are indebted to the remarkable efforts of the fellows and attending physicians who contributed to the current edition of this manual and worked enthusiastically to provide high-quality, contemporary, concise chapters.

—TJB, JBM & JMS

Contents

PART III. ADRENAL DISORDERS

PART IV. GONADAL DISORDERS

PART V. DISORDERS OF BONE AND MINERAL METABOLISM

PART VI. DISORDERS OF FUEL METABOLISM

PART VII. NEOPLASMS AND MULTI-SYSTEM DISORDERS

Sellar and Suprasellar Masses

Sobia Sadiq and Julie M. Silverstein

GENERAL PRINCIPLES

- The pituitary gland is located at the base of the brain and lies in a bony hollow in the sphenoid bone called the sella turcica ("Turkish saddle"). The gland is surrounded by dura and the pituitary stalk passes through an opening in a flat portion of the dura called the diaphragma sellae. The optic chiasm is anterior to the stalk and is located 5 to 10 mm above the diaphragma sellae.[1]
- The hypothalamus, which is located below the third ventricle and above the optic chiasm and pituitary gland, regulates the hormones produced by the anterior pituitary which include prolactin, thyroid-stimulating hormone (TSH), growth hormone (GH), adrenocorticotropic hormone (ACTH), luteinizing hormone (LH), and follicle-stimulating hormone (FSH). The posterior pituitary produces oxytocin and antidiuretic hormone (ADH).
- Pituitary adenomas are the most common sellar neoplasms.[2] Other masses include benign lesions such as Rathke cleft cysts, craniopharyngiomas, pituicytomas and meningiomas, malignant tumors such as germ cell tumors, chordomas, primary lymphoma and metastatic disease, and nonneoplastic lesions such as hypophysitis and sarcoidosis.
- Sellar and suprasellar masses can cause symptoms related to mass effect such as headache or vision loss, symptoms secondary to hormone oversecretion in the case of functional pituitary tumors, and symptoms related to hypopituitarism.

Classification

- Based on size, pituitary adenomas are classified as microadenomas (<10 mm in greatest diameter), macroadenomas (≥10 mm in greatest diameter), or giant adenomas (≥4 cm in greatest diameter). Depending on cell of origin, they can be hormone producing or functionally inactive; see Table 1-1.[3,4]
- The World Health Organization (WHO) classifies pituitary tumors based on pituitary adenohypophyseal cell lineage, immunomarkers, and transcription factors. Transcription factors PIT-1 (pituitary-specific POU-class homeodomain), SF-1 (steroidogenic factor 1), and T-PIT (T-box family member TBX19) regulate differentiation of acidophilic (somatotrophs, lactotrophs, and thyrotrophs), gonadotroph, and corticotroph cell lineages, respectively, from Rathke pouch. Additional transcription factors include ERα (estrogen receptor α), GATA2 (family of zinc-finger transcriptional regulatory proteins), and SF-1 (steroidogenic factor 1). Table 1-2 provides a summary of this classification and identifies tumor types with an increased risk of recurrence.[5]

Epidemiology

- Most sellar region masses are pituitary adenomas (85%), followed by craniopharyngiomas (3%), Rathke cleft cysts (2%), meningiomas (1%), and metastases (0.5%); other lesions such as hypophysitis, pituicytoma, spindle cell oncocytoma, and granular cell tumors of the neurohypophysis are rare.[6]

TABLE 1-1	FUNCTIONAL CLASSIFICATION OF PITUITARY ADENOMAS[3,4]		
Adenoma type	Incidence (%)	Hormones produced	Clinical relevance
Lactotroph	32–66	Prolactin (PRL)	Hyperprolactinemia, hypogonadism, and galactorrhea
Null cell and gonadotroph	14–54	Null cell: none Gonadotroph: FSH/LH, α-subunit	[a]Usually no hormonal dysfunction
Somatotroph	8–16	Growth hormone (GH)	Acromegaly or gigantism
Corticotroph	2–6	ACTH	Cushing disease
Thyrotroph	<1	TSH	Hyperthyroidism or silent when inactive TSH subunits are secreted
Plurihormonal adenomas	15	Multiple hormones, GH/ PRL most common	Mixed syndromes
"Silent" adenomas	Rare	Positive hormone(s) staining, but clinically silent	No hormonal dysfunction

[a]Although rare, gonadotroph adenomas can be associated with elevated estrogen levels in premenopausal women and elevated testosterone levels in men.

FSH, follicle-stimulating hormone; LH, luteinizing hormone; ACTH, adrenocorticotropic hormone; TSH, thyroid-stimulating hormone.

- Pituitary tumors account for 15% of intracranial masses[2] and prevalence ranges from 1 in 865 to 1 in 2,688 persons.[4]
- Based on autopsy studies and MRI data, pituitary tumors occur in 10% to 20% of the general population. Increased use of MRI has been associated with an increased incidence of pituitary incidentalomas.[7] In a cohort of adults undergoing MRI imaging for other reasons, microincidentalomas were found in 10% to 38% and macroincidentalomas in 0.16%.[8]

Etiology

- The majority of pituitary adenomas occur sporadically and are not part of syndromic disorders.[9]
- Mutations in **AIP** (encoding aryl-hydrocarbon receptor-interacting protein) are the most frequently observed germline mutations.[9]

Adenoma type	Morphologic variant	Immunomarkers	Transcription factors	[a]Risk of recurrence
Somatotroph	Densely granulated adenoma[b]	GH ± PRL ± α-subunit	PIT-1	Increased in sparsely granulated somatotroph adenomas
	Sparsely granulated adenoma	GH ± PRL	PIT-1	
	Mammosomatotroph adenoma	GH + PRL (same cells) ± α-subunit	PIT-1, ERα	
	Mixed somatotroph-lactotroph adenoma	GH + PRL (different cells) ± α-subunit	PIT-1, ERα	
Lactotroph	Sparsely granulated adenoma[b]	PRL	PIT-1, ERα	Increased in lactotroph adenomas in men
	Densely granulated adenoma	PRL	PIT-1, ERα	
	Acidophilic stem cell adenoma	PRL, GH	PIT-1, ERα	
Thyrotroph		β-TSH, α-subunit	PIT-1	
Corticotroph	Densely granulated adenoma[b]	ACTH	T-PIT	Increased in silent corticotroph and Crooke's cell adenomas
	Sparsely granulated adenoma	ACTH	T-PIT	
	Crooke's cell adenoma	ACTH	T-PIT	
Gonadotroph		β-FSH, β-LH, α-subunit	SF-1, GATA2, ERα	
Null cell		None	None	
Plurihormonal	Plurihormonal PIT-1 + adenoma	GH, PRL, β-TSH ± α-subunit	PIT-1	Increased in plurihormonal PIT-1 + adenomas
	Adenomas with unusual immunohistochemical combinations	Various combinations: ACTH/GH, ACTH/PRL	N/A	

[a]Risk of recurrence higher in any type of adenoma with elevated proliferative activity (based on mitosis and Ki-67 index).
[b]Most common.
GH, growth hormone; PRL, prolactin; PIT-1, pituitary-specific POU-class homeodomain transcription factor; ER, estrogen receptor; TSH, thyroid-stimulating hormone; ACTH, adrenocorticotropic hormone; T-PIT, T-box family member TBX19 transcription factor; FSH, follicle-stimulating hormone; LH, luteinizing hormone; SF-1, steroidogenic factor 1; GATA2, member of the GATA family of zinc-finger transcriptional regulatory proteins.
Adapted from Lopes MBS. The 2017 World Health Organization classification of tumors of the pituitary gland: a summary. *Acta Neuropathol* 2017;134:521–535, with permission from Springer.

- **Multiple endocrine neoplasia type 1 (MEN-1)** is characterized by pituitary, parathyroid, and pancreatic tumors.
- **Carney complex** is characterized by pituitary adenomas, cardiac myxomas, schwannomas, thyroid adenomas, and pigmented skin and mucosal lesions.

DIAGNOSIS

Clinical Presentation

The clinical presentation of sellar and suprasellar masses depends on whether the tumor is hormonally functional or nonfunctional (pituitary adenomas) and on whether there is mass effect or hemorrhage.

Hormonal Hypersecretion (Functional Adenomas)
- **Prolactinomas** (see Chapter 2, Prolactinoma)
  - Hyperprolactinemia causes hypogonadism in men and premenopausal women. Men present with decreased libido and impotence. Women often present with abnormal menses or infertility and galactorrhea.
  - There is often a delay in the diagnosis in postmenopausal women due to lack of clinical manifestations.
- **Somatotroph adenomas** (see Chapter 3, Acromegaly)
  - Acromegaly is characterized by skeletal overgrowth and soft tissue enlargement.
  - Acromegaly occurs due to elevated GH in the postpubertal phase of life. Gigantism results from GH excess occurring before fusion of the epiphyseal growth plates in children or adolescents.
  - Acromegalic patients have an increase in mortality related to cardiovascular, respiratory, gastrointestinal, and metabolic disorders.
  - The onset of acromegaly is insidious and often results in a delay in diagnosis.
- **Corticotroph adenomas** (see Chapter 15, Cushing Syndrome)
  - ACTH-secreting tumors cause Cushing disease.
  - Obesity (predominantly central fat distribution), hypertension, glucose intolerance or diabetes, hirsutism, and gonadal dysfunction are common.
  - Hypercortisolism produces skin thinning, easy bruising, abdominal striae, and proximal muscle weakness (inability to climb stairs or rise from a deep chair).
  - Psychiatric abnormalities including depression, lethargy, paranoia, and psychosis can also occur.
  - Long-standing Cushing disease can cause osteoporosis and aseptic necrosis of the femoral and humeral heads.
  - Patients may present with poor wound healing and frequent superficial fungal infections.
  - The classic symptoms and signs of hypercortisolism are not always present and are often not specific.
- **Thyrotroph adenomas**
  - TSH-secreting pituitary adenomas are rare and represent 0.5% to 3% of all pituitary tumors.[10]
  - Most patients present with large and invasive tumors with signs and symptoms of mass effect such as temporal visual field defects.
  - Goiter is usually present but the severity of symptoms related to hyperthyroidism is usually less than would be expected based on the elevated thyroid hormone levels.[10]
- **Gonadotroph adenomas**
  - The vast majority of the immunohistochemically confirmed gonadotroph adenomas are nonfunctioning and present only with mass effects.[11]

○ Clinically functioning gonadotroph adenomas associated with elevated circulating gonadotropins are rare and cause menstrual irregularity and the ovarian hyperstimulation syndrome in premenopausal females, testicular enlargement in males, and precocious puberty in children.[11]

Hormonal Hyposecretion

- **Hypopituitarism** can be a result of any hypothalamic or pituitary lesion (see Chapter 6, Hypopituitarism).
- Gonadotrophs are most commonly affected. Patients present with hypogonadism with low or inappropriately normal FSH and/or LH levels (secondary hypogonadism).
- Corticotrophs and thyrotrophs are most resistant to mass effects. TSH or ACTH deficiency usually indicates panhypopituitarism.
- GH deficiency is often present when two or more other hormones are deficient.
- Prolactin deficiency is rare and occurs when the anterior pituitary is completely destroyed such as in apoplexy.

Mass Effect

- Any sellar or suprasellar mass, if large enough and depending on location, may cause signs and symptoms of mass effect.
- Headaches are common and may not correlate with the size of the lesion.
- Visual defects are also common.
  ○ Upward compression and pressure on the optic chiasm may result in bitemporal hemianopsia, loss of red perception, scotomas, and blindness.
  ○ Lateral invasion into the cavernous sinuses can cause cranial nerve III, IV, V, and VI palsies leading to diplopia, ptosis, ophthalmoplegia, and facial numbness.
- Direct hypothalamic involvement may cause diabetes insipidus (DI) (see Chapter 4, Diabetes Insipidus), appetite/behavioral disorders (obesity, hyperphagia, anorexia, adipsia, and compulsive drinking), and sleep and temperature dysregulation.
- Cerebrospinal fluid (CSF) rhinorrhea, caused by inferior extension of an adenoma, is a very rare presentation.
- Uncinate seizures, personality disorders, and anosmia can occur if temporal and frontal brain lobes are invaded by an expanding parasellar mass.
- Masses causing deviation of the pituitary stalk can cause hyperprolactinemia from "stalk effect" (see Chapter 2, Prolactinoma).

Pituitary Apoplexy

- Apoplexy occurs in 2% to 12% of patients with pituitary adenomas and is a clinical syndrome characterized by symptoms and signs related to hemorrhage and/or infarction of a pituitary tumor.[12]
- Patients usually present with the sudden onset of a severe headache, vomiting, ocular palsies from progressive cranial nerve damage, visual field loss, and less commonly change in consciousness, cardiovascular collapse, and coma.
- Pituitary imaging reveals intra-adenoma hemorrhage and stalk deviation.
- Acute adrenal insufficiency may occur and patients should be started on glucocorticoid therapy. In addition, long-term hypopituitarism may develop.

Differential Diagnosis

- Table 1-3 lists the most common sellar and suprasellar masses. As stated above, pituitary adenomas are the most common type. Some of the other lesions in the sella are described below.
- **Craniopharyngiomas** are calcified, cystic, suprasellar tumors arising from remnants of Rathke's pouch and include two major histologic variants.[1]

TABLE 1-3 · SELLAR AND SUPRASELLAR MASSES

Pituitary adenomas
Somatotroph adenoma
Lactotroph adenoma
Thyrotroph adenoma
Corticotroph adenoma
Gonadotroph adenoma
Null-cell adenoma
Plurihormonal and double adenomas

Cysts
Rathke cleft (pars intermedia) cysts
Epidermoid cysts
Dermoid cysts
Arachnoid cysts

Hematolymphoid tumors
Lymphoma

Neuronal/paraneuronal tumors
Gangliocytoma
Neurocytoma
Paraganglioma
Neuroblastoma

Craniopharyngioma
Adamantinomatous craniopharyngioma
Papillary craniopharyngioma

Pituitary blastoma
Secondary tumors
Metastatic malignant tumors (breast
   cancer, lung cancer, and GI and
   GU cancers)

Germ cell tumors
Germinoma
Yolk sac tumor
Embryonal carcinoma
Choriocarcinoma
Teratoma
Mixed germ cell tumor

Miscellaneous lesions
Aneurysms
Hypophysitis
Infections
Giant cell granulomas
Sarcoidosis
Others

Tumors of the posterior pituitary
Pituicytoma
Granular cell tumor
Spindle cell oncocytoma
Ependymoma

Pituitary carcinoma
Mesenchymal/stromal tumors
Meningioma
Schwannoma
Chordoma
Solitary fibrous tumor/
   hemangiopericytoma

Adapted from *Lopes MBS.* The 2017 World Health Organization classification of tumors of the pituitary gland: a summary. *Acta Neuropathol* 2017;134:521–535.

- The most common type is **adamantinomatous craniopharyngioma,** which is characterized by tumors with cystic and/or solid components and calcifications. This type is more common in the pediatric population.
  - **Papillary craniopharyngiomas** are less common but more common in adults and are solid or mixed solid/cystic tumors less likely to be associated with calcifications. The discovery of mutations in *BRAF* (V600E), a proto-oncogene that plays a role in the MAPK/ERK (mitogen-activated protein kinases/extracellular signal-regulated kinases) signaling pathway, holds promise for *BRAF* inhibitors to treat these tumors.[13]
  - Craniopharyngiomas have a bimodal peak of incidence, occurring predominantly in children between the ages of 5 and 14 years; a second peak occurs in late middle age between 50 and 74 years.[14]

- ○ Large craniopharyngiomas can obstruct CSF flow and cause increased intracranial pressure.[14] Adults may present with neurologic symptoms, anterior pituitary hormone deficits, and DI.
- **Cysts: Rathke cleft cysts**, also known as pars intermedia cysts, are benign, noncalcified lesions that mimic hormonally inactive adenomas or craniopharyngiomas. They are the most common type of cystic mass. Other cysts include epidermoid, dermoid, and arachnoid cysts.
- **Pituitary blastoma** is a rare malignant neoplasm of the pituitary occurring most commonly in children less than 2 years old as part of the DICER1 syndrome, caused by mutations in the *DICER1* gene and also known as pleuropulmonary blastoma familial tumor and dysplasia syndrome.[5]
- **Pituitary granulomas**
  - ○ **Neurosarcoidosis** in the sellar region is rare and accounts for 1% of sellar masses. Sarcoidosis has a predilection for the cranial nerves, hypothalamus, pituitary gland, and stalk.[12] The most common hormonal abnormalities are hypogonadotropic hypogonadism (89%), DI (65%), and hyperprolactinemia (49%).[15]
  - ○ **Langerhans cell histiocytosis (LCH)** is characterized by infiltration of pathologic dendritic cells (Langerhans cells).[16] It can be uni- or multifocal and affect multiple sites, such as bone, skin, lung, pituitary, hypothalamus, liver, and spleen. LCH occurs more often in children and is almost always associated with DI. It may also cause anterior pituitary dysfunction and a thickened pituitary stalk on MRI.
  - ○ **Hand–Schüller–Christian disease** is a type of LCH that includes the triad of central DI, exophthalmos, and lytic bone lesions.[17] Other features of the disease include axillary skin rash and a history of recurrent pneumothorax. Children can present with growth retardation and anterior pituitary hormone deficits.
  - ○ **Erdheim–Chester disease**, a non-LCH, more commonly presents in middle-aged adults and is characterized by infiltration of giant cells and lipid-laden macrophages.[17] Clinical presentation is difficult to distinguish from LCH.
- **Hypophysitis** is characterized by either focal or diffuse infiltration of the pituitary by inflammatory cells and has an estimated annual incidence of 1 in 7 to 9 million.[18] Lesions mimic pituitary adenomas on MRI imaging.
  - ○ **Lymphocytic hypophysitis**, characterized by diffuse lymphocyte infiltration, is the most common variant and has a female predominance of 3:1.[18] It occurs mostly in women in late pregnancy or during the postpartum period and may be associated with other autoimmune diseases such as autoimmune thyroiditis. The diagnosis is confirmed by histology or resolution of the mass over time. Partial recovery of pituitary function and resolution of the sellar mass can occur spontaneously or with use of corticosteroids and hormone replacement.
  - ○ **Granulomatous hypophysitis** occurs more frequently in women but is not associated with pregnancy and is characterized by infiltration of multinucleated giant cells and histiocytes that form granulomas.[18]
  - ○ **IgG4-related hypophysitis** is more common in men and most often presents with panhypopituitarism and DI.[19] IgG4-related disease is a systemic disease characterized by infiltration of plasmocytes and can affect any organ system.
  - ○ **Immunotherapy-associated hypophysitis** (see Chapter 6, Hypopituitarism, and Chapter 40, Endocrine Effects of Oncology Drugs) occurs in up to 10% to 15% of patients receiving immune checkpoint inhibitors such as anticytotoxic T-lymphocyte–associated antigen 4 (CTLA-4) and programmed cell death 1 (PD-1) and PD-1 ligand (PD-L1) receptor monoclonal and presents on average 2 to 3 months after starting therapy.[18]
- **Pituitary hyperplasia** usually presents as generalized enlargement of the pituitary. Examples include lactotroph hyperplasia during pregnancy, thyrotroph hyperplasia secondary

to long-standing primary hypothyroidism, gonadotroph hyperplasia in long-standing primary hypogonadism, and very rarely, somatotroph hyperplasia in ectopic secretion of GH-releasing hormone.[20]

- **Pituitary metastasis** is rare and comprises <1% of intracranial metastasis. The most common types of malignancies to metastasize to the pituitary gland include breast and lung cancers. Other types include, but are not limited to, gastrointestinal, prostate, melanoma, pharynx, pancreas, thyroid, larynx, renal, liver, and ovarian cancers. Most patients present with DI and/or oculomotor nerve palsies.[21]
- **Pituitary carcinoma** is rare. Most tumors are functionally active (most commonly lactotroph adenomas) but they may also be clinically nonfunctioning. The diagnosis of carcinoma can only be established when the lesion metastasizes.

Diagnostic Testing

- All patients, regardless of symptoms, should undergo a basic laboratory evaluation to determine whether a tumor is functional (pituitary adenomas) and/or causing hypopituitarism.[8]
- Testing should include measurement of prolactin, insulin-like growth factor 1 (IGF-1) to screen for acromegaly, GH, 8 a.m. cortisol, ACTH, FSH, LH, TSH, free thyroxin (T4), 8 a.m. fasting total, and free testosterone (men) and estradiol in premenopausal women who have had a hysterectomy. Patients suspected of having Cushing disease or subclinical Cushing disease should undergo testing as described below and in Chapter 15, Cushing Syndrome.

Hormonal Hypersecretion
- **Prolactinoma**
  - Serum prolactin levels are usually proportional to tumor mass size. Values are generally >200 ng/mL in macroprolactinomas.
  - Hyperprolactinemia between 20 and 200 ng/mL can be due to microprolactinomas, stalk compression from a sellar mass, medications, or due to the "hook effect" (see Chapter 2, Prolactinoma).
- **Acromegaly**
  - Normal GH secretion is pulsatile, diurnal, and affected by a variety of factors.
  - Since acromegaly can be mild or subclinical, all patients presenting with a pituitary adenoma should be screened initially with an IGF-1 level. A GH level should also be ordered in patients suspected of having acromegaly but is not always elevated. Current guidelines recommend an elevated IGF-1 and failure to suppress GH during an oral glucose tolerance test (OGTT) to confirm the diagnosis.[22,23] An OGTT may not be necessary however, in patients with clearly elevated IGF-1 and GH levels and clinical features of acromegaly (see Chapter 3, Acromegaly).
- **Cushing disease**
  - Patients with clinical signs or symptoms of Cushing syndrome or suspected of having subclinical Cushing disease, should be screened with either a 24-hour urine-free cortisol, a low-dose dexamethasone suppression test, or late-night salivary cortisol levels.
  - A nonsuppressed ACTH level in the setting of biochemically confirmed Cushing syndrome suggests either a pituitary source (Cushing disease) or ectopic ACTH syndrome. A pituitary MRI, high-dose dexamethasone suppression test, and/or inferior petrosal sinus sampling (IPSS) can be used to differentiate between the two (see Chapter 15, Cushing Syndrome).
- **TSH-secreting adenomas**
  - Elevated thyroid hormone levels in the setting of an elevated or inappropriately normal TSH suggests the diagnosis of a thyrotroph adenoma. An elevated pituitary glycoprotein hormone α-subunit may be present.

- Falsely elevated TSH levels can be caused by circulating antibodies against TSH or heterophilic antibody interference and can be ruled out by serial dilution.
- Dynamic testing, such as triiodothyronine (T3) suppression and thyrotropin-releasing hormone (TRH) stimulation can be used to differentiate a TSH-secreting adenoma from thyroid hormone resistance syndromes.

- **Gonadotroph adenomas**
  - Most nonfunctioning pituitary adenomas arise from gonadotroph cells.
  - Although circulating LH and FSH levels may be elevated in a minority of patients, this is rarely clinically significant. In rare cases, testosterone levels in men and estradiol levels in premenopausal women may be elevated.

Hormonal Hyposecretion (Hypopituitarism)

- **Corticotropin deficiency (secondary adrenal insufficiency)**
  - ACTH deficiency produces hypotension, shock, nausea, vomiting, fatigue, and hyponatremia (see Chapter 12, Adrenal Insufficiency).
  - A subnormal morning cortisol level in the setting of a low or normal ACTH suggests secondary adrenal insufficiency.
  - Dynamic testing to evaluate the hypothalamic–pituitary–adrenal (HPA) axis can be done with a cosyntropin stimulation test or insulin-induced hypoglycemia.
  - Cosyntropin stimulation testing may be normal in recent-onset corticotropin deficiency because it takes time for adrenals to atrophy after acute disruption of ACTH secretion.
- **Thyrotropin deficiency (secondary hypothyroidism)**
  - A low serum T4 in the setting of an inappropriately low/normal TSH suggests secondary hypothyroidism.
  - A free T4 level should be used to monitor thyroid hormone replacement for secondary hypothyroidism.
- **GH deficiency**
  - Measurement of basal GH does not reliably distinguish between normal and subnormal GH secretion.
  - Patients with multiple pituitary hormone deficits (3 or 4) and a low IGF-1 are likely GH deficient and a low serum IGF-1 in a patient with pituitary disease may suggest the diagnosis of GH deficiency.
  - Stimulation tests to aid in the diagnosis are described in Chapter 6, Hypopituitarism.
- **Gonadotropin deficiency (secondary hypogonadism)**
  - Secondary hypogonadism may be due to hyperprolactinemia or damage to gonadotrophs from a sellar mass.
  - Normal menses in premenopausal women not on birth control suggests an intact pituitary–gonadal axis. In female patients with abnormal menses, serum LH/FSH, prolactin and estradiol levels should be checked.
  - Low serum testosterone in the setting of an inappropriately low or normal LH in males suggests the diagnosis.

Imaging

- Pituitary MRI
  - MRI with precontrast T1- and T2-weighted coronal and sagittal sections with thin slices and gadolinium-enhanced coronal and sagittal T1-weighted dynamic imaging is the best study to visualize pituitary tumors.[24] With dynamic imaging, coronal sequences are obtained every 30 seconds for 3 minutes following intravenous contrast (gadolinium) injection.[25]
  - On T1-weighted sections, most adenomas enhance more slowly than normal pituitary tissue after administration of contrast and thus appear as a hypoenhancing mass.

- MRI also detects tumor effects on surrounding structures including the cavernous sinuses, optic apparatus, sphenoid sinus, and hypothalamus.
  - T2-weighted images are important for diagnosing high-signal hemorrhage.
  - A thickened stalk may indicate the presence of hypophysitis, a granuloma, metastasis, or an atypical chordoma.
  - Cystic masses such as Rathke cleft cysts usually appear hyperintense on T1-weighted images.
- Pituitary CT allows better visualization of bony structures, including the sellar floor and clinoid bones. Calcifications associated with craniopharyngiomas, which may not be visible on MRI, can be seen on CT.

Diagnostic Procedures

All patients, including those without visual complaints, with tumors abutting or compressing the optic chiasm should undergo a formal visual field exam. Referral to an ophthalmologist should be considered in patients with abnormal testing and/or visual complaints.

TREATMENT

- Mainstay for treatment of pituitary tumors is **transsphenoidal surgical resection**.
- Indications for **surgery** include[8]:
  - Visual field deficit or other visual abnormalities, such as ophthalmoplegia or neurologic compromise due to compression.
  - Lesion abutting or compressing the optic nerves or chiasm on MRI.
  - Pituitary apoplexy with visual disturbance.
  - Hypersecreting tumors other than prolactinomas (see relevant chapters).
  - Surgery can be considered in the additional following situations:
    - Clinically significant growth of a pituitary incidentaloma
    - Loss of endocrine function
    - A lesion close to the optic chiasm in a female planning pregnancy
    - Unremitting headache
  - The most common transient complications include CSF leak, DI, syndrome of inappropriate antidiuretic hormone (SIADH), and delayed hyponatremia. Other complications include iatrogenic hypopituitarism, stroke, and permanent DI.
- **Pituitary irradiation** is usually reserved for large tumors with incomplete resection, for patients who have a contraindication for surgery, for some patients with hyperfunctioning tumors not cured by surgery, and for patients intolerant to medical therapy.
  - Stereotactic radiotherapy delivers high-dose radiation to the tumor while sparing surrounding tissue as compared to conventional radiation. They have similar long-term efficacy.
  - Major complications include delayed hypopituitarism which occurs in up to 20% by 5 years and 80% by 10 to 15 years,[4] optic nerve damage, and brain necrosis.
- **Medical therapy** for management of hormone-producing pituitary tumors is outlined in Chapters 2 (Prolactinoma), 3 (Acromegaly), and 15 (Cushing Syndrome).

MONITORING/FOLLOW-UP

- Hormonal monitoring and imaging follow-up recommendations for patients with hormone-producing tumors are outlined in Chapters 2 (Prolactinoma), 3 (Acromegaly), and 15 (Cushing Syndrome).
- Follow-up for patients with non–pituitary sellar masses depends on the type, size, invasiveness, and location of the tumor.

Pituitary Incidentalomas

- All patients with **asymptomatic pituitary macroadenomas** should have periodic assessments of their endocrine function. In a meta-analysis of patients with macroincidentalomas, hormone deficiency developed in 2.4% of patients per year.[8]
- Patients with **asymptomatic or incidental pituitary microadenomas** do not need reevaluation for hypopituitarism unless there is tumor growth.[8]
- Tumor growth without treatment occurs in approximately 10% of microadenomas and 24% of macroadenomas.[8] Growth occurs slowly as demonstrated by a meta-analysis showing that tumor growth in macroadenomas, microadenomas, and cystic lesions was 12.5, 3.3, and 0.05 per 100 person-years, respectively.[26]
- Patients with **asymptomatic pituitary microadenomas** should have a repeat MRI in 1 year, yearly for 3 years, and then less frequently. Patients with **asymptomatic macroadenomas** should have a follow-up MRI in 6 months, yearly for 3 years, and then periodically afterward.[8]
- Visual field testing should be performed in patients with a pituitary incidentaloma that enlarges and abuts or compresses the optic nerves or chiasm.
- Patients who develop signs or symptoms related to the adenoma or show an increase in size should undergo more frequent testing.

REFERENCES

1. Javorsky BR, Aron DC, Findling JW, Tyrrell JB. Hypothalamus and pituitary gland. In: Gardner DG, Shoback D, eds. *Greenspan's Basic & Clinical Endocrinology*. 10th ed. McGraw-Hill Education; 2018.
2. Famini P, Maya MM, Melmed S. Pituitary magnetic resonance imaging for sellar and parasellar masses: ten-year experience in 2598 patients. *J Clin Endocrinol Metab* 2011;96(6):1633–1641.
3. Shao S, Li X. Clinical features and analysis in 1385 Chinese patients with pituitary adenomas. *J Neurosurg Sci* 2013;57(3):267–275.
4. Molitch ME. Diagnosis and treatment of pituitary adenomas: a review. *JAMA* 2017;317(5):516–524.
5. Lopes MBS. The 2017 World Health Organization classification of tumors of the pituitary gland: a summary. *Acta Neuropathol (Berl)* 2017;134:521–535.
6. Kleinschmidt-DeMasters BK. Histological features of pituitary adenomas and sellar region masses. *Curr Opin Endocrinol Diabetes Obes* 2016;23(6):476–484.
7. Iglesias P, Arcano K, Triviño V, et al. Prevalence, clinical features, and natural history of incidental clinically non-functioning pituitary adenomas. *Horm Metab Res* 2017;49(09):654–659.
8. Freda PU, Beckers AM, Katznelson L, et al; Endocrine Society. Pituitary incidentaloma: an endocrine society clinical practice guideline. *J Clin Endocrinol Metab* 2011;96(4):894–904.
9. Lecoq A-L, Kamenický P, Guiochon-Mantel A, Chanson P. Genetic mutations in sporadic pituitary adenomas–what to screen for? *Nat Rev Endocrinol* 2015;11(1):43–54.
10. Amlashi FG, Tritos NA. Thyrotropin-secreting pituitary adenomas: epidemiology, diagnosis, and management. *Endocrine* 2016;52(3):427–440.
11. Ntali G, Capatina C, Grossman A, Karavitaki N. Clinical review: Functioning gonadotroph adenomas. *J Clin Endocrinol Metab* 2014;99(12):4423–4433.
12. Pekic S, Popovic V. Diagnosis of endocrine disease: expanding the cause of hypopituitarism. *Eur J Endocrinol* 2017;176(6):R269–R282.
13. Larkin S, Karavitaki N. Recent advances in molecular pathology of craniopharyngioma. F1000Research [Internet]. July 24, 2017;6. https://www.ncbi.nlm.nih.gov/pmc/articles/PMC5531159/. Accessed November 9, 2017.
14. Müller HL. Craniopharyngioma. *Endocr Rev* 2014;35(3):513–543.
15. Anthony J, Esper GJ, Ioachimescu A. Hypothalamic-pituitary sarcoidosis with vision loss and hypopituitarism: case series and literature review. *Pituitary* 2016;19(1):19–29.
16. Yeh EA, Greenberg J, Abla O, et al. Evaluation and treatment of langerhans cell histiocytosis patients with central nervous system abnormalities: current views and new vistas. *Pediatr Blood Cancer* 2017;65(1):e26784. http://onlinelibrary.wiley.com/journal/10.1002/(ISSN)1545-5017. Accessed November 9, 2017.

17. Yin J, Zhang F, Zhang H, et al. Hand-Schüller-Christian disease and Erdheim-Chester disease: coexistence and discrepancy. *Oncologist* 2013;18(1):19–24.
18. Faje A. Hypophysitis: evaluation and management. *Clin Diabetes Endocrinol* 2016;2:15.
19. Baptista B, Casian A, Gunawardena H, D'Cruz D, Rice CM. Neurological manifestations of IgG4-related disease. *Curr Treat Options Neurol* 2017;19(4):14.
20. De Sousa SMC, Earls P, McCormack AI. Pituitary hyperplasia: case series and literature review of an under-recognized and heterogeneous condition. *Endocrinol Diabetes Metab Case Rep* 2015;2015:150017.
21. He W, Chen F, Dalm B, Kirby PA, Greenlee JD. Metastatic involvement of the pituitary gland: a systematic review with pooled individual patient data analysis. *Pituitary* 2015;18(1):159–168.
22. Katznelson L, Laws ER, Melmed S, et al. Acromegaly: an endocrine society clinical practice guideline. *J Clin Endocrinol Metab* 2014;99(11):3933–3951.
23. Katznelson L, Atkinson JL, Cook DM, et al. American Association of Clinical Endocrinologists medical guidelines for clinical practice for the diagnosis and treatment of acromegaly–2011 update. *Endocr Pract* 2011;17(Suppl 4):1–44.
24. Paschou SA, Vryonidou A, Goulis DG. Pituitary incidentalomas: A guide to assessment, treatment and follow-up. *Maturitas* 2016;92:143–149.
25. Zamora C, Castillo M. Sellar and parasellar imaging. *Neurosurgery* 2017;80(1):17–38.
26. Fernández-Balsells MM, Murad MH, Barwise A, et al. Natural history of nonfunctioning pituitary adenomas and incidentalomas: a systematic review and metaanalysis. *J Clin Endocrinol Metab* 2011;96(4):905–912.

Prolactinoma

2

Sobia Sadiq and Julie M. Silverstein

GENERAL PRINCIPLES

Classification

- Prolactinomas are prolactin-secreting pituitary tumors.
- Classification is based on size, local invasion, and metastatic spread.
  - Microprolactinomas are tumors <10 mm in greatest diameter and are confined to the sella.
  - Macroprolactinomas are tumors ≥10 mm in greatest diameter and can invade local structures such as the cavernous and sphenoid sinuses and compress the optic chiasm.
  - Malignant prolactinomas are extremely rare and are defined by the presence of metastases (e.g., bone, lymph nodes, lung, liver, or spinal cord).

Epidemiology

- Prolactinomas account for close to 50% of pituitary adenomas,[1] 50% to 60% of functional pituitary tumors,[2] and present most frequently in women between the ages of 20 and 50 years old.[1]
- Microprolactinomas occur more often in women with a F:M ratio of 20:1.[3] Macroprolactinomas occur with similar frequency in men and women,[3] but 80% of prolactinomas in men are macroadenomas.[4]

Pathophysiology

Prolactin is released from the anterior pituitary in response to nipple stimulation, estrogen, thyrotropin-releasing hormone (TRH), and vasoactive intestinal peptide (VIP). Dopamine produced by the hypothalamus inhibits prolactin release thus regulating prolactin levels. Prolactin stimulates milk production and inhibits release of gonadotropin-releasing hormone (GnRH) and gonadotropins.

Associated Conditions

- Prolactinoma is the most frequent pituitary tumor in multiple endocrine neoplasia syndrome type 1 (MEN1).
- Prolactinomas may secrete other hormones. The most frequent mixed tumors are growth hormone (GH)/prolactin-secreting adenomas.

DIAGNOSIS

Clinical Presentation

Prolactinomas cause symptoms on the basis of hormonal secretion and mass effect.

- Symptoms due to hyperprolactinemia
  - Hyperprolactinemia interrupts the hypothalamic production of GnRH, inhibiting the release of luteinizing hormone (LH) and follicle-stimulating hormone (FSH) thereby resulting in hypogonadism and infertility.[2] Direct compression of gonadotrophs may

also cause hypogonadism and can occur with tumors of any size. Hypogonadism may be reversible with normalization of prolactin.

○ Premenopausal women frequently present with galactorrhea, amenorrhea, and infertility. Galactorrhea occurs via direct action of prolactin on the estrogenized breast.

○ Postmenopausal women rarely present early in the course of disease since menses are no longer present and galactorrhea is rarely present due to low estrogen levels. Hyperprolactinemia is often not recognized in postmenopausal patients until a prolactinoma has become sufficiently large to produce symptoms of mass effect such as headache or visual field defects.

○ Men present with signs and symptoms of secondary hypogonadism including decreased libido, impotence, infertility, loss of body hair, and gynecomastia. More subtle manifestations include decreased cognitive function and energy, and loss of muscle and bone mass. Men almost never have galactorrhea.

• Symptoms due to mass effect
  ○ Include headache from tumor expansion and visual field defects from compression of the optic chiasm. Rarely, patients may present with pituitary tumor apoplexy.[2]
  ○ Ophthalmoplegia and rhinorrhea are signs of more advanced disease. Ophthalmoplegia may occur when tumors expand laterally and invade the cavernous sinus. Rhinorrhea may occur if the tumor invades the sphenoid or ethmoid sinuses or after rapid drug-induced tumor shrinkage.
  ○ Secondary hypothyroidism and adrenal insufficiency may occur as a result of direct compression of thyrotrophs or corticotrophs by a macroprolactinoma. Unlike hypogonadism, if these hormonal deficiencies are present as a result of a macroprolactinoma, they are generally not reversible.

History

The history should focus on symptoms of hormonal overproduction and mass effect. It should also include a thorough investigation for alternate causes of hyperprolactinemia. Symptoms or history of hypothyroidism, adrenal insufficiency, renal disease, or cirrhosis should be sought. Current medications should be carefully reviewed. Any family history of pituitary tumors or syndromes of endocrine neoplasia should be noted.

Physical Examination

The physical examination should evaluate for bitemporal visual field defects and signs of hypopituitarism. Since nipple stimulation can raise prolactin levels, evaluation for galactorrhea is rarely indicated.

Diagnostic Criteria

• **The first requirement for a diagnosis of prolactinoma is a persistently elevated prolactin level.** In commonly used assays, normal prolactin levels are <25 ng/mL for women and <20 ng/mL for men.[2]

• The likelihood of prolactinoma can be roughly estimated based on the degree of elevation in the prolactin.[5]
  ○ Levels above normal but <100 ng/mL: possible prolactinoma
  ○ Levels 100 to 200 ng/mL: likely prolactinoma
  ○ Levels >200 ng/mL: usually diagnostic of a macroprolactinoma

• Alternate causes of mild to moderate prolactin elevations should be considered and if possible excluded (see section on Differential Diagnosis).

• Once persistent hyperprolactinemia is established and alternate causes excluded, a pituitary protocol brain MRI with gadolinium should be performed to define tumor size and anatomy. Microprolactinomas may be too small to be seen on MRI.

TABLE 2-1	DIFFERENTIAL DIAGNOSIS OF HYPERPROLACTINEMIA: MNEMONIC HIGH PROLACTINS

Hypothyroidism
Idiopathic
Glucocorticoid insufficiency
Hyperplasia of lactotrophs
Physiologic (nipple stimulation)
Renal failure
Opiates/other drugs
Liver failure
Adenoma
Convulsion
Trauma (chest wall)
Irradiation
No abnormality (macroprolactinemia)
Stalk effect

Differential Diagnosis

- The differential diagnosis for hyperprolactinemia can be remembered using the mnemonic **HIGH PROLACTINS** (Table 2-1).
- **Primary hypothyroidism** is associated with prolactin levels >25 ng/mL in 10% of patients with hypothyroidism from TRH stimulation of lactotrophs.[6] Prolactin levels typically return to normal with thyroid hormone replacement.
- **Idiopathic hyperprolactinemia** is characterized by prolactin levels between 20 and 100 ng/mL in patients in whom no cause can be found. Some of these patients have undetectable lactotroph microadenomas. Long-term follow-up has revealed that in one-third of these patients prolactin levels return to normal and in one-half prolactin levels remain stable.[7]
- **Glucocorticoids** have a suppressive effect on prolactin gene transcription and release. Although rare, hyperprolactinemia can occur in patients with adrenal insufficiency. Levels return to normal with glucocorticoid replacement.[4]
- **Lactotroph hyperplasia** from estrogen stimulation during pregnancy is associated with gradually increasing prolactin levels with levels up to 10 times above the upper limit of normal by the third trimester.[8]
- **Physiologic causes** include pregnancy as above, nipple stimulation, and physical stress such as exercise and hypoglycemia.
- **Renal or hepatic failure** may be associated with hyperprolactinemia due to decreased prolactin clearance.
- **Opiates/other drugs** (see Table 2-2).[2,9]
- **Adenomas** (prolactinomas).
- Prolactin levels are often elevated after epileptic seizures (**convulsion**).
- **Chest wall injuries**, irritating lesions (e.g., herpes zoster), and spinal cord injuries can activate neural reflexes similar to nipple stimulation and increase prolactin levels.
- **Irradiation** to the hypothalamus and pituitary, such as in patients treated for head and neck tumors, can cause hyperprolactinemia due to damage of dopamine-secreting neurons and thus loss of tonic inhibition of prolactin secretion.[10]
- Prolactin can circulate as a monomer or in aggregates (usually bound to IgG). **Macroprolactinemia** ("big prolactin") is characterized by elevated measurements of prolactin due to circulating prolactin aggregates and is felt to be a benign variant. In long-term follow-up of such patients, few had initial symptoms and none had symptom progression.[11] Macroprolactinemia

TABLE 2-2	MEDICATIONS THAT CAUSE HYPERPROLACTINEMIA	
Antipsychotics	**Antidepressants**	**Antiemetics**
Typical antipsychotics	Tricyclic antidepressants	Metoclopramide
Phenothiazines	Monoamine oxidase	Domperidone
Certain atypical antipsychotics	(MAO) inhibitors	**Other**
Risperidone	Fluoxetine (no other	Estrogens
Molindone	SSRIs)[a]	Cocaine
Quetiapine	**Antidepressants**	Heroin
Olanzapine	**Antihypertensive**	Alcohol
Opiates	**medications**	Anesthetics
Morphine	Verapamil	Marijuana
Methadone	Methyldopa	
	Reserpine	
	H₂ receptor blockers[a]	
	Cimetidine	
	Ranitidine	

[a]Case reports exist but data are not well established.
Data from *Wong A, Eloy JA, Couldwell WT, Liu JK*. Update on prolactinomas. Part 1: Clinical manifestations and diagnostic challenges. *J Clin Neurosci* 2015;22:1564.; *Molitch ME*. Drugs and prolactin. *Pituitary* 2008;11:210.

can be distinguished from monomeric hyperprolactinemia by polyethylene glycol precipitation. Some, but not all, laboratories routinely test for macroprolactinemia.
- Sellar and suprasellar masses as well as infiltrative and granulomatous disorders, can cause compression of the pituitary stalk (**"stalk effect"**) and/or damage to dopamine-secreting neurons leading to hyperprolactinemia by the same mechanism as with irradiation described above.

Diagnostic Testing

Laboratories
- After the diagnosis of hyperprolactinemia is made, the initial laboratory analyses should include:
  ○ Measurement of thyroid stimulating hormone and a comprehensive metabolic panel to exclude renal and liver disease.
  ○ A pregnancy test in premenopausal females.
  ○ Serum levels of insulin-like growth factor 1 (IGF-1), 8 a.m. cortisol, adrenocorticotropic hormone (ACTH), LH, FSH, testosterone (men only), and free thyroxine should be measured to assess pituitary function.
- Mild to moderate prolactin elevations (<200 ng/mL) in the setting of a pituitary macroadenoma may be due to **hook effect**. When an immunoradiometric assay is used to measure prolactin, hook effect can occur when large amounts of prolactin saturate the antibodies thus leading to a falsely low prolactin. This artifact can be excluded by performing an additional prolactin determination on diluted serum. If the diluted specimen yields a value that is higher, the diagnosis of macroprolactinoma can be made. Although the hook effect is no longer a problem in some laboratories, it is important to be familiar with local laboratory assays.

Imaging
- MRI with gadolinium enhancement provides the best anatomic detail of the hypothalamic–pituitary area.

• Visual field testing should be obtained if tumor is adjacent to or compressing the optic chiasm.

TREATMENT

• **All macroprolactinomas require treatment** whether or not compressive symptoms are present.
• **Not all microprolactinomas require treatment** and should be treated only when symptoms caused by hyperprolactinemia or rapidly increasing prolactin levels indicative of an enlarging tumor are present. As such, microprolactinomas in postmenopausal women rarely require treatment.
• Prolactinomas are unique among pituitary tumors in that **first-line treatment is medical, not surgical**.
• Since the mid-1980s, **dopamine agonists** have been the mainstay of management.[8]
• Most patients will respond to therapy within weeks of initiation as evidenced by symptoms and prolactin levels. Normalization of prolactin levels and reduction in tumor size occur in 60% to 70% of patients with macroadenomas.[5]
• The goals of treatment are to restore normal gonadal function and fertility, stop galactorrhea, and reduce tumor size. In asymptomatic patients with microadenomas, observation with serial monitoring every 6 to 12 months is a reasonable approach.[1] Rising prolactin levels or symptoms of hyperprolactinemia warrant a repeat MRI and initiation of treatment.
• In women not desiring pregnancy with microprolactinomas and oligomenorrhea or amenorrhea without bothersome galactorrhea, estrogen in the form of oral contraceptives or other estrogen plus progestin regimens are therapeutic options.[7]

Medications

• **Cabergoline,** a non-ergot D_2 receptor agonist, is the preferred dopamine agonist due to its higher efficacy and greater tolerability as compared to bromocriptine.[11,12] Cabergoline has a long half-life and is administered at doses ranging between 0.25 and 1 mg twice a week as compared to bromocriptine which is administered daily. Approximately 15% to 20% of patients, especially those with macroadenomas, may require higher than conventional doses (≥2 mg/wk and up to 11 mg/wk) to achieve control.[1]
  ○ Cabergoline normalizes prolactin in 95% of patients with microprolactinomas and approximately 80% of patients with macroprolactinomas. In addition, studies show that in approximately two-thirds of patients with macroprolactinomas, tumor size decreases by 90%.[10]
  ○ For patients with microprolactinomas, cabergoline can be started at 0.25 mg twice weekly and titrated based on subsequent prolactin levels checked 4 weeks after each dose adjustment. Since the goal of therapy is reversal of symptoms related to hyperprolactinemia, achieving a normal prolactin level may not be necessary. For patients with macroprolactinomas, a reasonable approach is to start 0.25 mg twice weekly and increase by 0.25 mg twice weekly until the patient is taking 1 mg twice weekly. After 4 weeks, the dose can be titrated by 0.25 to 0.5 mg a week until prolactin levels normalize.
  ○ Side effects which include headaches, dizziness, nausea, constipation, and abdominal pain usually disappear over time. Patients should be advised to take cabergoline before going to bed. Compulsive behaviors such as excessive gambling and hypersexuality and symptoms of psychosis or exacerbation of pre-existing psychosis are known but rare adverse effects of dopamine agonists.[1] Cerebrospinal fluid (CSF) rhinorrhea may occur following initiation of medical therapy, most commonly in the setting of invasive prolactinomas that shrink rapidly in response to dopamine agonist therapy.[13]

- A threefold to sixfold increased risk of cardiac valvular abnormalities has been found among patients with Parkinson disease who receive very high doses of cabergoline (3 to 5 mg/day) for more than 6 months; this adverse effect does not occur among patients with prolactinomas treated with conventional doses.[1,14] In a study of 192 patients in the United Kingdom, no associations were observed between cumulative doses of cabergoline used and the age-corrected prevalence of any valvular abnormality.[14]
- Echocardiograms should be obtained yearly in the subset of patients exceeding a weekly dose of 2 mg since the threshold dose for developing valvular abnormalities is unknown.[1]
- **Bromocriptine** is an ergot derivative D_2 receptor agonist. Therapeutic doses range between 2.5 and 15 mg/day (median 7.5 mg/day), but doses as high as 20 to 30 mg/day may be necessary in approximately 30% of patients.[14] Due to its relatively short half-life, bromocriptine is dosed twice or thrice daily.
  - Bromocriptine normalizes prolactin levels, restores gonadal function, and reduces tumor mass in approximately 80% to 90% of microprolactinomas and 70% of macroprolactinomas.[14]
  - Side effects are similar to those of cabergoline but tend to be more frequent and more severe and include nausea, vomiting, headache, and dizziness. Approximately 25% of patients develop postural hypotension after treatment initiation, which can result in dizziness or even syncope.[15] Side effects generally occur after the initial dose and with dosage increases.

Surgical Management

- Transsphenoidal surgery is a therapeutic option and leads to normalization of prolactin in 65% to 85% of patients with microadenomas and 30% to 40% of patients with macroadenomas with recurrence rates of 20% over 10 years.[1]
- Indications for surgery include increasing tumor size despite optimal medical therapy, pituitary apoplexy, intolerance, resistance, or contraindications to dopamine agonists, persistent optic chiasm compression, and CSF leak during administration of dopamine agonists.[8] In addition, surgery may be indicated in patients with cystic pituitary macroadenomas because they tend to be less responsive to dopamine agonist therapy.
- Pituitary surgery aimed at debulking tumor to reduce the risk of potential expansion during pregnancy may be indicated in women with macroprolactinomas desiring pregnancy.

Radiotherapy

Radiotherapy is generally reserved for patients whose hyperprolactinemia and tumor cannot be controlled with dopamine agonists or surgery.

SPECIAL CONSIDERATIONS

Resistant and Malignant Prolactinoma

- Dopamine agonist resistance, the mechanism of which is not clear, is defined by a failure to normalize prolactin with maximally tolerated doses of dopamine agonists and a failure to achieve at least a 50% reduction in tumor size. Men are more likely than women to be resistant to dopamine agonists and resistance is more likely to occur in macroadenomas.
- Patients on bromocriptine can be switched to cabergoline since approximately 80% of patients resistant to bromocriptine may normalize prolactin on cabergoline. Woman intolerant to the side effects of oral bromocriptine can be tried on intravaginal bromocriptine.[10]
- Dose increases of cabergoline up to 11 mg/wk may overcome resistance. Transsphenoidal surgery should be offered to symptomatic patients intolerant or resistant to high doses of cabergoline.

- Malignancy is defined by metastatic spread outside of the pituitary and can occur both within and outside the central nervous system. The alkylating agent, temozolomide, has been used for aggressive prolactinomas and pituitary carcinomas with limited success.[1]

Pregnancy

- During pregnancy, the normal pituitary increases in size, owing to marked lactotroph hyperplasia due to the effect of estrogen on prolactin synthesis. The risk of tumor expansion is small (<3%) for microprolactinomas but significant (30%) for macroprolactinomas.[16]
- Patients with prolactinomas wishing to become pregnant should be referred to specialists in high-risk obstetrics and endocrinology.
- Bromocriptine and cabergoline have been studied in 6,000 and >900 pregnancies, respectively, and are safe when taken during the first few weeks of gestation.[4] Because experience with cabergoline in pregnancy is more limited than bromocriptine, bromocriptine is still the first treatment choice for pregnancy induction.
- In women with microprolactinomas desiring fertility, bromocriptine should be titrated to normalize prolactin levels and restore regular menses. Barrier contraception should be recommended until menstrual cycles become regular so that a pregnancy test can be performed immediately if a cycle is missed. Once pregnancy is confirmed, bromocriptine should be discontinued in order to limit fetal exposure to the drug.
- In women with macroprolactinomas, control of tumor size should ideally be attained prior to conception because of the growth potential of these tumors during pregnancy. These patients should be treated with a dopamine agonist for a sufficient period to cause substantial tumor shrinkage in addition to regular menses. Only then should contraception be discontinued. If the tumor does not shrink sufficiently in size, pre-pregnancy transsphenoidal surgical debulking can be considered. Once pregnancy is achieved, dopamine agonist therapy should be discontinued followed by close surveillance for symptoms of tumor enlargement.
- Symptomatic tumor enlargement, likely from estrogen stimulation of lactotrophs and withdrawal of dopamine agonists, occurs in 2.4% of microprolactinomas, 21% of macroprolactinomas with no prior radiation or surgical treatment, and 4.7% of macroprolactinomas previously treated with radiation or surgery.[4] If symptomatic tumor enlargement occurs, reinstitution of dopamine agonist therapy is recommended over transsphenoidal surgery because of the increased risk of fetal loss during the first and second trimesters with any type of surgery.
- Guidelines recommend against serial prolactin measurements and routine MRIs during pregnancy in asymptomatic women. Pregnant women with severe headaches and/or visual field changes should undergo formal visual field assessment followed by an MRI without gadoliunium.[12]

MONITORING/FOLLOW-UP

- For patients on dopamine agonist therapy, prolactin levels should be checked 4 weeks after each dose adjustment and once stable can be checked yearly. Repeat MRI should be performed 3 months after initiation of therapy for patients with macroadenomas and patients with rising prolactin levels despite dopamine agonist therapy. For all others, guidelines recommend repeating an MRI after 1 year of therapy.[10] There are no clear guidelines on how often subsequent imaging should be performed and further imaging may not be necessary in patients with microprolactinomas since prolactin levels have been shown to correlate with tumor size.
- Visual field testing should be repeated at regular intervals if a visual field defect was present at diagnosis or if there is risk of tumor impingement on the optic chiasm.

- In men and women with secondary hypogonadism, reassessment of the hypothalamic–pituitary gonadal axis should be performed after normalization of prolactin. If secondary hypogonadism persists after 6 months, patients not desiring fertility should be considered for sex hormone replacement.
- According to the endocrine society guidelines, dopamine agonist therapy can be tapered with eventual discontinuation in patients who have been treated with dopamine agonists for at least 2 years, have a normal prolactin, and have no visible tumor on MRI.[12] Prospective studies show that up to 50% of patients with macroprolactinomas with normal prolactin levels and ≥50% tumor reduction will not recur after withdrawal from cabergoline[4] suggesting that patients with visible tumor but significant shrinkage can also be tapered and possibly weaned off of medical therapy.

REFERENCES

1. Molitch ME. Diagnosis and treatment of pituitary adenomas: a review. *JAMA* 2017;317:516–524.
2. Wong A, Eloy JA, Couldwell WT, Liu JK. Update on prolactinomas. Part 1: Clinical manifestations and diagnostic challenges. *J Clin Neurosci* 2015;22:1562–1567.
3. Iglesias P, Díez JJ. Macroprolactinoma: a diagnostic and therapeutic update. *QJM* 2013;106:495–504.
4. Molitch ME. Endocrinology in pregnancy: management of the pregnant patient with a prolactinoma. *Eur J Endocrinol* 2015;172:R205–R213.
5. Javorsky BR, Aron DC, Findling JW, Tyrrell JB. Hypothalamus and pituitary gland. In: Gardner DG, Shoback D, eds. *Greenspan's Basic & Clinical Endocrinology*. 10th ed. McGraw-Hill Education; 2018.
6. Chanson P, Maiter D. Prolactinoma. In: Melmed S, ed. *The Pituitary*. 4th ed. Academic Press; 2017:467–514.
7. Huang W, Molitch ME. Evaluation and management of galactorrhea. *Am Fam Physician* 2012;85:1073–1080.
8. Glezer A, Bronstein MD. The pituitary gland in pregnancy. In: Melmed S, ed. *The Pituitary*. 4th ed. Academic Press; 2017:397–411.
9. Molitch ME. Drugs and prolactin. *Pituitary* 2008;11:209–218.
10. Ipekci SH, Cakir M, Kiyici A, Koc O, Artac M. Radiotherapy-induced hypopituitarism in nasopharyngeal carcinoma: the tip of an iceberg. *Exp Clin Endocrinol Diabetes* 2015;123(7):411–418.
11. Wallace IR, Satti N, Courtney CH, et al. Ten-year clinical follow-up of a cohort of 51 patients with macroprolactinemia establishes it as a benign variant. *J Clin Endocrinol Metab* 2010;95:3268–3271.
12. Melmed S, Casanueva FF, Hoffman AR, et al. Diagnosis and treatment of hyperprolactinemia: an endocrine society clinical practice guideline. *J Clin Endocrinol Metab* 2011;96:273–288.
13. Lam G, Mehta V, Zada G. Spontaneous and medically induced cerebrospinal fluid leakage in the setting of pituitary adenomas: review of the literature. *Neurosurg Focus* 2012;32(6):E2.
14. Drake WM, Stiles CE, Bevan JS, et al. A follow-up study of the prevalence of valvular heart abnormalities in hyperprolactinemic patients treated with cabergoline. *J Clin Endocrinol Metab* 2016;101(11):4189–4194.
15. Gillam MP, Molitch ME, Lombardi G, Colao A. Advances in the treatment of prolactinomas. *Endocr Rev* 2006;27:485–534.
16. Klibanski A. Prolactinomas. *N Engl J Med* 2010;362:1219–1226.

Acromegaly

3

Karin Hickey and Julie M. Silverstein

GENERAL PRINCIPLES

- Acromegaly is a disorder characterized by overproduction of growth hormone (GH) and insulin-like growth factor 1 (IGF-1) and is most commonly caused by a pituitary adenoma.
- Overproduction of GH and IGF-1 results in progressive skeletal, skin, and organ growth and metabolic derangements, which are associated with significant morbidity and premature mortality if left untreated.

Definition

- **Acromegaly** is GH oversecretion occurring in the postpubertal phase of life.
- When GH oversecretion occurs before puberty, it may cause rapid growth and hypogonadism with failure of growth-plate closure, resulting in **gigantism**.

Epidemiology

- The prevalence ranges between 2.8 and 13.7 cases per 100,000 people and the annual incidence rates range between 0.2 and 1.1 cases per 100,000 people.[1]
- The median age at diagnosis is in the fifth decade of life with a median diagnostic delay of 4.5 to 5 years.[1] Incidence is similar in men and women.

Pathophysiology

- Acromegaly is most commonly due to a pure somatroph pituitary adenoma (60%). Adenomas that secrete a combination of GH and prolactin are less common (25%), while adenomas that secrete GH and thyroid-stimulating hormone (TSH) are rare.[2]
- Molecular studies of the pathogenesis of somatotroph adenomas are ongoing. A mutation in the Gsα protein has been found in up to 40% of somatotroph adenomas.[2]
- GH secretion, stimulated by growth hormone–releasing hormone (GHRH) from the hypothalamus, causes IGF-1 secretion from the liver. Normally, GH secretion is inhibited by both somatostatin from the hypothalamus and IGF-1 from peripheral tissue.
- Autonomous GH secretion from somatotroph adenomas increases IGF-1 secretion, which leads to growth of bone and cartilage, impaired glucose tolerance, and changes in protein and fat metabolism.

DIAGNOSIS

The diagnosis of acromegaly involves first recognizing the phenotype and then performing the appropriate hormonal workup. Lastly, imaging of the pituitary is performed.

Clinical Presentation

Patients with acromegaly present with **skeletal overgrowth and soft tissue enlargement**. Changes can be subtle over time and may best be recognized by comparing previous photographs of the patient. Symptoms related to hormonal deficiencies may arise as a result of compression of the remaining pituitary gland by the enlarging mass.

History
- Patients may report an increase in hat, ring, or shoe size.
- Headache is the second most common symptom, even when the adenoma is small.
- The voice tends to be deeper, related to sinus and laryngeal hypertrophy.
- Malodorous sweating, especially at night, may occur.
- Paresthesias related to carpal tunnel syndrome and other peripheral neuropathies occur, as do visual disturbances related to increased skeletal growth in the skull or to compression of the optic chiasm by the pituitary adenoma.
- Arthralgias and myalgias occur in 30% to 70% of patients with large joints affected more prominently. Spinal osteoarthritis with resulting backache, usually in the lumbar spine, also occurs. Rarely, spinal involvement leads to nerve compression leading to lumbar spinal stenosis or sciatica.[3]
- Dyspnea at rest or with exertion can happen with more advanced disease due to remodeling of myocardium.
- Endocrine symptoms related to compression of the remaining pituitary gland can be those of hypothyroidism (cold intolerance, fatigue, weight gain), hypogonadism (reduced libido, infertility, irregular menses), and hyperprolactinemia (irregular menses, galactorrhea).

Physical Examination
- Hypertension occurs in approximately 50% of patients.[4]
- Hands and feet are broad with wide, thick, and stubby fingers and toes.
- The nose is widened and thickened, the forehead and cheekbones are prominent, and facial lines are more visible. Mandibular overgrowth leads to prognathism, teeth separation, and jaw malocclusion.
- Skin can be sweaty and oily (70%), as well as coarse and thick. Skin tags can be numerous, and can grow in size.
- While arthropathy is common, objective findings are not prominent. Decreased joint mobility may be seen in later disease, but joint effusions and signs of inflammation are rare.

Differential Diagnosis
- Other causes of increased GH must be excluded. Exogenous use of GH should be considered in adolescent patients and body builders.
- Pituitary somatotroph carcinoma is exceptionally rare.
- Extrapituitary GH oversecretion is rare but can occur with ectopic pituitary adenomas in the sphenoid sinus or nasopharyngeal cavity or, much more rarely, by a peripheral tumor such as a pancreatic neuroendocrine tumor. GHRH hypersecretion that causes pituitary somatotrophs to oversecrete GH has been seen with pancreatic and bronchial carcinoid tumors.
- Genetic syndromes associated with acromegaly include familial isolated pituitary adenoma which is caused by mutations in the aryl-hydrocarbon receptor-interacting protein (AIP) gene in 20% of cases, McCune–Albright, Carney complex, and multiple endocrine neoplasia type 1 (MEN1).[5]

Diagnostic Testing

Laboratories
- The initial laboratory tests for a patient suspected of having acromegaly should be **IGF-1 and GH levels**. Current guidelines recommend an elevated IGF-1 and failure to suppress GH during an oral glucose tolerance test (OGTT) to confirm the diagnosis.[6,7]

However, an OGTT may not be needed if GH and IGF-1 levels are elevated in a patient with clear signs and symptoms of acromegaly.

- During an **OGTT**, blood is drawn at baseline for glucose and GH, 75 g of oral glucose is administered, and then blood is drawn for GH and glucose every 30 minutes for 2 hours. Although guidelines recommend using a nadir GH cutoff of <0.4 ng/mL using ultrasensitive assays to confirm the diagnosis of acromegaly,[6,7] studies show that if the GH level falls to <0.3 ng/mL during the OGTT, acromegaly is excluded.[4] False positives may occur in patients with diabetes, chronic hepatitis, renal failure, and anorexia. In addition, patients with mild acromegaly can have suppressed GH levels (<0.3 ng/mL) during an OGTT.[8]
- Assessment of the remainder of pituitary hormones, including measurement of prolactin, TSH, free thyroxine (T4), 8 a.m. cortisol, luteinizing hormone (LH), follicle-stimulating hormone (FSH), and testosterone (males only) should also take place. If indicated by symptoms and/or if the 8 a.m. cortisol is <15 mcg/dL, a cosyntropin stimulation test to diagnose adrenal insufficiency may be needed.

Imaging
- The initial imaging study should be an MRI of the brain, with and without gadolinium contrast, to evaluate for pituitary adenoma.
- Radiographs of the extremities and cranium will show abnormalities related to bone and cartilage overgrowth.
- Echocardiography may show hypertrophy of the interventricular septum and left ventricular posterior wall as well as diastolic, and less often systolic, dysfunction.

TREATMENT

- The goals of treatment include relief of symptoms, reduced tumor volume, and improvement of long-term morbidity and mortality. A GH level <1 ng/mL and an IGF-1 level in the normal range is the treatment goal.[6,9]
- An algorithm of the three major treatment modalities is presented in Figure 3-1.[6]

Surgical Management
- Surgery results in the most rapid reduction in GH levels and is the first-line treatment for microadenomas and most macroadenomas. Its efficacy depends on the size of the adenoma, tumor invasion, and the experience of the surgeon.
- Control rates quoted in studies are best achieved with an experienced neurosurgeon, performing at least 50 pituitary operations per year.[10]
- Transsphenoidal surgery is appropriate for intrasellar microadenomas, noninvasive macroadenomas, when the tumor is causing compressive symptoms, and for debulking of invasive tumors. Craniotomy is rarely required. Control rates for macroadenomas are lower (45% to 68%) than for microadenomas (81% to 100%).[5] Tumors with cavernous sinus involvement or transcapsular intra-arachnoid invasion have even lower cure rates.

Medications
- Pharmacologic treatment is used when surgery alone has not reduced GH and IGF-1 levels to normal. GH-lowering drugs are also used as primary therapy when surgery is contraindicated or in the case of large GH-secreting macroadenomas which are not likely to be completely removed by surgery. Medication may also be used as a bridge until radiation therapy has had its full effect.
- In general, all medical therapy for acromegaly should stop if a woman becomes pregnant, due to lack of available safety information.
- Please see Table 3-1 for medications used in the management of acromegaly.[11–14]

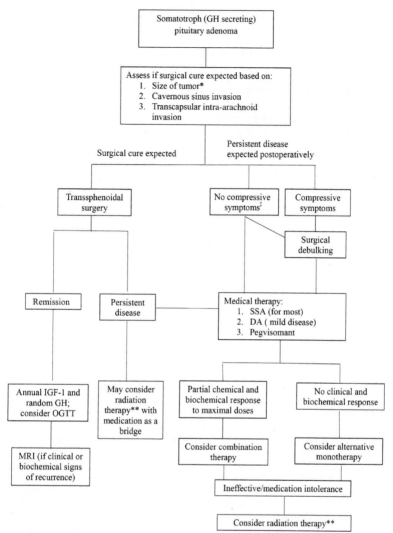

FIGURE 3-1 Algorithm for the management of acromegaly. IGF-1, insulin-like growth factor 1; GH, growth hormone; OGTT, oral glucose tolerance test; SSA, somatostatin analog; DA, dopamine agonist.
*Influence of tumor size on surgical outcome is uncertain; in general, tumors less than 2 cm have a greater chance of surgical success.
**Stereotactic radiosurgery (SRS) preferred over conventional radiotherapy (CRT).
‡In patients without compressive symptoms not expected to be cured surgically, primary medical therapy or surgical debulking followed by medical therapy can be considered.
Adapted from Katznelson L, Laws E, Sholomo M, et al. Acromegaly: an endocrine society clinical practice guideline. *J Clin Endocrinol Metab* 2014;99(11):3933–3951.

TABLE 3-1 MEDICAL THERAPY FOR ACROMEGALY

Agent	Description	Indication	Dosing	Efficacy	Side effects
First-generation SRLs					
Octreotide LAR	Long-acting octreotide Affinity for SSTR2, SSTR3, and SSTR5 Administered via IM injection q4wk	Primary therapy in nonsurgical candidates Persistent disease after surgery Bridge therapy until radiotherapy's full effect	10–40 mg IM q4wk Start 20 mg q4wk, increase by 10 mg q3mo based on IGF-1 levels	Normal IGF-1 in 38–85% GH <2.5 ng/mL in 33–75%	Hyperglycemia in up to 42% Most commonly nausea, diarrhea, abdominal pain, or distention Less commonly hair loss, cholelithiasis, bradycardia
Lanreotide depot	Long-acting lanreotide Affinity for SSTR2, SSTR3, and SSTR5 Administered via deep SC injection q4wk	Same as for octreotide LAR	60–120 mg SC q4wk Start 90 mg SC q4wk, titrate by 30 mg q3mo based on IGF-1 levels May give 120 mg SC q6–8wk if controlled on 60 or 90 mg SC	Normal IGF-1 in 39–80% GH <2.5 ng/mL in 38–80%	Same as for octreotide LAR
Second-generation SRL					
Pasireotide LAR	Long-acting pasireotide Affinity for SSTR1, SSTR2, SSTR3, and SSTR5 Administered via IM injection q4wk	Consider in patients not responsive to first-generation SRLs Role as primary therapy in nonsurgical candidates, for persistent disease after surgery or as bridge therapy until radiotherapy's full effect is not certain	20–60 mg IM q4wk Start 40 mg IM q4wk, titrate by 20 mg q3mo based on IGF-1 levels	Biochemical control in 31.3% compared to 19.2% of patients on octreotide LAR 20% biochemical control in patients resistant to first-generation SRLs	Hyperglycemia in 57.3–65% Other side effects similar to first-generation SRLs

(continued)

TABLE 3-1 MEDICAL THERAPY FOR ACROMEGALY *(Continued)*

Agent	Description	Indication	Dosing	Efficacy	Side effects
GH receptor antagonist					
Pegvisomant	GH antagonist leading to decreased production of IGF-1 Administered via SC injection qday	Second line in patients with persistent disease after surgery Can be used as first-line therapy Not recommended in patients with enlarging pituitary adenomas or in whom tumor growth is a concern	10–30 mg SC qday Start 40 mg SC × 1, then 10 mg SC qday, increase by 5 mg qday q4–6wk based on IGF-1 levels	Normalization of IGF-1 in 60% May improve fasting glucose, insulin, and HgbA1C levels	Transaminitis in 2.5%, monitor LFTs qmonth during first 6 months, then q4–6 mo Skin rash and lipohypertrophy at injection sites Periodic MRI to monitor tumor GH levels increase and should not be monitored
Dopamine agonists					
Cabergoline	Affinity for D2R Inhibits secretion of GH by stimulating dopaminergic receptors expressed on somatotropinomas Dosed orally twice weekly	Mild to moderate elevations in IGF-1/GH (<1.5 × ULN) Treatment of prolactin/GH co-secreting tumors	Dose 0.3–7 mg/wk Start 0.25 mg twice weekly × 1 month, titrate based on IGF-1 levels	Biochemical control in 30% as monotherapy Biochemical control as add-on to SRL in 40–50%	Nausea, headache, constipation, postural hypotension, dizziness, nasal stuffiness Psychosis and impulse control disorders (rare)

D2R, dopamine D2 receptor; GH, growth hormone; HgbA1C, glycosylated hemoglobin A1C; IGF-1, insulin-like growth factor 1; IM, intramuscular; LFTs, liver function tests; LAR, long-acting release; SRL, somatostatin receptor ligand; SSTR, somatostatin receptor subtype.

Data from Paragliola RM, Corsello SM, Salvatori R. Somatostatin receptor ligands in acromegaly: clinical response and factors predicting resistance. *Pituitary* 2017;20:109–115; Gadelha MR, Wildemberg LE, Bronstein MD, Gatto F, Ferone D. Somatostatin receptor ligands in the treatment of acromegaly. *Pituitary* 2017;20:100–108; Kuhn E, Chanson P. Cabergoline in acromegaly. *Pituitary* 2017;20:121–128; and Sandret L, Maison P, Chanson P. Place of cabergoline in acromegaly: a meta-analysis. *J Clin Endocrinol Metab* 2011;9(65):1327–1335.

- **Somatostatin receptor ligands (SRLs):** Somatostatin receptor subtype 2 (SSTR2) is expressed in >95% of GH-producing adenomas, SSTR5 is present in >85%, and SSTR1 and SSTR3 are present in 40% of tumors.[11] SRLs, including **octreotide, lanreotide,** and **pasireotide,** act as agonists to somatostatin receptors (SSTRs) on the tumor to decrease GH secretion.
- **First-generation SRLs: Octreotide and lanreotide** bind with high affinity to SSTR2 and have weak to moderate affinity for SSTR3 and SSTR5.[11] They are recommended as first-line therapy for patients who will likely not be cured by surgery or who are poor surgical candidates.[6] They may also be used as a temporizing measure before surgery to improve comorbidities, to control symptoms before radiation therapy achieves full effects, or after surgery when full biochemical control is not achieved.
  - Biochemical control is achieved in 20% to 54% of patients.[15] Variable efficacy rates reported in studies are likely secondary to differences in treatment history and definitions of biochemical control across studies. Studies that include patients known to respond to somatostatin analogs report higher response rates compared to studies that include only treatment-naïve patients.
  - Reduction of tumor size from 10% to >45% is seen in 36.6% of patients treated with first-generation SRLs.[7]
  - The initial does of **octreotide LAR** (long-acting release) is 20 mg intramuscular (IM) once a month. The dose is increased at 3-month intervals until plasma IGF-1 levels are normal or until a maximal dose of 40 mg is reached.
  - The initial dose of **lanreotide depot** is 90 mg via deep subcutaneous (SC) injection once a month. The dose is adjusted at 3-month intervals until IGF-1 levels are normal or a maximal dose of 120 mg is reached. Patients controlled on 60 or 90 mg SC may be switched to 120 mg SC every 6 to 8 weeks.
  - IGF-1 levels should be checked just prior to dosing of octreotide or lanreotide with dose adjustments every 3 months.
  - Side effects are mild and usually transient and include nausea, diarrhea, abdominal bloating, and cramping. These effects occur early and usually improve during the first few months of treatment. Gallstones develop with increased frequency but usually do not cause acute cholecystitis. Rarely, pancreatitis can occur. Hyperglycemia may also occur or worsen.
- **Second-generation SRL: Pasireotide,** in contrast to first-generation SRLs, targets multiple SSTR subtypes with highest affinity for SSTR5 followed by SSTR2, SSTR3, and SSTR1.[16] Because of its subtype binding affinity, it is approved for treatment of both acromegaly and Cushing disease.
  - In clinical trials, **pasireotide LAR** has been shown to be more effective than octreotide LAR as first-line medical treatment and effective in patients resistant to first-generation SRLs.[11] Further studies are needed to determine which patients would benefit the most from treatment with **pasireotide LAR.**
  - The initial dose of pasireotide is 40 mg IM every 28 days and can be titrated by 20 mg based on IGF-1 levels and symptoms to a maximum dose of 60 mg if IGF-1 levels have not normalized after 3 months. Similar to octreotide and lanreotide, IGF-1 levels should be checked just prior to dosing with dose adjustments every 3 months.
  - Pasireotide's safety profile is similar to first-generation SRLs except that **hyperglycemia** occurs more frequently due to its unique SRL binding profile.[16]
- **GH receptor antagonist: Pegvisomant** blocks GH action in peripheral tissues by antagonizing the GH receptor. This agent can be used when adequate biochemical control is not achieved with other treatment modalities, as first-line therapy in patients not controlled by surgery, or in combination with a somatostatin analog.
  - Although initial studies reported normalization of IGF-1 levels in >90% of patients, in clinical practice approximately 62% of patients achieve biochemical control.[14] Pegvisomant does not target the GH-secreting pituitary tumor, consequently GH levels rise and should not be monitored. Pegvisomant is not felt to cause notable tumor

growth.[17,18] However, serial imaging with MRI scan is nonetheless recommended to evaluate tumor size.[6]

- The initial dose is 40 mg SC as a loading dose and then 10 mg SC daily. The dose is increased in 5-mg increments at 4-week intervals until plasma IGF-1 is normal or a maximal dose of 30 mg is reached.
- Liver enzymes should be monitored once a month during the first 6 months of treatment and every 4 to 6 months thereafter. AST or ALT levels above three times the upper limit of normal may occur in 2.5% of patients.[17]

- **Dopamine agonists** inhibit secretion of GH by stimulating dopaminergic receptors expressed on somatotropinomas and can be used as first-line medical therapy in patients with mild elevations in GH and IGF-1 (<1.5 × upper limit of normal) with or without hyperprolactinemia.[6] **Cabergoline** is more effective and better tolerated than bromocriptine. Approximately 30% of patients achieve biochemical control with cabergoline monotherapy.[13]
  - The initial dosing of cabergoline is 0.25 mg twice per week. Doses as high as 7 mg per week may be needed.
  - Side effects include nausea and orthostatic hypotension, so the medication should be started at low doses and gradually titrated up. With long-term therapy at high doses, there may be an increased risk of cardiac valvular abnormalities.

- **Combination therapy:** In cases when monotherapy does not result in biochemical control, combination therapy may be considered. In patients not controlled on somatostatin analog monotherapy, the addition of cabergoline or pegvisomant leads to normalization of IGF-1 in 30% to 60%[16] and 58% to 100%[19] of patients, respectively. The combination of pegvisomant and cabergoline is also sometimes used.

- **Potential therapies:** Therapies in development include oral octreotide, a long-acting subcutaneous injectable form of octreotide, an SRL highly selective for GH suppression and a GH receptor blocker.[20]

Other Nonpharmacologic Therapies

- **Radiation therapy** is considered second or third line in patients who have not fully responded to surgery or medical therapy.[7]
- Both conventional radiotherapy (CRT) and stereotactic radiotherapy (e.g., Gamma Knife, CyberKnife, linear accelerator, and proton beam) have been used to treat somatotroph adenomas. Treatment with stereotactic radiosurgery (SRS), which delivers a high dose of radiation to a defined target, leads to tumor control in 93% to 100% of patients and biochemical control in 44% to 52% of patients at 5 years. SRS leads to less damage of surrounding brain tissue and thus fewer adverse consequences as compared to CRT but is limited by tumor size and proximity to the optic nerves. CRT leads to tumor control in 80% to 100% and biochemical control in 60% to 80% of patients but has a slower onset of action and full response to treatment may not be seen for up to 15 years.[21]
- Hypopituitarism occurs in >50% of patients with both CRT and SRS within 5 to 10 years of treatment.[6] There may be an increased risk of secondary tumors and stroke over time with both forms of radiotherapy.[21]

COMPLICATIONS

- The standardized mortality ratio for patients with acromegaly is 1.7 compared to the general population with most deaths caused by cardiovascular, respiratory, and cerebrovascular disease.[22]
- **Cardiovascular morbidity** is increased related to hypertension, left ventricular hypertrophy, diastolic and systolic dysfunction, and arrhythmias. Cardiac valvulopathy is also

common. Patients should undergo cardiovascular risk assessment with measurements of blood pressure and lipid profile. An electrocardiogram and/or echocardiogram and referral to a cardiologist in patients with known cardiac disease prior to surgery should be considered.[7]

- **Respiratory complications** of acromegaly include sleep apnea (>50% of patients)[4] and respiratory insufficiency. Though this may improve with treatment of acromegaly, some will continue to require nocturnal positive end-expiratory pressure.
- Insulin resistance develops as a result of both pancreatic β-cell dysfunction and insulin resistance in the liver, skeletal muscle, and adipose tissue. **Type 2 diabetes mellitus** occurs in 19% to 56% of patients and thus all patients should be screened for diabetes.[23]
- **Pituitary dysfunction**, including secondary hypothyroidism, hypogonadism, and adrenal insufficiency and hypoprolactinemia may occur due to local tumor effects and must be adequately screened for as described in Chapter 1 (Sellar and Suprasellar Masses) and Chapter 6 (Hypopituitarism).
- The risk of **colonic polyps** is increased in patients with acromegaly, which may be associated with an increased risk of colorectal cancer although patients with acromegaly do not have an increased risk of death due to cancer. Colonoscopy at the time of diagnosis is recommended with follow-up testing as per clinical guidelines for the general population.[7,24]
- Risk of **thyroid nodules** and **thyroid cancer** is higher in patients with acromegaly. Thyroid ultrasonography is recommended in patients with palpable thyroid nodules but is not advocated for widespread screening.[6]
- Acromegaly has been shown to be associated with **higher femoral neck bone density** and an **increased risk of vertebral fractures** likely due to effects of elevated GH and IGF-1 on bone turnover.[25] Bone densitometry should be performed in patients with a history of fracture and considered in patients at high risk for fracture, such as patients with hypogonadism.

MONITORING/FOLLOW-UP

- **Biochemical testing**
  - In patients who have undergone surgery, a postoperative day 1 GH level <2 ng/mL has been shown to correlate with long-term remission. IGF-1 levels should be measured 12 weeks after surgery and repeated 9 to 12 weeks later if still elevated since there may be a delay in normalization of IGF-1.[7]
  - An IGF-1 in the normal range and a random GH <1 ng/mL by ultrasensitive assay define control.[9]
  - An OGTT can also be used to assess outcome. Although many authors recommend using a nadir GH level <0.3 ng/mL to define control, current guidelines recommend a nadir GH level <0.4 ng/mL.[6]
  - Only IGF-1 levels are monitored with GH receptor antagonist therapy and the OGTT should not be used in patients receiving somatostatin analogs.
  - A full assessment of pituitary function should occur 4 to 6 weeks after surgery.
  - Ongoing assessment for pituitary dysfunction is needed after radiation therapy.
- Imaging follow-up
  - An MRI can be performed at 3 to 4 months after surgery to establish a baseline[7] with the timing of subsequent MRI scans depending on disease control. If disease control is achieved by surgery, MRI may only be needed every 2 to 3 years. In patients who are not adequately controlled, MRI should likely be followed yearly.
  - With GH receptor antagonist therapy, an MRI should be performed 6 months after initiation of therapy and then yearly because of the potential risk of tumor enlargement.

OUTCOME/PROGNOSIS

- If left untreated, acromegalic patients live on average 10 years less than control patients. Death is most commonly due to cardiovascular disease.
- Surgery done by an experienced surgeon has the most favorable outcome.

REFERENCES

1. Lavrentaki A, Paluzzi A, Wass JA, Karavitaki N. Epidemiology of acromegaly: review of population studies. *Pituitary* 2017;20(1):4–9.
2. Melmed S. Acromegaly pathogenesis and treatment. *J Clin Invest* 2009;119:3189–3202.
3. Chanson P, Salenave S, Kamenicky P, Cazabat L, Young J. Acromegaly. *Best Pract Res Clin Endocrinol Metab* 2009;23:555–574.
4. Melmed S. Acromegaly. In: Melmed S, ed. *The Pituitary*. 4th ed. Cambridge, MA: Academic Press; 2017.
5. Capatina C, Wass JAH. 60 years of neuroendocrinology: acromegaly. *J Endocrinol* 2015; 226(2):T141–T160.
6. Katznelson L, Laws E, Sholomo M, et al. Acromegaly: an endocrine society clinical practice guideline. *J Clin Endocrinol Metab* 2014;99(11):3933–3951.
7. Katznelson L, Atkinson JL, Cook DM, et al. American association of clinical endocrinologists medical guidelines for clinical practice for the diagnosis and treatment of acromegaly-2011 update. *Endocrine Practice* 2011;17(Suppl 4):1–44.
8. Ribeiro-Oliveira A, Faje AT, Barkan AL. Limited utility of oral glucose tolerance test in biochemically active acromegaly. *Eur J Endocrinology* 2011;164(1):17–22.
9. Guistina A, Chanson P, Bronstein D, et al. A consensus on criteria for cure of acromegaly. *J Clin Endocrinol Metab* 2010;95:3141–3148.
10. Casanueva FF, Barkan AL, Buchfelder M, et al. Criteria for the definition of Pituitary Tumor Centers of Excellence (PTCOE): a pituitary society statement. *Pituitary* 2017;20:489–498.
11. Gadelha MR, Wildemberg LE, Bronstein MD, Gatto F, Ferone D. Somatostatin receptor ligands in the treatment of acromegaly. *Pituitary* 2017;20:100–108.
12. Paragliola RM, Corsello SM, Salvatori R. Somatostatin receptor ligands in acromegaly: clinical response and factors predicting resistance. *Pituitary* 2017;20:109–115.
13. Sandret L, Maison P, Chanson P. Place of cabergoline in acromegaly: a meta-analysis. *J Clin Endocrinol Metab* 2011;96(5):1327–1335.
14. Kuhn E, Chanson P. Cabergoline in acromegaly. *Pituitary* 2017;20:121–128.
15. Shanik MH, Cao PD, Ludlam WH. Historical response rates of somatostatin analogues in the treatment of acromegaly: a systematic review. *Endocr Pract* 2016;22(3):350–356.
16. Cuevas-Ramos D, Fleseriu M. Pasireotide: a novel treatment for patients with acromegaly. *Drug Des Devel Ther* 2016;10:227–239.
17. Van der Lely AJ, Biller BM, Brue T, et al. Long-term safety of pegvisomant in patients with acromegaly: comprehensive review of 1288 subjects in ACROSTUDY. *J Clin Endocrinol Metab* 2012;97(5):1589–1597.
18. Buhk JH, Jung S, Psychogios MN, et al. Tumor volume of growth hormone-secreting pituitary adenomas during treatment with pegvisomant: a prospective multicenter study. *J Clin Endocrinol Metab* 2010;95(2):552–558.
19. Lim DST, Fleseriu M. The role of combination medical therapy in the treatment of acromegaly. *Pituitary* 2017;20:136–148.
20. Melmed S. New therapeutic agents for acromegaly. *Nat Rev Endocrinol* 2016;12(2):90–98.
21. Gheorghiu ML. Updates in outcomes of stereotactic radiation therapy in acromegaly. *Pituitary* 2017;20:154–168.
22. Sherlock M, Reulen RC, Alonso AA, et al. ACTH deficiency, higher doses of hydrocortisone replacement, and radiotherapy are independent predictors of mortality in patients with acromegaly. *J Clin Endocrinol Metab* 2009;94:4216–4223.
23. Pivonello R, Auriemma RS, Grasso LF, et al. Complications of acromegaly: cardiovascular, respiratory and metabolic comorbidities. *Pituitary* 2017;20:46–62.
24. Melmed S, Casanueva FF, Klibanski A, et al. A consensus on the diagnosis and treatment of acromegaly complications. *Pituitary* 2013;16:294–302.
25. Mazziotti G, Biagioli E, Maffezzoni F, et al. Bone turnover, bone mineral density, and fracture risk in acromegaly: a meta-analysis. *J Clin Endocrinol Metab* 2015;100(2):384–394.

Diabetes Insipidus

4

Laura N. Hollar and Julie M. Silverstein

GENERAL PRINCIPLES

Definition

- Diabetes insipidus (DI) is a disorder of water balance caused by the nonosmotic renal loss of water leading to the excretion of a large volume of dilute urine.
- Polyuria is defined as 24-hour urine output >40 to 50 mL/kg/day in adults.[1,2]

Classification

- **Central DI** is caused by complete or partial deficiency of antidiuretic hormone (ADH) secretion from the posterior pituitary gland.
- **Nephrogenic DI** is caused by complete or partial renal resistance to ADH.
- **Primary polydipsia** is due to suppression of ADH secretion caused by excessive fluid intake due to a defect in thirst mechanism (dipsogenic) or cognitive abnormalities (polygenic).[2,3]

Epidemiology

- All forms of DI are rare with an estimated prevalence of central DI of 1 in 25,000.[4,5] No gender predilection has been seen. Most cases present in adulthood, although familial central DI and nephrogenic DI usually present during childhood.
- Transient central DI occurs in 10% to 30% of patients after transsphenoidal pituitary surgery while only 2% to 7% of patients develop permanent dysfunction.[6] Approximately 67.5% to 80% of patients with clinical evidence of postoperative DI need treatment with desmopressin (DDAVP, an ADH analog) at least once after surgery.[7,8]

Etiology

- See Table 4-1 for a list of causes of DI.[9]
- Central DI is caused by destruction of ADH-producing cells in the hypothalamus and posterior pituitary gland. The destruction can be traumatic, infectious, neoplastic, or infiltrative in origin resulting in complete or partial lack of ADH secretion.
- Nephrogenic DI is caused by either congenital or acquired impaired renal responsiveness to ADH.

Pathophysiology

- ADH is synthesized in the supraoptic and paraventricular nuclei of the hypothalamus and transported to the posterior pituitary gland for storage and secretion. Osmoreceptors in the hypothalamus are very sensitive to changes in plasma osmolality, primarily determined by the sodium concentration. Baroreceptors also elicit ADH release with a decrease in blood volume of 5% to 10%.[5]
- ADH release is inhibited until the osmolality rises above a threshold, after which ADH secretion rises rapidly in proportion to the plasma osmolality.

TABLE 4-1	CAUSES OF DIABETES INSIPIDUS
Central DI	Head trauma (may remit after 6 months)
	Postsurgical (develops 1–6 days after surgery and often disappears, recurs, or becomes chronic)
	Tumors—craniopharyngioma, pinealoma, meningioma, germinoma, glioma, benign cysts, leukemia, lymphoma, metastatic breast or lung
	Infections—TB, syphilis, mycoses, toxoplasmosis, encephalitis, meningitis
	Granulomatous disease—sarcoidosis, histiocytosis X, Wegener granulomatosis
	Cerebrovascular disease—aneurysms, thrombosis, Sheehan syndrome, cerebrovascular accident
	Idiopathic—sporadic or familial (rare autosomal dominant trait)
Nephrogenic DI	Congenital—rare inherited disorder caused by inherited mutations in the AVP receptor (X-linked recessive) or in the water channel of the renal tubule (autosomal recessive)
	Acquired—much more common and less severe
	Medications—lithium, amphotericin B, demeclocycline, cisplatin, aminoglycosides, rifampin, foscarnet, methoxyflurane, vincristine
	Electrolyte disorders—hypercalcemia, hypokalemia
	Chronic tubulointerstitial diseases—polycystic kidney disease, medullary sponge kidney, obstructive uropathy, papillary necrosis
	Sickle cell disease and trait
	Multiple myeloma, amyloidosis
	Sarcoidosis

AVP, arginine vasopressin; DI, diabetes insipidus; TB, tuberculosis.
Reprinted from Fried LF, Palevsky PM. Hyponatremia and hypernatremia. *Med Clin North Am* 1997; 81:585–609, with permission from Elsevier.

- ADH primarily acts on the distal tubules and collecting ducts of the kidneys to increase water reabsorption.
- The effects of ADH are mediated via a G-protein–coupled V_2 receptor that signals the translocation of aquaporin-2 channels into the apical membrane of the principal cells in the collecting duct. In conjunction with aquaporin-3 and aquaporin-4 channels on the basolateral surface of these cells, water is then allowed to flow freely down the osmotic gradient from the relatively dilute tubular fluid to the highly concentrated renal medulla. Therefore, decreased production or activity of ADH results in impaired water reabsorption in the nephron, leading to a dilute urine and loss of free water.[10]
- An intact thirst mechanism is very effective in preventing hypernatremia (hypertonic dehydration). An increase in basal plasma osmolality of as little as 1% to 2% is sufficient to induce thirst. Once this threshold is reached, even a small increase in hypertonicity stimulates a very large increase in water intake.[2]

DIAGNOSIS

Patients with DI present with increased thirst and polyuria, with urine volume typically exceeding 3 L/day. Symptoms of hypernatremia (e.g., weakness, altered mental status, coma, or seizures) may develop with significant or rapid dehydration.

Clinical Presentation

History
- A thorough history including the patient's age, rate of onset, duration and degree of polyuria or nocturia, family history, history of head trauma/surgery, dietary habits, fluid intake, the presence/absence of thirst, the presence of headaches or vision changes, medication history, the presence of psychiatric illness, and a history of diabetes mellitus and/or renal failure is essential for diagnosis and to differentiate DI from other causes of polyuria.
- Patients with DI often crave cold liquids.

Physical Examination
Orthostatic hypotension and skin tenting may be signs of volume depletion.

Diagnostic Criteria

- Diagnosis of DI is made when polyuria is present in the setting of an inappropriately low urine osmolality (<300 mOsm/kg) for a given plasma osmolality. The urine specific gravity is usually <1.001 to 1.010.[11]
- Plasma sodium may be normal or elevated (i.e., in someone who does not have an intact thirst mechanism).

Differential Diagnosis

- Several conditions can present with polyuria. Simultaneous measurement of urine and plasma osmolality is essential to differentiate the various causes.
- **Hypotonic polyuria** (Uosm <300 mOsm/kg) can be either physiologic (due to an increase in free water intake leading to appropriate suppression of ADH, free water diuresis, and a normal serum osmolality) or pathologic (due to a decrease in the production or action of ADH).
- **A fully concentrated urine (urine osmolality 800 to 1,200 mOsm/kg) in the setting of hypernatremia essentially rules out DI** and other causes should be considered (e.g., insensible water losses from skin, lungs, and GI tract and/or salt loading from feedings, medications, or intravenous fluids).
- **Nonhypotonic polyuria** (Uosm >300 mOsm/kg) is caused by **solute diuresis,** most commonly due to diuretics and hyperglycemia. Glucosuria in the setting of a urine specific gravity >1.010 is characteristic of polyuria due to hyperglycemia. If glucosuria is absent, other less common types of solute diuresis (such as relief from urinary obstruction, recovery from renal failure, or administration of large amounts of sodium, mannitol, or radiocontrast dye) should be considered.
- If hyponatremia is present, polyuria is most likely due to **primary polydipsia**.
- **Chronic hypokalemia and hypercalcemia** can cause partial nephrogenic DI. On the other hand, hypokalemia can also be a consequence of DI, and hypercalcemia can be caused by volume depletion. Patients with chronic kidney disease may also develop partial DI as a consequence of defects in the renal concentrating capacity.

Diagnostic Testing

- **The water deprivation test** is the standard method for differentiating polyuria caused by primary polydipsia, central and nephrogenic DI.

○ **This test is unnecessary and potentially dangerous in the setting of hypertonic hypernatremia**, in which primary polydipsia is not a consideration. Likewise, DI is virtually ruled out if the patient has hypotonic hyponatremia. Therefore, a water deprivation test **should only be performed in a patient with hypotonic polyuria with a normal plasma sodium/osmolality**.

○ **Water deprivation test procedure:**

  ▪ Discontinue drugs that influence ADH secretion or action. Caffeine, alcohol, and tobacco should be avoided for at least 24 hours.

  ▪ Patient's water intake is restricted starting after dinner unless the patient is producing >10 L of urine/day, in which case the deprivation test is only done during the day under close supervision. Body weight, plasma osmolality, serum sodium, urine osmolality, and urine volume should be followed hourly.

  ▪ Fluids are withheld until one of the following occurs:
    1. Urine osmolality reaches a normal value ruling out DI (>600 to 800 mOsm/kg) *OR*
    2. Body weight decreases by 5% and plasma sodium and osmolality reach the upper limits of normal (sodium >145 mEq/L and osmolality >295 mOsm/kg) *OR*
    3. A stable hourly urine osmolality occurs (variation of <5% over 3 hours) despite rising plasma osmolality.

  ▪ If #2 or #3 above occurs, DDAVP 4 mcg SC or IV is administered and urine osmolality is measured at 30, 60, and 120 minutes.

○ Interpretation of the test

  ▪ In healthy individuals, water deprivation increases plasma osmolality, stimulating ADH secretion and water retention by the kidney (hence increasing urine osmolality).[2]

  ▪ In complete DI, with absent or ineffective ADH, the urine osmolality remains less than plasma osmolality (generally <300 mOsm/kg).

  ▪ In partial DI and primary polydipsia, urine osmolality will be greater than plasma osmolality, but the urine will remain submaximally concentrated (>300 to <800 mOsm/kg).

  ▪ If urine osmolality increases >50% from the level achieved during water deprivation after administration of DDAVP, the diagnosis of central DI is established.

  ▪ Plasma vasopressin can be measured before and after water deprivation but is not readily available in all laboratories.[2] The levels should be analyzed as a function of the concurrent plasma and urine osmolality. Patients with central DI and primary polydipsia have basal levels of plasma ADH that are subnormal. Patients with nephrogenic DI have normal to elevated basal levels. During water deprivation, ADH levels rise in primary polydipsia and nephrogenic DI but remain subnormal in central DI.[4]

○ Pitfalls of water deprivation test:

  ▪ The diagnosis of partial DI may be difficult, since there may be enough ADH secretion to partially concentrate the urine.

  ▪ ADH secretion or action can be normal in patients with primary polydipsia, but the associated chronic polyuria can lead to "washout" of the medullary interstitium. This results in loss of the transtubular osmolar gradient required to maintain the maximum urinary concentrating ability of the kidneys, making it difficult to differentiate from partial DI.[3]

• **Hypertonic saline test** may be used if the water restriction test is inconclusive or cannot be performed.[2]

  ○ Hypertonic (3%) saline is infused at 0.05 to 0.1 mL/kg/min for 1 to 2 hours, and plasma osmolality and sodium are measured every 30 minutes.

  ○ ADH is measured once the serum sodium and osmolality are above the upper limits of normal (sodium >145 mEq/L and osmolality >295 mOsm/kg).

○ Nomograms have been established to differentiate between primary polydipsia, partial central DI, and partial nephrogenic DI. However, this test **may be contraindicated in patients at risk for complications of volume overload** (e.g., those with underlying heart disease).

TREATMENT

- **Replacement of water deficit:**
  ○ Water deficit should be calculated and replaced orally with water whenever possible. Hypotonic saline can be given intravenously in a patient who cannot tolerate oral intake.
  ○ If hypernatremia has developed rapidly over a period of hours, the water deficit can be corrected to decrease the plasma sodium at 1 mEq/L/hr. If hypernatremia developed slowly, the rate should be no more than 0.5 mEq/L/hr, up to a maximum of 8 to 10 mEq/L/day, using the smallest volume of fluid possible to avoid cerebral edema.[12]
  ○ The water deficit can be calculated from the serum sodium using the following formula:

  $$\text{Water deficit (L)} = \text{Total Body Water}^* \times ([Na+]serum - 140) \div 140$$

  For example, if a 70-kg man has serum sodium of 150 mEq/L, the calculated water deficit is 3 L [{0.6 × 70 × (150 − 140)} ÷ 140]. To decrease the sodium at a rate of 0.5 mEq/L/hr, 3 L of D5W can be administered over 20 hours [(150 − 140 mEq/L) ÷ 0.5 mEq/L/hr] at a rate of 150 mL/hr (3 L ÷ 20 hours).

  ○ Alternatively, the change in serum sodium for each liter of fluid given can be approximated from the following equation:

  $$\text{Change in serum Na+} = ([Na+]infusate - [Na+]serum) \div (\text{Total Body Water}^* + 1)$$

  For the same person, the calculated decrease in sodium per liter of D5W would be $(0 - 150) \div (0.6 \times 70 + 1) = -3.5$ mEq/L. To decrease the sodium at an initial rate of 0.5 mEq/L/hr, D5W should be infused at approximately 143 mL/hr (0.5 mEq/L/hr ÷ 3.5 mEq/L × 1,000 mL). This formula is particularly useful when choosing a hypotonic fluid other than D5W.

  Total body water = Total body weight in kg × 0.6 in men/0.5 in women

  ○ Both of these strategies only approximate the expected change in sodium and the rate of infusion needs to be adjusted to account for other ongoing free water losses.
  ○ The fluid infusion rate may need to be decreased if DDAVP is used to treat DI and plasma sodium and volume status should be assessed every 2 to 4 hours.
- **Treatment of central DI:**
  ○ **DDAVP**, an ADH analog, is a potent antidiuretic with no vasopressor activity and a longer duration of action than ADH. It is the most common agent used to treat central DI. It is available in parenteral, oral, intranasal, and sublingual (Canada only) preparations.
  ○ DDAVP given intravenously or subcutaneously has a rapid onset of action and is usually given at a dose of 1 to 2 mcg once or twice daily.
  ○ Intranasal DDAVP also has a rapid onset of action and can be given at a dose of 1 to 4 sprays/day (1 spray = 10 mcg) in 1 to 3 divided doses/day.
  ○ Oral DDAVP has an onset of action of 30 to 60 minutes and can be given at a dose of 0.1 to 0.4 mg one to four times a day.
  ○ Use of oral DDAVP has been shown to be very effective, but may be limited in some patients owing to variable gut absorption and reduced bioavailability.
  ○ Conversion from intranasal to parenteral preparation is easily accomplished by reducing the dose by a factor of 10; conversion from intranasal to oral requires that the dose be titrated due to the variable bioavailability with oral preparations.

- **Treatment of acute postsurgical central DI**
  - Patients who are alert and have an intact thirst mechanism should be able to maintain adequate fluid intake to prevent hypernatremia. Although these patients may not need drug therapy, they need to be closely monitored and therapy should be considered in patients who develop bothersome polyuria.
  - If DDAVP is indicated, a simple and safe method of dosing a patient who has an intact thirst mechanism and is tolerating oral intake is to start with 0.05 to 0.1 mg of oral DDAVP and assess for response (decreased urine output, increased urine osmolality, and decreased thirst). If the response is not appropriate within a few hours, the dose should be increased by 0.1 mg every few hours until an appropriate response (urine output <300 mL/hr) is achieved. The patient should continue to receive DDAVP on an as-needed basis until a stable regimen is determined.
  - Throughout the dose titration, patients should be given free access to water and told to drink only when thirsty to avoid water intoxication and hyponatremia.
  - If oral intake is inadequate, intravenous administration of hypotonic fluid (D5W, 45% NaCl or 0.2% NaCl) should be used. Normal saline should be avoided in patients with DI unless needed for initial volume resuscitation/hypovolemia (solute load to kidneys worsens renal water loss).
- **Treatment of chronic central DI:**
  - Chronic DI in patients with an intact thirst mechanism should be treated with a fixed dosing regimen of DDAVP. The lowest possible dose based on symptoms should be used to minimize the risk of hyponatremia. Patients are usually able to correct their free water losses by increasing their fluid intake as directed by their thirst mechanism.
  - Bedtime dosing of DDAVP helps to reduce disabling nocturia.
  - Management is extremely difficult in adipsic patients with DI. In general, they are managed with a fixed dose of DDAVP and adequate hydration. They are instructed to adjust their fluid intake based on indirect indicators of water balance (e.g., daily weight measurements) or serum sodium when feasible.
- **Treatment of nephrogenic DI:**
  - In acquired nephrogenic DI, correction of associated electrolyte disorders or discontinuation of offending drugs can improve DI. However, in most patients the underlying cause cannot be corrected and treatment must be used.[2,5]
  - Dietary sodium restriction and a thiazide diuretic (e.g., hydrochlorothiazide 25 mg once or twice daily) can be used to control nephrogenic DI. Thiazides cause an overall reduction in electrolyte–free water excretion by stimulating proximal tubular sodium and water reabsorption, hence diminishing sodium/water delivery to the ADH-sensitive sites in the collecting tubules.
  - Amiloride, a potassium-sparing diuretic, may enhance the effect of thiazide diuretics by increasing sodium excretion and the resulting antipolyuric response to volume depletion. It can be used in lithium-induced DI because it acts by blocking sodium channels in the collecting ducts through which lithium enters and interferes with the tubular response to ADH.
  - Indomethacin, a nonsteroidal anti-inflammatory drug (NSAID) with antidiuretic action, has been shown to effectively treat lithium-induced nephrogenic DI.[1]
  - DDAVP at high doses may be effective in partial nephrogenic DI.[5]

SPECIAL CONSIDERATIONS

- **DI after pituitary surgery:**
  - Central DI, the most common complication of pituitary surgery, usually develops on postoperative days 1 to 3 and is most often transient lasting 1 to 7 days.[8]
  - Although rare, DI after transsphenoidal surgery can be associated with a triphasic pattern characterized by early DI, followed by normal urine output (or syndrome of inappropriate

antidiuretic hormone secretion) due to release of stored hormone (lasts 24 hours to several days), followed by permanent DI (occurs once the hormone stores are depleted).[6]

- ○ Microadenoma (secondary to stalk manipulation and exploration), intraoperative CSF leak, nonpituitary sellar lesions (e.g., craniopharyngiomas or Rathke cleft cysts), young age, male sex, suprasellar extension, and Cushing disease have been shown to be predictors for DI after pituitary surgery.[7]
- ○ Postoperative pituitary patients require close monitoring of their fluid intake and output, electrolytes, and urine specific gravity.
- ○ For management, see section "acute postsurgical central DI" above.

COMPLICATIONS

- Overtreatment and undertreatment can result in hyponatremia and hypernatremia, respectively.
- It is essential for a patient with DI to have access to water. If a patient loses access to water, as may occur during a medical emergency or surgery, he or she is at high risk for dehydration and hypernatremia. Under these circumstances, urine output and serum sodium concentration should be followed closely and hypotonic fluid and as-needed DDAVP should be administered.

MONITORING/FOLLOW-UP

- Patients with central DI treated with DDAVP on a fixed dosing schedule should be monitored for the development of hyponatremia.
- Adipsic patients can use weight monitoring to estimate water loss/retention.
- Occasional withdrawal of DDAVP is reasonable to confirm recurrence of polyuria.

PATIENT EDUCATION

All patients with DI should be educated about the signs and symptoms of hyper/hyponatremia and advised to wear or carry a medical alert tag or card.

REFERENCES

1. Kalra S, Zargar AH, Jain SM, et al. Diabetes insipidus: the other diabetes. *Indian J Endocrinol Metab* 2016;20(1):9–21.
2. Roberston GL. Diabetes insipidus: differential diagnosis and management. *Best Pract Res Clin Endocrinol Metab* 2016;30:205–218.
3. Fenske W, Allolio B. Current state and future perspectives in the diagnosis of diabetes insipidus: a clinical review. *J Clin Endocrinol Metab* 2012;97:3426–3437.
4. Zerbe RL, Robertson GL. A comparison of plasma vasopressin measurements with a standard indirect test in the differential diagnosis of polyuria. *N Engl J Med* 1981;305:1539–1546.
5. Moeller HB, Rittig S, Fenton RA. Nephrogenic diabetes insipidus: essential insights into the molecular background and potential therapies for treatment. *Endocr Rev* 2013;34(2):278–301.
6. Prete A, Corsello SM, Salvatori R. Current best practice in the management of patients after pituitary surgery. *Ther Adv Endocrinol Metab* 2017;8(3):33–48.
7. Nemergut EC, Zuo Z, Jane JA Jr, Laws ER Jr. Predictors of diabetes insipidus after transsphenoidal surgery: a review of 881 patients. *J Neurosurg* 2005;103:448–454.
8. Ausiello JC, Bruce JN, Freda PU. Postoperative assessment of the patient after transsphenoidal pituitary surgery. *Pituitary* 2008;11:391–401.
9. Fried LF, Palevsky PM. Hyponatremia and hypernatremia. *Med Clin North Am* 1997;81:585–609.
10. Bichet DG. Chapter 8: the posterior pituitary. In: Melmed S, ed. The Pituitary. 4th ed. Cambridge, MA: Academic Press; 2017.
11. Robertson GL. Differential diagnosis of polyuria. *Annu Rev Med* 1988;39:425–442.
12. Adrogue HJ, Madias NE. Hypernatremia. *N Engl J Med* 2000;342:1493–1499.

Syndrome of Inappropriate Antidiuretic Hormone

Johnathon S. Parham and
Julie M. Silverstein

GENERAL PRINCIPLES

Definitions

The syndrome of inappropriate antidiuretic hormone secretion (SIADH) is a disorder in which water excretion is impaired by the unregulated secretion of antidiuretic hormone (ADH) from the posterior pituitary leading to free water retention and varying degrees of dilutional hyponatremia.[1]

Epidemiology

Hyponatremia is the most common electrolyte abnormality in hospitalized patients, with a prevalence estimated to be as high as 38% in some series.[2]

Etiology

- The causes of SIADH are summarized in Table 5-1.[2]
- Prognosis is dependent on the underlying etiology as well as the severity of the hyponatremia and associated symptoms. SIADH usually resolves with therapy for the underlying etiology.

Pathophysiology

- ADH, also known as arginine vasopressin (AVP), is a key component of the homeostatic mechanisms that regulate water balance.
- In normal individuals, ADH is released from cells in the neurohypophysis in response to increased serum osmolality or decreased intravascular volume. ADH exerts its activity in the kidneys via the vasopressin V_2 receptor to increase water permeability at the distal tubule and collecting duct of the nephron, enhancing water reabsorption at these sites.[2]
- With excess ADH, hypo-osmolar hyponatremia develops because water cannot be excreted normally. Therefore, the hallmark of SIADH is an inappropriately elevated urine osmolality in the setting of a low plasma osmolality.[2]

DIAGNOSIS

Clinical Presentation

- As with other causes of hyponatremia, the rate of fall of serum sodium is often more strongly correlated with morbidity and mortality than is the actual magnitude of the decrease.
- It is rare to have symptoms with serum sodium levels of ≥ 125 mEq/L, but with acute hyponatremia (<48 hours) patients may complain of malaise and nausea.[3]
- At serum sodium levels of <125 mEq/L, patients may present with neuropsychiatric signs and symptoms, ranging from difficulty concentrating, muscular weakness, headache, nausea, lethargy, ataxia, and altered mood to cerebral edema, increased intracranial pressure (ICP), confusion, seizures, and coma. This is termed hyponatremic encephalopathy and reflects osmotic water shifts into the brain.[2,3]

TABLE 5-1	COMMON CAUSES OF THE SYNDROME OF INAPPROPRIATE ANTIDIURETIC HORMONE SECRETION (SIADH)

CNS

Mass lesions (tumors, brain abscesses, hematoma)

Inflammatory/infectious diseases (encephalitis, meningitis, systemic lupus erythematous, multiple sclerosis)

Degenerative/demyelinating diseases (Guillain–Barré syndrome, spinal cord lesions)

Subarachnoid hemorrhage

CVA

Hydrocephalus

Head trauma

Delirium tremens

Acute psychosis

Drug related

Bromocriptine

Carbamazepine

Chlorpropamide

Clofibrate

Cyclophosphamide

Desmopressin (DDAVP)

Ecstasy

Haloperidol (Haldol)

Nicotine

Opiates

Phenothiazines

Selective serotonin reuptake inhibitors (SSRIs)

Tricyclic antidepressants (TCAs)

Vinblastine

Vincristine

Pulmonary

Infections (tuberculosis, acute bacterial and viral pneumonia, aspergillosis, empyema, PCP)

Mechanical/ventilatory causes (acute respiratory failure, COPD, positive-pressure ventilation)

Bronchiectasis

Cystic fibrosis

Neoplasms (ectopic ADH secretion)

Duodenal carcinoma

Lymphoma

Mesothelioma

Olfactory neuroblastoma

Pancreatic carcinoma

Prostate carcinoma

Small cell carcinoma of lung

Thymoma

(continued)

TABLE 5-1	COMMON CAUSES OF THE SYNDROME OF INAPPROPRIATE ANTIDIURETIC HORMONE SECRETION (SIADH) (Continued)

Miscellaneous
HIV/AIDS
Idiopathic
Nausea
Pain

CNS, central nervous system; CVA, cerebrovascular accident; PCP, *Pneumocystis jirovecii* pneumonia; COPD, chronic obstructive pulmonary disease.

Adapted from Robinson AG, Verbalis JG. Posterior pituitary. In: Melmed S, Polonsky KS, Larsen PR, Kronenberg HM, eds. *Williams Textbook of Endocrinology*. 13th ed. Philadelphia, PA: Elsevier; 2016:313–324.

- Risk factors for developing cerebral edema from hyponatremia include age less than 16, women, hypoxemia, and ecstasy use.
- Signs of either volume depletion or overload are not consistent with SIADH and should prompt an evaluation for other causes of hyponatremia.[4]

Diagnostic Criteria

- SIADH is a diagnosis of exclusion, and therefore, other causes of hyponatremia must be ruled out.
- Essential diagnostic criteria include[1,2,5]:
  - **Low plasma osmolality:** a plasma osmolality <275 mOsm/kg is consistent with SIADH, and rules out hypertonic or isotonic causes of hyponatremia.
  - **Inappropriately elevated urine osmolality and urine sodium concentration:** a urine osmolality >100 mOsm/kg and urine sodium concentration >30 mEq/L are consistent with SIADH.
  - **Euvolemia:** volume depletion or overload should prompt an evaluation for an alternative diagnosis. SIADH should be considered if hypo-osmolar hyponatremia persists once clinical euvolemia is restored.
  - **Normal adrenal and thyroid function tests.**
  - **No evidence of advanced kidney disease.**
  - **No recent use of diuretic agents.**
- Supplemental diagnostic criteria that are not needed to make a diagnosis of SIADH, but could be useful in situations of uncertainty, include:
  - **Abnormal water load test**, which is defined as the inability to excrete at least 80% of a water load (20 mL/kg water ingested in 10 to 20 minutes) after 4 hours and/or the failure to dilute urinary osmolality to <100 mOsm/kg. This test should be administered after the serum sodium level is >125 mEq/L through water restriction and/or saline administration.
  - No significant correction of plasma sodium with volume expansion, but improvement after fluid restriction.
  - **Serum uric acid levels <4 mg/dL** are common in SIADH, as volume expansion and ADH acting on V_1 receptors increase the clearance of uric acid.[2]

Differential Diagnosis

- SIADH is a diagnosis of exclusion that should be differentiated from other known causes of euvolemic hypotonic hyponatremia. **Euvolemic hypotonic hyponatremia** is characterized by low to normal total body sodium and normal to elevated total body water.[1]

- The most common cause of euvolemic hypotonic hyponatremia is SIADH, but other causes of euvolemic hypotonic hyponatremia that must be excluded include[2]:
  - **Hypothyroidism,** a rare cause of hyponatremia, leads to low sodium by uncertain mechanisms. Proposed mechanisms include dysregulation of ADH release or clearance, or both, as well as effects on vascular tone, cardiac output, and renal blood flow.
  - **Adrenal insufficiency** is also an unusual cause of hyponatremia. ADH is an adrenocorticotropic hormone (ACTH) secretagogue and is subject to negative feedback by glucocorticoids. Hyponatremia from adrenal insufficiency is thought to be caused by the loss of negative feedback on ADH secretion.
  - **Primary polydipsia** may lead to hyponatremia if free water intake exceeds the capacity of the kidneys to excrete free water.
  - **Potomania** was classically described in binge beer drinkers, but is now found more commonly in people with unusual dietary habits or eating disorders (e.g., anorexia nervosa). These patients develop hypotonic hyponatremia in the setting of dilute urine because of low solute intake and excretion. Free water clearance is dependent on solute excretion by the kidneys. If solute intake is decreased because of a restricted diet, solute excretion will also be decreased, and the kidneys will not be able to clear as much free water.
  - **Thiazide diuretics** typically cause hypotonic hyponatremia associated with hypovolemia, but patients can be euvolemic if free water intake is increased to compensate for thirst and volume depletion.
  - **Reset osmostat** is a variant of SIADH in which there is a shift in the set point for ADH release to a lower plasma osmolality. Therefore, the patient may have inappropriately concentrated urine in the setting of hypotonic hyponatremia, but will be able to dilute urine normally in response to a water load and concentrate urine in response to dehydration.
  - **Nephrogenic syndrome of inappropriate antidiuresis** is a rare X-linked genetic syndrome in which all of the criteria for SIADH are met, but in which ADH levels are undetectable. It results from gain-of-function mutations in the renal vasopressin V_2 receptor causing increased water resorption.[6]
  - A debated and not widely accepted cause of hyponatremia is **cerebral salt wasting syndrome (CSWS)** which is thought to cause hyponatremia as a result of natriuresis secondary to intracranial disease. This natriuresis results in hyponatremia, volume contraction, and clinically evident hypovolemia. As of yet only a few cases have ever met historically accepted criteria for CSWS and it remains an exceedingly rare cause of hyponatremia.[7]

TREATMENT

- SIADH is usually self-limited, and the primary management strategy is to correct the underlying etiology. However, immediate treatment strategies are based on the severity of the hyponatremia and any associated symptoms.
- Patients with chronic or asymptomatic hyponatremia may have mild and subtle neurologic symptoms and should be considered for treatment.[2]
- Rate of correction:
  - Overly aggressive correction of hyponatremia may result in the development of **osmotic demyelination syndrome** (ODS), a potentially devastating neurologic condition; therefore, correction of hyponatremia should always be done with caution. If the rate of development of hyponatremia is rapid (<48 hours), an equally rapid rate of correction is felt to be safe. However, resolving the symptoms should be the primary goal, whereas correction to normonatremia should be performed more judiciously.[8] In cases where the acuity or chronicity of the hyponatremia is not known, the rate

TABLE 5-2	GENERAL RECOMMENDATIONS FOR EMPLOYMENT OF FLUID RESTRICTION

General recommendations

Restrict all intake that is consumed by drinking, not just water

Aim for a fluid restriction that is 500 mL/day below the 24-hour urine volume

Do not restrict sodium or protein intake unless indicated

Monitoring

Monitor [Na$^+$] every 8 to 12 hours initially

Continue fluid restriction until [Na$^+$] is within the normal range

For transient SIADH, fluids can be liberalized every 2 to 3 days based on [Na$^+$]

Patients with chronic SIADH should be maintained on fluid restriction, monitored for symptoms, and have [Na$^+$] measured periodically

Predictors of the likely failure of fluid restriction

High urine osmolality (≥500 mOsm/kg H$_2$O)

Sum of the urine Na$^+$ and K$^+$ concentrations exceeds the serum Na$^+$ concentration

24-hour urine volume <1,500 mL/day

[Na$^+$], serum sodium concentration

Adapted from Robinson AG, Verbalis JG. Posterior pituitary. In: Melmed S, Polonsky KS, Larsen PR, Kronenberg HM, eds. *Williams Textbook of Endocrinology*. 13th ed. Philadelphia, PA: Elsevier; 2016: 313–324.

---

of correction should be limited to 1 to 2 mEq/L/hr for the first 3 to 4 hours, and by no more than 0.5 mEq/L/hr thereafter, for a maximum correction of 10 mEq/L per 24 hours.[8]

  ◦ Risk factors for ODS include serum [Na+] ≤105 mEq/L, hypokalemia, advanced liver disease, malnutrition, or alcoholism.[2] Correction should be monitored closely in these patients, and re-lowering of sodium with desmopressin and/or free water should be considered if overly rapid correction occurs in patients at high risk for ODS.[9]

• With any chosen therapeutic strategy, plasma sodium and volume status should be assessed frequently (initially every 1 to 2 hours, and then every 4 hours when the correction rate is stable) to monitor and make adjustments to therapy.

Nonpharmacologic Therapies

Fluid restriction is the mainstay of therapy for most patients with SIADH so that free water excretion in the urine exceeds dietary intake. Fluid restriction is summarized in Table 5-2.[2] It may take 3 to 4 days to start working and can be difficult to use in the inpatient setting, where volumes of fluids are typically administered as a part of ongoing therapies. It should not be used in hypovolemic patients.

Medications

First Line

• **Intravenous saline** can improve SIADH-induced hyponatremia if the osmolality of the intravenous fluid is greater than the osmolality of the urine. This usually requires the use of hypertonic saline. *Hypertonic saline should be reserved ONLY for treatment of acute or severely symptomatic hyponatremia.*[10] Many strategies have been employed to calculate the initial rate of hypertonic saline. One simple formula to estimate the increase in plasma sodium for 1 L of fluid:

$$\text{Change in } [Na+]_{plasma} = ([Na+]_{infusate} - [Na+]_{plasma}) \div (\text{total body water} + 1)$$

where $[Na+]_{infusate} = $ mEq/L of sodium in the infusate (e.g., 3% saline is 513 mEq/L), and total body water = body weight (kg) $\times$ (0.6 for men or 0.5 for women).

For example, if a 70-kg man is having seizures and has a plasma sodium of 110 mEq/L, the calculated increase in sodium per liter of 3% saline would be $(513 - 110) \div (0.6 \times 71) = 9.4$ mEq/L. To increase the sodium at an initial rate of 2 mEq/L/hr, 3% saline should be infused at 213 mL/hr (2 mEq/L/hr $\div$ 9.4 mEq/L $\times$ 1,000 mL). If one can estimate the expected change of sodium in 1 L of intravenous fluid, a rate can be calculated for that infusion to avert overcorrecting too quickly. Stop 3% saline promptly once severe signs and symptoms of cerebral edema resolve.

- **Oral salt tablets** increase serum sodium by the same mechanism as hypertonic saline. Salt tablets are usually reserved for treatment of chronic or asymptomatic hyponatremia.[8]

Second Line

- **Loop diuretics** can enhance the effect of solute loading with oral salt or intravenous saline by increasing free water excretion and impairing the renal responsiveness to ADH.[8]
- **Demeclocycline** acts on the renal collecting tubules to diminish responsiveness to ADH, resulting in increased free water excretion. The dose of 300 to 600 mg twice daily is typically reserved for chronic or asymptomatic SIADH-induced hyponatremia.[8] The major side effect is nephrotoxicity, so renal function should be monitored closely.
- **Vasopressin receptor antagonists** exert their activity on renal V_{1a} and V_2 receptors resulting in a selective water diuresis without affecting sodium excretion.[8,10,11] Examples include intravenous conivaptan and oral tolvaptan. Multiple studies have shown these agents to effectively increase serum sodium level when compared to placebo. Intravenous conivaptan can exert its effect in as little as 1 to 2 hours, permitting a more rapid initial elevation on serum sodium and has been shown to be used safely in neurosurgical patients with SIADH.[12] While this may be an initial benefit in patients who are symptomatic, careful monitoring must be maintained to avoid overly rapid correction of hyponatremia. Thirst, hypokalemia, and headaches are common side effects. These agents should be initiated in the hospital to monitor the active phase of correction. Vaptans are contraindicated in hypovolemic hyponatremia. In recent studies, prolonged administration of tolvaptan maintained an increase in serum sodium with an acceptable margin of safety.[13]

REFERENCES

1. Adrogué HJ, Madias NE. The challenge of hyponatremia. *J Am Soc Nephrol* 2012;23(7):1140–1148.
2. Robinson AG, Verbalis JG. Posterior pituitary. In: Melmed S, Polonsky KS, Larsen PR, Kronenberg HM, eds. *Williams textbook of Endocrinology.* 13th ed. Philadelphia, PA: Elsevier; 2016:313–324.
3. Ball SG, Baylis PH. Vasopressin, diabetes insipidus, and syndrome of inappropriate antidiuresis. In: DeGroot LJ, Jameson JL, eds. *Endocrinology.* 5th ed. Philadelphia, PA: Elsevier; 2006:537–556.
4. Sterns RH, Nigwekar SU, Hix JK. The treatment of hyponatremia. *Semin Nephrol* 2009;29(3):282–299.
5. Ellison DH, Berl T. Clinical practice. The syndrome of inappropriate antidiuresis. *N Engl J Med* 2007;356(20):2064–2072.
6. Decaux G, Vandergheynst F, Bouko Y, Parma J, Vassart G, Vilain C. Nephrogenic syndrome of inappropriate antidiuresis in adults: High phenotypic variability in men and women from a large pedigree. *J Am Soc Nephrol* 2007;18(2):606–612.

7. Verbalis JG, Greenberg A, Burst V, et al. Diagnosing and treating the syndrome of inappropriate antidiuretic hormone secretion. *Am J Med* 2016;129(5):537.e9–e23.

8. Furst H, Hallows KR, Post J, et al. The urine/plasma electrolyte ratio: A predictive guide to water restriction. *Am J Med Sci* 2000;319(4):240–244.

9. Cawley MJ. Hyponatremia: Current treatment strategies and the role of vasopressin antagonists. *Ann Pharmacother* 2007;41(5):840–850.

10. Potts M, DeGiacomo A, Deragopian L, Blevins L. Use of intravenous conivaptan in neurosurgical patients with hyponatremia from syndrome of inappropriate antidiuretic hormone secretion. *Neurosurgery* 2011;69(2):268–273.

11. Sterns RH, Silver SM. Cerebral salt wasting versus SIADH: what difference? *J Am Soc Nephrol* 2008;19(2):194–196.

12. Vaidya C, Ho W, Freda BJ. Management of hyponatremia: Providing treatment and avoiding harm. *Cleve Clin J Med* 2010;77(10):715–726.

13. Berl T, Quittnat-Pelletier F, Verbalis JG, et al. Oral tolvaptan is safe and effective in chronic hyponatremia. *J Am Soc Nephrol* 2010;21(4):705–712.

Hypopituitarism

6

Julia P. Dunn and Julie M. Silverstein

GENERAL PRINCIPLES

Definition

Hypopituitarism is peripheral hormonal hyposecretion due to either insufficient or ineffective production of pituitary hormones and includes secondary adrenal insufficiency (AI), secondary hypothyroidism, secondary hypogonadism, growth hormone deficiency (GHD), and diabetes insipidus (see Chapter 4, Diabetes Insipidus).

Epidemiology

- Congenital and genetic disorders that cause hypopituitarism often present in early childhood or with delayed/absent puberty.
- Acquired disorders can present throughout a person's life. The prevalence in adults is approximately 45 per 100,000.[1]
- Pituitary microadenomas rarely cause anterior hormone deficiency. Deficiency of at least one pituitary hormone occurs in approximately 60% to 85% of patients with pituitary macroadenomas.[2]
- New anterior pituitary insufficiency occurs in 5% to 7% of patients after transsphenoidal surgery for pituitary adenomas.[3]

Etiology

- Hypopituitarism can result from any hypothalamic or pituitary lesion or insult.[4]
- Any sellar or parasellar mass can cause hypopituitarism (see Chapter 1, Sellar and Suprasellar Masses). Additional etiologies are summarized in Table 6-1.[5]
- Reported frequencies of specific etiologies vary by study population,[1,6,7] but in general, most adult hypopituitarism can be attributed to:
  - Pituitary adenomas (55%)
  - Craniopharyngiomas (4% to 12%)
  - Nonpituitary CNS tumors (3% to 4%)
  - Nonpituitary irradiation (1%)
  - Traumatic brain injury (TBI) (2% to 4%)
  - Empty sella (1% to 7%)
  - Sheehan syndrome (1% to 6%)
  - Inflammatory/infiltrative disorders (1% to 2%)
  - Hypophysitis (2%)
  - Idiopathic (8% to 10%)
- Patients treated with **irradiation** for both pituitary and nonpituitary conditions are at increased risk for hypopituitarism that can develop up to 20 years after treatment. The risk is increased with higher radiation doses and longer follow-up.[8]
  - GHD occurs in almost 100% of patients by 5 years although incidence depends on criteria used for diagnosis.

TABLE 6-1 NONNEOPLASTIC CAUSES OF HYPOPITUITARISM

Treatment of sellar or parasellar disease
Surgery
Radiotherapy
Radiosurgery

Infiltrative disease
Hypophysitis
Hemochromatosis
Sarcoidosis/granulomatous disorders
Langerhans cell histiocytosis

Vascular
Pituitary tumor apoplexy
Sheehan syndrome
Carotid artery aneurysm
Subarachnoid hemorrhage

Genetic
Combined pituitary hormone
  deficiencies
Isolated pituitary hormone
  deficiencies

Developmental
Midline cerebral and cranial
  malformations
Pituitary hypoplasia or aplasia
Ectopic pituitary

Traumatic
Head injury
Perinatal trauma

Infections
Bacterial/viral/fungal
Tuberculosis
Syphilis

Medications
Immune checkpoint inhibitors
Opiates
Glucocorticoids/megestrol acetate
Suppressive thyroxine treatment
Sex steroid treatment
GnRH agonists
Antiseizure medications
Dopamine

Systemic disease
Obesity
Anorexia nervosa
Chronic illness
Chronic intense exercise

Empty or partially empty sella

Idiopathic

GnRH, gonadotropin-releasing hormone.
Data from Carmichael JD. Anterior pituitary failure. In: Melmed S, ed. *The Pituitary*. 4th ed. London: Academic Press; 2017:329–364.

- ○ Secondary hypogonadism occurs in 60%, secondary hypothyroidism in 30%, and secondary AI in 60% by 10 years. Hyperprolactinemia occurs primarily in women who received doses of >40 Gy.
- In **stereotactic radiosurgery**, the incidence of new-onset hypopituitarism is higher in patients with functional pituitary adenomas as compared to nonfunctioning pituitary adenomas due to the higher doses of radiation used.
  - ○ The rate of hypopituitarism has been reported in 0% to 40% (mean 8.8%), 0% to 69% (mean 24.3%), and 0% to 40% (mean 16.4%) of patients with nonfunctioning pituitary adenomas, Cushing disease, and acromegaly, respectively.[9]
  - ○ GHD occurs in 85% to 100% of patients who receive cranial irradiation for nonpituitary brain tumors in childhood by 5 years with more rapid onset if higher doses are used.[10]
  - ○ Forty-one percent of adults receiving cranial radiotherapy for nonpituitary brain tumors develop hypopituitarism after a mean time of 3.2 years.[11] Nasopharyngeal

carcinoma patients receive high-dose irradiation to the skull base and 62% develop hypopituitarism after 5 years.[12]

- In **TBI**, the reported prevalence of TBI-induced hypopituitarism is 15% to 68%.[13]
  - Risk is higher in severe TBI (35%) versus mild to moderate TBI (11% to 17%) and is more likely to occur with repetitive trauma (e.g., boxing, football) and may present years after trauma.[14]
  - Long-term deficits occur in 23% to 32% of moderate–severe TBI patients.
  - GHD occurs in 20%, secondary hypogonadism in 11%, AI in 7%, secondary hypothyroidism in 6%, and DI in 3%.[13,15]
  - The incidence of pituitary deficiencies is highest (>60%, most common hypogonadism) in the first 3 months after TBI.
- **Subarachnoid hemorrhage** causes chronic hypopituitarism in 38% of patients with GHD occurring in >20%, secondary hypogonadism in 6%, secondary AI in 6%, secondary hypothyroidism in 9%, and DI in 3%.[15]
- After both TBI and subarachnoid hemorrhage, recovery or new pituitary deficiencies can occur between 3 and ≥12 months post event.[15,16]
- **Immune checkpoint inhibitors** (see Chapter 40, Endocrine Effects of Oncology Drugs) can cause hypopituitarism.
  - Anti-cytotoxic T-lymphocyte–associated antigen 4 (CTLA-4) and programmed cell death 1 (PD-1) and PD-1 ligand (PD-L1) receptor monoclonal antibodies (mAbs) are used in the treatment of melanoma and other malignancies and are associated with several endocrine toxicities including hypophysitis.
  - The incidence of hypophysitis is highest with ipilimumab, (CTLA-4 mAb) as compared to other anti–CTLA-4 mAbs such as tremelimumab and anti–PD-1/PD-L1 mAbs (e.g., nivolumab, pembrolizumab, atezolizumab, avelumab, and durvalumab).
  - Ipilimumab, used to treat late-stage melanoma, renal cell, prostate, and lung carcinoma, causes autoimmune hypophysitis in 5% to 17%.[17]
  - Patients present with headache, weakness, and other symptoms of hormone deficiency.
  - Pituitary enlargement and/or the appearance of a mass is seen on MRI.
  - Unlike other causes of hypopituitarism, secondary AI, hypothyroidism, and hypogonadism are common with preservation of growth hormone (GH).
  - Secondary hypothyroidism and hypogonadism may resolve but AI persists in most patients long term. High-dose glucocorticoids can lead to symptomatic improvement but have not been shown to reverse AI as compared to physiologic replacement doses.[18]
- Hemorrhagic fever with renal syndrome is a severe systemic illness caused by *Hantavirus*, which can be transmitted by rodents. In the United States, *Hantavirus* is more common west of the Mississippi River, particularly in the southwest. This syndrome has led to hypopituitarism in 18% of patients at 2-year follow-up.[19]

DIAGNOSIS

The diagnosis and treatment of secondary hypogonadism, AI, and hypothyroidism are discussed in detail in their respective chapters. The diagnosis and treatment of adult growth hormone deficiency (AGHD) are discussed separately below.

Clinical Presentation

- Depending on etiology, presentation can be abrupt such as with apoplexy and after surgery or insidious, developing over years with vague symptoms (e.g., fatigue, cognitive decline, reduced exercise capacity) such as after irradiation.
- Gonadotrophs are most commonly affected and typically occur in isolation when not mass related (e.g., chronic disease).

- Corticotrophs and thyrotrophs are most resistant to mass effects and the last to lose function. Secondary hypothyroidism or AI usually indicates panhypopituitarism.
- GHD is often present when two or more other hormones are deficient.
- Prolactin deficiency is rare and occurs when the anterior pituitary is destroyed, as in apoplexy.

Diagnostic Criteria

- In general, diagnosis of a central deficiency is made by persistently low levels of peripheral hormone with low or inappropriately normal levels of pituitary trophic hormone.[4]
- When testing is available and not contraindicated, central deficiency can be confirmed by the failure of pituitary trophic hormone rise with stimulation.
- Imaging to rule out a sellar mass, preferably with MRI of the pituitary with and without gadolinium, is recommended even if there is a possible nonmass etiology.

TREATMENT

- Acutely ill patients with secondary AI should be treated with stress-dose glucocorticoids.
- Patients presenting with pituitary apoplexy should be started on glucocorticoid replacement while testing for AI is pending.
- AI may mask partial DI and onset of DI symptoms can become evident after initiation of glucocorticoid replacement.[20]

SPECIAL CONSIDERATIONS

- Female patients with hypopituitarism require close monitoring during pregnancy as medication dose adjustments are necessary.
- Hydrocortisone or prednisone can be used during pregnancy. Dexamethasone is not inactivated by the placenta and should therefore not be used. Glucocorticoid dosage may need to be increased during the third trimester of pregnancy.
- Patients with both primary and secondary hypothyroidism generally require a 30% increase in the dose of their levothyroxine. Free T4 levels should be monitored every 4 to 6 weeks during pregnancy and the dose adjusted to maintain the free T4 within the high-normal range.
- GH replacement is not recommended during pregnancy.

ADULT GROWTH HORMONE DEFICIENCY

Clinical Presentation

- Symptoms of AGHD are nonspecific but can include muscle weakness, reduced exercise capacity, fatigue, and decreased quality of life.
- AGHD is also associated with dyslipidemia, insulin resistance, an increase in inflammatory markers, decreased muscle strength, decreased lean body and bone mass, and increased risk of cardiovascular disease.[21,22]

Diagnosis

- Testing for AGHD can be considered in the following situations:
  - Patients with history of childhood-onset GHD who have achieved adult height.
  - Patients with history of hypothalamic or pituitary disease or surgery and/or radiation to the pituitary or hypothalamus.
  - Patients with history of head trauma (e.g., TBI or subarachnoid hemorrhage).
  - Patients with history of other pituitary hormone deficiencies.

- An insulin-like growth factor type 1 (IGF-1) within the normal range does not rule out GHD and a random GH measurement is not diagnostic of AGHD because of its pulsatile pattern.
- **GH stimulation testing in adults:**
  - Several agents, which stimulate GH secretion in normal individuals, can be used to establish the diagnosis of GHD.
  - The **insulin tolerance test (ITT)** is felt to be the gold standard for evaluation of AGHD[3] but is rarely done because of safety concerns. 0.05- to 0.15-IU/kg regular insulin is administered IV to decrease glucose levels below 40 mg/dL. Blood sampling for GH levels is done fasting and 20, 30, 40, and 60 minutes after hypoglycemia has occurred. GH <3 to 5 μg/L after hypoglycemia has a sensitivity of 96% and specificity of 92% for the diagnosis of AGHD.[23]
  - The **growth hormone–releasing hormone (GHRH)-arginine test** is commonly performed outside of the United States (as of publication, GHRH is not commercially available in the United States). GHRH directly stimulates GH secretion from the pituitary and arginine potentiates the response of the pituitary to GHRH by inhibiting somatostatin. An IV bolus of 1 μg/kg of GHRH is given followed by an arginine (30 g) infusion for 30 minutes. GH levels are sampled in the blood at baseline and every 30 minutes for 120 minutes. Since the GH response is blunted in obese individuals, GH cutoffs depend on BMI (<11.0 μg/L for BMI ≥30 kg/m², <8.0 μg/L for BMI 25 to 30 kg/m², and <4.0 μg/L for BMI <25 kg/m²).[24]
  - The **glucagon stimulation test** can be used when GHRH is not available and the ITT is either contraindicated or not practical.[21] The exact mechanism of GH stimulation is not known but may be due to secondary endogenous insulin release in response to hyperglycemia. 1-mg IM glucagon (1.5 mg if patient weighs >90 kg) is administered and serum GH and glucose levels are measured at baseline and every 30 minutes for 4 hours. A peak GH <3 μg/L in lean patients (BMI ≤25 kg/m²) is felt to be consistent with GHD. A GH cutoff of <1 μg/L has been proposed for patients with BMIs >25 kg/m² to decrease overdiagnosis of AGHD.[24]
  - The Endocrine Society recommends that the following be used to diagnose AGHD.[21]
    - For patients with a clinical context making GHD a possibility (e.g., history of pituitary irradiation), no stimulation test is needed in patients with ≥3 hormone deficiencies and a low-age and gender-matched IGF-1 as the likelihood of concomitant GHD is high.
    - One stimulation test is recommended to make the diagnosis in patients with <3 hormone deficiencies.
    - Since adult-onset idiopathic GHD is rare, two stimulatory tests should be performed to make the diagnosis.

Treatment

- Because of the controversies regarding the treatment of adults with GHD, the decision to start a patient on GH replacement requires thoughtful and individualized consideration of the risks and benefits.
- The recommended starting dose of GH is age dependent (0.4 to 0.5 mg/day, age <30 years; 0.2 to 0.3 mg/day, age 30 to 60; and 0.1 to 0.2 mg/day, age >60 years) because older patients are more susceptible to GH-related side effects. The dose can be titrated up or down based on an individual patient's clinical and biochemical response.[25] Women on oral estrogen may require higher doses because of suppression of IGF-1 production from the liver.
- Side effects include paresthesia, joint stiffness, peripheral edema, arthralgia, myalgia, carpal tunnel, hyperglycemia, and retinopathy (rare).

- GH replacement has been shown to increase lean body mass,[26] increase BMD,[27] decrease the risk of fracture,[28] and improve quality of life.[29,30]
- Some, but not all studies show an increase in strength and/or exercise capacity associated with an increase in muscle mass.[31]
- Despite increasing LDL[25,26] and decreasing inflammatory markers,[22] it is not clear if GH improves surrogate markers of cardiovascular disease and/or decreases the risk of developing the metabolic syndrome.[32,33]
- GH replacement may transiently increase glucose levels[34] but has not been shown to increase the risk of diabetes.[35]
- Despite the theoretical concern that GH replacement may increase the risk of malignancy or pituitary tumor regrowth/recurrence, several studies have shown that long-term GH treatment in adults does not increase the risk of de novo cancers and/or increase the risk of recurrent pituitary tumors.[25] GH treatment is, however, contraindicated in patients with active malignancy.
- Although some studies suggest that the increased mortality in hypopituitary patients is related to AGHD,[36,37] there are no prospective long-term randomized studies comparing GH treatment and placebo on cardiovascular hard outcomes and mortality.

REFERENCES

1. Regal M, Paramo C, Sierra SM, Garcia-Mayor RV. Prevalence and incidence of hypopituitarism in an adult Caucasian population in northwestern Spain. *Clin Endocrinol (Oxf)* 2001;55(6):735–740.
2. Vieira LN, Boguszewski CL, Araujo LA, et al. A review on the diagnosis and treatment of patients with clinically nonfunctioning pituitary adenoma by the Neuroendocrinology Department of the Brazilian Society of Endocrinology and Metabolism. *Arch Endocrinol Metab* 2016;60(4):374–390.
3. Dallapiazza RF, Jane JA Jr. Outcomes of endoscopic transsphenoidal pituitary surgery. *Endocrinol Metab Clin North Am* 2015;44(1):105–115.
4. Fleseriu M, Hashim IA, Karavitaki N, et al. Hormonal replacement in hypopituitarism in adults: An endocrine society clinical practice guideline. *J Clin Endocrinol Metab* 2016;101(11):3888–3921.
5. Carmicahel J. Chapter 10: Anterior pituitary failure. In: Melmed S, ed. *The Pituitary*. 4th ed. Academic Press; 2017:329–364.
6. Abs R, Bengtsson BA, Hernberg-Stahl E, et al. GH replacement in 1034 growth hormone deficient hypopituitary adults: demographic and clinical characteristics, dosing and safety. *Clin Endocrinol (Oxf)* 1999;50(6):703–713.
7. Doknic M, Pekic S, Miljic D, et al. Etiology of hypopituitarism in adult patients: The experience of a single center database in the serbian population. *Int J Endocrinol* 2017;2017:6969286.
8. Darzy KH, Shalet SM. Hypopituitarism following radiotherapy. *Pituitary* 2009;12(1):40–50.
9. Ding D, Starke RM, Sheehan JP. Treatment paradigms for pituitary adenomas: defining the roles of radiosurgery and radiation therapy. *J Neurooncol* 2014;117(3):445–457.
10. Clayton PE, Shalet SM. Dose dependency of time of onset of radiation-induced growth hormone deficiency. *J Pediatr* 1991;118(2):226–228.
11. Agha A, Sherlock M, Brennan S, et al. Hypothalamic-pituitary dysfunction after irradiation of nonpituitary brain tumors in adults. *J Clin Endocrinol Metab* 2005;90(12):6355–6360.
12. Lam KS, Tse VK, Wang C, Yeung RT, Ho JH. Effects of cranial irradiation on hypothalamic-pituitary function—a 5-year longitudinal study in patients with nasopharyngeal carcinoma. *Q J Med* 1991;78(286):165–176.
13. Tritos NA, Yuen KC, Kelly DF. American Association of Clinical Endocrinologists and American College of Endocrinology disease state clinical review: a neuroendocrine approach to patients with traumatic brain injury. *Endocr Pract* 2015;21(7):823–831.
14. Tanriverdi F, Unluhizarci K, Coksevim B, Selcuklu A, Casanueva FF, Kelestimur F. Kickboxing sport as a new cause of traumatic brain injury-mediated hypopituitarism. *Clin Endocrinol (Oxf)* 2007;66(3):360–366.

15. Giordano G, Aimaretti G, Ghigo E. Variations of pituitary function over time after brain injuries: the lesson from a prospective study. *Pituitary* 2005;8(3–4):227–231.

16. Lauzier F, Turgeon AF, Boutin A, et al. Clinical outcomes, predictors, and prevalence of anterior pituitary disorders following traumatic brain injury: a systematic review. *Crit Care Med* 2014;42(3):712–721.

17. Dillard T, Yedinak CG, Alumkal J, Fleseriu M. Anti-CTLA-4 antibody therapy associated autoimmune hypophysitis: serious immune related adverse events across a spectrum of cancer subtypes. *Pituitary* 2010;13(1):29–38.

18. Albarel F, Gaudy C, Castinetti F, et al. Long-term follow-up of ipilimumab-induced hypophysitis, a common adverse event of the anti-CTLA-4 antibody in melanoma. *Eur J Endocrinol* 2015;172(2):195–204.

19. Stojanovic M, Pekic S, Cvijovic G, et al. High risk of hypopituitarism in patients who recovered from hemorrhagic fever with renal syndrome. *J Clin Endocrinol Metab* 2008;93(7):2722–2728.

20. Iwasaki Y, Kondo K, Hasegawa H, Oiso Y. Osmoregulation of plasma vasopressin in three cases with adrenal insufficiency of diverse etiologies. *Horm Res* 1997;47(1):38–44.

21. Molitch ME, Clemmons DR, Malozowski S, Merriam GR, Vance ML. Evaluation and treatment of adult growth hormone deficiency: an Endocrine Society clinical practice guideline. *J Clin Endocrinol Metab* 2011;96(6):1587–1609.

22. Melmed S, ed. *The Pituitary*. 4th ed. Academic Press; 2017.

23. Yuen KC, Tritos NA, Samson SL, Hoffman AR, Katznelson L. American Association of Clinical Endocrinologists and American College of Endocrinology disease state clinical review: update on growth hormone stimulation testing and proposed revised cut-point for the glucagon stimulation test in the diagnosis of adult growth hormone deficiency. *Endocr Pract* 2016;22(10):1235–1244.

24. Yuen KCJ. Growth hormone stimulation tests in assessing adult growth hormone deficiency. In: De Groot LJ, Chrousos G, Dungan K, et al., eds. *Endotext*. South Dartmouth, MA: MDText. com, Inc.; 2000.

25. Gasco V, Caputo M, Lanfranco F, Ghigo E, Grottoli S. Management of GH treatment in adult GH deficiency. *Best Pract Res Clin Endocrinol Metab* 2017;31(1):13–24.

26. Maison P, Griffin S, Nicoue-Beglah M, Haddad N, Balkau B, Chanson P. Impact of growth hormone (GH) treatment on cardiovascular risk factors in GH-deficient adults: a metaanalysis of blinded, randomized, placebo-controlled trials. *J Clin Endocrinol Metab* 2004;89(5):2192–2199.

27. Barake M, Klibanski A, Tritos NA. Effects of recombinant human growth hormone therapy on bone mineral density in adults with growth hormone deficiency: a meta-analysis. *J Clin Endocrinol Metab* 2014;99(3):852–860.

28. Mazziotti G, Bianchi A, Bonadonna S, et al. Increased prevalence of radiological spinal deformities in adult patients with GH deficiency: influence of GH replacement therapy. *J Bone Miner Res* 2006;21(4):520–528.

29. Koltowska-Haggstrom M, Mattsson AF, Shalet SM. Assessment of quality of life in adult patients with GH deficiency: KIMS contribution to clinical practice and pharmacoeconomic evaluations. *Eur J Endocrinol* 2009;161(Suppl 1):S51–S64.

30. Mo D, Blum WF, Rosilio M, Webb SM, Qi R, Strasburger CJ. Ten-year change in quality of life in adults on growth hormone replacement for growth hormone deficiency: an analysis of the hypopituitary control and complications study. *J Clin Endocrinol Metab* 2014;99(12):4581–4588.

31. Rubeck KZ, Bertelsen S, Vestergaard P, Jorgensen JO. Impact of GH substitution on exercise capacity and muscle strength in GH-deficient adults: a meta-analysis of blinded, placebo-controlled trials. *Clin Endocrinol (Oxf)* 2009;71(6):860–866.

32. Claessen KM, Appelman-Dijkstra NM, Adoptie DM, et al. Metabolic profile in growth hormone-deficient (GHD) adults after long-term recombinant human growth hormone (rhGH) therapy. *J Clin Endocrinol Metab* 2013;98(1):352–361.

33. Attanasio AF, Mo D, Erfurth EM, et al. Prevalence of metabolic syndrome in adult hypopituitary growth hormone (GH)-deficient patients before and after GH replacement. *J Clin Endocrinol Metab* 2010;95(1):74–81.

34. Woodmansee WW, Hartman ML, Lamberts SW, Zagar AJ, Clemmons DR. Occurrence of impaired fasting glucose in GH-deficient adults receiving GH replacement compared with untreated subjects. *Clin Endocrinol (Oxf)* 2010;72(1):59–69.

35. Attanasio AF, Jung H, Mo D, et al. Prevalence and incidence of diabetes mellitus in adult patients on growth hormone replacement for growth hormone deficiency: a surveillance database analysis. *J Clin Endocrinol Metab* 2011;96(7):2255–2261.

36. Stochholm K, Gravholt CH, Laursen T, et al. Mortality and GH deficiency: a nationwide study. *Eur J Endocrinol* 2007;157(1):9–18.
37. Svensson J, Bengtsson BA, Rosen T, Oden A, Johannsson G. Malignant disease and cardiovascular morbidity in hypopituitary adults with or without growth hormone replacement therapy. *J Clin Endocrinol Metab* 2004;89(7):3306–3312.

Nodular Thyroid Disease and Goiter

7

Sina Jasim and Amy E. Riek

GENERAL PRINCIPLES

- There are two causes of goiter, or thyroid enlargement. **Goiter can result from generalized thyroid enlargement without nodules or from nodular thyroid disease including multinodular goiter (MNG) or a solitary thyroid nodule.** Small thyroid nodules can also be present without overall thyroid enlargement.
- The primary concern with diffuse goiter is thyroid function and whether it is causing obstructive symptoms because of compression of nearby structures (esophagus, trachea).
- The major concern with thyroid nodules is possible malignancy.

Epidemiology

- Goiter is more common in females, and it is also more common in iodine-deficient areas. In the United States, sporadic goiter affects more than 5% of adult population.[1]
- **Thyroid nodules are very common** in clinical practice. The prevalence of palpable thyroid nodules in iodine-sufficient areas is around 5% in women and 1% in men,[2,3] but most nodules are not palpable. In those with a solitary nodule on examination of the thyroid, neck ultrasound (US) can identify additional nodules up to 50% of the time.[4] With the increased frequency of imaging for evaluation of nonthyroid lesions of the neck, the incidental finding of thyroid nodules has dramatically increased. High-resolution US detects thyroid nodules in 19% to 68% with higher frequencies in women and the elderly.[5]
- **A vast majority of thyroid nodules are benign, but 5% to 10% are likely malignant**, highlighting the clinical importance of evaluating for this risk when evaluating a thyroid nodule. Thyroid nodules carry a similar risk of malignancy regardless of whether the patient has a solitary nodule or multiple nodules.[6]

Etiology

- Diffuse goiter can be seen in Graves disease (see Chapter 8 Hyperthyroidism) or chronic lymphocytic (Hashimoto) thyroiditis. In iodine-deficient areas, diffuse goiter is common as the thyroid grows in response to excess thyroid stimulating hormone (TSH) resulting from inadequate iodine supply to produce thyroid hormone.
- Thyroid nodules result from benign cysts or adenomas or from malignancy, typically of primary thyroid origin but also occasionally primary thyroid lymphoma or metastatic disease from other sites. Multiple factors, including genetic, environmental, and demographic factors interact in the development and pathogenesis of thyroid nodules.

DIAGNOSIS

Clinical Presentation

- Clinical evaluation includes assessment of **symptoms, family history of thyroid disorders or thyroid cancer, and history of head and neck radiation**.

- Goiter can be asymptomatic or, at times, present with compressive neck symptoms such as cough, shortness of breath, and swallowing difficulty. Retrosternal extension can cause tracheal deviation or compression and thoracic outlet obstruction.
- **Most thyroid nodules are nonfunctional** but some can autonomously produce excess thyroid hormone causing clinical hyperthyroidism (see Chapter 8 Hyperthyroidism).
- **Thyroid nodules typically present as a painless lump in the neck by routine examination.** If pain is present, it is likely due to hemorrhage into a thyroid cyst. Thyroid nodules are increasingly found during imaging for evaluation of nonthyroid lesions of the neck or chest. Of note, focal [18F] fluorodeoxyglucose positron emission tomography ([18]FDG-PET) uptake within a sonographically confirmed thyroid nodule increases malignancy risk in that nodule to about 35%.[7]
- **Concerning history for thyroid cancer** includes extremes of age (younger than 14 or older than 70 years), rapid nodule growth, hoarseness of the voice, history of childhood head and neck radiation, or family history of thyroid cancer or syndromes associated with thyroid cancer such as Cowden disease, Carney complex, familial adenomatous polyposis (FAP), Werner syndrome/progeria, or multiple endocrine neoplasia type 2 (MEN2).[8]
- **Concerning findings on physical examination** include fixation of the nodule to surrounding tissue, cervical lymphadenopathy, or vocal cord paralysis.

Diagnostic Testing

Laboratories

- **TSH should be measured in all patients.** Suppressed TSH suggests a diagnosis of Graves disease or one or more toxic nodules (producing thyroid hormone), which do not require biopsy. Hyperthyroidism due to a thyroid nodule should be confirmed with thyroid scintigraphy prior to decision making regarding biopsy (see Imaging below).
- The routine measurement of serum thyroglobulin (Tg) is not indicated in a patient with thyroid nodules.
- Serum calcitonin is not routinely measured but may be considered in clinical scenarios where it might change management, such as suspicious cytology not consistent with papillary thyroid carcinoma or family history of medullary thyroid carcinoma.

Imaging

- **Thyroid ultrasonography (US)**
  - High-resolution US is a widely used, inexpensive, and sensitive (~95%) method in the detection of small, nonpalpable thyroid nodules.
  - **Diagnostic thyroid/neck US should be performed in patients with clinically or incidentally found thyroid nodule(s)** in order to evaluate the thyroid parenchyma, gland and nodule size and location, sonographic features of the nodules, and cervical lymph nodes. Up to 50% of patients with single nodules on physical examination will show additional nodules.[5]
  - The sonographic features of the thyroid nodule(s) classify the risk of malignancy to help direct decision making for fine-needle aspiration (FNA) biopsy and further management.
  - **Sonographic features of nodules that are associated with higher risk of thyroid cancer** include the presence of microcalcifications, hypoechoic echogenicity, irregular margins, and larger anterior–posterior than transverse dimension (see Table 7-1).[9,10]
  - **Anterior cervical lymph node compartments (central and lateral) should be evaluated by US during thyroid nodule evaluation.** If sonographically suspicious cervical lymph nodes are detected, FNA of the suspicious lymph node should be performed for cytology, and washout submitted for Tg measurement to confirm thyroid origin of cells.[9]

TABLE 7-1 COMPARISON OF THYROID NODULE ULTRASOUND FEATURES INDICATING FINE-NEEDLE ASPIRATION

American thyroid association 2015 guidelines (risk of malignancy)	AACE/ACE 2016 guidelines (risk of malignancy)	Indications for FNA
A. Benign (<1%) Purely cystic nodules **B. Very low suspicion (<3%)** Spongiform or partially cystic nodules without features described in higher-risk categories **C. Low suspicion (5–10%)** Isoechoic or hyperechoic solid nodule or partially cystic nodule with eccentric solid component without: • Microcalcifications • Irregular margin • Extrathyroidal extension • Taller than wide shape (on transverse view)	**Low-risk lesion (1%)*** • Cysts (fluid component >80%) • Mostly cystic nodules (>50%) and not associated with suspicious US signs • Isoechoic spongiform nodules, either confluent or with regular halo	A. No biopsy B. ≥2 cm (*AACE) C. ≥1.5 cm
Intermediate suspicion (10–20%) Hypoechoic solid nodule with smooth margins without: • Microcalcifications • ETE • Or taller than wide shape	**Intermediate-risk thyroid lesion (5–15%)** Slightly hypoechoic/isoechoic nodules, with ovoid to round shape, smooth or ill-defined margins. May be present: • Intranodular vascularization • Elevated stiffness at elastography • Macro or continuous rim calcifications • Indeterminate hyperechoic spots	≥2 cm (AACE) ≥1 cm (ATA)

(continued)

TABLE 7-1	COMPARISON OF THYROID NODULE ULTRASOUND FEATURES INDICATING FINE-NEEDLE ASPIRATION (Continued)	
American thyroid association 2015 guidelines (risk of malignancy)	AACE/ACE 2016 guidelines (risk of malignancy)	Indications for FNA
High suspicion (>70–90%) Solid hypoechoic nodule or solid hypoechoic component of partially cystic nodule with one or more of the following features: • Irregular margins (infiltrative, microlobulated) • Microcalcifications • Taller than wide shape • Rim calcifications • Evidence of ETE	**High-risk thyroid lesion (50–90%)** Nodules with at least one of the following features: • Marked hypoechogenicity • Spiculated or lobulated margins • Microcalcifications • Taller than wide shape (AP > TR) • Extrathyroidal growth • Pathologic adenopathy	≥1 cm

AACE/ACE, American Association of Clinical Endocrinologists/American College of Endocrinology; AP, anteroposterior; ATA, American Thyroid Association; ETE, extrathyroidal extension; FNA, fine-needle aspiration; TR, transverse; US, ultrasonography.

Haugen BR, Alexander EK, Bible KC, et al. 2015 American Thyroid Association management guidelines for adult patients with thyroid nodules and differentiated thyroid cancer: The American Thyroid Association Guidelines Task Force on Thyroid Nodules and Differentiated Thyroid Cancer. *Thyroid* 2016;26(1):1–133; and Gharib H, Papini E, Garber JR, et al. American Association of Clinical Endocrinologists, American College of Endocrinology, and Associazione Medici Endocrinologi medical guidelines for clinical practice for the diagnosis and management of thyroid nodules–2016 update. *Endocr Pract* 2016;22(5):622–639.

- **CT and MRI**
  - These imaging modalities are not routinely used, but are useful in the evaluation of patients with compressive symptoms and large goiter with suspected retrosternal extension.
  - Noncontrast CT is preferred to avoid possible iodine-induced thyrotoxicosis in the setting of an MNG.[11]
- **Thyroid scintigraphy (radionuclide scan)**
  - A thyroid scan is only useful in the setting of one or more thyroid nodules associated with low TSH.
  - Nodules with increased uptake compared to the surrounding thyroid tissue (hot nodules) have a lower risk of malignancy, so biopsy and cytologic evaluation are not indicated.

Diagnostic Procedures
- **For thyroid nodules meeting biopsy criteria, FNA with cytologic evaluation is the procedure of choice. FNA should be performed based on the sonographic pattern of the nodule and respective size cutoff described in Table 7-1.** FNA is typically performed by four to six passes with a 25- to 27-gauge needle, often with US guidance.
- Patients with multiple thyroid nodules have the same risk of malignancy as those with solitary nodules.[6] In these patients, **each nodule ≥1 cm should be evaluated independently.** If multiple sonographically similar very low or low suspicion pattern nodules are present, FNA should be performed on the largest nodules (≥2 cm).
- **Cytologic adequacy** requires the presence of at least six groups of well-visualized follicular cells, each group containing at least 10 well-preserved epithelial cells, preferably on a single slide.[12]
- Thyroid nodule FNA cytology should be reported using diagnostic groups outlined in the **Bethesda System for Reporting Thyroid Cytopathology.** These categories and associated risk of malignancy are[13]:
  - **Nondiagnostic/unsatisfactory**
  - **Benign:** 0% to 3% malignant
  - **Atypia of undetermined significance/follicular lesion of undetermined significance** (AUS/FLUS): 5% to 15% malignant
  - **Follicular neoplasm/suspicious for follicular neoplasm** (FN/SFN), a category that also encompasses the diagnosis of Hürthle cell neoplasm/suspicious for Hürthle cell neoplasm: 15% to 30% malignant
  - **Suspicious for malignancy** (SUSP): 60% to 75% malignant
  - **Malignant:** 97% to 99% malignant
- **Molecular diagnostic testing** of thyroid nodules is becoming increasingly incorporated into clinical practice with FNA and is evolving rapidly. These genetic panels are used in combination with indeterminate cytology results (AUS/FLUS and FN/SFN) to increase or decrease the likelihood of malignancy in order to facilitate surgical decision making. See Table 7-2 for the most common available tests and their diagnostic characteristics.[14–19] Of note, **molecular diagnostic tests require dedicated cellular material, which is collected during FNA but only resulted in the case of indeterminate cytology (see Surgical Management below).**

TREATMENT

Surgical Management

- **Goiter**
  - **Near-total or total thyroidectomy should be performed for large or retrosternal diffuse goiters with obstructive symptoms. Lobectomy can be considered for removal of a benign nodule that is large (>4 cm) or causing compressive symptoms.**
  - Surgery is the preferred therapy in patients with nontoxic, nonobstructive goiter that continues to grow and may potentially cause obstructive symptoms or cosmetic concerns.

	Afirma gene expression classifier (Veracyte)	ThyGenX/ThyraMIR (Interpace diagnostics)	ThyroSeq v2 (CBLPath/university of pittsburgh medical center)
Methodology	mRNA expression microarray (167 genes) with benign or suspicious classification by proprietary algorithm	Next-generation sequencing for genetic alterations (8 genes) with reflex if negative to miRNA expression analysis (10 miRNAs) that classifies positive or negative	Next-generation sequencing for DNA and RNA alterations (56 genes)
Collection requirements	2 dedicated FNA passes	1 dedicated FNA pass	1–2 drops from first FNA pass
Negative predictive value	94–95%	94% if both negative	96–97%
Positive predictive value	36–37%	81% if ThyGenX positive, 74% if ThyraMIR positive	71–83%
Clinical utility	Strong "rule out" test if negative; validated in blinded multicenter prospective trial; high false-positive rate in Hürthle cell lesions	Strong "rule out" and "rule in" test when combined; validated in blinded multicenter prospective trial; ability to risk stratify positive ThyGenX results based on mutation	Strong "rule out" and "rule in" test; ability to risk stratify positive results based on mutation

FNA, fine-needle aspiration.

○ **An asymptomatic, euthyroid patient with a nonobstructive goiter may require no intervention** and can be monitored for further growth, obstruction, or autonomy.
- **Thyroid nodules are surgically resected if indicated based upon cytology results as follows:**
  ○ **Nondiagnostic: FNA should be repeated** and will result in a diagnostic specimen in 60% to 80% of cases. Management and follow-up of recurrent nondiagnostic FNA results depend on growth rate, radiologic features, and individual risk factors, but any concerning features should prompt surgical removal.
  ○ **Benign: No further treatment is necessary**, and routine TSH suppression therapy is not indicated. Surgical removal or percutaneous ethanol injection (PEI) can be considered for recurrent cystic thyroid nodules with benign cytology.
  ○ **AUS/FLUS:** This category is considered to be **indeterminate**, and patient preference and feasibility, as well as risk factors and sonographic appearance should be taken into account when discussing management options, which include:
    - **Repeat FNA** (results in more definitive cytologic diagnosis in 70% to 90% of cases)
    - **Molecular testing** (see Table 7-2 for the most commonly available tests)
    - **Continued surveillance**
    - **Diagnostic surgical excision** (lobectomy is generally the preferred initial surgical approach for indeterminate nodules, although total thyroidectomy can be considered for nodules that are cytologically or sonographically suspicious for malignancy, concerning molecular diagnostics, or large [>4 cm] in size, and in patients with radiation exposure or history of familial thyroid carcinoma)[7]
  ○ **FN/SFN:** This category is also considered to be **indeterminate**, with similar considerations as AUS/FLUS, though malignancy risk is higher. Management options include:
    - **Diagnostic surgical excision**
    - **Molecular tewsting**
  ○ **Malignant or SUSP: Surgical resection is generally recommended.** See Chapter 10 Thyroid Cancer for further details and follow-up.

Medications

- Thyroid hormone suppressive therapy was widely used in the past for treating benign goiters; more so in diffuse than in nodular types. Its use remains controversial, and neither the AACE[10] nor the ATA[9] guidelines recommend it.

Other Nonpharmacologic Therapies

- Radioiodine is not routinely used in treating nontoxic goiter, particularly in the United States.
- Several interventions are performed in selected experienced centers and for selected patients for thyroid nodules when surgery is not an option:
  ○ PEI
  ○ Laser ablation, cryoablation, or radiofrequency ablation

MONITORING/FOLLOW-UP

- Due to the low false-negative rate of FNA results (1.1%), the **follow-up for nodules with benign cytology is determined by risk stratification based on sonographic features:**
  ○ **High suspicion:** repeat US and FNA within 12 months.
  ○ **Low-to-intermediate suspicion:** repeat US in 12 to 24 months. If sonographic evidence of growth, defined by 20% growth in two or more dimensions of at least

2 mm or 50% increase in volume, or new suspicious sonographic features, repeat FNA could be considered.

○ **Very low suspicion:** consider follow-up with US at least 2 years later.

○ **Nodules with two benign FNA results:** no further follow-up for malignancy is necessary.

• **Follow-up of thyroid nodules that did not initially meet criteria for FNA is similarly based upon sonographic features:**

○ **High suspicion:** repeat US in 6 to 12 months.

○ **Low-to-intermediate suspicion:** consider repeat US at 12 to 24 months.

○ **Very low suspicion solid nodules or pure cysts >1 cm:** consider follow-up with US at least 2 years later.

○ **Very low suspicion solid nodules or pure cysts ≤1 cm:** no routine imaging follow-up is necessary.

REFERENCES

1. Malboosbaf R, Hosseinpanah F, Mojarrad M, Jambarsang S, Azizi F. Relationship between goiter and gender: a systematic review and meta-analysis. *Endocrine* 2013;43(3):539–547.
2. Tunbridge WM, Evered DC, Hall R, et al. The spectrum of thyroid disease in a community: the Whickham survey. *Clin Endocrinol (Oxf)* 1977;7(6):481–493.
3. Vander JB, Gaston EA, Dawber TR. The significance of nontoxic thyroid nodules. Final report of a 15-year study of the incidence of thyroid malignancy. *Ann Intern Med* 1968;69(3): 537–540.
4. Tan GH, Gharib H, Reading CC. Solitary thyroid nodule. Comparison between palpation and ultrasonography. *Arch Intern Med* 1995;155(22):2418–2423.
5. Tan GH, Gharib H. Thyroid incidentalomas: management approaches to nonpalpable nodules discovered incidentally on thyroid imaging. *Ann Intern Med* 1997;126(3):226–231.
6. Papini E, Guglielmi R, Bianchini A, et al. Risk of malignancy in nonpalpable thyroid nodules: predictive value of ultrasound and color-Doppler features. *J Clin Endocrinol Metab* 2002;87(5):1941–1946.
7. Soelberg KK, Bonnema SJ, Brix TH, Hegedüs L. Risk of malignancy in thyroid incidentalomas detected by 18F-fluorodeoxyglucose positron emission tomography: a systematic review. *Thyroid* 2012;22(9):918–925.
8. Richards ML. Familial syndromes associated with thyroid cancer in the era of personalized medicine. *Thyroid* 2010;20(7):707–713.
9. Haugen BR, Alexander EK, Bible KC, et al. 2015 American Thyroid Association management guidelines for adult patients with thyroid nodules and differentiated thyroid cancer: The American Thyroid Association Guidelines Task Force on Thyroid Nodules and Differentiated Thyroid Cancer. *Thyroid* 2016;26(1):1–133.
10. Gharib H, Papini E, Garber JR, et al. American Association of Clinical Endocrinologists, American College of Endocrinology, and Associazione Medici Endocrinologi medical guidelines for clinical practice for the diagnosis and management of thyroid nodules–2016 update. *Endocr Pract* 2016;22(5):622–639.
11. Rieu M, Bekka S, Sambor B, Berrod JL, Fombeur JP. Prevalence of subclinical hyperthyroidism and relationship between thyroid hormonal status and thyroid ultrasonographic parameters in patients with non-toxic nodular goitre. *Clin Endocrinol (Oxf)* 1993;39(1):67–71.
12. Baloch ZW, Tam D, Langer J, Mandel S, LiVolsi VA, Gupta PK. Ultrasound-guided fine-needle aspiration biopsy of the thyroid: role of on-site assessment and multiple cytologic preparations. *Diagn Cytopathol* 2000;23(6):425–429.
13. Cibas ES, Ali SZ. The Bethesda System for reporting thyroid cytopathology. *Thyroid* 2009;19(11):1159–1165.
14. Nikiforov YE. Role of molecular markers in thyroid nodule management: then and now. *Endocr Pract* 2017;23(8):979–988.
15. Zhang M, Lin O. Molecular Testing of Thyroid Nodules: A review of current available tests for fine-needle aspiration specimens. *Arch Pathol Lab Med* 2016;140(12):1338–1344.
16. Alexander EK, Kennedy GC, Baloch ZW, et al. Preoperative diagnosis of benign thyroid nodules with indeterminate cytology. *N Engl J Med* 2012;367(8):705–715.

17. Labourier E, Shifrin A, Busseniers AE, et al. Molecular testing for miRNA, mRNA, and DNA on fine-needle aspiration improves the preoperative diagnosis of thyroid nodules with indeterminate cytology. *J Clin Endocrinol Metab* 2015;100(7):2743–2750.

18. Nikiforov YE, Carty SE, Chiosea SI, et al. Highly accurate diagnosis of cancer in thyroid nodules with follicular neoplasm/suspicious for a follicular neoplasm cytology by ThyroSeq v2 next-generation sequencing assay. *Cancer* 2014;120(23):3627–3634.

19. Nikiforov YE, Carty SE, Chiosea SI, et al. Impact of the multi-gene ThyroSeq next-generation sequencing assay on cancer diagnosis in thyroid nodules with atypia of undetermined significance/follicular lesion of undetermined significance cytology. *Thyroid* 2015;25(11):1217–1223.

Hyperthyroidism

8

Kevin T. Bauerle and William E. Clutter

GENERAL PRINCIPLES

Epidemiology

Hyperthyroidism, or thyrotoxicosis, is fivefold more common in women and has an overall prevalence of 1.2%.

Etiology

- **Graves disease** is the most common cause of hyperthyroidism and is mediated by **thyroid-stimulating immunoglobulins (TSIs)** which bind to the thyroid-stimulating hormone (TSH) receptor and mimic the effects of TSH. Graves disease is more common in women. Patients have a **diffuse, nontender goiter**. Increased blood flow sometimes causes a thyroid bruit. The natural history of Graves disease may be marked by exacerbations and remissions of hyperthyroidism. Graves disease includes two unique extrathyroidal signs caused by the underlying autoimmune disease, not by thyroid hormone excess:
  - **Graves orbitopathy (GO)**, characterized by inflammation and edema of retro-orbital tissues (extraocular muscles and fat), causes forward protrusion of the globe (proptosis or exophthalmos).
  - **Pretibial myxedema**, a rare plaque-like thickening of the skin over the shins, is due to accumulation of glycosaminoglycans in the dermis.
- **Toxic multinodular goiter** (MNG) is the most common cause of hyperthyroidism in older patients, and its prevalence increases in setting of iodine deficiency. It is characterized by areas of autonomous function within an MNG that develop in response to somatic mutations in genes regulating thyroid hormone synthesis and secretion.
- Other rarer causes of hyperthyroidism include:
  - **Iodine-induced hyperthyroidism.** Precipitated by drugs such as **amiodarone** or radiographic contrast media. Occurs in up to 3% of patients treated with amiodarone in North America and typically in the setting of underlying thyroid pathology, such as MNG.
  - **Toxic adenomas.** Similar to toxic MNG, hyperthyroidism develops due to autonomous function of a single nodule.
  - **Thyroiditis.** Transient hyperthyroidism results from release of preformed thyroid hormone by inflamed thyroid tissue.
- **Subacute thyroiditis.** Caused by granulomatous inflammation in the setting of a viral syndrome, resulting in a painful and tender goiter.
- **Painless thyroiditis.** Caused by an autoimmune process resulting in a nontender goiter. Most often observed in the postpartum period.
- **Factitious hyperthyroidism.** Occasionally reported with surreptitious ingestion of thyroid hormone for the purposes of weight loss.
- Very high levels of **human chorionic gonadotropin (hCG)** (which weakly cross-reacts with the TSH receptor) secreted by trophoblastic tumors can cause hyperthyroidism.
- **TSH-secreting pituitary adenoma.** See Chapter 1 for further discussion (Table 8-1).

TABLE 8-1	CAUSES OF HYPERTHYROIDISM

Graves disease
Toxic multinodular goiter
Toxic adenoma
Iodine and iodine-containing drugs (e.g., amiodarone, iodinated contrast agents)
Painless thyroiditis
Subacute thyroiditis
Factitious hyperthyroidism
Ectopic thyroid tissue (struma ovarii)
Chorionic gonadotropin induced (choriocarcinoma, hydatidiform mole)
TSH-secreting pituitary adenoma

TSH, thyroid-stimulating hormone.

DIAGNOSIS

Clinical Presentation

- **Symptoms** include heat intolerance, weight loss, weakness, palpitations, oligomenorrhea, and anxiety (Table 8-2). **Signs** include brisk tendon reflexes, fine tremor, proximal weakness, stare, and eyelid lag. Cardiac abnormalities include sinus tachycardia, atrial fibrillation, and exacerbation of coronary artery disease or heart failure. **In the elderly,**

TABLE 8-2	MANIFESTATIONS OF HYPERTHYROIDISM

Symptoms
Heat intolerance, increased sweating
Weight loss (often with increased appetite)
Anxiety, irritability
Palpitations
Oligomenorrhea
Increased stool frequency
Dyspnea
Fatigue, weakness

Signs
Brisk reflexes, fine tremor
Lid lag, stare
Sinus tachycardia
Atrial fibrillation
Warm, moist skin
Palmar erythema, onycholysis
Hair loss
Muscle weakness and wasting
Exacerbation of heart failure or coronary artery disease
Periodic paralysis (primarily in Asian men)

TABLE 8-3	MANIFESTATIONS OF GRAVES DISEASE

Diffuse goiter
Ophthalmopathy
   Retrobulbar pressure or pain
   Periorbital edema, scleral injection
   Exophthalmos (proptosis)
   Extraocular muscle dysfunction
   Exposure keratitis
   Optic neuropathy (rare)
Pretibial myxedema (localized dermopathy)

hyperthyroidism may present with only atrial fibrillation, heart failure, weakness, or weight loss.

- Graves disease may cause additional findings that are not due to hyperthyroidism (Table 8-3). Symptoms of orbitopathy include increased lacrimation, foreign body sensation, conjunctival redness, and periorbital edema. Fibrosis of extraocular muscles can cause diplopia. Rarely, proptosis threatens vision by corneal exposure (due to incomplete lid closure) or compression of the optic nerve.

Differential Diagnosis

The cause of hyperthyroidism should be determined because this affects the choice of therapy (Table 8-4). Differential diagnosis is based on:

- **The presence of orbitopathy or pretibial myxedema with or without a symmetrically enlarged thyroid** is highly suggestive of Graves disease and no further testing is warranted.
- **The presence of multiple nodules or a single nodule** is suggestive of a toxic MNG or adenoma, respectively. This diagnosis should be confirmed with a nuclear medicine thyroid scan with technetium or ^{123}I demonstrating a single or multiple areas of radioisotope uptake.
- A **painful, tender thyroid** indicates subacute thyroiditis and is supported by an elevated ESR and serum thyroglobulin levels.
- **The absence of palpable thyroid enlargement** almost always represents Graves disease, but the possibility of factitious hyperthyroidism, painless thyroiditis, iodine-induced hyperthyroidism, or substernal extension of the goiter in a patient with a difficult thyroid examination should be considered. In overt thyrotoxicosis, measurement of receptor antibodies or TSIs can be particularly helpful as these have a sensitivity and specificity that

TABLE 8-4	DIFFERENTIAL DIAGNOSIS OF HYPERTHYROIDISM

Type of goiter	Diagnosis
Diffuse, nontender goiter	Graves disease or painless thyroiditis
Multiple thyroid nodules	Toxic multinodular goiter
Single thyroid nodule	Thyroid adenoma
Tender painful goiter	Subacute thyroiditis
Normal thyroid gland	Graves disease, painless thyroiditis, or factitious hyperthyroidism

TABLE 8-5	DIFFERENTIAL DIAGNOSIS OF HYPERTHYROIDISM BASED ON RAIU
Increased RAIU	**Decreased RAIU**
Graves disease	Subacute thyroiditis
Toxic multinodular goiter	Painless thyroiditis
Thyroid adenoma	Iodine-induced hyperthyroidism
	Factitious hyperthyroidism

RAIU, radioactive iodine uptake.

exceed 95%. If either TSI or TRAb is positive, a diagnosis of Graves disease is confirmed. If antibody testing is negative, additional testing, including **24-hour radioactive iodine uptake** (RAIU, see Table 8-5) measurement, can be used to distinguish different etiologies of hyperthyroidism:

○ **Pregnancy within the past year and elevated thyroglobulin levels** are supportive of a diagnosis of a painless postpartum thyroiditis. If the patient is not nursing, RAIU measurement can support this diagnosis by showing a reduced uptake. TPO Ab are often positive as well.

○ **Recent contrast administration or amiodarone therapy** is also important to consider, especially in individuals with thyroid gland pathology. In these cases, RAIU is likely to be diminished.

○ RAIU will also be reduced in individuals taking exogenous thyroid hormone.

Diagnostic Testing

Laboratories

- Hyperthyroidism should be suspected in any patient with compatible symptoms, as it is a readily treatable disorder that may become very debilitating.
- **Plasma TSH is the best initial diagnostic test**, as a TSH level >0.4 µU/mL excludes a diagnosis of hyperthyroidism, **except** in the case of a TSH-secreting pituitary adenoma.
  ○ A subnormal TSH should be followed by measurement of triiodothyronine (T_3) and free thyroxine (T_4). In most patients with overt hyperthyroidism, both T_3 and free T_4 (FT_4) levels will be elevated. A small subset of individuals may have isolated elevation of T_3 (T_3 toxicosis).
  ○ **Subclinical hyperthyroidism** is defined as a subnormal TSH in the setting of normal thyroid hormone levels. Symptoms of hyperthyroidism are often absent.
  ○ Other causes of TSH suppression:
    ▪ Critical illness resulting in **severe nonthyroidal illness.** Patients have normal or low plasma free T_4 and low plasma T_3.
    ▪ **Central hypothyroidism.** FT_4 levels are low or low-normal, and clinical signs of hyperthyroidism are absent.
    ▪ When the etiology of hyperthyroidism is not clear based on clinical assessment, antibody testing and nuclear medicine studies may be useful. These tests are further discussed below.

TREATMENT

- Treatment of hyperthyroidism involves management of symptoms related to increased adrenergic tone as well as management of thyrotoxicosis with radioactive iodine (RAI), thionamides, or subtotal/total thyroidectomy.

- Some forms of hyperthyroidism (subacute or postpartum/painless thyroiditis) are transient and require only symptomatic therapy. These forms of hyperthyroidism may be followed by a period of hypothyroidism before return to a euthyroid state.[1]

Medications

- β-**Adrenergic antagonists** (such as **atenolol** 25 to 100 mg daily) are used to relieve symptoms such as palpitations, tremor, and anxiety, until hyperthyroidism is controlled by thionamides or definitive therapy, or until transient hyperthyroidism resolves. The dose is adjusted to alleviate symptoms and tachycardia, and then reduced gradually as hyperthyroidism is controlled.
- Thianomides
  - **Methimazole** and **propylthiouracil** (**PTU**) inhibit thyroid hormone synthesis by blocking thyroid peroxidase.[2] PTU also inhibits extrathyroidal conversion of T_4 to T_3 by type 1 deiodinase.
  - **Methimazole is preferred** over PTU except in the first trimester of pregnancy or in the treatment of thyroid storm (see below).[3]
  - Unlike RAI and surgery, which represent definitive therapy of hyperthyroidism, these drugs have no permanent effect on thyroid function.
  - A trial of methimazole for 12 to 18 months is a reasonable approach in any patient, especially if definitive therapy is refused. If a euthyroid state is not achieved, definitive therapy should be performed.
  - The following scenarios favor the use of thionamides over definitive therapy:
    - Elderly patients or those with severe hyperthyroidism–associated symptoms or cardiac disease requiring rapid biochemical control prior to the use of definitive therapy.
    - Presence of moderate to severe active GO that may be exacerbated by RAI therapy.
    - Pregnancy.
    - High likelihood of inducing disease remission with a short course of therapy. **Remission may occur in up to one-third of patients** on thionamide therapy and is more frequent in younger women with mild disease, recent-onset hyperthyroidism, small goiter, and low TRAb titer.
  - **Initiation of therapy.** Before starting therapy, patients must be warned of side effects. Usual starting doses are PTU, 100 to 200 mg tid, or methimazole, 10 to 40 mg daily.
  - **Side effects** are most likely to occur within the first few months of therapy.
    - Minor side effects include rash, urticaria, fever, arthralgias, and transient leukopenia.
    - **Agranulocytosis** occurs in about 0.3% of patients treated with thionamides.
    - Other life-threatening side effects include **hepatitis** (more common with PTU), vasculitis, and drug-induced lupus erythematosus. These complications usually resolve if the drug is stopped promptly.
    - **Patients must be warned to discontinue the drug immediately and contact physician if jaundice or symptoms suggestive of agranulocytosis develop (e.g., fever, chills, sore throat).**
  - **Follow-up.** FT_4 levels are initially evaluated at 4-week intervals, and dose should be increased if FT_4 is not normalized. TSH may remain suppressed well after normalization of FT_4. Dose is then adjusted to maintain plasma free T_4 within the normal range.
  - Discontinuation of thionamide therapy should be considered at the end of 12 to 18 months, if the patient is biochemically euthyroid and on low-dose therapy. Measurement of thyrotropin receptor antibodies (TRAb) is helpful in predicting the likelihood of recurrence of hyperthyroidism. High TRAb levels predict a relapse rate that exceeds 80%, and definitive therapy should be discussed with the patient. On the other hand, low titers have a relapse rate of ~30%, and thionamides can be safely stopped in this group.[4]

Other Nonpharmacologic Therapies

- A single dose of iodine-131 permanently controls hyperthyroidism in about 80% to 90% of patients, and further doses can be given if necessary. A **pregnancy test** is done immediately before therapy in potentially fertile women. A 24-hour RAIU is usually measured and used to calculate the dose.
- Most patients with Graves disease are treated with ~10 to 15 mCi, while treatment of toxic MNG requires higher doses.
- Thionamides interfere with RAI therapy and should be discontinued 3 to 4 days before treatment. In individuals with cardiac disease or severe symptoms of hyperthyroidism, thionamides may be resumed 3 to 7 days after RAI therapy.
- RAI is **contraindicated in pregnant or lactating women**.
- RAI is the **preferred definitive treatment** modality in:
  - poor surgical candidates
  - patients with prior neck surgery or irradiation
- Patients are evaluated at 4- to 6-week intervals with FT_4 measurement. A transition to hypothyroidism (reflected by a subnormal FT_4) typically occurs between 2 and 6 months posttreatment. **If thyroid function stabilizes within the normal range**, this interval may be increased gradually to annual monitoring. **If hypothyroidism develops**, thyroxine therapy is started and titrated to restore biochemical euthyroidism.
- **If clinical hyperthyroidism persists after 6 months, RAI treatment is repeated.**
- **Side effects:**
  - Permanent hypothyroidism in patients treated for Graves disease occurs in over half of patients within the 1st year and continues to develop at a rate of approximately 3% per year thereafter.
  - A slight exacerbation of hyperthyroidism following treatment (because of release of stored thyroid hormone) is clinically important in **patients with severe cardiac disease**, and such patients should be treated initially with thionamides to restore euthyroidism.
  - Worsening of active GO (see below for further discussion).[4,5]

Surgical Management

Subtotal/total thyroidectomy provides long-term control of hyperthyroidism in most patients, but may trigger a perioperative exacerbation of hyperthyroidism.

- For treatment of Graves disease, **euthyroidism** should be achieved with a thionamide prior to surgery as above and **supersaturated potassium iodide (SSKI)**, 80 mg (2 drops) orally bid is added 1 to 2 weeks before surgery. Both drugs are stopped postoperatively. A β-blocker may also be used in preparation for the surgery if tachycardia is prominent. For treatment of a toxic nodule or toxic MNG, SSKI is not required.
- Total thyroidectomy or near-total thyroidectomy are preferred in management of toxic MNG or Graves disease, while lobectomy may be sufficient in those with a single toxic adenoma.
- Following total thyroidectomy, thyroxine replacement is initiated at a dose of 1.6 μg/kg. For subtotal thyroidectomy or lobectomy, thyroxine replacement can be withheld until a persistent TSH elevation is observed.
- Preferred **definitive treatment** modality in:
  - Patients with moderate to severe active GO seeking definitive therapy
  - Documented or suspected coexistent malignancy
  - Symptomatic compression by large goiters or nodules >4 cm
- **Complications** of thyroidectomy include hypoparathyroidism, recurrent laryngeal nerve injury, and perioperative death.[4,6]

SPECIAL CONSIDERATIONS

- **Amiodarone-induced thyrotoxicosis (AIT)** occurs via two mechanisms. While AIT1 is precipitated by excess iodine resulting in increased thyroid hormone synthesis and treated most appropriately with high doses of methimazole (40 mg daily), AIT2 represents a destructive thyroiditis and is effectively treated with moderate doses of oral glucocorticoids (prednisone 40 to 60 mg daily). Methimazole therapy has been shown to be effective as an initial treatment without distinguishing between AIT1 and AIT2 in an iodine-replete area. Nevertheless, consideration should be given to concurrent use of glucocorticoids and methimazole in severely thyrotoxic individuals at high risk for related complications. Alternatively, if methimazole therapy alone demonstrates no improvement, glucocorticoids may be added later as an adjunctive therapy. Given the long half-life of amiodarone, there is no indication for discontinuation of therapy during a period of thyrotoxicosis.[7]
- Subclinical hyperthyroidism **increases the risk of atrial fibrillation in the elderly, particularly those >65**, and predisposes to **osteoporosis** in **postmenopausal women**.
  - Treatment with definitive therapy or thionamides is indicated in individuals with a **TSH <0.1 and an additional risk factor for complications of subclinical hyperthyroidism (age >65, cardiovascular disease, or osteoporosis)**.
  - Treatment may also be considered in younger patients with a TSH <0.1 and symptoms of hyperthyroidism and those with a milder degree of TSH suppression with coexistent osteoporosis or cardiovascular disease.[4,8]
- **Urgent therapy** is warranted when hyperthyroidism exacerbates heart failure or coronary artery disease and in rare patients with severe hyperthyroidism complicated by fever and delirium (thyroid storm). Treatment is aimed at blocking adrenergic symptoms of hyperthyroidism and inhibiting synthesis, release, and peripheral conversion of T4 to T3 and includes:
  - **PTU, 200 mg orally q6h.**
  - **SSKI, 5 drops orally q6h**, should be started after the first dose of PTU, to inhibit thyroid hormone secretion.
  - **Propranolol**, 60 to 80 mg orally q6h (or an equivalent dose of a parenteral β-antagonist), should be provided to control tachycardia.
  - **Hydrocortisone 100 mg IV q8h** may be useful in patients with life-threatening hyperthyroidism.
  - Plasma free T_4 is measured every 3 to 7 days, and the doses of PTU and iodine are gradually decreased when FT_4 approaches the normal range.
  - If patient is intolerant of thionamides, surgery is the treatment of choice.[4,9]
- **Hyperthyroidism in pregnancy.** Hyperthyroidism increases the risk of miscarriage, preeclampsia, premature labor, and low birth weight. If hyperthyroidism is suspected, plasma TSH should be measured. Plasma TSH declines in early pregnancy owing to the thyroid-stimulating effects of hCG, but rarely to <0.1 μU/mL. If TSH is <0.1 μU/mL, the diagnosis should be confirmed by measurement of plasma FT_4.
  - PTU is the preferred thionamide during the first trimester because of lower risk of birth defects. After the first trimester, methimazole is preferred because of a lower risk of liver failure and an overall lower risk of birth defects after the 10th week of gestation. The dose should be adjusted at 4-week intervals to maintain the plasma free T_4 near the upper limit of the normal range. Overtreatment should be avoided to prevent fetal hypothyroidism.
  - TSIs can cause fetal or neonatal hyperthyroidism. In pregnant women who have previously been treated with RAI or thyroidectomy, measurement of plasma TSI in the third trimester helps assess the risk of neonatal hyperthyroidism.
  - Newborns should be monitored carefully for hyperthyroidism.
  - Women treated with methimazole may safely breastfeed.[10]

- **Treatment of GO.** Mild or moderate orbitopathy often improves spontaneously and may require no treatment. Symptoms of conjunctival irritation respond to lubricant eye drops and ointment at bedtime, which also protect against exposure keratitis. More severe orbitopathy, with the risk of visual loss, should be treated with glucocorticoids in consultation with an experienced ophthalmologist. It is important to distinguish between inactive and active GO, which is characterized by pain, redness, swelling, chemosis, and progression of proptosis and eye movement limitations. Importantly, RAI has been shown to exacerbate active GO and is contraindicated in patients with moderate to severe GO. RAI may be used in patients with mild active GO, though oral glucocorticoid therapy should be considered in those with risk factors for exacerbation of GO (advanced age, smoking, elevated TRAb titer). Prolonged hypothyroidism after RAI treatment should be avoided, as this may also exacerbate GO.[4,11]

REFERENCES

1. Brent GA. Clinical practice. Graves' disease. *N Engl J Med* 2008;358(24):2594–2605.
2. Drugs for thyroid disorders. *Treat Guidel Med Lett* 2009;7(84):57–64.
3. Cooper DS, Rivkees SA. Putting propylthiouracil in perspective. *J Clin Endocrinol Metab* 2009;94(6):1881–1882.
4. Ross DS, Burch HB, Cooper DS, et al. 2016 American Thyroid Association guidelines for diagnosis and management of hyperthyroidism and other causes of thyrotoxicosis. *Thyroid* 2016;26(10):1343–1421.
5. Ross DS. Radioiodine therapy for hyperthyroidism. *N Engl J Med* 2011;364(6):542–550.
6. Querat C, Germain N, Dumollard JM, et al. Surgical management of hyperthyroidism. *Eur Ann Otorhinolaryngol Head Neck Dis* 2015;132(2):63–66.
7. Osman F, Franklyn JA, Sheppard MC, Gammage MD. Successful treatment of amiodarone-induced thyrotoxicosis. *Circulation* 2002;105(11):1275–1277.
8. Santos Palacios S, Pascual-Corrales E, Galofre JC. Management of subclinical hyperthyroidism. *Int J Endocrinol Metab* 2012;10(2):490–496.
9. Nayuk B, Burman K. Thyrotoxicosis and thyroid storm. *Endocrinol Metab Clin North Am* 2006;35(4):663–686, vii.
10. Alexander EK, Pearce EN, Brent GA, et al. 2017 guidelines of the American Thyroid Association for the diagnosis and management of thyroid disease during pregnancy and the postpartum. *Thyroid* 2017;27(3):315–389.
11. Bahn RS. Graves' ophthalmopathy. *N Engl J Med* 2010;362(8):726–738.

Hypothyroidism

Sudhir Singh and William E. Clutter

GENERAL PRINCIPLES

Hypothyroidism is common, especially in women, with a prevalence of about 2% (compared with 0.1% for men). Prevalence of subclinical hypothyroidism is between 4% and 8.5% in those without known thyroid disease and it increases with age and in women.[1] Congenital hypothyroidism is one of the most common preventable causes of mental retardation.

Etiology

- **Primary hypothyroidism** (due to disease of the thyroid itself) accounts for more than 95% of cases (Table 9-1).
  - **Chronic lymphocytic thyroiditis (Hashimoto disease)** is by far the most common cause.
  - **Iatrogenic hypothyroidism** due to thyroidectomy or radioactive iodine (RAI, iodine-131) therapy is also common.
  - **Transient hypothyroidism** occurs in painless (or postpartum) thyroiditis and subacute thyroiditis, usually after a period of hyperthyroidism.
  - **Drugs that may cause hypothyroidism**[2] (usually in patients with underlying autoimmune thyroiditis) include iodine-containing drugs such as **amiodarone**, lithium, interferon-α and interferon-β, interleukin-2, checkpoint inhibitor immunotherapy (e.g., ipilimumab, pembrolizumab, and nivolumab)[3] thalidomide, bexarotene, and sunitinib.[4] Thionamide drugs used to treat hyperthyroidism can cause hypothyroidism.
  - **Infiltrative diseases like Riedel thyroiditis, hemochromatosis, scleroderma, leukemia, and amyloidosis can occasionally cause hypothyroidism.**
- **Secondary hypothyroidism** due to thyroid-stimulating hormone (TSH) deficiency is uncommon but may occur in any disorder of the pituitary or hypothalamus. It rarely occurs without other evidence of pituitary disease.
- Rare hemangiomas that express thyroid hormone deiodinase type 3 (which converts thyroxine [T_4] to inactive reverse triiodothyronine [rT_3]) may cause hypothyroidism, a syndrome called **consumptive hypothyroidism.**

Pathophysiology

- **Hashimoto thyroiditis** (chronic lymphocytic thyroiditis) is much more common in women, and increases in prevalence with age. Lymphocytic infiltration of the thyroid gradually destroys thyroid follicles and impairs thyroid hormone production, prompting a compensatory rise in TSH. Depending on the extent of follicular damage and lymphocytic infiltration, an **atrophic, impalpable thyroid** or a **firm, nontender diffuse goiter** can be found. Hashimoto disease is also the most common cause of euthyroid goiter in the United States. Hypothyroidism may be preceded by a period of **subclinical hypothyroidism**, with gradually rising TSH and declining L-thyroxine levels. Antithyroid antibodies (**antithyroid peroxidase [anti-TPO]** and **antithyroglobulin**) are generally present, and help to distinguish Hashimoto from other causes of hypothyroidism, but thyroid dysfunction is caused by cellular immunity. Patients with Hashimoto thyroiditis may have autoimmune disease of other endocrine glands (such as type 1 diabetes,

TABLE 9-1	CAUSES OF HYPOTHYROIDISM

Primary hypothyroidism
Chronic lymphocytic (Hashimoto) thyroiditis
Radioactive iodine treatment or external neck radiation
Thyroidectomy
Transient (during recovery from painless thyroiditis or subacute thyroiditis)
Drugs
Severe iodine deficiency (not seen in the United States)
Congenital hypothyroidism (thyroid dysgenesis or genetic defects in thyroid
  hormone synthesis)

Secondary (central) hypothyroidism
Any pituitary or hypothalamic disease

Other
Consumptive hypothyroidism due to vascular tumors expressing deiodinase

Addison disease, or systemic autoimmune disorders), and often have a family history of either Hashimoto or Graves disease.

- **Iatrogenic hypothyroidism** is a common complication after treatment with RAI therapy and after total thyroidectomy. Occasionally, patients develop hypothyroidism even after hemithyroidectomy.
- Most cases of **congenital hypothyroidism** are caused by dysplasia or aplasia of the thyroid, with little or no detectable thyroid tissue. Rarely, genetic defects of hormone synthetic enzymes or maternal treatment with antithyroid drugs or iodine causes congenital hypothyroidism with a goiter.

DIAGNOSIS

Clinical Presentation

- Hypothyroidism causes a variety of symptoms, many of which are nonspecific; please see Table 9-2. It usually develops gradually, and the onset of symptoms is insidious.

TABLE 9-2	SYMPTOMS AND SIGNS OF HYPOTHYROIDISM

Symptoms	Signs
Cold intolerance	Delayed tendon reflex relaxation
Lethargy, fatigue	Facial and periorbital puffiness
Weight gain (modest)	Bradycardia
Dry skin, hair loss	Poor memory, dementia
Constipation	Nonpitting edema (myxedema)
Myalgias, arthralgias	Pleural and pericardial effusions
Menorrhagia	Carpal tunnel syndrome
Hoarseness	Deafness
	Hypoventilation
	Hypothermia

- The most specific findings are **cold intolerance** (feeling cold when others are comfortable) and **delayed relaxation of tendon reflexes**. Other symptoms include mild weight gain (due to decreased metabolic rate), fatigue, somnolence, constipation, menorrhagia and impaired fertility, myalgias, and hoarseness. Other signs include bradycardia, facial and periorbital edema, dry skin, and nonpitting edema (myxedema). **Hypothyroidism does not cause marked obesity.**
- Rare manifestations include hypoventilation, hypothermia, pericardial or pleural effusions, deafness, and carpal tunnel syndrome.
- Laboratory findings may include **hyponatremia** and elevated plasma levels of cholesterol, low-density lipoprotein (LDL), triglycerides, and creatine kinase. Primary hypothyroidism may cause hyperprolactinemia. The ECG may show low voltage and T-wave abnormalities.

Diagnostic Testing

Hypothyroidism is common, readily treatable, and should be suspected in any patient with compatible symptoms, especially in the presence of a diffuse goiter or a history of RAI therapy or thyroid surgery.

- **In suspected primary hypothyroidism, plasma TSH is the best initial diagnostic test. A normal value excludes primary hypothyroidism, and a markedly elevated value (>20 μU/mL) confirms the diagnosis.**
- Mild elevation of plasma TSH (<20 μU/mL) may be caused by **nonthyroidal illness**, but usually indicates **mild (or subclinical) primary hypothyroidism.**
  ○ These patients may have nonspecific symptoms compatible with hypothyroidism and a mild increase in serum cholesterol and LDL cholesterol. They develop clinical hypothyroidism at a rate of about 2% to 5% per year.[1]
  ○ In patients with mildly elevated plasma TSH, the test should be repeated with measurement of plasma free T_4 to confirm the diagnosis.
- **If secondary hypothyroidism is suspected because of evidence of pituitary disease** (e.g., a known sella turcica or hypothalamic mass), **plasma free T_4 should be measured.** A low value is diagnostic of secondary hypothyroidism in this setting.
  ○ **Plasma TSH levels are usually within the reference range in secondary hypothyroidism and cannot be used alone to make this diagnosis.**
  ○ Patients with secondary hypothyroidism should be evaluated for other pituitary hormone deficits and the pituitary should be imaged with magnetic resonance imaging (MRI).

TREATMENT

- **Levothyroxine** is the drug of choice. The average replacement dose is 1.6 to 1.8 mcg/kg orally daily, and most patients require doses between 75 and 150 mcg daily. In elderly patients, the average replacement dose is lower. The need for lifelong treatment should be emphasized.
  ○ Levothyroxine should be taken 30 to 60 minutes before a meal. It should not be taken together with **medications that inhibit its absorption** including **calcium carbonate, proton pump inhibitors, iron supplements**, cholestyramine, sucralfate, or aluminum hydroxide.
  ○ **Other drug interactions that increase thyroxine clearance and dose requirement** include estrogen, rifampin, some anticonvulsants (carbamazepine, phenytoin, and phenobarbital), and some anticancer drugs (imatinib and bexarotene). **Amiodarone** blocks conversion of T_4 to triiodothyronine (T_3), and increases levothyroxine dose requirements.
- **Initiation of therapy.** Young, otherwise healthy adults should be started on 1.6 to 1.8 mcg/kg daily. Symptoms begin to improve within a few weeks. In otherwise healthy

elderly patients, the initial dose should be 50 mcg daily. Patients with **cardiac disease** should be started on 25 to 50 mcg daily and monitored carefully for exacerbation of cardiac symptoms.

- **Dose adjustment and follow-up:**
  - **In primary hypothyroidism, the goal of therapy is to maintain plasma TSH within the normal range.** Plasma TSH should be measured 6 to 8 weeks after initiation of therapy. The dose of levothyroxine should be adjusted in 12.5- to 25-mcg increments at intervals of 6 to 8 weeks until plasma TSH level is normal. Thereafter, if TSH is stable, annual TSH measurement is adequate to monitor therapy. TSH should be measured frequently in the following conditions:
    - **First trimester of pregnancy**, since the thyroxine dose requirement increases at this time (see Pregnancy section under Special Considerations):
      - If patient is started on a new medication interfering with absorption and metabolism of thyroid hormone
      - Weight changes
      - Diagnosis of new disease conditions like celiac disease and nephrotic syndrome[5]
  - **In secondary hypothyroidism, plasma TSH cannot be used to adjust therapy.** The goal of therapy is to maintain plasma free T4 near the middle of the reference range. The dose of levothyroxine should be adjusted at 6 to 8 week intervals until this goal is achieved. Thereafter, annual measurement of plasma free T4 is adequate to monitor therapy.
  - **Side effects:** Overtreatment produces iatrogenic hyperthyroidism, indicated by a subnormal TSH level, and should be avoided since it increases the risk of osteoporosis and atrial fibrillation.
    - Coronary artery disease may be exacerbated by treatment of hypothyroidism. The dose of levothyroxine should be increased slowly, with careful attention to worsening angina, heart failure, or arrhythmias.
    - Concomitant adrenal failure should be treated before levothyroxine treatment is started.

SPECIAL CONSIDERATIONS

- **Mild (or subclinical) hypothyroidism**
  - Patients with mild hypothyroidism should be treated with levothyroxine in following situations[6]:
    - pregnancy, or
    - the plasma TSH is >10 μU/mL
  - There is no consensus guideline for treatment of mild (or subclinical) hypothyroidism in patients with TSH level between 4.5 and 10 μU/mL. Treatment can be considered in following conditions[7]:
    - If patients have symptoms compatible with hypothyroidism
    - Presence of a goiter
    - Hypercholesterolemia that warrants treatment
  - Untreated patients should be monitored annually, and levothyroxine should be started if symptoms develop or serum TSH increases to >10 μU/mL.
- **Pregnancy**[8]
  - **Thyroxine dose requirement increases by an average of 50% in the first half of pregnancy** due to accelerated conversion of T_4 to reverse T_3 by placental deiodinase type 3.
  - In women with primary hypothyroidism, **plasma TSH level should be measured as soon as pregnancy is confirmed and monthly thereafter through** midgestation and at least once near 30 weeks of gestation. The levothyroxine dose should be increased by 20% to 30% to maintain plasma TSH level within the lower half of the trimester-specific

range when available. If it is not available, it is reasonable to target TSH level <2.5 mU/L. An alternative approach is to instruct patients to increase their levothyroxine dose by one to two pills per week as soon as pregnancy is confirmed, and to monitor and adjust the dose as above.

- ○ For pregnant patients with subclinical hypothyroidism with TSH concentration >2.5 mU/L, TPO antibody should be checked. If found to be positive, treatment with levothyroxine should be considered.
- ○ After delivery, the prepregnancy dose should be resumed.
- **Problems with treatment:** Treatment of most cases of hypothyroidism is straightforward. Occasionally, it is difficult to achieve a levothyroxine dose that normalizes TSH level, or a dose that was adequate no longer maintains a normal TSH level. Common explanations include:
  - ○ **Poor or erratic medication compliance.** Directly observed therapy at weekly intervals may be necessary in some cases.
  - ○ **Drug interactions** (see Treatment section in this chapter).
  - ○ **Pregnancy**, in which the dose requirement increases in the first trimester.
  - ○ **Gradual failure of remaining thyroid function** after RAI treatment of hyperthyroidism.
  - ○ **Significant weight changes.**
- **Diagnosis of hypothyroidism in severely ill patients: In severe nonthyroidal illness**, the diagnosis of hypothyroidism may be difficult.[9] Plasma free T_4 measured by routine assays may be low.
  - ○ **Plasma TSH is the best initial diagnostic test. A normal TSH value is strong evidence that the patient is euthyroid**, except when there is evidence of pituitary or hypothalamic disease or in patients treated with **dopamine** or high doses of **glucocorticoids**.
  - ○ **Marked elevation of plasma TSH (>20 μU/mL) establishes the diagnosis of primary hypothyroidism.**
  - ○ **Moderate elevations of plasma TSH (<20 μU/mL) may occur in euthyroid patients with nonthyroidal illness and are not specific for hypothyroidism.** Plasma free T_4 should be measured if TSH is moderately elevated, or if secondary hypothyroidism is suspected, and patients should be treated for hypothyroidism if plasma free T_4 is low. Thyroid function in these patients should be reevaluated after recovery from illness.
- **Emergent therapy for hypothyroidism is rarely necessary:** Most patients with hypothyroidism and concomitant illness can be treated in the usual manner. However, hypothyroidism may impair survival in critical illness by contributing to **hypoventilation, hypotension, hypothermia, bradycardia, or hyponatremia**. Little evidence supports the contention that severe hypothyroidism alone causes coma or shock; most reports of **myxedema coma** predate recognition that nonthyroidal illness itself lowers thyroid hormone levels.
  - ○ Hypoventilation and hypotension should be treated intensively, along with any concomitant diseases. Confirmatory tests (plasma TSH and free T_4) should be obtained before thyroid hormone therapy is started.
  - ○ **Levothyroxine, 50 to 100 mcg IV, can be given q6 to 8h for 24 hours**, followed by 75 to 100 mcg IV daily until oral intake is possible. Replacement therapy should be continued in the usual manner if the diagnosis of hypothyroidism is confirmed. This method rapidly alleviates thyroxine deficiency while minimizing the risk of exacerbating underlying coronary disease or heart failure.
  - ○ **Such rapid correction is warranted only in extremely ill patients. Vital signs and cardiac rhythm should be monitored carefully to detect early signs of exacerbation of heart disease.**
  - ○ **Hydrocortisone**, 50 mg IV q8h, is usually recommended during rapid replacement of thyroid hormone, because such therapy may precipitate adrenal crisis in patients with adrenal failure.

THYROIDITIS

There are several types of thyroiditis that may cause hyperthyroidism, hypothyroidism, or a euthyroid goiter.[10]

- **Autoimmune or Hashimoto thyroiditis (refer to pathophysiology section)**
- **Painless thyroiditis** (also known as postpartum or silent thyroiditis) is an autoimmune disorder that is most common in the first 6 months of the postpartum period.
  - It is characterized by a small, nontender diffuse goiter, and transient hyperthyroidism followed by hypothyroidism.
  - Hypothyroidism is usually transient, but may be permanent.
  - Hyperthyroidism results from follicular damage and release of stored hormone by a lymphocytic infiltrate. Consequently, **radioactive iodine uptake (RAIU) is very low**. Anti-TPO antibodies may be present.
  - The diagnosis should be suspected in women with symptoms of hyper- or hypothyroidism within 6 months of delivery. Plasma TSH and free T_4 should be measured to confirm the functional state. The hyperthyroid phase can be distinguished from Graves disease by measurement of RAIU (if the patient is not nursing), and repeating thyroid function tests after several weeks to assess for spontaneous improvement.
  - Symptoms of hyperthyroidism should be treated with a β-**adrenergic antagonist**. Thionamides are not useful, since thyroid hormone synthesis is already suppressed.
- Symptomatic hypothyroidism is treated with replacement therapy with levothyroxine for 2 to 3 months followed by discontinuation for 4 to 6 weeks and measurement of plasma TSH level.
- **Subacute thyroiditis** is characterized by a painful, tender goiter and transient hyperthyroidism resulting from release of stored thyroid hormone, followed by transient hypothyroidism. It is the most common cause of thyroid pain. It frequently occurs after an upper respiratory tract infection and is thought to have a viral etiology.
  - Symptoms of hyperthyroidism occur in 50% of patients and can be treated with a β-adrenergic antagonist.
  - Pain should be treated with nonsteroidal anti-inflammatory drugs (NSAIDs); corticosteroid treatment may be needed in severe cases.
  - Thionamides or RAI is not useful.
  - Transient hypothyroidism may be treated with levothyroxine for 3 to 6 months.
- **Riedel thyroiditis** is a very rare fibrosing thyroiditis that may be part of a systemic fibrosing process. Patients present with a painless, hard, fixed goiter. Patients are initially euthyroid, but hypothyroidism eventually develops. Treatment is primarily surgical, although therapy with glucocorticoids and methotrexate may be tried early in the course of the disease.
- **Immunoglobulin G4–related thyroid disease (IgG4-RTD):** IgG4-related disease affects many organ systems, including endocrine organs, particularly thyroid. Four subcategories of IgG4-RTD have been identified—Riedel thyroiditis, fibrosing variant of Hashimoto thyroiditis, IgG4-related Hashimoto thyroiditis, and Graves disease with elevated IgG4 levels. Genetic factors, antigen–antibody reactions, and allergic phenomenon have been suspected to cause the disease although the exact etiology is not known. IgG4-RTD is diagnosed based on clinical features, serologic evidence, and histologic features. Management comprises medical and surgical options. Steroids are the first-line treatment. Tamoxifen and rituximab can be considered in steroid-resistant cases. Surgical treatment is usually reserved for Riedel thyroiditis variant to relieve obstruction.[11]

REFERENCES

1. Surks MI, Ortiz E, Daniels GH, et al. Subclinical thyroid disease: Scientific review and guidelines for diagnosis and management. *JAMA* 2004;291(2):228–238.

2. Barbesino G. Drugs affecting thyroid function. 2010. http://www.liebertpub.com/thy. doi:10.1089/thy.2010.1635
3. Corsello SM, Barnabei A, Marchetti P, De Vecchis L, Salvatori R, Torino F. Endocrine side effects induced by immune checkpoint inhibitors. *J Clin Endocrinol Metab* 2013;98(4):1361–1375.
4. Mannavola D, Coco P, Vannucchi G, et al. A novel tyrosine-kinase selective inhibitor, sunitinib, induces transient hypothyroidism by blocking iodine uptake. *J Clin Endocrinol Metab* 2007;92(9):3531–3534.
5. Roberts CG, Ladenson PW. Hypothyroidism. *Lancet* 2004;363(9411):793–803.
6. Garber JR, Cobin RH, Gharib H, et al. Clinical practice guidelines for hypothyroidism in adults: cosponsored by the American Association of Clinical Endocrinologists and the American Thyroid Association. *Thyroid* 2012;22(12):1200–1235.
7. Gharib H, Tuttle RM, Baskin HJ, Fish LH, Singer PA, McDermott MT. Subclinical thyroid dysfunction: A joint statement on management from the American Association of Clinical Endocrinologists, the American Thyroid Association, and the Endocrine Society. *J Clin Endocrinol Metab* 2005;90(1):581–585; discussion 586–587.
8. Alexander EK, Pearce EN, Brent GA, et al. 2017 guidelines of the American Thyroid Association for the diagnosis and management of thyroid disease during pregnancy and the postpartum. *Thyroid* 2017;27(3):315–389.
9. Adler SM, Wartofsky L. The nonthyroidal illness syndrome. *Endocrinol Metab Clin North Am* 2007;36(3):657–672.
10. Pearce EN, Farwell AP, Braverman LE. Thyroiditis. *N Engl J Med* 2003;348(26):2646–2655.
11. Kottahachchi D, Topliss DJ. Immunoglobulin G4-related thyroid diseases. *Eur Thyroid J* 2016;5(4):231–239.

Thyroid Cancer

Kevin T. Bauerle and Amy E. Riek

GENERAL PRINCIPLES

Approximately 95% of thyroid malignancies are differentiated thyroid carcinomas (DTCs) arising from follicular cells (**papillary or follicular carcinomas**). These cancers retain many properties of normal thyroid cells: they **take up iodine** and **synthesize thyroglobulin (Tg)**, although less efficiently than normal thyroid tissue. **Their growth and function are stimulated by thyroid-stimulating hormone (TSH).** These three properties are used in treatment and follow-up of thyroid carcinoma.[1-3] This chapter will discuss the classification, management, and follow-up of DTC. A brief discussion regarding the much less common anaplastic and medullary thyroid cancers will follow (see Special Considerations).

Classification

- **Papillary thyroid carcinoma (PTC)** (84%) is the most common type of DTC. PTC is a slow-growing tumor that may remain localized for years. It characteristically metastasizes first to cervical lymph nodes. Microscopic foci of papillary carcinoma are common at autopsy and thought to be present in as many as 30% of adults.
- **Follicular thyroid carcinoma (FTC) (and the Hürthle cell subset)** (12%) can be more aggressive, and may metastasize early to lung and bone. Many thyroid cancers have mixed papillary and follicular morphology; these behave like papillary carcinoma.[1-3]
- **Poorly differentiated thyroid carcinoma (PDTC)** (<3%) is significantly more aggressive with higher metastatic rate than well-differentiated disease and characterized pathologically by particular architecture and high-grade features (convoluted nuclei, high mitotic activity, and/or tumor necrosis). These lesions are less likely to secrete Tg and concentrate radioactive iodine (RAI). Clinically, PDTC falls on the spectrum between PTC and anaplastic thyroid cancer and warrants more aggressive initial interventions and follow-up.[3-5]

Epidemiology

- Thyroid cancer represents **3.4% of all new cases of cancer**, but only 0.3% of cancer deaths in the United States. Lifetime risk is 1.2%.
- **Incidence has tripled** over the past 40 years, but much of this is due to detection bias as imaging has become more widespread.
- Women are about three times more likely to get thyroid cancer, and the median age at diagnosis is 51.
- Overall **prognosis is excellent**, with 98.2% of patients surviving 5 years.[1-3]

Risk Factors

- Female gender
- Age (peak 40s to 50s for women, 60s to 70s for men)
- Family history of thyroid cancer
- Low-iodine diet

- Radiation exposure including medical treatments (particularly in childhood and/or with head/neck treatment) and radiation fallout from power plant accidents or nuclear weapons.
- Familial adenomatous polyposis, Cowden disease, and Carney complex, type 1 increase the risk of DTC. Isolated PTC can also run in families, though the genetic patterns are not well defined.[1-3]

DIAGNOSIS

Clinical Presentation

Differentiated thyroid cancer usually presents as an **asymptomatic single nodule**. It is not painful or tender, and does not cause hyper- or hypothyroidism. Clinical findings that increase the probability of malignancy in a nodule are listed in Chapter 7 Nodular Thyroid Disease and Goiter.

Diagnostic Testing

The diagnostic procedure of choice is fine-needle aspiration (FNA) biopsy with cytologic assessment. Ultrasound (US) guidance is often used to guide the biopsy.[3] See Chapter 7 Nodular Thyroid Disease and Goiter for ultrasound criteria guiding the choice for FNA and for cytologic criteria and molecular diagnostics guiding the choice for surgical resection.

TREATMENT

Surgical Management

- **Preoperative ultrasound** should be performed in all patients with malignant or suspicious for malignant FNA results as this identifies 20% to 31% of involved lymph nodes (present in 20% to 25% of patients). FNA of lymph nodes should be performed if lymph node involvement is unclear. CT can be considered if US reveals bulky or extensive nodal disease.
- **Initial surgical planning**
  ○ **Total or near-total thyroidectomy** should be performed if the tumor is >4 cm or if there is gross extrathyroidal extension, lymph node involvement, or distant metastases.
  ○ **Thyroid lobectomy or total/near-total thyroidectomy** can be considered if the tumor is 1 to 4 cm and if there is no extrathyroidal extension, lymph node, or distant metastases. Risk factors (age, contralateral nodules, radiation history, family history, etc.) and patient preference should be taken into account.
  ○ **Thyroid lobectomy** is indicated as the surgical approach if the tumor is <1 cm with no extrathyroidal extension, lymph node, or distant metastases.[3] However, recent data suggest that **continued active surveillance is a reasonable option in low-risk patients with papillary microcarcinoma** (defined as <1 cm with no high-grade features on cytology, extrathyroidal extension, or evidence of lymph node or distant metastases). In this patient population, a Japanese study of over 2,000 patients who self-selected active surveillance versus immediate surgery demonstrated no difference in oncologic outcome over a median 47 months of follow-up, with no subjects developing distant metastases or dying of thyroid cancer. However, those in the immediate surgery group had a higher rate of unfavorable outcomes related to surgical complications, prompting consideration of active surveillance in this subset.[6]
  ○ **Lymph node dissection**
    ▪ **No lymph node dissection** is indicated if the tumor is <4 cm, noninvasive, clinically node negative, and in most follicular cancers.

- **Central compartment dissection** should be performed if there are clinically involved central nodes.
- **Prophylactic central compartment dissection** can be considered if the tumor is >4 cm, lateral nodes are clinically involved, or if pathology results will be used to plan further treatment.
- **Lateral compartment dissection** should be performed if biopsy-proven lateral node metastases are present.
- **Completion thyroidectomy** should be offered to those lobectomy patients for whom total thyroidectomy would have been recommended if final pathology had been known at the time of initial surgery. Central compartment dissection should be included if lymph nodes are clinically involved. Of note, completion may be unnecessary for lower-risk lesions.
- The following information from the **surgical pathology report** should be noted in order to risk stratify for further treatment decision making:
  - Tumor size
  - Resection margins
  - Capsular invasion
  - Vascular invasion with number of involved vessels
  - Number of lymph nodes examined and involved
  - Size of largest metastatic focus to lymph nodes
  - Presence of extranodal extension of metastases
  - Pathologic variants with unfavorable prognosis (tall cell, columnar cell, hobnail PTC, insular, widely invasive FTC)
  - Pathologic variants with favorable prognosis (noninvasive follicular variant of papillary, minimally invasive FTC)
- Further treatment is determined primarily by the **risk of recurrence** of the cancer based on imaging and pathology results. While TNM staging by the Union for International Cancer Control (UICC) and the American Joint Committee on Cancer (AJCC) based on age, tumor size, histology, and extrathyroidal spread is established for DTC, this staging system explains only 5% to 30% of the mortality related to thyroid cancer. Thus, **we favor using the risk stratification from the 2015 American Thyroid Association guidelines**, which incorporates additional features (e.g., more specific histologic features, molecular profile, extent of vascular invasion, size of metastases). This system divides patients into three categories of recurrence risk: low, intermediate, and high (Table 10-1) and has stronger correlation with outcomes. Across multiple validation studies, the likelihood of patients having no evidence of disease after total thyroidectomy and RAI remnant ablation for these risk groups is 78% to 91%, 52% to 64%, and 31% to 32%, respectively.[3] **Of note, a distinction has recently been made for the particularly low-risk pathologic result of noninvasive follicular thyroid neoplasm with papillary-like nuclear features (NIFTP), which should be reported to patients as benign.** This pathologic classification can be used for a lesion of any size, but requires complete encapsulation (fully examined by pathology) of a follicular variant PTC, and while it should be resected with lobectomy, does not require completion thyroidectomy or RAI.[7]

Other Nonpharmacologic Therapies

- Following total or near-total thyroidectomy, replacement thyroid hormone is typically withheld pending the pathology results, as potential further treatment with RAI requires an elevated level TSH to optimize iodine uptake and the effectiveness of treatment.
- While the decision for use of subsequent RAI therapy following surgical therapy is largely based on the risk of recurrence (discussed below), postoperative disease status should also be considered.

TABLE 10-1	AMERICAN THYROID ASSOCIATION RISK OF RECURRENCE CLASSIFICATIONS[3]		
	Low risk (must have all)	Intermediate risk (any)	High risk (any)
Local or distant metastases	None or ≤5 cervical nodal micrometastases <2 mm in largest dimension (if PTC)	>5 cervical nodal metastases with all <3 cm in largest dimension	Any nodal metastases ≥3 cm or distant metastases
Local invasion	None (if PTC); none or capsular only (if FTC)	Microscopic invasion into perithyroidal soft tissues	Macroscopic invasion of tumor into perithyroidal soft tissues
Vascular invasion	None (if PTC); <4 foci (if FTC)	Present (if PTC)	>4 foci (if FTC)
Surgical resection	Grossly complete	N/A	Grossly incomplete
Histologic variant	Nonaggressive	Aggressive (e.g., tall cell, hobnail, columnar cell)	N/A
Post-RAI treatment WBS result	No metastatic foci outside the thyroid bed	Metastatic foci in the neck	N/A
Postoperative Tg level	<10 ng/mL	<10 ng/mL	Suggestive of distant metastases (≥10 ng/mL)

FTC, follicular thyroid carcinoma; PTC, papillary thyroid carcinoma; RAI, radioactive iodine; Tg, thyroglobulin; WBS, whole body scan.

- Assessment of postoperative disease status is primarily based on biochemical assessment of disease. **Tg** is a protein produced by normal thyroid follicular cells at levels detectable in the serum, and most DTC retains this capability, making it a useful tumor marker following thyroidectomy. It is stimulated by TSH, either endogenous or recombinant, so is expected to be 5- to 10-fold higher with TSH stimulation.
- **Serum Tg should be measured at least 3 to 4 weeks postoperatively** when it reaches its nadir, but may still be detectable in patients with remnant thyroid tissue, either benign or malignant. The postoperative level is primarily useful in establishing a baseline level following surgical management and providing guidance for patients in whom RAI is being considered. The risk of recurrent or persistent disease is directly correlated with postoperative Tg level. Therefore, Tg levels should be considered in the context of risk stratification when guiding decision making for RAI. In general, a Tg of >10 ng/mL (stimulated or nonstimulated) is suggestive of persistent or recurrent disease and increases the likelihood of failing initial RAI treatment, having distant metastases, and dying of thyroid cancer. For this reason, additional therapies may be considered in an ATA low- or intermediate-risk individual with a postoperative Tg of 5 to 10 ng/mL. Conversely, a TSH-stimulated Tg of <1 to 2 ng/mL is a strong predictor of remission.

- Several factors can affect Tg results. Many laboratories utilize immunometric assays, which should be calibrated to the international standard, but wide variation still exists. Therefore, **serial Tg levels should be monitored over time with the same laboratory assay.** Immunoassays are also prone to interference with **anti-Tg antibodies**, which can cause falsely lower Tg levels. All Tg immunoassays are typically accompanied by an antibody level, and if antibodies are present, the Tg levels should not be utilized for treatment decisions. Alternatively, some laboratories are moving to newer **liquid chromatography–tandem mass spectrometry (LC-MS/MS) assays that are not subject to Tg antibody interference**, though they have a higher limit of quantification (usually 0.5 ng/mL).[3,8]

- **Radioiodine** is a uniquely targeted thyroid cancer treatment as the thyroid is one of few tissues in the body that takes up iodine. It is generally administered in remnant ablative doses (usually 30 mCi) to facilitate detection of recurrent disease or in therapeutic doses (usually 100 to 150 mCi) to improve disease-free survival by destroying persistent disease. While RAI is relatively safe, cumulative doses exceeding 500 to 600 mCi result in a significant increase in the risk of secondary malignancies and should be avoided. RAI should also be avoided in women who are pregnant, and pregnancy should be avoided for up to a year after RAI administration. Men receiving cumulative RAI doses >400 mCi should be warned of potential risk of infertility with high doses of RAI. **Levothyroxine should be withdrawn for 3 to 4 weeks prior to RAI therapy, with verification of TSH >30 mIU/L prior to treatment.** Recombinant human thyrotropin (rhTSH) stimulation is an alternative option for those with low-risk disease or those with intermediate-risk disease without substantial lymph node involvement prior to remnant ablation. Patients should also follow a low-iodine diet for 1 to 2 weeks prior to treatment as this increases the likelihood of remnant ablation success. For decision making regarding RAI, factors affecting recurrence risk, disease follow-up implications, and patient preference should be considered, but general guidelines are as follows:
  - **Low-risk patients** after thyroidectomy or lobectomy only: **RAI is not recommended**, but if used, ablative dose is recommended.
  - **Intermediate-risk patients** after total thyroidectomy: **RAI should be considered** at ablative dose for lower-risk features and therapeutic dose for higher-risk features.
  - **High-risk patients** after total thyroidectomy: **RAI is recommended** at therapeutic dose.

- **A post–RAI-therapy whole body scan (WBS) should be performed 3 to 7 days after treatment** to confirm the presence of RAI-avid structural disease. Of note, it is not unexpected for the posttreatment WBS to show uptake in the thyroid bed as complete thyroidectomy is technically difficult and unnecessary, particularly if RAI is administered.

- Initial management of **RAI-avid metastatic disease:**
  - **Aerodigestive disease and locoregional involvement:** This is best managed by surgical excision. RAI may be used as an adjunctive therapy.
  - **Pulmonary micrometastasis** (<2 mm in size): RAI is provided in doses of 100 to 200 mCi every 6 to 12 months as long as clinical response is noted and disease concentrates RAI. Pulmonary macronodular metastases may be treated with surgical resection (in the case of a single nodule) or RAI, though this is rarely curative.
  - **Bone metastases:** These may be treated with RAI at a dose of 100 to 200 mCi, but this is rarely curative. External beam radiation, surgery, and antiresorptive agents should be considered (see below).
  - **Brain metastases:** These are primarily treated with surgery and stereotactic radiation. RAI may be considered but prior treatment with radiation and glucocorticoids should be considered to negate the effects of RAI-induced inflammation or TSH-driven increase in tumor size.

○ Systemic kinase inhibitor therapy is often reserved for individuals with widespread, progressive disease that is RAI refractory.[3]

• Management of **RAI-refractory metastatic disease:**

○ **RAI-refractory metastatic disease may fail to concentrate RAI at the time of diagnosis or may lose the ability to concentrate RAI over time.** It is also important to recognize that some lesions may concentrate RAI while others may not and that RAI-refractory disease may also be defined as those lesions that concentrate RAI but progress over time despite RAI therapy. No further RAI treatment is warranted in these patients.

○ Patients with stable, asymptomatic, and minimally progressive disease can be followed with serial imaging every 3 to 12 months and continued TSH suppression (see below).

○ Prior to consideration of systemic treatments, metastatic lesions to the brain, lung, liver, or bone that are producing symptoms or at high risk of local complications may be treated with surgery, stereotactic radiation, or thermal ablation.

○ Systemic therapies with kinase inhibitors should be considered in those with diffuse disease progression not amenable to local therapy, symptomatic disease such as wide-spread adenopathy or dyspnea, or imminently threatening disease expected to require intervention or result in morbidity/mortality in <6 months. A brief discussion of these agents is found below.[3,9,10]

Medications

• All patients who have undergone total thyroidectomy and some who have undergone lobectomy will require thyroid hormone replacement, typically with levothyroxine. For those at higher risk of recurrence, **levothyroxine at a dose that suppresses plasma TSH to below the normal range is used.** Recommended target TSH ranges by risk groups are as follows:

○ High-risk patients: <0.1 mU/L

○ Intermediate-risk patients: 0.1 to 0.5 mU/L

○ Low-risk patients: 0.5 to 2.0 mU/L for those managed with lobectomy or with thyroidectomy. In the latter group, Tg should be undetectable. If Tg is measurable after thyroidectomy (with or without remnant ablation), moderate TSH suppression (0.1 to 0.5 mU/L) should be considered.

• **The kinase inhibitors sorafenib and lenvatinib have been approved for use in RAI-refractory DTC.** These agents are associated with a number of side effects including hepatotoxicity, hypertension, cardiotoxicity, QTc prolongation, as well as increases in TSH levels requiring titration of thyroxine therapy to maintain TSH levels at goal. In the case of patients who progress through first-line kinase inhibitors, therapeutic clinical trials, second-line kinase inhibitors, or cytotoxic chemotherapy may also be considered.

• **Bone-directed antiresorptive agents such as denosumab and zoledronic acid should be considered in patients with diffuse RAI-refractory bone metastases,** as these have been shown to delay skeletal adverse events in patients with other tumor types. It is also well recognized that bone metastases tend to respond poorly to RAI and kinase therapy. In the case of localized bone disease or only a few lesions, surgery, thermoablation, or radiation continue to be the preferred therapy.[3,9,10]

MONITORING/FOLLOW-UP

• **Serum Tg and anti-Tg antibodies should be monitored every 6 to 12 months after initial therapy** and possibly more frequently in high-risk patients. If structural disease is absent and unstimulated serum Tg is <0.2 ng/mL, Tg measurements can be lengthened to every 1 to 2 years in low- to intermediate-risk patients. In individuals not treated with remnant ablation or total thyroidectomy, optimal cutoffs have not been established. Nevertheless, a rising Tg over time may be suspicious for growing cancer.

- **Neck ultrasound should be obtained 6 to 12 months after initial therapy to evaluate thyroid bed and cervical nodes.** Follow-up ultrasounds should be based on the risk of recurrent disease and Tg status. Suspicious lymph nodes >8 to 10 mm may be biopsied for cytology with Tg measurement in needle washout. Smaller nodes may be followed over time.
- **Diagnostic WBS with I-123 or low-activity I-131 should be performed 6 to 12 months after adjuvant RAI treatment in high- or intermediate-risk patients with higher-risk features.** Diagnostic WBS is not required for low- or intermediate-risk patients with lower-risk features if neck ultrasound shows no structural disease and serum Tg is undetectable.
- **Fluorodeoxyglucose-positron emission tomography (FDG-PET) scan should be obtained in patients with elevated Tg and negative WBS and in the patients diagnosed with poorly differentiated thyroid cancers** because they may trap RAI ineffectively or have an impaired ability to make or secrete Tg.
- **TSH suppression goals should be modified over time based on structural/functional (ultrasound or RAI imaging) and biochemical (Tg) evidence of disease** as well as long-term risk of hyperthyroidism, including exacerbation of cardiovascular disease in elderly men and loss of bone mass in postmenopausal women.
  - If structural disease persists by neck ultrasound or RAI imaging, TSH should be targeted to <0.1 mU/L.
  - If there is evidence of disease biochemically (Tg >1 to 2 ng/mL), moderate suppression of TSH (0.1 to 0.5 mU/L) should be considered, taking into account the original ATA risk classification as well as Tg level and trend.
  - In low- to intermediate-risk patients without structural or biochemical evidence of disease, TSH may be targeted to the lower half of normal range.
  - In high-risk patients without structural or biochemical evidence of disease, TSH suppression to 0.1 to 0.5 mU/L should be maintained for up to 5 years.
- **Management of recurrence**
  - Compartmental neck dissection is preferred in those patients with biopsy-proven LN recurrence or persistent disease with involved nodes measuring >8 to 10 mm in the shortest diameter.
  - RAI therapy may be provided to individuals where LNs are identified on diagnostic WBS. It may be used as an alternative therapy in those with minimal disease burden, when disease is not amenable to surgical intervention, or as an adjunctive therapy in combination with surgery.
  - Ethanol ablation may be considered in individuals who are poor surgical candidates and have smaller nodes.[3]

OUTCOME/PROGNOSIS

- **PTC** has an excellent prognosis with a 10-year survival that exceeds 95%. Recurrence rates vary significantly based on initial ATA risk stratification.
- **FTC** has a widely variable prognosis, depending upon the size of the tumor, the age of the patient, and the extent of angioinvasion, which predicts risk of metastatic disease. Specifically, FTC with only capsular invasion or no capsular invasion but only minor vascular invasion has a recurrence rate <7%, while FTC with greater vascular invasion increases the risk of distant metastases to 30% to 55%.
- **PDTC** has an intermediate prognosis between DTC and anaplastic thyroid carcinoma (ATC) and is associated with 72% 5-year survival and 46% 10-year survival. Tumors tend not to be less responsive to radioiodine, and systemic treatments are commonly necessary.[1–5]

SPECIAL CONSIDERATIONS

- **Anaplastic thyroid cancer**
  - **ATC** (1% of thyroid cancers) is a rare, rapidly progressive thyroid cancer with a dismal prognosis (median survival of ~6 months). Tumors tend to have a limited response to radioiodine, as well as traditional chemotherapy and radiotherapy.
  - ATC is **significantly more aggressive** at the time of diagnosis:
    - About 40% of patients present with extrathyroidal extension of disease and/or lymph node (LN) metastases.
    - About 50% of patients present with widely metastatic disease.
  - **Core or open biopsy**, rather than FNA, is often required for diagnosis. Since ATC often arises in the patients with a prior history of PTC or coexisting PTC, it may be distinguished from poorly differentiated DTC based on the absence of Tg and thyroid transcription factor (TTF) 1 staining. Approximately 40% to 50% of patients have a history of DTC or coexistent DTC noted on pathology.
  - **Preoperative imaging** to be obtained following diagnosis should be aimed at identifying metastatic disease and determining the extent of disease burden in the neck, including:
    - Neck ultrasound
    - Neck and chest CT
    - FDG-PET/CT
    - Mirror or fiberoptic evaluation of vocal cords
    - MRI brain
  - **If grossly negative margins can be achieved**, **surgical resection** should be attempted. In patients with intrathyroidal disease +/− lymph nodes, lobectomy or near-total thyroidectomy and lymph node dissection should be performed. If there is extrathyroidal extension, an en bloc resection should be performed.
  - **In those with good functional status and unresectable disease or gross remnant disease present following resection, radiation therapy with or without concurrent chemotherapy should be considered. Surgical resection should then be reconsidered** if response to therapy improves the likelihood of successful surgical resection of locoregional disease.
  - **Tracheostomy** may be required to prevent asphyxia related to disease burden, and **gastrostomy** may be required for nutritional support.
  - Definitive radiation therapy with or without concurrent chemotherapy should be offered to patients with good functional status following surgical resection. **Acceptable chemotherapy regimens include** some combination of taxane, anthracycline, and/ or platinum.
  - In patients who present with widely metastatic disease, palliation of symptoms should be prioritized. Radiation therapy or surgery may be necessary if focal disease is imminently threatening. Otherwise, if an aggressive course is preferred, systemic therapy can be attempted. Radiation may be particularly useful for relief of bone pain in those with bone metastases.
  - **Palliative radiation therapy** should be offered to those with local symptoms, poor functional status, and unresectable disease.
  - Levothyroxine replacement should be titrated to maintain clinical and biochemical euthyroidism, unless for the treatment of coexistent DTC.
  - During active therapy, patients should be monitored closely for malnutrition, impaired enteral feeding, airway compromise, and neutropenia.
  - Frequent serial imaging should be obtained in patients who demonstrate a response to initial therapy.
  - RAI scanning and therapy are not advised for ATC unless the patient survives 1 to 2 years and has coexistent DTC.[11,12]

- Medullary thyroid cancer
  - **Medullary carcinoma of the thyroid (MTC)** (4% of thyroid cancers) arises from neuroendocrine C cells (parafollicular cells). Approximately 75% of medullary carcinoma are sporadic. MTC is a component of multiple endocrine neoplasia **(MEN) 2A and 2B**. Of note, **familial MTC syndrome**, characterized by MTC without hyperparathyroidism or pheochromocytoma, is now considered a variant of MEN 2A. These syndromes are caused by mutations of different regions of the *RET* proto-oncogene and are discussed further in Chapter 37 Multiple Endocrine Neoplasia Syndromes. The remainder of this discussion will focus on sporadic MTC.
  - The 10-year survival rate of those with MTC ranges from 75% to 85%.
  - Diagnosis is often achieved on **cytology of FNA (50% to 80% sensitivity)** or on surgical pathology following lobectomy for indeterminate cytology. Measurement of serum calcitonin is not recommended given the high prevalence of falsely elevated serum calcitonin levels.
  - Approximately 75% of patients present with lymph node involvement, while 5% to 10% demonstrate distant metastases.
  - Following diagnosis, **calcitonin and carcinoembryonic antigen (CEA) levels should be measured** and *RET* germline mutational analysis be performed.
  - If *RET* mutational analysis is positive or unknown, **screening for coexistent MEN2A and MEN2B conditions should be performed**. This should include serum calcium to detect primary hyperparathyroidism and plasma fractionated metanephrines to screen for pheochromocytoma.
  - If serum calcitonin exceeds 500 pg/mL, body imaging should be pursued prior to surgical management to evaluate for the presence of metastatic disease. **Total thyroidectomy with cervical lymph node dissection** is the mainstay of treatment. Following surgical resection, external beam radiation therapy should be considered for individuals with residual tumor, extrathyroidal extension, or bulky nodal disease. Those with progressive metastatic disease should be considered for enrollment in clinical trial or tyrosine kinase inhibitor therapy.
  - Serum calcitonin should be measured 3 months after surgery. If undetectable or normal, serial neck ultrasounds and calcitonin measurements can be obtained every 6 to 12 months.
  - If calcitonin is <150 pg/mL and there is no evidence of structural disease on imaging or examination, the frequency of neck imaging and biochemical assessment should be increased. If structural disease recurrence is confirmed, repeat neck dissection should be considered.
  - If calcitonin is >150 pg/mL, distant metastases are more likely, and neck and body imaging should be performed.
  - Treatment of recurrent disease may include observation, surgical resection, radiation therapy, systemic therapy, or other localized therapies.[13,14]

REFERENCES

1. Fagin JA, Wells SA. Biologic and clinical perspectives on thyroid cancer. *N Engl J Med* 2016; 375(11):1054–1067.
2. Jemal A, Ward EM, Johnson CJ, et al. Annual report to the nation on the status of cancer, 1975–2014, Featuring Survival. *JNCI J Natl Cancer Inst* 2017;109(9):1–22.
3. Haugen BR, Alexander EA, Bible KC, et al. 2015 American Thyroid Association management guidelines for adult patients with thyroid nodules and differentiated thyroid cancer. *Thyroid* 2016;26:1–33.
4. Burman KD. Is poorly differentiated thyroid cancer poorly characterized? *J Clin Endocrinol Metab* 2014;99(4):1167–1169.
5. Roman S, Sosa JA. Aggressive variants of papillary thyroid cancer. *Curr Opin Oncol* 2013;25(1): 33–38.

6. Oda H, Miyauchi A, Ito Y, et al. Incidences of unfavorable events in the management of low-risk papillary microcarcinoma of the thyroid by active surveillance versus immediate surgery. *Thyroid* 2015;26(1):150–155.

7. Nikiforov YE, Sethala RR, Tallini G, et al. Nomenclature revision for encapsulated follicular variant of papillary thyroid carcinoma: a paradigm shift to reduce overtreatment of indolent tumors. *JAMA Oncol* 2016;2(8):1023–1029.

8. Mazzaferri EL, Robbins RJ, Spencer CA, et al. A consensus report of the role of serum thyroglobulin as a monitoring method for low-risk patients with papillary thyroid carcinoma. *J Clin Endocrinol Metab* 2003;88(4):1433–1441.

9. Pfister DG, Fagin JA. Refractory thyroid cancer: a paradigm shift in treatment is not far off. *J Clin Oncol* 2008;26(29):4701–4704.

10. Bible KC, Ryder M. Evolving molecularly targeted therapies for advanced-stage thyroid cancers. *Nat Rev Clin Oncol* 2016;13(7):403–416.

11. Smallridge RC, Ain KB, Asa SL, et al. American Thyroid Association guidelines for management of patients with anaplastic thyroid cancer. *Thyroid* 2012;22(11):1104–1139.

12. Smallridge RC. Approach to the patient with anaplastic thyroid carcinoma. *J Clin Endocrinol Metab* 2012;97(8):2566–2572.

13. Wells SA Jr, Asa SL, Dralle H, et al. Revised American Thyroid Association guidelines for the management of medullary thyroid carcinoma. *Thyroid* 2015;25(6):567–610.

14. Sippel RS, Kunnimalaiyaan M, Chen H. Current management of medullary thyroid cancer. *Oncologist* 2008;13(5):539–547.

11

Adrenal Incidentaloma

Ritika Puri and Charles A. Harris

GENERAL PRINCIPLES

Definition

- Adrenal incidentaloma is an adrenal mass discovered incidentally on a radiologic study performed for indications other than evaluation for adrenal disease.[1]
- The patient may or may not have symptoms and signs associated with the mass.
- Further workup of adrenal incidentaloma is warranted to rule out malignant potential and hormonal activity of the mass.

Epidemiology

- In a meta-analysis by Kloos et al. of autopsy series, prevalence of adrenal incidentaloma ranged from 1.05% to 8.7%. There was a significant increase in prevalence with increasing age. No significant difference was noted between men and women.[2]
- Adrenal mass in children, adolescents, pregnant women, and adults less than 40 years of age has a higher likelihood of malignancy.
- In a radiologic study using high-resolution computerized tomography (CT), Bovio et al. reported a prevalence of 4.4%.[3]
- The prevalence has most likely increased due to the rate of CT scans in the United States having doubled between 1997 and 2007.[4]

Etiology

- Nonfunctioning adenomas are most common (82.4%), followed by subclinical Cushing syndrome (SCS) (5.3%), pheochromocytomas (5.1%), adrenocortical carcinomas (ACCs) (4.7%), metastatic lesions (2.5%), and aldosterone-producing adenomas (1%).[1]
- Table 11-1 lists several common differential diagnoses associated with adrenal incidentalomas.

DIAGNOSIS

Clinical Presentation

A thorough history and physical examination should be completed to elicit any subtle signs or symptoms that may suggest hormonal dysfunction or malignancy:

- **Cushing syndrome** (weight gain, moon facies, central obesity, supraclavicular fat pads, thinned skin, easy bruising, striae, acne, proximal muscle weakness, irregular menses, hirsutism, hypertension, diabetes, and vertebral compression fractures). Patients may present with overt Cushing syndrome or with SCS without typical stigmata of hypercortisolism.
- **Pheochromocytoma** (hypertension, paroxysms of headache, palpitations, anxiety attacks, perspiration, and/or pallor). About 15% patients with pheochromocytoma do not have hypertension.
- **Aldosterone-secreting adenoma** (hypertension or hypokalemia).
- **Malignancy** (weight loss, history of primary nonadrenal cancers, lymphoma).
- Patients suspected of **metastasis** will usually have a known history of malignancy.

TABLE 11-1	DIFFERENTIAL DIAGNOSIS OF ADRENAL INCIDENTALOMA

Benign	Malignant
Nonhormone secreting	Adrenocortical carcinoma
Nonfunctioning adenoma	Metastatic neoplasm
Lipoma/myelolipoma	Lymphoma
Cyst	Malignant pheochromocytoma
Ganglioneuroma	
Hematoma	
Infection (tuberculosis, fungal)	
Hormone secreting	
Pheochromocytoma	
Aldosterone-secreting adenoma	
Subclinical Cushing syndrome	

- **ACC** may be hormonally active in two-thirds of cases and usually manifest with rapidly progressing signs and symptoms of hypercortisolemia, virilization, and less frequently with aldosteronism or feminization.

Diagnostic Criteria

In evaluating such a mass, the major concerns to address are:

- Is the mass benign or malignant?
- Is the mass hormonally active?

Diagnostic Testing

Laboratories

- Nearly all patients with adrenal incidentalomas should be screened for autonomous cortisol production, pheochromocytoma, and hyperaldosteronism (if hypertensive). Patients with virilization should be screened for ACC.
- **Cortisol-producing adrenal adenoma:** A 2009 guidelines from the American Association of Clinical Endocrinologists/American Association of Endocrine Surgeons (AACE/AAES) recommend a 1-mg overnight dexamethasone suppression test to screen for autonomous cortisol production.[5] If clinical suspicion is high, salivary cortisol and urine-free cortisol can be used.
- **Subclinical pheochromocytoma:** Screen with plasma metanephrine and normetanephrine or 24-hour urine metanephrine and normetanephrine. However, one must be aware that plasma levels are associated with a higher false-positive rate whereas urine measurements have higher false-negative rate.
- **Hyperaldosteronism:** Aldosterone-to-renin ratio (plasma aldosterone concentration [PAC]/plasma renin activity ratio [PRA]) >20 and PAC >15 ng/dL is highly sensitive for primary hyperaldosteronism (however the cutoff values are laboratory dependent).[1,5]
- Dehydroepiandrosterone sulfate (DHEA-S) level should be determined if virilizing signs or symptoms are present.
- Patients with bilateral adrenal masses should be assessed clinically, biochemically, and radiologically in the same way as unilateral masses. In addition, serum 17-hydroxyprogesterone should be measured to exclude congenital adrenal hyperplasia and evaluation for adrenal insufficiency should be considered.[6]

- Any positive results on these screening tests should prompt further evaluation. Please refer to chapters on Conn syndrome (Chapter 14), Cushing syndrome (Chapter 15), and Pheochromocytoma (Chapter 16) for more detailed discussions of these tests and their interpretation.

Imaging

Three important criteria to differentiate benign lesion from malignant are size, CT attenuation value on unenhanced CT, and contrast washout pattern.

- **Size:** In general, adrenal tumors <3 cm are benign and tumors >6 cm are malignant. Diagnostic criteria are not as clear for lesions measuring 4 to 6 cm. If they are hormonally inactive and have a clear benign appearance on CT scan, such lesions can be monitored. Masses >6 cm, regardless of appearance on CT scan, are more likely to be malignant, and surgical referral is warranted. All masses >4 cm with indeterminate imaging characteristics need to be referred for surgery.
- **Noncontrast CT attenuation** value of <10 Hounsfield units (HU) is suggestive of a benign lesion and is superior to adrenal size in differentiating between benign and malignant tumor.[7,8] In a study by Hamrahian et al. it is proposed that for masses <4 cm, cutoff of 20 HU is acceptable.[7]
- **Pattern of enhancement and de-enhancement** on adrenal protocol CT scan can assist in determining the nature of the adenoma. Rapid contrast washout, that is, absolute contrast washout of more than 60% at 15 minutes is suggestive of benign adenoma.[8,9]
- **Magnetic resonance imaging** (MRI) appears to be as effective as CT scanning in distinguishing benign and malignant masses,[10] with benign adenomas exhibiting signal drop on chemical shift imaging with intensity similar to T2-weighted images of the liver. Pheochromocytomas generally exhibit hyperintensity on T2-weighted imaging. Again, masses >6 cm in diameter by MRI are more likely to be malignant, even if they have a benign appearance on MRI, and should prompt surgical referral.

Diagnostic Procedures

- Biopsy of the adrenal mass is generally not advised, as it is rarely helpful, except if there is suspicion for metastasis or infection. In a patient with known extra-adrenal primary malignancy, biopsy may help distinguish recurrence and metastasis from other etiologies of adrenal mass.[11]
- Biopsy should be done only after pheochromocytoma has been ruled out by biochemical testing, as biopsy of a pheochromocytoma can precipitate a hypertensive emergency and hemorrhage.

TREATMENT

- Adrenal mass with concerning radiographic characteristics and most masses ≥4 cm should be resected.
- Prior to surgical excision of an adrenal mass it is important to exclude pheochromocytoma and to assess for excess cortisol secretion.
- All pheochromocytomas should undergo surgical resection. Pheochromocytomas have a 10% to 15% recurrence rate and require long-term follow-up with biochemical testing.
- Patients with overt Cushing syndrome should undergo surgical resection.
- In patients with SCS, clear guidelines for surgical versus medical management are not available due to lack of long-term morbidity and mortality data. Surgical resection should be reserved for patients with worsening clinical comorbidities such as hypertension, diabetes, dyslipidemia, osteoporosis.[5,12] Per European Society of Endocrinology (ESE) and European Network for the Study of Adrenal Tumors (ENSAT) guidelines, individualized approach

should be adopted to consider these patients for surgery based on comorbidities, age, degree of cortisol excess, general health, and patient's preference.[6,13]

- Patients with cortisol-producing adenomas should be treated with exogenous glucocorticoids after the surgery due to the concern of adrenal crisis. After surgery, patients should undergo corticotropin stimulation test to evaluate for adrenal insufficiency. Hypersecretion of cortisol from one gland causes atrophy of contralateral adrenal gland which may take 6 to 18 months to recover after unilateral adrenalectomy. In general, the hypothalamus–pituitary–adrenal (HPA) axis recovers faster in patients with SCS when compared to patients with overt Cushing syndrome.

- Aldosterone-producing adenomas should be differentiated from primary adrenal hyperplasia as aldosterone-producing adenoma is best treated surgically, while primary adrenal hyperplasia is medically managed with mineralocorticoid antagonists.

- Any lesion suspected of being ACC should be resected. Two-thirds of ACC are hormone producing. All patients should undergo biochemical evaluation prior to resection.

- Adrenal metastatic lesions can be resected for symptomatic palliation in selected patients. Overall prognosis in these patients is poor.

- See Figure 11-1 for algorithm for managing adrenal incidentalomas.

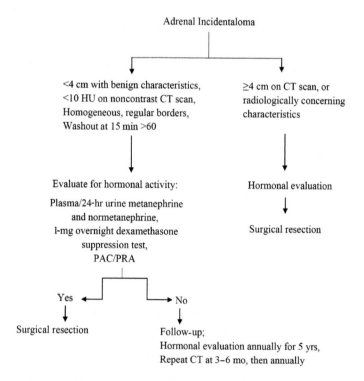

HU = Hounsfield units; PAC = plasma aldosterone concentration; PRA = plasma renin activity.

FIGURE 11-1 Algorithm for management of adrenal incidentaloma.

MONITORING/FOLLOW-UP

- If the history, physical examination, and hormonal and radiologic evaluations are not suggestive of malignant potential or increased hormonal activity, then it is reasonable to conclude that the incidentaloma is benign, but follow-up is necessary.
- Patients with adrenal incidentalomas <4 cm and radiologic findings consistent with a benign lesion should have repeat CT scan in 3 to 6 months and then annually for 1 to 2 years.[5,14] Nodules that remain stable in size are very unlikely to be malignant, and the risk of further imaging outweighs the benefits.[15]
- Hormonal evaluation should be done at the time of diagnosis and then annually for up to 5 years.
- If the tumor grows more than 1 cm or becomes hormonally active, surgical excision should be considered.

REFERENCES

1. Young WF Jr. Management approaches to adrenal incidentalomas: a view from Rochester, Minnesota. *Endocrinol Metab Clin North Am* 2000;29(1):159–185, x.
2. Kloos RT, Gross MD, Francis IR, Korobkin M, Shapiro B. Incidentally discovered adrenal masses. *Endocr Rev* 1995;16(4):460–484.
3. Bovio S, Cataldi A, Reimondo G, et al. Prevalence of adrenal incidentaloma in a contemporary computerized tomography series. *J Endocrinol Invest* 2006;29(4):298–302.
4. Brenner DJ, Hall EJ. Computed tomography-an increasing source of radiation exposure. *N Engl J Med* 2007;357(22):2277–2284.
5. Zeiger MA, Thompson GB, Duh QY, et al. The American Association of Clinical Endocrinologists and American Association of Endocrine Surgeons medical guidelines for the management of adrenal incidentalomas. *Endocr Pract* 2009;15(Suppl 1):1–20.
6. Fassnacht M, Arlt W, Bancos I, et al. Management of adrenal incidentalomas: European Society of Endocrinology Clinical Practice Guideline in collaboration with the European Network for the Study of Adrenal Tumors. *Eur J Endocrinol* 2016;175(2):G1–G34.
7. Hamrahian AH, Ioachimescu AG, Remer EM, et al. Clinical utility of noncontrast computed tomography attenuation value (Hounsfield units) to differentiate adrenal adenomas/hyperplasias from nonadenomas: Cleveland Clinic experience. *J Clin Endocrinol Metab* 2005;90(2):871–877.
8. Boland GW, Lee MJ, Gazelle GS, et al. Characterization of adrenal masses using unenhanced CT: An analysis of the CT literature. *AJR Am J Roentgenol* 1998;171(1):201–204.
9. Caoili EM, Korobkin M, Francis IR, et al. Adrenal masses: characterization with combined unenhanced and delayed enhanced CT. *Radiology* 2002;222(3):629–633.
10. Yip L, Tublin ME, Falcone JA, et al. The adrenal mass: correlation of histopathology with imaging. *Ann Surg Oncol* 2010;17(3):846–852.
11. Lenert JT, Barnett CC Jr, Kudelka AP, et al. Evaluation and surgical resection of adrenal masses in patients with a history of extra-adrenal malignancy. *Surgery* 2001;130(6):1060–1067.
12. De Leo M, Cozzolino A, Colao A, Pivonello R. Subclinical Cushing's syndrome. *Best Pract Res Clin Endocrinol Metab* 2012;26(4):497–505.
13. Starker LF, Kunstman JW, Carling T. Subclinical Cushing syndrome: a review. *Surg Clin North Am* 2014;94(3):657–668.
14. Nieman LK. Approach to the patient with an adrenal incidentaloma. *J Clin Endocrinol Metab* 2010;95(9):4106–4113.
15. Cawood TJ, Hunt PJ, O'Shea D, Cole D, Soule S. Recommended evaluation of adrenal incidentalomas is costly, has high false-positive rates and confers a risk of fatal cancer that is similar to the risk of the adrenal lesion becoming malignant; time for a rethink? *Eur J Endocrinol* 2009;161(4):513–527.

Adrenal Insufficiency

12

Rong Mei Zhang and Kim Carmichael

GENERAL PRINCIPLES

- Adrenal insufficiency (AI) is due to disruption of the hypothalamus–pituitary–adrenal (HPA) axis regulation of steroidogenesis.
- Addison first described this syndrome in 1855 characterized by wasting and hyperpigmentation.[1]

Classification

- **Primary AI (Addison disease)** corresponds to adrenal dysfunction from any cause.
- **Secondary AI** refers to adrenocorticotropic hormone (ACTH) deficiency due to hypothalamic or pituitary dysfunction.

Epidemiology

Primary AI has a prevalence of 93 to 144 per million and peaks in the fourth decade.[1] Secondary AI has a prevalence of 150 to 280 per million with a peak age of onset in the sixth decade.[1] Both conditions are more prevalent in women.

Etiology

For a complete list of AI causes, see Table 12-1.

- **Primary AI**
  - Tuberculosis was the most common etiology for primary AI and is still a factor in the developing world.[1]
  - Autoimmune adrenalitis has emerged as the leading cause of primary AI.[1] It can be isolated or be part of an autoimmune polyglandular syndrome (APS, types I and II) (see Chapter 39).
  - Congenital adrenal hyperplasia causes abnormalities of adrenal steroid biosynthesis enzymes causing impaired cortisol synthesis (see Chapter 13).
  - Other etiologies include[2]:
    - Infiltrative conditions (hemochromatosis, amyloid, infiltrative infections)
    - Bilateral adrenal hemorrhage
    - Metastatic cancer
    - Medications
- **Secondary AI**
  - Iatrogenic
    - Sudden cessation of exogenous glucocorticoid therapy via any route is the most frequent cause of secondary AI, and can suppress the HPA axis with rates of 2% (low dose) to 21% (high dose).[3] Recovery of the HPA axis ranges from 9 to 12 months.[1]
    - Megestrol acetate (Megace) can suppress the HPA axis, and patients need exogenous glucocorticoids until HPA axis recovery after discontinuation.[4]
  - Hypothalamic–pituitary
    - A pituitary mass may cause panhypopituitarism.

TABLE 12-1 CAUSES OF ADRENAL INSUFFICIENCY

Primary (adrenal)

Autoimmune (70–90%)
Isolated adrenal insufficiency (associated with HLA-DR3)
Polyglandular autoimmune syndrome type I (mutation in the *AIRE* gene)
Polyglandular autoimmune syndrome type II (associated with HLA-DR3)

Infectious and infiltrative
Tuberculosis (7–20%)
Disseminated pseudomonas, histoplasmosis
HIV and its opportunistic infections (CMV, *Mycobacterium avium* complex, *Cryptococcus*, *Pneumocystis carinii* pneumonia, toxoplasmosis)
Syphilis
Amyloidosis
Sarcoidosis

Metastatic carcinoma
Lung, breast, colon cancer, melanoma

Medications
Rifampin, phenytoin, barbiturates, ketoconazole, etomidate, tyrosine kinase inhibitors

Adrenal hemorrhage/infarction
Meningococcal sepsis with Waterhouse–Friderichsen syndrome
Primary antiphospholipid syndrome
Disseminated intravascular coagulopathy

Genetic disorders
Adrenoleukodystrophy (mutation in the *ABCD1* gene)
Congenital adrenal hyperplasia (deficiencies in steroidogenic acute regulatory protein, 21-hydroxylase, 11β-hydroxylase, 3β-hydroxyl-Δ-5-steroid dehydrogenase)
Mutations in *DAX-1* and *SF-1* transcription factors
Smith–Lemli–Opitz syndrome (*DHCR7* gene mutation)
Kearns–Sayre syndrome (mitochondrial DNA deletions)
Familial glucocorticoid deficiency (*type 1 MC2R, type 2 MRAP* gene mutations)

Secondary (pituitary or hypothalamus)

Iatrogenic
Abrupt withdrawal of megestrol (a progestin with some glucocorticoid activity)
Prolonged use of exogenous glucocorticoids (inhaled, oral, topical)
Pituitary surgery or radiation
Head trauma

Pituitary/hypothalamic tumors
Pituitary adenoma
Craniopharyngioma
Rathke cleft cyst
Pituitary stalk lesions

Infectious and infiltrative
Tuberculosis
Histoplasmosis
Neurosarcoidosis
Hemochromatosis
Lymphocytic hypophysitis
Metastasis (lung, breast)

Infarction, hemorrhage/apoplexy
Sheehan syndrome
Large intracranial artery aneurysms

Genetic pituitary abnormalities
HESX, PROP1, LIM, SRY
Isolated ACTH deficiency
Familial cortisol-binding globulin deficiency

Relative adrenal insufficiency
Critical illness
Liver disease (cirrhosis, acute liver failure, transplant)

ACTH, adrenocorticotropic hormone; CMV, cytomegalovirus.

- ▪ Other causes include lymphocytic hypophysitis, infectious and infiltrative diseases, pituitary infarction or hemorrhage, and head trauma.
- ▪ Isolated ACTH deficiency is rare.

DIAGNOSIS

Diagnosis of AI is difficult and depends on clinical suspicion corroborated by biochemical evidence.

Clinical Presentation

The clinical presentation is variable and depends on the level of HPA axis affected and the rate or extent of adrenal function lost.

- **Acute AI (adrenal crisis):** Acute AI occurs with primary AI and can cause decreased mineralocorticoid activity and adrenergic response with cytokine-mediated glucocorticoid resistance.[5] It is critical to recognize because this is an endocrine emergency. **Clinical features** include:
  - ○ Precipitated by acute stress.
  - ○ Shock with severe volume depletion and hypotension out of proportion to the severity of illness.
  - ○ Nausea, vomiting with prior weight loss and anorexia, abdominal pain, fatigue, fever, confusion, coma, electrolyte abnormalities (hyperkalemia, hyponatremia, hypoglycemia), eosinophilia.
- **Chronic primary AI** is insidious.[2] A significant illness can transform chronic primary AI into an adrenal crisis, so early recognition is essential. In its early stage, **symptoms are nonspecific:**
  - ○ Malaise, weakness, myalgias, weight loss
  - ○ Nausea, vomiting, anorexia, and abdominal pain, dizziness
  - ○ Depression, loss of libido
  - ○ Increased sensitivity to noises, smells, and taste
- Primary AI causes glucocorticoid and mineralocorticoid deficiency.
  - ○ Lack of feedback inhibition on the pituitary by cortisol leads to increased ACTH, which stimulates the melanocortin receptor to upregulate melanin synthesis, and causes **hyperpigmentation of the skin and mucosa.**
  - ○ Mineralocorticoid deficiency results in renal salt wasting causing salt craving, hyponatremia, hyperkalemia, volume depletion, and hypotension.
  - ○ Loss of adrenal androgen is more apparent in women, which induces loss of axillary and pubic hair, decreased libido, and impaired well-being.
- Patients with autoimmune adrenalitis may have other autoimmune diseases such as hypo- or hyperthyroidism, type 1 diabetes, alopecia areata, or vitiligo.
- Longstanding AI can cause impaired memory, depression, and psychosis.
- **Secondary AI:** Patients with secondary AI present with similar symptoms as chronic primary AI.
  - ○ Secondary AI patients experience other pituitary hormone deficiency symptoms (amenorrhea, decreased libido, or hypothyroidism), or mass effect (headaches, visual field defects) from a pituitary or hypothalamic tumor.
  - ○ Secondary AI patients do not manifest hyperpigmentation because their ACTH is not elevated, and they have less prominent electrolyte abnormalities, volume depletion, and hypotension due to an intact renin–angiotensin–aldosterone (RAA) system.

Diagnostic Testing

A multistep approach is needed to determine if inadequate cortisol secretion is due to decreased adrenal secretion or lack of ACTH.

Laboratories

Testing for Inadequate Cortisol Secretion: Inappropriately low cortisol production is the sine qua non finding in AI of any cause.

- Basal cortisol measurements
  - 8 a.m. cortisol levels of ≥19 mcg/dL rule out AI, whereas cortisol ≤3 mcg/dL is indicative of AI. All other values need dynamic testing.[6]
  - Estrogen therapy raises cortisol by increasing corticosteroid-binding globulin while both are decreased in cirrhosis.[1]
  - Hypoproteinemia may falsely lower serum cortisol levels.[7]
- Corticotropin stimulation tests
  - The corticotropin stimulation test is the most widely used dynamic test to assess adrenal function[6,8] and has higher sensitivity in primary AI.[9]
  - The corticotropin (standard 250 mcg or low-dose 1 mcg) can be given intravenously (IV) or intramuscularly with cortisol measured baseline and 30 and 60 minutes after corticotropin.
  - Cortisol levels >18 mcg/dL exclude primary AI and severe chronic secondary AI.
  - The low-dose stimulation test is proposed as a more sensitive test for mild secondary AI or with steroid use. Superiority of the low-dose test remains controversial and technical concerns limit its use.[10]
  - The stimulation tests may be normal in recent-onset secondary AI.
  - Testing for AI after pituitary surgery should be done 4 to 6 weeks postoperatively.
  - Chronic partial secondary AI may not be detected by the corticotropin test. An insulin tolerance test (ITT) may be needed in these patients (see subsequent text).
  - Most steroid replacements interfere with the radioimmunoassay for cortisol except dexamethasone. Patients on replacement should delay their dose until after the stimulation test.
  - If adrenal crisis is suspected, IV saline and dexamethasone 4-mg IV q6h should be started until the stimulation test is performed.
- **ITT** is the gold standard for secondary AI since hypoglycemia is a stressor that causes rapid activation of the HPA axis.[6]
  - IV insulin (0.1 to 0.15 U/kg) is given with glucose and cortisol is measured at 0, 30, 45, 60, 90, and 120 minutes.
  - Hypoglycemia of <40 mg/dL with neuroglycopenic symptoms is essential.
  - Normal response is a cortisol >20 mcg/dL.
  - Close supervision is mandatory. Cardiovascular disease or seizures are contraindications.
- **Evaluating the HPA axis during critical illness is challenging.**[11]
  - Inappropriately low cortisol levels can be seen during critical illness with a structurally normal HPA axis (relative AI).
  - Severe illness causes decreased cortisol-binding proteins, leading to an increase in the ratio of free to bound cortisol.
  - In septic shock or ARDS, corticotropin stimulation testing should not be performed as a basis for glucocorticoid therapy.
  - Surviving Sepsis Guidelines make no recommendation on the use of cortisol or stimulation test to guide steroid therapy due to cortisol variability in severe illness.[12] Further studies are required to determine the utility of these tests in critical illness.
- Differentiating primary and secondary AI can be done with a baseline ACTH concentration.[13,14] The cosyntropin stimulation test does not differentiate between primary and secondary disease. An ACTH level should be drawn with the basal cortisol level; an elevated baseline ACTH level with a low basal serum cortisol suggests primary AI. Secondary AI patients have low cortisol with a low or low-normal ACTH level.

- The CRH stimulation test differentiates pituitary from hypothalamic cause of AI.[15]
  - ACTH peaks at 15 to 30 minutes and cortisol peaks at 30 to 45 minutes following CRH in AI from a hypothalamic etiology.
  - CRH stimulation testing has limited usefulness due to its cost, availability, and limited data.
- **Renin and aldosterone concentrations:** Mineralocorticoids are usually affected in primary AI. Aldosterone levels are low with an elevated renin.[1] In secondary AI, the renin–angiotensin–aldosterone system functions normally.
- **Autoantibodies:** Adrenal antibodies are detected in ≥90% of patients with autoimmune adrenalitis and can predate symptoms of AI.[16]
  - **Adrenal cortex antibody and 21-hydroxylase antibody** are commonly tested. The presence of both antibodies makes the diagnosis likely up to 99%.[17]
  - Elevated 17-hydroxyprogesterone can detect congenital adrenal hyperplasia.[18]
  - Evaluation of other organ dysfunctions associated with autoimmune AI includes calcium, islet cell antibodies, TSH, B12, CBC, hepatic, and gonadal function.
  - In boys with AI and negative autoimmune adrenalitis evaluation, very–long-chain fatty acids should be measured to exclude adrenoleukodystrophy as AI may present before neurologic symptoms.[18]

Imaging

- **Radiologic imaging should be performed except in known autoimmune AI or adrenomyeloneuropathy.**[2]
- **MRI imaging** of the hypothalamic–pituitary region is superior to CT in secondary AI. Analysis of sagittal and coronal sections provides the most information.
- CT should be obtained for bone invasion or calcifications in persons with craniopharyngioma.
- CT and MRI are often used to image the adrenal glands. In autoimmune adrenalitis, imaging reveals small or absent adrenal glands. Enlarged or calcified adrenals suggest an infectious, hemorrhagic, or malignant diagnosis.

Diagnostic Procedures

Adrenal biopsy is not required unless the presentation is concerning for metastases with an unidentified primary or infiltrative disorder, but only after pheochromocytoma has been excluded.

TREATMENT

- **Acute treatment:** Adrenal crisis is a life-threatening condition requiring immediate treatment. Therapy should not be delayed to perform diagnostic studies.
  - Volume replacement using normal saline is essential.
  - While blood for cortisol, ACTH, and chemistry is drawn, "stress-dose" steroids should be given.
  - If the diagnosis is unclear, dexamethasone should be given followed by corticotropin stimulation testing.
  - In patients with a history of AI, dexamethasone (4-mg IV q12h) or hydrocortisone (50- to 100-mg IV q6–8h) can be given.
  - Once improved, taper steroids over 1 to 3 days to an oral maintenance dose.
  - Mineralocorticoid replacement is not useful in acute AI, as it takes several days for its effects to become apparent; IV saline will suffice.
  - Adrenal crisis symptoms resolve over 1 to 2 hours after glucocorticoid therapy.
- **Maintenance treatment:** Maintenance therapy requires physiologic oral glucocorticoid doses. Patients with primary or secondary AI require glucocorticoid replacement (5 to

8 mg/m^2/day) with **hydrocortisone** (15 to 30 mg/day) or **prednisone** (4.0 to 7.5 mg/day) in one to three divided doses. It is **best to give a single morning dose** to mimic the physiologic diurnal variation. In a split-dose regimen, the larger dose is given in the morning and the smaller dose in the afternoon.

○ Treatment should be tailored to the lowest dose to avoid complications of excess replacement (weight gain, osteoporosis, immunocompromise) while also avoiding AI. Treatment surveillance is based on symptoms of over replacement or under replacement. No laboratory assessment is reliable for monitoring replacement quantity.

○ Patients with primary AI should also receive mineralocorticoid replacement with **fludrocortisone** (0.05 to 0.2 mg daily). Fludrocortisone dose is titrated by symptoms, blood pressure, potassium level and renin activity level. Renin activity level should be in the mid-upper normal range.

○ **Dehydroepiandrosterone** (DHEA) replacement (25 to 50 mg) may have positive effects on well-being, lean body mass, and femoral bone. A 6-month trial with monitoring of morning DHEA-S is appropriate, with discontinuation if no clinical benefit is achieved.[18,19]

SPECIAL CONSIDERATIONS

Treatment for specific situations:

- **Stress dosing**
  ○ Patients should increase their daily glucocorticoid dose during acute illness.
  ○ In addition to aggressive hydration, the usual daily dose can be doubled and then doubled again if symptoms of AI persist. An injectable dexamethasone or hydrocortisone kit can be prescribed for home use. Patients may return to their daily replacement doses on resolution within 1 to 3 days.
  ○ The patient should be immediately brought to a hospital for IV steroids if health status is uncertain.
- **Perioperative dosing:** During the peri- or postoperative period, inadequate steroid coverage can cause signs of impending adrenal crisis.
  ○ Minor procedures and most radiologic studies require the usual daily dose.
  ○ For moderate procedures requiring general anesthesia, patients should continue their daily steroid dose preoperatively and hydrocortisone 25-mg IV q8h during the procedure.
  ○ For major operations, patients should receive their daily dose preoperatively and hydrocortisone 50-mg IV q8h during the procedure.
  ○ Glucocorticoid can be tapered to baseline over 1 to 2 days.[20]
- **Secondary AI:** There is no need for mineralocorticoid replacement, but other pituitary hormone deficiencies may be present.
- **Thyroid disease**
  ○ The patient with AI and hypothyroidism must first receive glucocorticoid replacement before thyroid hormone to avoid precipitating adrenal crisis.
  ○ Glucocorticoid replacement should be doubled or tripled in these patients since hyperthyroidism increases cortisol clearance.[2]
- **Pregnancy**
  ○ Increased cortisol, cortisol-binding globulin, progesterone, and renin are physiologic changes in late pregnancy. Glucocorticoid doses need to be increased in the third trimester by 20% to 40%. Dexamethasone is not recommended due to lack of placental inactivation.[18]
  ○ Saline hydration and hydrocortisone 25-mg IV q6 should be administered during labor. At delivery or if labor is prolonged, hydrocortisone should be administered 100-mg q6h IV or via continuous infusion. After delivery, the dose can be tapered to the maintenance dose within 2 to 3 days.

- **AI after exogenous steroids**
  - Recovery of adrenal atrophy from steroid treatment is variable.
  - Steroids should be slowly tapered with close monitoring of AI symptoms. Dynamic testing can be performed when titrated to a low steroid dose with delayed administration on the day of testing to avoid assay interference.
- **Patient education**
  - All patients should obtain a **medical-alert identification AI**.
  - The patient and family should be instructed on how to inject steroids (e.g., dexamethasone or hydrocortisone) in an emergency.
  - Bring patients to immediate medical attention if adrenal crisis symptoms present.

REFERENCES

1. Chamandari E, Nicolaides N, Chrousos G. Adrenal insufficiency. *Lancet* 2014;383:21–27.
2. Arlt W, Allolio B. Adrenal insufficiency. *Lancet* 2003;361(9372):1881–1893.
3. Broersen LH, Pereira AM, Jørgensen JO, Dekkers OM. Adrenal insufficiency in corticosteroids use: systematic review and meta-analysis. *J Clin Endocrinol Metab* 2015;100:2171–2180.
4. Chidakel AR, Zweig SB, Schlosser JR, Homel P, Schappert JW, Fleckman AM. High prevalence of adrenal suppression during acute illness in hospitalized patients receiving megestrol acetate. *J Endocrinol Invest* 2006;29(2):136–140.
5. Allolio B. Extensive expertise in endocrinology. Adrenal crisis. *Eur J Endocrinol* 2015;172:115–124.
6. Grinspoon SK, Biller BM. Clinical review 62: Laboratory assessment of adrenal insufficiency. *J Clin Endocrinol Metab* 1994;79:923–931.
7. Hamrahian AH, Oseni TS, Arafah BM. Measurements of serum free cortisol in critically ill patients. *N Engl J Med* 2004;350:1629–1638.
8. May ME. Adrenocortical insufficiency—clinical aspects. In: Vaughan ED Jr, Carey RM, eds. *Adrenal Disorders*. New York: Thieme Medical; 1989:171–189.
9. Dori RI, Qualls CR, Crapo LM. Diagnosis of adrenal insufficiency. *Ann Int Med* 2003;139:194–204.
10. Wade M, Baid S, Calis K, Raff H, Sinaii N, Nieman L. Technical details influence the diagnostic accuracy of the 1 microg ACTH stimulation test. *Eur J Endocrinol* 2010;162:109–113.
11. Marik PE, Pastores SM, Annane D, et al. Recommendations for the diagnosis and management of corticosteroid insufficiency in critically ill adult patients: consensus statements from an international task force by the American College of Critical Care Medicine. *Crit Care Med* 2008;36:1937–1949.
12. Rhodes A, Evans LE, Alhazzani W, et al. Surviving sepsis campaign: international guidelines for management of sepsis and septic shock: 2016. *Intensive Care Med* 2017;43:304–377.
13. Wallace I, Cunningham S, Lindsay J. The diagnosis and investigation of adrenal insufficiency in adults. *Ann Clin Biochem* 2009;46(Pt 5):351–367.
14. Blevins LS Jr, Shankroff J, Moser HW, Ladenson PW. Elevated plasma adrenocorticotropin concentration as evidence of limited adrenocortical reserve in patients with adrenomyeloneuropathy. *J Clin Endocrinol Metab* 1994;78(2):261–265.
15. Orth DN. Corticotropin-releasing hormone in humans. *Endocr Rev* 1992;13:164–191.
16. Betterle C, Dal Pra C, Mantero F, Zanchetta R. Autoimmune adrenal insufficiency and autoimmune polyendocrine syndromes: autoantibodies, autoantigens, and their applicability in diagnosis and disease prediction. *Endocr Rev* 2002;23(3):327–364.
17. Falorni A, Laureti S, Nikoshkov A, et al. 21-hydroxylase autoantibodies in adult patients with endocrine autoimmune diseases are highly specific for Addison's disease. Belgian Diabetes Registry. *Clin Exp Immunol* 1997;107(2):341–346.
18. Bornstein SR, Allolio B, Arlt W, et al. Diagnosis and treatment of primary adrenal insufficiency: an endocrine society clinical practice guideline. *J Clin Endocrinol Metab* 2016;101:364–389.
19. Gurnell EM, Hunt PJ, Curran SE, et al. Long-term DHEA replacement in primary adrenal Insufficiency: a randomized, controlled trial. *J Clin Endocrinol Metab* 2008;93:400–409.
20. Coursin DB, Wood KE. Corticosteroid supplementation for adrenal insufficiency. *JAMA* 2002;287(2):236–240.

Adult Congenital Adrenal Hyperplasia

13

Laura N. Hollar and Kim Carmichael

GENERAL PRINCIPLES

- Congenital adrenal hyperplasia (CAH) consists of a group of autosomal recessive genetic disorders characterized by functional abnormalities in enzymes of the adrenal steroid biosynthesis pathway, leading to impaired cortisol biosynthesis and a compensatory increase in serum adrenocorticotropic hormone (ACTH).[1-3]
- Clinical and biochemical phenotype depends upon the severity and type of enzyme deficiency, resulting in various alterations in glucocorticoid, mineralocorticoid, and sex steroid synthesis.[1] Classic presentations include a severe form with neonatal salt wasting due to concurrent aldosterone deficiency and a form with apparently normal aldosterone biosynthesis that leads to atypical genitalia.[2] Milder, nonclassic forms may present with adult androgen excess.[4]
- Classic CAH is responsible for most cases of pseudohermaphroditism in females and about 50% of all cases of ambiguous genitalia.

Epidemiology

- About 95% of cases result from **21-hydroxylase deficiency** and 5% to 8% from **11β-hydroxylase deficiency**.[5,6] Rare forms of CAH include 17α-hydroxylase/17,20-lyase deficiency, 3β-hydroxysteroid dehydrogenase type 2 deficiency (3B-HSD2), P450 oxidoreductase (POR) deficiency, and lipoid adrenal hyperplasia or cholesterol side-chain cleavage (SCC) enzyme deficiency.[1]
- Refer to Table 13-1 for information on prevalence.
- The majority of cases of classic CAH are discovered during childhood; however, better understanding of the genetics and pathophysiology of CAH has led to frequent discoveries of its milder, nonclassic forms during adulthood.[1]
- The overall incidence of nonclassic CAH is not known but appears to be 0.1% to 0.2% in the general population.

Etiology

- **Deficient cortisol production** is the key aberration in CAH, and mastery of the adrenal steroid biosynthesis pathway is essential to understanding the pathogenesis of the disease and the rationale behind treatment (please see Figure 13-1).
- The types of CAH are determined by the distinct point at which adrenal steroidogenesis is interrupted. See Table 13-1 for CAH classification and information on specific mutations, the associated enzyme deficiency, and phenotypic presentation.[1,5]
- Mutations associated with large reductions in enzyme activity result in severe deficiencies of aldosterone and cortisol, whereas mutations associated with milder reductions result in less severe hormone abnormalities and a nonclassic course.
- Some patients with nonclassic CAH have one allele with a "severe" mutation and one allele with a "mild" mutation. Thus, the severity of the phenotype in compound heterozygotes is determined by the less severe mutation.[1]
- The reduction in cortisol levels stimulates ACTH release by the pituitary, in turn causing increased production of cortisol precursors, such as progesterone and 17-hydroxyprogesterone (17-OHP), which may be metabolized to androgen precursors (see Fig. 13-1).

TABLE 13-1 CONGENITAL ADRENAL HYPERPLASIA CLASSIFICATION

	21-Hydroxylase deficiency	11β-Hydroxylase deficiency	17α-Hydroxylase/17, 20-lyase deficiency	3β-Hydroxysteroid dehydrogenase type 2 deficiency	P450 oxidoreductase deficiency	Lipoid adrenal hyperplasia or SCC enzyme deficiency
Incidence	Classic: 1:14,000 Nonclassic: 1:200–1,000	Classic: 1:100,000 Nonclassic: unknown	1:50,000	Rare	Rare	Rare
Affected gene	CYP21A2	CYP11B1	CYP17A1	HSD3B2	P450 oxidoreductase (POR)	Steroidogenic acute regulatory protein (StAR)
Hormonal alterations	↑17-OHP, 21-deoxycortisol, androstenedione, and renin ↓Cortisol and aldosterone	↑DOC, 11-deoxycortisol, androstenedione, 17-OHP ↓Cortisol, aldosterone, corticosterone, renin	↑DOC, corticosterone, and progesterone ↓Cortisol, aldosterone, 17-OHP, 170-hydroxy-pregnenolone, DHEA, androstenedione	↑17-hydroxypregnenolone, DHEA, renin ↓Cortisol, aldosterone, progesterone, 17-OHP, androstenedione, DOC, 11-deoxycortisol	↑Pregnenolone, progesterone, 17-OHP, DOC, corticosterone ↓DHEA and androstenedione	↑Renin ↓All steroids
Clinical presentation	Classic: neonatal salt wasting, virilization Nonclassic: mild androgen excess	Classic: virilization, hypertension, hypokalemia Nonclassic: rare, androgen excess	Adolescent female with absent secondary sex characteristics and hypergonadotropic hypogonadism, hypertension, hypokalemia	Classic: neonatal salt wasting, underdeveloped XY genitalia, mild virilization XX genitalia Nonclassic: extremely rare	Atypical genitalia, XX virilization does not progress, Maternal virilization, skeletal manifestations	Classic: neonatal salt wasting, female genitalia Nonclassic: AI, variable gonadal function and genitalia

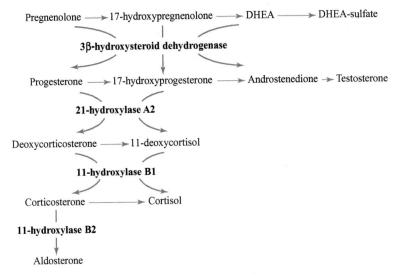

FIGURE 13-1 The adrenal steroid biosynthesis pathway.

Classification

- Three-fourths of patients with classic CAH are *"salt wasters,"* as they have no 21-hydroxylase activity and produce insufficient aldosterone to retain sodium.
- The remaining one-fourth of patients, who produce low but detectable enzyme activity, retain enough ability to produce aldosterone, and although virilized, do not waste sodium and so are known as *"simple virilizers."*
- Those who retain 20% to 60% of enzymatic activity typically present in adulthood with more subtle, nonclassic forms, and acute adrenal crisis is uncommon.[3]
- Patients with classic 21-hydroxylase deficiency are at high risk for development of adrenal insufficiency without exogenous glucocorticoid administration.

DIAGNOSIS

Clinical Presentation

- **Classic 21-hydroxylase deficiency** presents at birth or within several weeks of birth with hypotension as a result of adrenal insufficiency.
- **Simple virilizing 21-hydroxylase deficiency** is usually diagnosed shortly after birth in females owing to external genital abnormalities (clitoral enlargement, fusion of the labial folds, formation of urogenital sinus), but for boys the diagnosis can be delayed for years until signs of androgen excess develop.
- The symptoms of nonclassic 21-hydroxylase deficiency may be subtle or even absent. It can present at any age after birth usually with hyperandrogenic symptoms such as cystic acne, hirsutism, infertility, and irregular menses. These symptoms can wax and wane over time. Males with nonclassic CAH may experience infertility and acne.[1,4]
- In children of both sexes, nonclassic CAH may be diagnosed during a workup for premature pubarche or accelerated linear growth with advanced bone age.
- The **differential diagnosis for nonclassic CAH in adults** is limited but includes **polycystic ovarian syndrome, virilizing adrenal or ovarian tumors, and exogenous anabolic steroid use.**

- In nonclassic CAH females, hyperandrogenic features dominate the physical examination. Hirsutism is the single most common symptom, followed by oligomenorrhea and acne.[1]
- Men might present with small testes compared to the phallus, oligospermia, infertility, and short stature. In classic CAH, the prevalence of testicular adrenal rest tumors is 21% to 28% and is found almost exclusively in severe mutation types.[1,7]
- Final adult height may be reduced owing to premature closure of epiphyses due to androgen excess.
- POR deficiency may have skeletal manifestations such as craniofacial abnormalities.[1]

Diagnostic Testing

- Screening newborns for CAH via measurement of 17-OHP minimizes delay in diagnosis and reduces morbidity from adrenal crisis. A few nonclassic CAH cases are detected by newborn screening, but most are missed because of borderline or normal 17-OHP.
- If neonatal screen is positive or CAH is suspected, a panel of steroids by mass spectrometry is indicated. However, diagnosis often requires a cosyntropin stimulation test, as described below.
- Mass spectrometry of urinary steroid metabolites provides an alternative to serum testing and can be especially useful in differentiating POR deficiency.[1,8]
- Genotyping confirms carrier states and is helpful for genetic counseling.
- **Classic 21-hydroxylase deficiency is characterized by significantly elevated levels of 17-OHP** in infancy, with varying degrees of virilization that may not become apparent until later in childhood.
- Early morning 17-OHP levels should be drawn during the follicular phase in women. A **17-OHP of <200 ng/dL makes CAH unlikely**, and a **value >400 ng/dL has been reported to have 100% specificity and 90% sensitivity**.[9]
- The gold standard for hormonal diagnosis is the cosyntropin stimulation test, which should be done for values between 200 ng/dL and 400 ng/dL.
  - 250 mcg of synthetic ACTH is administered IV and plasma concentrations of 17-OHP are measured at baseline and at 60 minutes after the drug is given; reference values for the local laboratory should be obtained. **Patients with classic CAH have values >300 ng/dL and nonclassic CAH will usually have 17-OHP values >1,000 ng/dL. If values are <50 ng/dL, CAH may be ruled out.**[1]
  - Plasma cortisol is measured at baseline and at 30 and 60 minutes after stimulation.
  - If the post-ACTH cortisol level is <20 mcg/dL, the patient should be made aware of the need to take additional glucocorticoids during times of physiologic stress. Please see Chapter 12 for details on diagnosing adrenal insufficiency.
  - Genotyping should only be done if cosyntropin stimulation results are equivocal and for purposes of genetic counseling.[1]
- First-degree family members of affected patients should be screened for CAH because of the potential absence of clinical signs and harm that may result if a patient does not receive therapy.

TREATMENT

- The goal of therapy in CAH is to both correct the deficiency in cortisol secretion and to suppress ACTH overproduction.
- Therapy consists of a balance between sufficient glucocorticoid replacement to suppress the overproduction of androgens and to prevent adrenal crises in classic cases, while avoiding complications related to glucocorticoid excess. Persons should carry medical alert identification and be educated on appropriate stress dosing.
- **Treatment for classic "salt-wasting" CAH** is glucocorticoid and mineralocorticoid replacement and sodium chloride supplementation.[1]

- **Treatment of adults with *nonclassic* 21-hydroxylase deficiency** should only be undertaken for infertility or hyperandrogenism that is unacceptable to the patient. There are no reports of death from adrenal insufficiency as a result of nonclassic CAH in the medical literature; therefore, stress-dose steroids are usually not required unless subnormal cortisol response was demonstrated during cosyntropin stimulation. See Chapter 12 for details on diagnosis and management of adrenal insufficiency.
- **Hydrocortisone is the preferred treatment in children** because of improved clinical outcomes with respect to final adult height.
  - Typical dose is 10 to 15 mg/m²/day of hydrocortisone in two or three divided doses.
  - After completion of linear growth, long-acting glucocorticoids are preferred.
- Aldosterone biosynthetic defect is clinically apparent only in the salt-wasting form. However, **subclinical aldosterone deficiency** is present in all forms and can be **evaluated by the aldosterone to plasma renin activity (PRA) ratio.**
  - All patients with elevated PRA or decreased aldosterone to PRA ratio benefit from mineralocorticoid therapy and adequate dietary sodium supplementation.[1]
  - Maintenance of sodium balance reduces vasopressin and ACTH levels, allowing the use of lower glucocorticoid doses.
  - Sensitivity to mineralocorticoids may vary over time, and the need for mineralocorticoid replacement should be reassessed periodically.
- Sex steroid replacement is started at the time of puberty in 17-OH deficiency, lipoid CAH, SCC deficiency, POR deficiency, and 3β-HSD2 deficiency.[1]
- Genital surgery continues to generate much controversy. The patient's family should be educated on the advantages and disadvantages of surgery as an option in patients with disorders of sex development.

COMPLICATIONS

- Unfortunately, treatment outcome in CAH is often suboptimal either due to incomplete suppression of hyperandrogenism or, conversely, due to overtreatment-induced hypercortisolism. Both of these can result in decreased final adult height, 1.7 to 2.0 SD below the average in the normal population.[2]
- Final adult height may be improved in children with advanced bone age, predicted to be at least 1 standard deviation below midparental target height, with the use of growth hormone and luteinizing hormone releasing hormone agonists.[10]
- See Chapter 12 for management of adrenal crisis in classic, salt-wasting CAH.

MONITORING/FOLLOW-UP

- Monitoring the effects of steroid replacement is crucial. 17-OHP levels are relatively resistant to suppression by glucocorticoids, and thus, a normal 17-OHP level often represents overtreatment. Overtreatment can cause iatrogenic Cushing syndrome and lead to reduced bone mineral density.
- 17-OHP levels should be maintained at the upper end of normal to mildly supranormal levels with androstenedione levels in the normal range.[1]
- Mineralocorticoid replacement may be monitored by following blood pressure and potassium levels.
- Elevated renin levels or hypotension may signify insufficient mineralocorticoid replacement.
- Adrenal imaging should be reserved only for those with an atypical clinical or biochemical course. There is insufficient data to recommend routine screening for adrenal masses.
- Pregnancy in classic CAH should be managed by an endocrinologist experienced in this area. While subfertility in women with nonclassic CAH is mild, there is some evidence

that treatment with glucocorticoids reduces miscarriage rates.[11] Treatment of prenatal CAH is regarded as experimental.[1]

- Discussion of prenatal counseling, diagnosis, and treatment of CAH is beyond the scope of this chapter, and the reader is referred to the following reviews.[12,13]

REFERENCES

1. El-Maouche D, Arlt W, Merke DP. Congenital adrenal hyperplasia. *Lancet* 2017;390:2194–2210.
2. Speiser PW, Azziz R, Baskin LS, et al. Congenital adrenal hyperplasia due to steroid 21-hydroxylase deficiency: an endocrine society clinical practice guideline. *J Clin Endocrinol Metab* 2010; 95:4133–4160.
3. Speiser PW, White PC. Congenital adrenal hyperplasia. *N Engl J Med* 2003;349:776–788.
4. Carmina E, Dewailly D, Escobar-Morreale HF, et al. Non-classic congenital adrenal hyperplasia due to 21-hydroxylase deficiency revisited: an update with a special focus on adolescent and adult women. *Hum Reprod Update* 2017;23(5):580–599.
5. Hannah-Shmouni F, Chen W, Merke DP. Genetics of congenital adrenal hyperplasia. *Endocrinol Metab Clin North Am* 2017;46(2):435–458.
6. Bulsari K, Falhammar H. Clinical perspectives in congenital adrenal hyperplasia due to 11β-hydroxylase deficiency. *Endocrine* 2017;55(1):19–36.
7. Dumic M, Duspara V, Grubic Z, Oguic SK, Skrabic V, Kusec V. Testicular adrenal rest tumors in congenital adrenal hyperplasia-cross-sectional study of 51 Croatian male patients. *Eur J Pediatr* 2017;176:1393–1404.
8. Hines JM, Bancos I, Bancos C, et al. High-resolution, accurate-mass (HRAM) mass spectometry urine steroid profiling in the diagnosis of adrenal disorders. *Clin Chem* 2017;63:1824–1835.
9. Azziz R, Hincapie LA, Knoxhenhauer ES, Dewailly D, Fox L, Boots LR. Screening for 21-hydroxylase-deficient nonclassic adrenal hyperplasia among hyperandrogenic women: a prospective study. *Fertil Steril* 1999;72(5):915–925.
10. Turcu AF, Auchus RJ. The next 150 years of congenital adrenal hyperplasia. *J Steroid Biochem Mol Biol* 2015;153:63–71.
11. Bidet M, Bellane Chatelet C, Galand Porter MB, et al. Fertility in women with nonclassical congenital adrenal hyperplasia due to 21-hydroxylase deficiency. *J Clin Endocrinol Metab* 2010;95:1182–1190.
12. Yau M, Khattab A, New MI. Prenatal diagnosis of congenital adrenal hyperplasia. *Endocrinol Metab Clin North Am* 2016;45:267–281.
13. Nimkarn S, New MI. Congenital adrenal hyperplasia due to 21-hydroxylase deficiency: a paradigm for prenatal diagnosis and treatment. *Ann N Y Acad Sci* 2010;1192:5–11.

Hyperaldosteronism

14

Ningning Ma and Thomas J. Baranski

GENERAL PRINCIPLES

Definition

Primary aldosteronism, also known as Conn syndrome, is defined as inappropriate (renin-independent) overproduction of aldosterone. Primary aldosteronism must be distinguished from secondary aldosteronism, which is appropriate (renin-dependent) increased production of aldosterone in response to relative hypovolemia as is seen in renovascular hypertension and with diuretic therapy.

Classification

Distinguishing between uni- and bilateral disease is of utmost importance because it determines therapy. Unilateral disease is confined to a single adrenal gland and is usually treated with surgery. Bilateral disease is present in both adrenal glands and is usually treated medically.

Epidemiology

The true prevalence of primary aldosteronism is not known. Older literature had suggested a low prevalence of <1% in hypertensive patients. More recent literature suggests a prevalence of up to 12% in hypertensive patients.[1,2]

Etiology

Primary aldosteronism can be caused by several adrenal disorders:

- Aldosterone-producing adenoma (APA)
- Adrenal gland hyperplasia (uni- or bilateral)
- Aldosterone-secreting adrenal cortical carcinoma (ACC)
- Aldosterone-secreting ovarian tumor
- Familial hyperaldosteronism (FH)

Pathophysiology

Aldosterone is produced in the zona glomerulosa and is synthesized and released in response to renin-dependent production of angiotensin II. Serum potassium, adrenocorticotropic hormone (ACTH), dopamine, and atrial natriuretic peptide (ANP) also affect its production and secretion. Aldosterone-induced sodium retention and potassium wasting do not lead to generalized edema or profound hypokalemia because of "aldosterone escape," in which an increase in urinary sodium and decrease in urinary potassium excretion counteract the acute effects of excess aldosterone. This phenomenon is thought to be mediated by increased secretion of ANP induced by hypervolemia, decreased abundance of the thiazide-sensitive NaCl cotransporter, and pressure natriuresis.

DIAGNOSIS

Clinical Presentation

The classic findings in primary aldosteronism are hypertension and hypokalemia. However, **the most common presentation of primary aldosteronism is normokalemic hypertension.**

Hypertension is usually, but not always, present,[3] but hypokalemia is present in less than half of confirmed cases.[1,4]

History

Symptoms related to hypokalemia, such as muscle weakness and cramping, can occur. Other symptoms are nonspecific and may include headache, fatigue, palpitations, and polyuria. A careful medication history is important, as many antihypertensives can interfere with diagnostic testing, as can licorice ingestion or chewing tobacco use. A family history of early-onset primary aldosteronism, hypertension, or cerebrovascular events should raise suspicion for FH.

Physical Examination

There are no specific physical findings in primary aldosteronism, though hypertension is present in the majority of cases.

Diagnostic Criteria

The diagnosis of primary aldosteronism is based on the demonstration of renin-independent overproduction of aldosterone.

Differential Diagnosis

- **Adrenal gland hyperplasia and APAs account for the majority of cases of primary aldosteronism.** Other causes are rare and account for <3% of cases.
- APAs account for approximately one-third of cases of primary aldosteronism. They are seen on occasion in multiple endocrine neoplasia type 1.
- Adrenal gland hyperplasia, also known as idiopathic hyperaldosteronism (IHA), accounts for approximately two-thirds of cases of primary aldosteronism and may affect one or both adrenal glands.
- Aldosterone-secreting ACC is rare, and only a subset of these tumors will secrete aldosterone. These tumors often come to attention as a result of pain from local invasion or cosecretion of cortisol and/or adrenal androgens, which lead to symptoms of Cushing syndrome and/or virilization.
- Aldosterone-secreting ovarian tumor as a cause of primary aldosteronism is extremely rare.
- Familial hyperaldosteronism
  - FH type 1, or glucocorticoid-remediable aldosteronism (GRA), is an autosomal-dominant disorder usually associated with bilateral adrenal hyperplasia. It is caused by recombination between the promoter regions of 11β-hydroxylase (*CYP11B1*) and the coding regions of 18-hydroxylase (*CYP11B2*), such that in the chimeric gene, ACTH (rather than renin or serum potassium) drives the expression of aldosterone synthase and aldosterone production. In contrast to most patients with primary aldosteronism who develop hypertension between the third and fifth decades, GRA patients develop hypertension at birth or in early childhood. Patients with GRA are usually normokalemic because their aldosterone release has the same circadian pattern as that of ACTH, and, therefore, aldosterone secretion is above normal for only part of the day. However, these patients can develop marked hypokalemia when treated with thiazide diuretics. Patients with GRA also tend to have an increased prevalence of early cerebrovascular complications, especially hemorrhagic strokes from ruptured intracerebral aneurysms.
  - FH type 2 is ACTH independent and leads to the occurrence of APA, IHA, or both, in an autosomal-dominant pattern. Although the exact genetic defect is unknown, a locus on chromosome 7p22 has been implicated.
  - FH type 3 results from gain-of-function mutations in the *KCNJ5* gene, resulting in increased calcium influx into zona glomerulosa cells, leading to secretion of aldosterone and possibly cell proliferation.

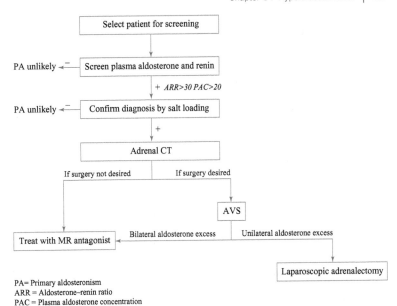

PA= Primary aldosteronism
ARR = Aldosterone–renin ratio
PAC = Plasma aldosterone concentration
CT = Computed tomography
AVS = Adrenal vein sampling
MR = Mineralocorticoid receptor

FIGURE 14-1 Approach to the patient with suspected primary aldosteronism.

○ Various other somatic mutations have been identified in APAs, including *ATP1A1*, *ATP2B3*, and *CACNA1D*. These currently have no clinical implication for treatment.

Diagnostic Testing

Diagnostic testing for primary aldosteronism aims to establish renin-independent aldosterone excess and determines whether the source is uni- or bilateral via the three-step algorithm shown in Figure 14-1[5]:

• Screening for renin-independent aldosterone production
• Confirmation of renin-independent aldosterone production
• Localization of aldosterone production

Laboratories
• **Screening for renin-independent hyperaldosteronism** is recommended in patient groups with a relatively high prevalence, including patients with:
  ○ Sustained blood pressure >150/100 on three measurements
  ○ Blood pressure >140/90 on three antihypertensive drugs (including a diuretic)
  ○ Controlled hypertension on four or more antihypertensives
  ○ Hypertension of any stage associated with spontaneous or diuretic-induced hypokalemia
  ○ Hypertension associated with adrenal incidentaloma
  ○ Hypertension with a family history of early-onset hypertension or cerebrovascular accident at an early age (<40 years)
  ○ Hypertension and sleep apnea
  ○ Hypertension and a first-degree relative with primary aldosteronism[5]

TABLE 14-1	MEDICATIONS THAT MAY AFFECT SCREENING FOR PRIMARY ALDOSTERONISM		
Medications	Effect on PAC	Effect on PRA	Effect on ARR
Diuretics	↑	↑ ↑	↓
β-Blockers, α₂-agonists, NSAIDs, renin inhibitors	↓	↓ ↓	↑
ACE inhibitors, ARBs, Ca-channel blockers, renin inhibitors	↓	↑ ↑	↓

PAC, plasma aldosterone concentration; PRA, plasma renin activity; ARR, aldosterone–renin ratio; NSAID, nonsteroidal anti-inflammatory drug; ACE, angiotensin-converting enzyme; ARB, angiotensin receptor blocker; Ca, calcium.

Adapted from Funder JW, Carey RM, Mantero F, et al. Case detection, diagnosis, and treatment of patients with primary aldosteronism: an endocrine society clinical practice guideline. *J Clin Endocrinol Metab* 2016;101(5):1889–1916.

- Screening for GRA via genetic testing should be considered in patients with confirmed primary aldosteronism and any of the following:
  ○ Onset prior to 20 years of age
  ○ Family history of primary aldosteronism
  ○ Personal or family history of stroke prior to age 40[5]
- Clinicians should ensure that potassium is replete, sodium intake is liberalized, and certain interfering substances are discontinued for at least 4 weeks before proceeding with screening. Interfering medications include diuretics (particularly mineralocorticoid receptor antagonists such as spironolactone) and products derived from licorice root, such as chewing tobacco.
- **The two tests ordered for biochemical screening for primary hyperaldosteronism are the plasma aldosterone concentration (PAC) and the plasma renin activity (PRA). The aldosterone–renin ratio (ARR) can be calculated from these two values and is equal to PAC/PRA. A PAC >20 ng/dL and an ARR >30 (units are ng/dL per ng/mL/hr) used together have a 90% sensitivity and specificity for primary hyperaldosteronism.**[6] Using these values as screening cutoffs is reasonable, though they are not universally agreed upon. Borderline results should be interpreted with caution; testing can be repeated if interference from medications is suspected or patients can proceed directly to confirmatory testing. **Use of the ARR alone without consideration of the PAC may be misleading.** For example, a subset of patients with essential hypertension may have elevated ratios by virtue of very low PRA without concomitant elevation in PAC.
- Many medications (particularly antihypertensives) can interfere with the PAC or ARR. The results of testing should always be interpreted after taking into account potential interference (Table 14-1).[5] For example, angiotensin-converting enzyme (ACE) inhibitors and angiotensin receptor blockers (ARBs) may raise the PRA and lead to a false-negative result for the ARR in patients with primary aldosteronism. However, an elevated ARR in the context of ACE inhibitor or ARB treatment is highly suggestive of primary aldosteronism. If a false screening result is suspected, interfering medications should be discontinued and hydralazine, verapamil, or α-adrenergic blockers such as doxazosin used to control blood pressure. An interpretation of the possible combinations of PAC and PRA can be found in Table 14-2.

TABLE 14-2	DIFFERENTIAL DIAGNOSIS FOR HYPERTENSION AND HYPOKALEMIA	
↑PAC and ↓PRA	↑PRA and ↑PAC	↓PRA and ↓PAC
Primary aldosteronism Aldosterone-producing adrenal adenomas Idiopathic hyperaldosteronism Glucocorticoid-remediable aldosteronism Primary adrenal hyperplasia	**Secondary aldosteronism** Renal artery stenosis Renin-secreting tumor Malignant hypertension Chronic renal disease Aortic coarctation Aortic stenosis	**Mineralocorticoid excess states** 17α-hydroxylase deficiency 11β-hydroxylase deficiency Deoxycorticosterone-secreting tumors

PAC, plasma aldosterone concentration; PRA, plasma renin activity.

- **Confirmation of renin-independent hyperaldosteronism** is made by documenting nonsuppression of aldosterone during sodium loading. Oral and intravenous sodium loading tests are the most commonly used confirmatory tests. The underlying principle is that an increase in intravascular volume should decrease renin release and subsequent aldosterone production in patients without primary aldosteronism. Sodium loading may lead to volume overload, especially in patients with compromised left ventricular function or renal failure, and must be closely monitored. Potassium should be adequately replaced prior to initiation of either test.
  - **Oral sodium loading test:** The patient is instructed to consume 6 g/day of sodium. Potassium must be measured daily and replaced as needed, because sodium loading in patients with primary aldosteronism leads to potassium wasting. A 24-hour urine collection is started no sooner than the 3rd day and assayed for urine aldosterone, sodium, and creatinine. Urine aldosterone excretion >12 to 14 mcg per 24 hours confirms nonsuppressibility of aldosterone. Adequacy of sodium loading is documented by urinary excretion of sodium >200 mEq/day.[5]
  - **Intravenous sodium loading test:** Two liters of normal saline are infused intravenously over 4 hours into the recumbent patient. Potassium repletion should be confirmed before but does not need to be monitored during saline infusion. A PAC >10 ng/dL at 4 hours confirms and a PAC <5 ng/dL refutes the diagnosis of primary aldosteronism. A PAC between 5 ng/dL and 10 ng/dL is considered a "gray zone."[5]
  - **Alternate tests:** The protocols for alternate tests including the fludrocortisone suppression test and captopril challenge test are detailed elsewhere.[5] The use of the fludrocortisone suppression test is limited by the need for inpatient admission for monitoring purposes. The captopril suppression test is an acceptable but less standardized alternative if sodium loading is contraindicated as in heart or renal failure.

Imaging and Diagnostic Procedures

Localization of aldosterone production is essential to direct therapy in patients with primary aldosteronism who desire a surgical cure, because only patients with unilateral disease are likely to derive benefit from surgery. As a rule, imaging is not a reliable way to distinguish unilateral from bilateral disease but should be performed to identify tumors likely to be malignant. Adrenal vein sampling (AVS) remains the localization procedure of choice for patients seeking a surgical cure.

- **Adrenal imaging:** A computed tomography (CT) of the adrenal glands should be performed to identify adrenocortical carcinoma, which tends to be large (>4 cm) and has a characteristic CT appearance. A magnetic resonance imaging (MRI) study can be substituted if CT is contraindicated. Imaging should not be used alone to localize aldosterone production because it cannot reliably distinguish between a unilateral and a bilateral source. For example, IHA and a nonfunctioning adrenal incidentaloma may coexist. In these cases, a unilateral adrenal mass would be detected on imaging, but the source of aldosterone excess would be bilateral. Conversely, APAs may be too small to be detected by CT. In that situation, the presence of "normal" adrenal glands might incorrectly imply a bilateral source of aldosterone excess. Concordance between CT and AVS is only approximately 50%.[7,8]

- **AVS:** AVS is expensive, invasive, and technically difficult, but is 95% sensitive and 100% specific for detection of unilateral disease.[7] Almost all patients will require AVS to localize the source of aldosterone excess. Patients with GRA are an exception to this rule since their disease is always bilateral. Some groups also make an exception for patients younger than age 35 with a solitary unilateral adenoma because nonfunctioning adenomas are less common in this age group.[7,9] AVS involves catheterization of the bilateral adrenal veins. A continuous cosyntropin infusion (50 mcg/hr) may be begun 30 minutes before catheterization and continued throughout the procedure. The infusion stimulates aldosterone and cortisol production, thereby minimizing the effect of stress-induced fluctuations on both aldosterone and cortisol production, avoiding the problem of sampling when an APA might be hormonally silent, and maximizing the cortisol gradient between the adrenal vein and vena cava, which is used to confirm successful placement of the catheter. Blood samples from bilateral adrenal veins and a single peripheral vein are then obtained for the measurement of plasma aldosterone and cortisol. Right and left adrenal aldosterone concentrations should be divided by their respective cortisol concentrations to correct for dilution effects. The right and left cortisolcorrected aldosterone levels can then be compared. A lateralization ratio of more than 4:1 is indicative of unilateral aldosterone excess. A ratio of <3:1 suggests a bilateral source. A ratio between 3:1 and 4:1 is inconclusive. An adrenal/peripheral vein cortisol ratio of 10:1 confirms successful adrenal vein catheterization.

- **Other tests:** Other ancillary tests can be used in cases where AVS is unsuccessful, though none have been validated. As such, many clinicians avoid them altogether and instead repeat AVS or decide between surgical and medical therapy on the basis of clinical evidence or imaging. The postural stimulation test (in which a paradoxical fall in PAC occurs from a supine 8 a.m. sample to a sample obtained after 4 hours of upright posture in the presence of an APA) is used rarely. Adrenal scintigraphy with a ^{131}I-labeled cholesterol analog and measurement of plasma 18-hydroxycorticosterone levels are no longer used in most centers.

TREATMENT

Surgical resection is the treatment of choice for unilateral disease. Medical therapy is the treatment of choice for bilateral disease or for patients with unilateral disease who are poor surgical candidates.

Medications

- **Spironolactone** (12.5 to 400 mg orally daily) is the primary mineralocorticoid receptor antagonist used in the treatment of primary aldosteronism. Although doses up to 400 mg daily have traditionally been used, recent guidelines suggest a maximum dose of 100 mg.[5] Spironolactone is rapidly effective in correcting hypokalemia, but its antihypertensive effects may not be apparent for several weeks. Antiandrogenic side effects, including gynecomastia, erectile dysfunction, impotence, and decreased libido in men and menstrual irregularities in women, limit its tolerability.

- **Eplerenone** (25 to 50 mg orally twice daily) is a newer highly selective mineralocorticoid receptor antagonist currently approved for treatment of essential hypertension. It has less potency than spironolactone but fewer side effects due to its extremely low-binding affinity for both the androgen and progesterone receptors.[10] The improved tolerability of eplerenone needs to be weighed against its greater cost and the lack of clinical trials thus far supporting its use in primary aldosteronism.
- **Amiloride** (5 to 20 mg orally daily) and **triamterene** (100 to 150 mg orally twice daily) are potassium-sparing diuretics that block the aldosterone-sensitive sodium channel in the collecting tubules. They are less efficacious than the mineralocorticoid receptor antagonists but can be considered as adjunct therapy or as monotherapy if other agents are poorly tolerated. Since these agents do not block the aldosterone receptor itself, they do not prevent the deleterious effects of aldosterone on the cardiovascular system. Side effects include dizziness, fatigue, and nausea.
- **Dexamethasone** (0.125 mg orally at bedtime, titrated as needed) and **prednisone** (2.5 mg orally at bedtime, titrated as needed) are the glucocorticoids of choice in the treatment of GRA and work by partially suppressing ACTH secretion by the pituitary. They should not be used for treatment of primary aldosteronism due to other causes. Dexamethasone and prednisone are preferable to hydrocortisone due to their longer half-lives and should be given at bedtime to suppress the early morning ACTH surge. The lowest effective dose should be used to minimize risk for iatrogenic Cushing syndrome. Treatment with a glucocorticoid alone may not be sufficient to normalize blood pressure and the addition of a mineralocorticoid receptor antagonist may be required.
- Other antihypertensive agents may need to be used in combination with a mineralocorticoid receptor antagonist if blood pressure remains uncontrolled.

Surgical Management

- Laparoscopic total adrenalectomy performed by an experienced surgeon is the treatment of choice for unilateral disease because it may eliminate the need for antihypertensive medication, reduce the number of antihypertensives needed, and correct endogenous aldosterone overproduction. Laparoscopic adrenalectomy is associated with shorter hospital stays and lower morbidity than an open approach. Partial adrenalectomy should not be performed because AVS cannot determine whether a single APA or unilateral hyperplasia is the cause of aldosterone excess.
- Preoperative management goals are adequate blood pressure control and correction of hypokalemia. Typically, an aldosterone receptor antagonist is recommended prior to surgery.
- Postoperative management can be guided by PAC, which should be measured to confirm surgical cure shortly after surgery. Serum potassium should be followed, as hypokalemia corrects quickly after adrenalectomy, and supplements should be discontinued. Mineralocorticoid antagonists should be discontinued and other antihypertensive therapy reduced as tolerated based on blood pressure. Maximum improvement in blood pressure is usually achieved in the first 6 months after surgery, but blood pressure can continue to fall for up to 1 year.[5] Because aldosterone production in the remaining adrenal gland can initially be suppressed, a sodium-rich diet and weekly monitoring of serum potassium levels are recommended for the 1st month after surgery.

COMPLICATIONS

- Studies have indicated that long-term exposure to aldosterone excess may lead to structural damage of both the cardiovascular system[11–13] and kidneys[14,15] that is independent of blood pressure. Patients with primary aldosteronism are not only at increased risk for surrogate end points such as left ventricular hypertrophy[16] and diastolic dysfunction,[17] but they are also at increased risk for cardiovascular events[18] as compared to patients with essential hypertension. Aldosterone has also been implicated in the development of endothelial dysfunction[19] and arterial stiffness.[20] Glomerular filtration rate and urinary albumin excretion are both higher in patients with primary aldosteronism than in patients with essential hypertension, and long-term follow-up of these patients suggests that these parameters are reversible with appropriate treatment of the aldosterone excess.[21,22]

OUTCOME/PROGNOSIS

- Although blood pressure improves and serum potassium levels normalize in most patients with surgically treated primary aldosteronism, the presence of pre-existing essential hypertension, end-organ damage, changes in vascular tone, or nephrosclerosis may contribute to postoperative hypertension, which persists in between 40% and 70% of patients despite complete correction of the hyperaldosteronism.[23–25]
- Factors that predict an increased chance for surgical cure include the following: presence of an APA, preoperative response to spironolactone, female gender, younger age (<44 years), shorter duration of hypertension (<5 years), preoperative use of fewer antihypertensives (≤2 agents), higher preoperative ARR, and a family history of hypertension in no more than one first-degree relative.[24–26]
- Clinical trials of treatment of aldosterone excess in primary aldosteronism on morbidity and/or mortality are not currently available.

REFERENCES

1. Mulatero P, Stowasser M, Loh KC, et al. Increased diagnosis of primary aldosteronism, including surgically correctable forms, in centers from five continents. *J Clin Endocrinol Metab* 2004;89(3):1045–1050.
2. Monticone S, Burrello J, Tizzani D, et al. Prevalence and clinical manifestation of primary aldosteronism encountered in primary care practice. *J Am Coll Cardiol* 2017;69(14):1811–1820.
3. Kono T, Ikeda F, Oseko F, Imura H, Tanimura H. Normotensive primary aldosteronism: report of a case. *J Clin Endocrinol Metab* 1981;52(5):1009–1013.
4. Rossi GP, Bernini G, Caliumi C, et al. A prospective study of the prevalence of primary aldosteronism in 1,125 hypertensive patients. *J Am Coll Cardiol* 2006;48(11):2293–2300.
5. Funder JW, Carey RM, Mantero F, et al. Case detection, diagnosis, and treatment of patients with primary aldosteronism: an endocrine society clinical practice guideline. *J Clin Endocrinol Metab* 2016;101(5):1889–1916.
6. Weinberger MH, Fineberg NS. The diagnosis of primary aldosteronism and separation of two major subtypes. *Arch Intern Med* 1993;153(18):2125–2129.
7. Young WF, Stanson AW, Thompson GB, Grant CS, Farley DR, van Heerden JA. Role for adrenal venous sampling in primary aldosteronism. *Surgery* 2004;136(6):1227–1235.
8. Nwariaku FE, Miller BS, Auchus R, et al. Primary hyperaldosteronism: effect of adrenal vein sampling on surgical outcome. *Arch Surg* 2006;141(5):497–502; discussion 502–503.
9. Tan YY, Ogilvie JB, Triponez F, et al. Selective use of adrenal venous sampling in the lateralization of aldosterone-producing adenomas. *World J Surg* 2006;30(5):879–885; discussion 886–887.
10. Parthasarathy HK, Ménard J, White WB, et al. A double-blind, randomized study comparing the antihypertensive effect of eplerenone and spironolactone in patients with hypertension and evidence of primary aldosteronism. *J Hypertens* 2011;29:980–990.
11. Rocha R, Funder JW. The pathophysiology of aldosterone in the cardiovascular system. *Ann N Y Acad Sci* 2002;970:89–100.
12. Savard S, Amar L, Plouin PF, Steichen O. Cardiovascular complications associated with primary aldosteronism: a controlled crosssectional study. *Hypertension* 2013;62:331–336.
13. Mulatero P, Monticone S, Bertello C, et al. Long-term cardio- and cerebrovascular events in patients with primary aldosteronism. *J Clin Endocrinol Metab* 2013;98:4826–4833.
14. Greene EL, Kren S, Hostetter TH. Role of aldosterone in the remnant kidney model in the rat. *J Clin Invest* 1996;98(4):1063–1068.
15. Hollenberg NK. Aldosterone in the development and progression of renal injury. *Kidney Int* 2004;66(1):1–9.

16. Rossi GP, Sacchetto A, Visentin P, et al. Changes in left ventricular anatomy and function in hypertension and primary aldosteronism. *Hypertension* 1996;27(5):1039–1045.

17. Rossi GP, Sacchetto A, Pavan E, et al. Remodeling of the left ventricle in primary aldosteronism due to Conn's adenoma. *Circulation* 1997;95(6):1471–1478.

18. Milliez P, Girerd X, Plouin PF, Blacher J, Safar ME, Mourad JJ. Evidence for an increased rate of cardiovascular events in patients with primary aldosteronism. *J Am Coll Cardiol* 2005;45(8):1243–1248.

19. Taddei S, Virdis A, Mattei P, Salvetti A. Vasodilation to acetylcholine in primary and secondary forms of human hypertension. *Hypertension* 1993;21(6 Pt 2):929–933.

20. Blacher J, Amah G, Girerd X, et al. Association between increased plasma levels of aldosterone and decreased systemic arterial compliance in subjects with essential hypertension. *Am J Hypertens* 1997;10(12 Pt 1):1326–1334.

21. Sechi LA, Novello M, Lapenna R, et al. Long-term renal outcomes in patients with primary aldosteronism. *JAMA* 2006;295(22):2638–2645.

22. Catena C, Colussi G, Nadalini E, et al. Cardiovascular outcomes in patients with primary aldosteronism after treatment. *Arch Intern Med* 2008;168:80–85.

23. Meyer A, Brabant G, Behrend M. Long-term follow-up after adrenalectomy for primary aldosteronism. *World J Surg* 2005;29(2):155–159.

24. Celen O, O'Brien MJ, Melby JC, Beazley RM. Factors influencing outcome of surgery for primary aldosteronism. *Arch Surg* 1996;131(6):646–650.

25. Sawka AM, Young WF, Thompson GB, et al. Primary aldosteronism: factors associated with normalization of blood pressure after surgery. *Ann Intern Med* 2001;135(4):258–261.

26. Williams TA, Lenders JW, Mulatero P, et al. Outcomes after adrenalectomy for unilateral primary aldosteronism: an international consensus on outcome measures and analysis of remission rates in an international cohort. *Lancet Diabetes Endocrinol* 2017;5(9):689–699.

Cushing Syndrome

15

Sobia Sadiq and Julie M. Silverstein

GENERAL PRINCIPLES

- Cushing syndrome (CS) is a clinical condition resulting from prolonged exposure to excessive glucocorticoids from either endogenous or exogenous sources.
- The most common cause of CS is from the administration of exogenous glucocorticoids.

Classification

Cushing syndrome can be divided into two categories based on pathophysiology: adreno-corticotropic hormone (ACTH) dependent or independent (Table 15-1).[1]

- **ACTH-dependent** hypercortisolism is the most common cause of endogenous CS and is most commonly due to an ACTH-secreting pituitary tumor. Other causes include ectopic ACTH syndrome and ectopic corticotropin-releasing hormone (CRH) syndrome.
  - When CS is secondary to an ACTH-secreting pituitary adenoma, it is called **Cushing disease (CD)**, which was originally described by Harvey Cushing in 1932.[2] ACTH secretion from the pituitary adenoma stimulates the overproduction of cortisol from the adrenal glands.
  - Ectopic-ACTH syndromes lead to bilateral adrenocortical hyperplasia and hyperfunction. Small cell lung cancer and neuroendocrine tumors of the lung, thymus, and pancreas are the most common causes of ectopic ACTH secretion.
  - In ectopic CRH syndrome, CRH secretion by the primary tumor causes hyperplasia of pituitary corticotrophs, consequent hypersecretion of ACTH, bilateral adrenal hyperplasia, and finally cortisol hypersecretion. It is extremely rare.[3]
- **ACTH-independent** forms of CS are due to exogenous glucocorticoids or primary adrenal disorders.
  - Iatrogenic CS can be secondary to oral, topical, inhaled, and injectable glucocorticoids. Megestrol acetate, which has intrinsic glucocorticoid activity, has been shown to cause glucocorticoid-like effects in up to 30% of patients treated for long periods of time.[4] The combination of ritonavir, a potent CYP3A4 enzyme inhibitor, and fluticasone can cause CS because of delayed clearance of fluticasone.
  - The most common cause of endogenous ACTH-independent CS is an adrenal adenoma. Other causes include adrenal carcinoma, primary pigmented nodular adrenocortical disease (PPNAD), and adrenocorticotropin-independent macronodular adrenocortical hyperplasia (AIMAH).

Epidemiology

Cushing syndrome is exceedingly rare with an estimated incidence of 0.2 to 5.0 per million people per year and a prevalence of 39 to 79 per million. The median age of onset is 41.4 years with a female-to-male ratio of 3:1.[1]

Associated Conditions

- **Carney complex** is an autosomal-dominant syndrome characterized by micronodular adrenal hyperplasia and pituitary adenomas, testicular and thyroid tumors, cardiac atrial

TABLE 15-1 CAUSES OF ENDOGENOUS CUSHING SYNDROME

Diagnosis	% of patients
ACTH dependent	70–80
Cushing disease (pituitary hypersecretion of ACTH)	60–70
Ectopic ACTH syndrome (nonpituitary tumors)	5–10
Ectopic CRH syndrome (nonhypothalamic tumors causing pituitary hypersecretion of ACTH)	<1
ACTH independent	20–30
Adrenal adenoma	10–22
Adrenal carcinoma	5–7
Micronodular hyperplasia	<2
Macronodular hyperplasia	<2

ACTH, adrenocorticotropic hormone; CRH, corticotropin-releasing hormone.
Adapted from Lacroix A, Feelders RA, Stratakis CA, Nieman LK. Cushing's syndrome. *Lancet* 2015;386:913–927.

myxomas, pigmented lentigines, blue nevi, and schwannomas. Mutations in the *PRKAR1A* gene cause most cases of Carney complex.

- **McCune–Albright syndrome** is characterized by hypercortisolism from hyperplastic adrenal macronodules, as well as café au lait spots and polyostotic fibrous dysplasia.
- Genetic disorders or gene defects associated with CS include[5]:
  - Cushing disease: multiple endocrine neoplasia (MEN1) syndrome
  - Ectopic-ACTH syndrome: *RET* gene mutations
  - Adrenal CS caused by adrenal adenomas: defects in *PRKACA, CTNNB1, GCPR, GNAS1,* and *PRKAR1A* genes
  - Adrenal cortical carcinoma: defects in *p53* (Li–Fraumeni syndrome), *GNAS, MEN1, IGF-II, H-19, CDKI* (Beckwith–Wiedemann syndrome), and adenomatous polyposis coli genes

DIAGNOSIS

Clinical Presentation

- Patients present with a wide spectrum of manifestations ranging from subclinical to overt symptoms, depending on the underlying etiology, and the duration and intensity of excess glucocorticoid production.
- The signs and symptoms of this syndrome are often nonspecific and there are inherent limitations in the diagnostic testing, making the diagnosis of CS one of the most challenging in endocrinology.
- Some of the findings suggestive of CS are presented below (also see Table 15-2).[6] However, it is important to note that none of them are truly pathognomonic of the syndrome, requiring a high degree of clinical suspicion to diagnose CS.
  - **Progressive central obesity** involving the abdomen, face, and neck (buffalo hump, moon facies, supraclavicular fat pads, and exophthalmos from retro-orbital fat deposition).
  - **Metabolic complications** include glucose intolerance (owing to stimulation of gluconeogenesis by cortisol and peripheral insulin resistance caused by obesity) and

TABLE 15-2	SYMPTOMS AND SIGNS IN PATIENTS WITH CUSHING SYNDROME	
Sign/symptom		% of patients
Truncal obesity		95
Facial fullness		90
Gonadal dysfunction (decreased libido)		90
Skin atrophy and bruising		80
Menstrual irregularity		80
Hypertension		75
Hirsutism, acne		75
Mood disorders		70
Muscle weakness		65
Diabetes or glucose intolerance		60
Osteopenia, osteoporosis, fractures		50

Adapted from Newell-Price J, Bertagna X, Grossman AB, Nieman LK. Cushing's syndrome. *Lancet* 2006;367:1605–1617.

hypertension (through poorly understood multifactorial etiologies), both of which confer increased cardiovascular risk, a major cause of morbidity and death in patients with CS.[1] Severe hypertension and hypokalemia are more commonly seen in patients with ectopic ACTH syndrome because the very high serum cortisol levels overwhelm the capacity of the 11β-hydroxysteroid dehydrogenase type 2 enzyme, which oxidizes cortisol to cortisone in renal tubules, thereby resulting in activation of mineralocorticoid receptors.[7]

○ **Hypercoagulability** due to elevated levels of factor VIII, factor IX, and von Willebrand factor and increased thrombin production increases the risk of arterial and venous thrombosis.[6]

○ **Dermatologic manifestations** include skin atrophy (thinning of the stratum corneum), fragile skin with easy bruisability, wide purple striae (due to the stretching of fragile skin), cutaneous fungal infections, and hyperpigmentation (in ectopic ACTH syndrome).

○ **Reproductive changes** in women include menstrual irregularities, hirsutism, oily facial skin with acne, and other signs of virilization (temporal balding, deepening voice), especially in women with adrenal carcinoma. In men, **secondary hypogonadism** with signs and symptoms of low testosterone can occur.

○ **Musculoskeletal manifestations** are proximal myopathy, muscle wasting (resulting from the catabolic effects of excess glucocorticoid on skeletal muscle), and osteoporosis (caused by decreased bone formation, increased bone resorption, and decreased intestinal and renal calcium reabsorption). Vertebral compression fractures, pathologic fractures of the rib or long bones, and aseptic necrosis of the femoral heads may also be present.

○ **Neuropsychiatric changes** can include labile mood, agitated depression, anxiety, panic attacks, mild paranoia, impaired short-term memory and cognition, psychosis, and insomnia.

Differential Diagnosis

• **Nonneoplastic physiologic hypercortisolism (pseudo-Cushing syndrome)** is characterized by mild hypercortisolism and may be difficult to distinguish from true CS.[8,9]

- Phenotype similar to CS: depression, chronic kidney disease, alcoholism, obesity, uncontrolled diabetes mellitus, psychiatric illness, and pregnancy.
  - Absence of clinical features of CS: physiologic stress (hospitalization, trauma, surgery, acute illness), malnutrition, anorexia nervosa, intense chronic exercise, hypothalamic amenorrhea, and states of elevated cortisol-binding protein (pregnancy, estrogen therapy).
  - The distinguishing feature of this disorder is that the laboratory and clinical findings of hypercortisolism disappear if the primary process is successfully treated.
- **Metabolic syndrome** which is characterized by central obesity, hypertension, and glucose intolerance may mimic CS.
- **Polycystic ovarian syndrome** may present with menstrual irregularities and hyperandrogenism (hirsutism, acne) which can be features of CS.
- **Factitious CS** secondary to surreptitious ingestion of corticosteroids is rare and may be difficult to diagnose. Patients often present with clinical features of CS, fluctuating 24-hour urine free cortisol (UFC) levels, and intermittently suppressed ACTH levels. Measurement of corticosteroids by high-performance liquid chromatography tandem mass spectrometry (HPLC-MS/MS) in plasma and urine can be used to confirm the presence of exogenous steroids.[10]

Diagnostic Testing
- Please see Figure 15-1 for diagnostic testing algorithm.[1,6,11]
- The biochemical diagnosis of CS involves **three critical steps:**
  1. Documenting the presence of hypercortisolism. (Does the patient have CS?)
  2. Determining if the cortisol excess is ACTH independent or ACTH dependent. (Does the patient have primary adrenal disease or an ACTH-secreting tumor?)
  3. Determining the source of the ACTH in the ACTH-dependent form. (Does the patient have CD or ectopic ACTH syndrome?)
- **Does the patient have CS?**
  - The **24-hour** UFC measurement is one of the most frequently utilized tests for the diagnosis of CS. The patient can be assumed to have CS if basal urinary cortisol excretion is three to four times higher than the normal range on at least two separate occasions. The evaluation can then proceed to the next step of establishing the cause for the hypercortisolism. If it is equivocally increased—that is, above the upper limit of normal (ULN), but not quite three to four times as much—the patient needs to be reevaluated after several weeks or undergo further testing (see subsequent text and Table 15-3).[9,12,13]
  - The **1-mg overnight dexamethasone suppression test** is another commonly used screening test. Unfortunately, this test is associated with a high false-positive rate (Table 15-4) and it should not be used as the sole criterion for making the diagnosis of CS. Some authors suggest obtaining a dexamethasone level at the same time as cortisol. A low dexamethasone level suggests noncompliance, individual variation in dexamethasone metabolism, or drug effects on dexamethasone metabolism.[9,14]
  - Some endocrinologists prefer to use the 48-hour, 2-mg/day **low-dose dexamethasone suppression test** (LDDST) as a screening test in patients who have conditions associated with overactivation of the hypothalamic–pituitary–adrenal (HPA) axis (e.g., in patients with certain psychiatric conditions, obesity, alcoholism, or diabetes mellitus) because in some studies it has been shown to have a higher specificity than the 1-mg test.[5]
  - The **late-evening salivary cortisol** is another validated screening test with distinct advantages: it is noninvasive, saliva is easily collected, cortisol is stable in saliva even at room temperature for several days, and it can be performed by the patient at home.[9,15]
  - The **CRH-dexamethasone test** may be useful to differentiate patients with Cushing's from those with nonneoplastic physiologic hypercortisolism. Compared to patients with CS, depressed patients continue to show a suppressed plasma cortisol (<1.4 mcg/dL) even after

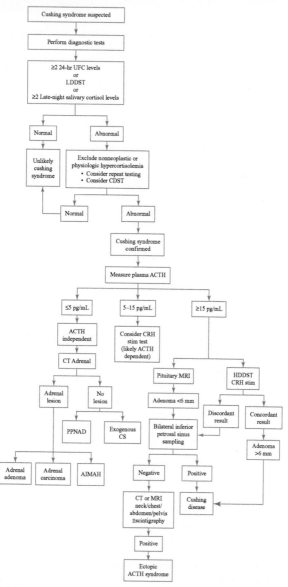

FIGURE 15-1 Diagnosis of Cushing syndrome. UFC, urine free cortisol; LDDST, low-dose dexamethasone suppression test; CDST, corticotropin-releasing hormone (CRH) dexamethasone suppression test; ACTH, adrenocorticotropic hormone; HDDST, high-dose dexamethasone suppression test; AIMAH, ACTH-independent macronodular adrenal hyperplasia; PPNAD, primary pigmented nodular adrenocortical disease; CS, Cushing syndrome. Adapted from Lacroix A, Feelders RA, Stratakis CA, Nieman LK. Cushing's syndrome. *Lancet* 2015;386:913–927; Newell-Price JDC. Cushing disease. In: Melmed S, ed. *The Pituitary.* 4th ed. Academic Press; 2017:515–571; Nieman LK, Biller BMK, Findling JW, et al. The diagnosis of Cushing's syndrome: an endocrine society clinical practice guideline. *J Clin Endocrinol Metab* 2008;93:1526–1540.

TABLE 15-3 BIOCHEMICAL TESTS FOR ESTABLISHING CUSHING SYNDROME

Test	Protocol	Measurements	Criteria	Sensitivity (%)	Specificity (%)
24-hr UFC	24-hr urine collection	Cortisol, creatinine	>3 × ULN	80–98	45–98
1-mg overnight LDDST	Dex, 1 mg PO at 11 p.m.	8 a.m. plasma cortisol	>1.8 mcg/dL	91–97	80–94
			>5 mcg/dL	85–90	95–99
2-day LDDST	Dex, 0.5 mg PO q6h for 48 hrs (last dose 6 a.m.)	8 a.m. plasma cortisol	>1.8 mcg/dL	91–98	70–95
Dex-CRH	Same as 2-day LDDST; CRH, 1 mcg/kg IV at 8 a.m.	Plasma cortisol 15 min after CRH injection	>1.4 mcg/dL	98–100	60–100
Late-evening salivary cortisol	11 p.m. sample	Salivary cortisol	>145 ng/dL	92–100	93–100
Midnight plasma cortisol	Indwelling catheter and hospitalization recommended	Midnight plasma cortisol	>7.5 mcg/dL (awake)	91–98	92–100
			>1.8 mcg/dL (sleeping)	100	30–62

UFC, urine free cortisol; ULN, upper limit of normal; LDDST, low-dose dexamethasone suppression test; Dex, dexamethasone; CRH, corticotropin-releasing hormone.
Data from Sharma ST. An individualized approach to the evaluation of Cushing syndrome. *Endocr Pract* 2017;23:726–737.

TABLE 15-4	CAUSES OF FALSE-POSITIVE AND FALSE-NEGATIVE BIOCHEMICAL TESTS FOR CUSHING SYNDROME	
Test	False positive	False negative
LDDST	Error with timing of dex administration Meds increasing metabolism of dex (phenytoin, rifampin, carbamazepine, pioglitazone) Meds increasing CBG (estrogen, mitotane) Decreased absorption of dex Nonneoplastic physiologic hypercortisolism	Chronic renal failure (GFR <30 mL/min) Meds decreasing metabolism of dex (amiodarone, ciprofloxacin, itraconazole, fluconazole, ritonavir, cimetidine, fluoxetine, diltiazem) Increased sensitivity of the HPA axis to dex
24-hr UFC	High fluid intake Interference with carbamazepine in the HPLC assay Nonneoplastic physiologic hypercortisolism	Cyclic Cushing's Early Cushing's Chronic renal failure Interference with fibrate class of drugs
Late-night salivary cortisol	Improper collection/storage Licorice Chewing tobacco/smoking Brushing teeth before obtaining sample Touching swab with hands	Cyclic Cushing's
Midnight plasma cortisol	Stress from hospitalization or blood draw Critically ill patients Patient not resting/sleeping Not drawn from indwelling line	Cyclic Cushing's

LDDST, low-dose dexamethasone suppression test; dex, dexamethasone; GFR, glomerular filtration rate; CBG, cortisol-binding globulin; HPA, hypothalamic–pituitary–adrenal; UFC, urine free cortisol; HPLC, high-performance liquid chromatography.
Adapted from Sharma ST. An individualized approach to the evaluation of Cushing syndrome. *Endocr Pract* 2017;23:726–737.

CRH infusion, which reflects preserved sensitivity of ACTH secretion to dexamethasone suppression.[8,9]

- **Does the patient have ACTH-independent or ACTH-dependent CS?**
  - Once the biochemical diagnosis of CS has been confirmed, an 8 a.m. plasma **ACTH and cortisol level** should be measured.
  - Undetectable or low levels of ACTH (<5 pg/dL) in a patient with a serum cortisol concentration >15 mcg/dL characterizes a primary adrenal source (ACTH-independent CS). If ACTH-independent CS is suspected, thin-section computed tomography (CT) or magnetic resonance imaging (MRI) of the adrenal glands looking for an adrenal mass is indicated.
  - ACTH levels >15 pg/dL typically indicate an ACTH-dependent cause, and the next step involves a search for the source of the high ACTH (pituitary vs. ectopic).

○ An ACTH level in the 5 to 15 pg/dL range is considered indeterminate and should be repeated. If the ACTH level remains consistently in the indeterminate range, a **CRH stimulation test** can be performed. If after infusion of 1 mcg/kg of CRH the peak ACTH response is blunted (<10 pg/dL), an ACTH-independent (adrenal) cause is likely. However, if there is >50% increase in ACTH from baseline after CRH infusion, an ACTH-dependent cause is then more likely.[16]

- **Does the patient have Cushing disease (CD) or ectopic ACTH syndrome?**
  ○ There can be considerable overlap in ACTH levels between patients with CD and ectopic ACTH syndrome, but the distinction between the two is critical as it significantly influences treatment. Several tests can be utilized to aid in the differentiation between pituitary CD and nonpituitary (ectopic) ACTH syndrome (Table 15-5).[17–19]
  ○ The **high-dose dexamethasone suppression test (HDDST)** takes advantage of the fact that high doses of glucocorticoids partially suppress ACTH secretion from most corticotroph pituitary adenomas whereas most nonpituitary tumors associated with ectopic ACTH are resistant to feedback inhibition (exceptions include carcinoid tumors of the bronchus, thymus, and pancreas). The high-dose test can be administered as a standard 2-day test (2 mg, every 6 hours × 8 doses) or as a single overnight 8-mg dose. If the UFC suppresses >90%, or the plasma cortisol suppresses >50% from baseline, CD is most likely.[1,2,9]
  ○ The **CRH** and **DDAVP stimulation tests** are additional noninvasive tests that can be used to distinguish CD from ectopic ACTH syndrome. Both agents stimulate an increase in ACTH and cortisol in most patients with CD. Because pituitary ACTH secretion is suppressed, most patients with ectopic ACTH syndrome do not respond.
  ○ An **MRI of the pituitary gland** should be obtained in all patients with ACTH-dependent CS. A pituitary mass >6 mm suggests CD. Based on autopsy and MRI studies, the prevalence of pituitary incidentalomas ranges from 10% to 28% in "healthy" individuals[20]; so the presence of a small pituitary adenoma does not confirm CD. In addition, 20% to 58% of patients with CD may not have a visible tumor on MRI.[17]
  ○ **Inferior petrosal sinus sampling (IPSS)** is an invasive procedure that involves measuring the central-to-peripheral ACTH gradient and is considered the gold standard to identify a pituitary versus an ectopic source of ACTH. It is recommended in patients with adenomas <6 mm in size and in patients with discordant test results (i.e., when there is cortisol suppression on HDDST [suggesting CD] in the setting of a negative pituitary MRI). See Table 15-5[17] and Figure 15-1[1,6,11] for more details.

TREATMENT

- Treatment is based on the source of the hypercortisolism, so the need for an accurate diagnosis cannot be overemphasized. The goal of treatment is to reverse the clinical manifestations of hypercortisolism by decreasing cortisol secretion to normal levels.
- In **exogenous CS**, gradual withdrawal of the glucocorticoids is important because most patients on long-term therapy will have some degree of HPA axis suppression with resultant adrenal insufficiency if therapy is abruptly discontinued.
- In **ACTH-independent CS**, adrenal imaging by either CT or MRI will demonstrate unil- or bilateral disease. Patients should be referred for **adrenalectomy**. After unilateral adrenalectomy, patients should receive glucocorticoid replacement until the HPA axis recovers from the prolonged suppressive effects of glucocorticoid excess. Patients with bilateral adrenalectomy require lifelong glucocorticoid and mineralocorticoid replacement.
- In **CD**, a **transsphenoidal microadenectomy** is the treatment of choice for patients with a clearly circumscribed microadenoma. In other cases, subtotal resection of the anterior pituitary may be performed. Options for patients with incomplete resection of the tumor or recurrence include repeat surgery, pituitary radiotherapy with either conventional radiation

TABLE 15-5 TESTS TO DIFFERENTIATE CUSHING DISEASE FROM ECTOPIC ACTH SYNDROME

Test	Cushing disease	Ectopic ACTH syndrome
Clinical presentation	Onset of symptoms gradual; slow progression over many years	Sudden onset of symptoms; rapidly progressive
Hypokalemia	Occurs <10% of cases	Common
24-hr UFC	<10 × ULN	Often >10 × ULN
ACTH level	Usually <200 pg/mL	Usually >200 pg/mL
MRI pituitary	Lesion >6 mm suggests CD	Incidental microadenoma may be present
8-mg overnight HDDST[18] Measure baseline plasma cortisol at 8 a.m.; give dex, 8 mg PO at 11 p.m.; re-draw cortisol 8 a.m. next day	>50% suppression of plasma cortisol SENS 95% SPEC 100% >80% suppression of plasma cortisol SENS 62% SPEC 100%	>50% suppression of plasma cortisol
CRH stimulation test Place an indwelling venous catheter 2 hrs prior to testing. Give CRH 1 mcg/kg IV bolus at 8 a.m.; draw plasma ACTH at −5, −1 min before CRH and +15, +30 min after CRH	≥35–50% increase in ACTH ≥20% increase in cortisol	<35% increase in ACTH <20% increase in cortisol
Desmopressin stimulation test[6,19] Measure baseline, 15, 30, 45, and 60 min serum ACTH and cortisol levels from an indwelling venous catheter after 10-µg IV desmopressin	>35–50% increase in ACTH SENS 84–89% SPEC 40–60%	<35% increase in ACTH
IPSS Simultaneous bilateral inferior petrosal sinus sampling and peripheral sampling for ACTH before and after 100 mcg IV CRH	Pre-CRH: ACTH IPS:P ≥ 2 Post-CRH: ACTH IPS:P ratio ≥3 SENS 97–100% SPEC 100%	Pre-CRH: ACTH IPS:P ratio <2 Post-CRH: ACTH IPS:P ratio <3

ACTH, adrenocorticotropic hormone; UFC, urine free cortisol; ULN, upper limit of normal; CD, Cushing disease; HDDST, high-dose dexamethasone suppression test; dex, dexamethasone; SENS, sensitivity; SPEC, specificity; CRH, corticotropin-releasing hormone; IPSS, inferior petrosal sinus sampling; IPS:P, inferior petrosal sinus to peripheral ratio.

Adapted from Sharma ST. An individualized approach to the evaluation of Cushing syndrome. *Endocr Pract* 2017;23:726–737; Aytug S, Laws ER Jr, Vance ML. Assessment of the utility of the high-dose dexamethasone suppression test in confirming the diagnosis of Cushing disease. *Endocr Pract* 2012;18:152–157; and Terzolo M, Reimondo G, Alì A, et al. The limited value of the desmopressin test in the diagnostic approach to Cushing's syndrome. *Clin Endocrinol (Oxf)* 2001;54:609–616.

or stereotactic radiation, bilateral adrenalectomy, or medical therapy. Pituitary irradiation may not control hypercortisolism for months to years, and patients require medical therapy until the full effects of the radiation are seen. Surgical cure with transsphenoidal adenectomy can be assessed by postoperative morning cortisol and ACTH levels, which are undetectable with successful complete resection of the tumor. After transsphenoidal resection of the adenoma, patients require glucocorticoid replacement until recovery of the HPA axis.

- **Ectopic ACTH-dependent CS** should be confirmed with imaging studies, including CT, MRI, and/or scintigraphy (e.g., ^{68}Ga-DOTATATE). Tumors that can be localized by imaging studies should be removed surgically. If the source is an occult tumor or if there is metastatic disease, medical therapy or bilateral adrenalectomy is recommended.[20]

Medications

Medications to decrease cortisol production or inhibit the action of cortisol can be used in patients when surgery is contraindicated, to control hypercortisolism prior to surgery, to treat persistent or recurrent disease, and as bridge therapy until radiation has had its full effect in patients with CD. Medical therapy is also used in patients with ectopic ACTH-dependent CS with inoperable or undetectable tumors. Medications include pituitary-targeted therapy (CD only), adrenal enzyme inhibitors, and glucocorticoid receptor antagonists.

- Pituitary-targeted medications
  - Approximately 80% of corticotroph pituitary adenomas express dopamine receptor D_2. **Cabergoline**, at doses between 1 and 7 mg/wk (median 2 to 3.5 mg/wk), has been shown to lead to biochemical control in 25% to 40% of patients with CD.[21] Up to one-third of patients, however, develop escape and may need to be switched to alternate therapy.[22] In addition, the combination of ketoconazole and cabergoline has been shown to control hypercortisolism in up to 80% of patients not controlled on monotherapy with ketoconazole or cabergoline alone.[23] For side effects, see Chapter 2 (Prolactinoma).
  - **Pasireotide**, a somatostatin receptor ligand also used in the treatment of acromegaly (see Chapter 3), binds four of the five somatostatin receptors with highest affinity for somatostatin receptor type 5 (SSTR5), which is predominantly expressed in corticotroph adenomas. It is approved in a twice-daily SC formulation for treatment of CD and can be considered for patients with mild elevations in 24-hour UFC with persistent or recurrent CD or for newly diagnosed patients who are not candidates for surgery. After 6 months of treatment, approximately 50% of patients with mild CD, defined by 24-hour UFC >1.5–2 × the ULN, 26% of patients with moderate CD (24-hour UFC >2–5 × ULN), and 8% of patients with severe CD (24-hour UFC >5 × ULN) normalized their 24-hour UFC.[24] Pasireotide may also be considered if a large tumor is present that is unlikely to be completely removed by surgery or if an experienced neurosurgeon is not available as it has been shown to lead to a >25% tumor reduction in patients.[25] Patients should be started on 600 or 900 mcg SC twice daily with dose adjustments in 300-mcg increments based on 24-hour UFC levels and clinical response. Reduction of cortisol levels occurs within the first 2 months and thus patients likely to respond can be identified early. Incidence of hyperglycemia-related adverse events in clinical trials was higher in patients with CD (68.4% to 73%) than in patients with acromegaly (57.3% to 67%), possibly due to differences in underlying disease pathophysiology.[26] For additional side effects see Chapter 3 (Acromegaly).
  - **Pasireotide** may be used in combination with **cabergoline** and/or **ketoconazole** in patients not responsive to monotherapy. In a prospective trial of 17 patients with CD, 29% normalized 24-hour UFC with pasireotide alone, 24% with combination of pasireotide

and cabergoline, and 35% with the combination of pasireotide, cabergoline, and keto-conazole.[27]

- **Steroidogenesis inhibitors**
  - **Adrenal steroidogenesis inhibitors** inhibit key enzymes involved in steroidogenesis and can be used to treat any cause of endogenous CS.
  - **Ketoconazole** is an antifungal agent that inhibits side-chain cleavage, 17,20-lyase, and 11β-hydroxylase enzymes. Studies show normalization of 24-hour UFC in 50% of patients.[28] Ketoconazole has a black box warning in the United States because of the risk of liver toxicity, its most serious side effect, and it is contraindicated in patients with liver disease. Liver enzymes (LFTs) should be monitored every week for 1 month after each dose change, then monthly for 3 months, and periodically afterward. In a study including 190 patients with CS, 13% of patients had LFT elevations <5 × ULN, 2.5% had elevations >5 × ULN, all LFTs returned to baseline after dose decrease or discontinuation, and there were no cases of fatal hepatitis.[29] Other side effects include gynecomastia, impotence, and gastrointestinal symptoms. Doses range from 200 to 1,200 mg orally daily in two to three divided doses.
  - **Metyrapone** inhibits 11β-hydroxylase and is not widely available in the United States. It leads to biochemical normalization in 52% of patients,[30] is fast acting, and safest to use in pregnancy. Major side effects include increased androgens, hypertension, and hypokalemia through increased 11-deoxycorticosterone. Doses range from 250 to 1,000 mg orally and it is given every 6 hours.
  - **Etomidate** blocks multiple enzymes in steroidogenesis such as side-chain cleavage, 17-hydroxylase, 11β-hydroxylase, 17,20-lyase enzymes, and aldosterone synthase and is the only agent available IV. It can be used to rapidly control hypercortisolism in patients with severe complications of CS such as psychosis, sepsis, or hypertension.
  - **Mitotane** inhibits cholesterol side-chain cleavage enzyme and 11β-hydroxylase. Mitotane induces permanent destruction of adrenocortical cells and therefore can be used to achieve medical adrenalectomy as an alternative to surgical adrenalectomy. It is most commonly used in the treatment of adrenocortical carcinoma. In a retrospective study conducted in France, remission occurred in 73% of patients with CD treated for a median duration of 6.7 months.[22] Glucocorticoid replacement is started at initiation of mitotane treatment and mineralocorticoid treatment may eventually be required. Side effects are generally dose dependent and include gastrointestinal symptoms, weakness, lethargy, leukopenia, gynecomastia, and hypercholesterolemia. Doses start at 0.5 g orally at bedtime and are increased slowly to 2 to 3 g/day in three to four divided doses. Mitotane levels can be monitored to assess efficacy.
  - The combination of **mitotane, metyrapone**, and **ketoconazole** for treatment of patients with severe ACTH-dependent CS not candidates for adrenalectomy was shown to lead to rapid decreases in cortisol and clinical improvement in a study that included 11 patients.[25]
- **Glucocorticoid receptor antagonists**
  - **Mifepristone (RU486)** is a glucocorticoid and progesterone receptor antagonist with three times the binding affinity for the glucocorticoid receptor than dexamethasone and more than 10 times the binding affinity than that of cortisol. In the United States, it is approved for treatment of CS (from any cause) in patients with diabetes or impaired glucose tolerance who have failed surgery or are not candidates for surgery. In our opinion, mifepristone can be considered in patients who do not have diabetes as well. It can also be considered in patients where rapid reductions in cortisol are needed such as in patients with ectopic ACTH syndrome with severe manifestations of hypercortisolism or to improve metabolic parameters in patients before surgery.
  - Mifepristone is associated with improvement in clinical manifestations of CS in 75% of patients, improvements in glucose tolerance in 60%, and improvement in blood pressure

in 40%.[25] In long-term follow-up of 36 patients with CD and MRI data in the pivotal SEISMIC trial, 4 (3 with macroadenomas) had tumor progression and 2 had tumor regression and thus MRI scans should be monitored for tumor growth.[31]

○ Mifepristone has a rapid onset of action (1 to 4 hours) and a long half-life (24 to 90 hours) and is thus dosed once daily. Patients should be started on 300 mg daily with the dose increased by 300-mg/day increments every 2 to 4 weeks based on clinical response to a maximum dose of 1,200 mg daily.

○ Because of its mechanism of action, ACTH and cortisol levels increase and cannot be monitored in patients with CD or ectopic CS. In patients with adrenal CS, a decrease in ACTH can be used as a surrogate marker of clinical response. Cortisol excess leads to activation of the mineralocorticoid receptor and results in increases in blood pressure, hypokalemia, and edema and many patients thus require high doses of an aldosterone receptor antagonist and potassium supplementation. Other side effects include nausea, fatigue, headaches, arthralgia, and endometrial hyperplasia and vaginal bleeding in women.

• **Investigational medications:** Medications currently being investigated include osilodrostat (LCI699), an inhibitor of 11β-hydroxylase and aldosterone synthase,[28] levoketoconazole, a 2S,4R enantiomer of ketoconazole,[28] and CORT125134, a selective glucocorticoid hormone antagonist.[32]

SPECIAL CONSIDERATIONS

• **Nelson syndrome** can occur due to loss of negative feedback in patients with refractory CD (pituitary adenoma) treated with bilateral adrenalectomy. It results in enlargement of residual tumor and extreme elevations in serum ACTH levels. Patients develop hyperpigmentation associated with the high ACTH levels. It is not clear whether or not pituitary irradiation before or after bilateral adrenalectomy prevents this syndrome.[33]

• There have been rare cases of CS during pregnancy. **Pregnant patients** may be treated effectively with transsphenoidal surgery (for CD) or bilateral adrenalectomy. In addition, metyrapone and cabergoline may be used to treat hypercortisolism during pregnancy.[34]

PROGNOSIS

• Mortality in CS is increased with a standard mortality ratio (SMR) roughly between 2.0 and 4.0[1] with most deaths resulting from cardiovascular/thromboembolic complications or bacterial/fungal infections. Effective therapy, either by surgical cure or by pharmacologic control of hypercortisolism, leads to gradual improvement in the symptoms and signs of CS over a period of 2 to 12 months. Hypertension, glucose intolerance, osteoporosis, and psychiatric symptoms generally improve but may not resolve completely.

• The remission rate after transsphenoidal surgery for CD is 78% with a mean follow-up duration of 64 months and the rate of recurrence is up to 32%.[35] Cure is likely if the patient develops hypocortisolism in the first few days to weeks after surgery. A postoperative nadir morning plasma cortisol <2 to 5 mcg/dL within a few days of surgery has a 90 to 100% positive predictive value for remission.[36,37] Since some patients with low postoperative cortisol levels recur, lifelong follow-up is needed.

• Recovery of the HPA axis in patients cured after transsphenoidal surgery may be delayed up to 2 years and patients thus require repeat testing of their HPA axis to determine the potential need for lifetime exogenous steroid replacement therapy. Patients with panhypopituitarism subsequent to surgery require lifetime monitoring and titration of hormone replacement therapy.

• Reported remission rates for radiosurgery in patients with CD vary between 0% and 100% (mean 51%) with the mean time interval to biochemical remission of 12 months.

Because of the higher doses used to treat functional tumors, the rate of hypopituitarism is higher (up to 69%) in patients with CD as compared to nonfunctional tumors.[38]
- Patients with ectopic ACTH secretion or adrenocortical carcinoma may have a poor prognosis associated with the underlying malignancy. These patients are rarely cured, but the hypercortisolism can be controlled with medications or bilateral adrenalectomy.

REFERENCES

1. Lacroix A, Feelders RA, Stratakis CA, Nieman LK. Cushing's syndrome. *Lancet* 2015;386: 913–927.
2. Pivonello R, De Martino MC, De Leo M, Lombardi G, Colao A. Cushing's syndrome. *Endocrinol Metab Clin North Am* 2008;37:135–149.
3. Shahani S, Nudelman RJ, Nalini R, Kim HS, Samson SL. Ectopic corticotropin-releasing hormone (CRH) syndrome from metastatic small cell carcinoma: a case report and review of the literature. *Diagn Pathol* 2010;5:56. http://www.diagnosticpathology.org. Accessed October 25, 2017.
4. Vassiliadi D, Tsagarakis S. Unusual causes of Cushing's syndrome. *Arq Bras Endocrinol Metabol* 2007;51:1245–1252.
5. Pappachan JM, Hariman C, Edavalath M, Waldron J, Hanna FW. Cushing's syndrome: a practical approach to diagnosis and differential diagnoses. *J Clin Pathol* 2017;70:350–359.
6. Newell-Price JDC. Cushing disease. In: Melmed S, ed. *The Pituitary*. 4th ed. Academic Press; 2017:515–571.
7. Carroll TB, Aron DC, Findling JW, Tyrrell JB. Glucocorticoids and adrenal androgens. In: Gardner DG, Shoback D, eds. *Greenspan's Basic & Clinical Endocrinology*. 10th ed. McGraw-Hill Education; 2018.
8. Findling JW, Raff H. Diagnosis of endocrine disease: differentiation of pathologic/neoplastic hypercortisolism (Cushing's syndrome) from physiologic/non-neoplastic hypercortisolism (formerly known as pseudo-Cushing's syndrome). *Eur J Endocrinol* 2017;176:R205–R216.
9. Nieman LK, Biller BMK, Findling JW, et al. The diagnosis of Cushing's syndrome: an Endocrine Society Clinical Practice Guideline. *J Clin Endocrinol Metab* 2008;93:1526–1540.
10. Thynne T, White GH, Burt MG. Factitious Cushing's syndrome masquerading as Cushing's disease. *Clin Endocrinol (Oxf)* 2014;80:328–332.
11. Nieman LK, Biller BMK, Findling JW, et al. Treatment of Cushing's Syndrome: an Endocrine Society Clinical Practice Guideline. *J Clin Endocrinol Metab* 2015;100:2807–2831.
12. Pecori Giraldi F, Ambrogio AG, De Martin M, Fatti LM, Scacchi M, Cavagnini F. Specificity of first-line tests for the diagnosis of Cushing's syndrome: assessment in a large series. *J Clin Endocrinol Metab* 2007;92:4123–4129.
13. Elamin MB, Murad MH, Mullan R, et al. Accuracy of diagnostic tests for Cushing's syndrome: a systematic review and metaanalyses. *J Clin Endocrinol Metab* 2008;93:1553–1562.
14. Ueland GÅ, Methlie P, Kellmann R, et al. Simultaneous assay of cortisol and dexamethasone improved diagnostic accuracy of the dexamethasone suppression test. *Eur J Endocrinol* 2017;176: 705–713.
15. Yorke E, Atiase Y, Akpalu J, Sarfo-Kantanka O. Screening for Cushing syndrome at the primary care level: what every general practitioner must know. *Int J Endocrinol* 2017;2017:1547358.
16. Invitti C, Pecori Giraldi F, de Martin M, Cavagnini F. Diagnosis and management of Cushing's syndrome: results of an Italian multicentre study. Study Group of the Italian Society of Endocrinology on the Pathophysiology of the Hypothalamic-Pituitary-Adrenal Axis. *J Clin Endocrinol Metab* 1999;84:440–448.
17. Sharma ST; AACE Adrenal Scientific Committee. An individualized approach to the evaluation of Cushing syndrome. *Endocr Pract* 2017;23:726–737.
18. Aytug S, Laws ER Jr, Vance ML. Assessment of the utility of the high-dose dexamethasone suppression test in confirming the diagnosis of Cushing disease. *Endocr Pract* 2012;18:152–157.
19. Terzolo M, Reimondo G, Alì A, et al. The limited value of the desmopressin test in the diagnostic approach to Cushing's syndrome. *Clin Endocrinol (Oxf)* 2001;54:609–616.
20. Iglesias P, Arcano K, Triviño V, et al. Prevalence, clinical features, and natural history of incidental clinically non-functioning pituitary adenomas. *Horm Metab Res* 2017;49:654–659.
21. Ferriere A, Cortet C, Chanson P, et al. Cabergoline for Cushing's disease: a large retrospective multicenter study. *Eur J Endocrinol* 2017;176:305–314.

22. Cuevas-Ramos D, Lim DST, Fleseriu M. Update on medical treatment for Cushing's disease. *Clin Diabetes Endocrinol* 2016;2:16. https://clindiabetesendo.biomedcentral.com. Accessed October 25, 2017.

23. Barbot M, Albiger N, Ceccato F, et al. Combination therapy for Cushing's disease: effectiveness of two schedules of treatment: should we start with cabergoline or ketoconazole? *Pituitary* 2014;17:109–117.

24. Colao A, Petersenn S, Newell-Price J, et al. A 12-month phase 3 study of pasireotide in Cushing's disease. *N Engl J Med* 2012;366:914–924.

25. Pivonello R, De Leo M, Cozzolino A, Colao A. The treatment of Cushing's disease. *Endocr Rev* 2015;36:385–486.

26. Silverstein JM. Hyperglycemia induced by pasireotide in patients with Cushing's disease or acromegaly. *Pituitary* 2016;19:536–543.

27. Feelders RA, de Bruin C, Pereira AM, et al. Pasireotide alone or with cabergoline and ketoconazole in Cushing's disease. *N Engl J Med* 2010;362:1846–1848.

28. Fleseriu M, Castinetti F. Updates on the role of adrenal steroidogenesis inhibitors in Cushing's syndrome: a focus on novel therapies. *Pituitary* 2016;19:643–653.

29. Castinetti F, Guignat L, Giraud P, et al. Ketoconazole in Cushing's disease: is it worth a try? *J Clin Endocrinol Metab* 2014;99:1623–1630.

30. Daniel E, Aylwin S, Mustafa O, et al. Effectiveness of metyrapone in treating Cushing's syndrome: a retrospective multicenter study in 195 patients. *J Clin Endocrinol Metab* 2015;100:4146–4154.

31. Fleseriu M, Findling JW, Koch CA, Schlaffer SM, Buchfelder M, Gross C. Changes in plasma ACTH levels and corticotroph tumor size in patients with Cushing's disease during long-term treatment with the glucocorticoid receptor antagonist mifepristone. *J Clin Endocrinol Metab* 2014;99: 3718–3727.

32. Hunt H, Donaldson K, Strem M, et al. Assessment of safety, tolerability, pharmacokinetics, and pharmacological effect of orally administered CORT125134: an adaptive, double-blind, randomized, placebo-controlled phase 1 clinical study. *Clin Pharmacol Drug Dev* 2018;7:408–421.

33. Ritzel K, Beuschlein F, Mickisch A, et al. Clinical review: Outcome of bilateral adrenalectomy in Cushing's syndrome: a systematic review. *J Clin Endocrinol Metab* 2013;98:3939–3948.

34. Caimari F, Valassi E, Garbayo P, et al. Cushing's syndrome and pregnancy outcomes: a systematic review of published cases. *Endocrine* 2017;55:555–563.

35. Pivonello R, De Martino MC, De Leo M, Simeoli C, Colao A. Cushing's disease: the burden of illness. *Endocrine* 2017;56:10–18.

36. Hameed N, Yedinak CG, Brzana J, et al. Remission rate after transsphenoidal surgery in patients with pathologically confirmed Cushing's disease, the role of cortisol, ACTH assessment and immediate reoperation: a large single center experience. *Pituitary* 2013;16:452–458.

37. Ayala A, Manzano AJ. Detection of recurrent Cushing's disease: proposal for standardized patient monitoring following transsphenoidal surgery. *J Neurooncol* 2014;119:235–242.

38. Ding D, Starke RM, Sheehan JP. Treatment paradigms for pituitary adenomas: defining the roles of radiosurgery and radiation therapy. *J Neurooncol* 2014;117:445–457.

Pheochromocytoma and Paraganglioma

16

Sudhir Singh and Cynthia J. Herrick

GENERAL PRINCIPLES

- Although adrenal (pheochromocytoma) and extra-adrenal (paraganglioma) tumors can present in a similar fashion, they are distinct in association with malignancy and genetic predisposition to various syndromes.
- The term pheochromocytoma comes from the Greek words phaios, meaning "dusky," and chromo, meaning "color." The first description of a pheochromocytoma is credited to Frankel, who reported finding bilateral adrenal tumors on autopsy in an 18-year-old woman in 1886.
- New evidence suggests that up to 40% of patients with pheochromocytoma/paraganglioma have a germline mutation and 10% to 15% are metastatic.[1] All patients should be considered for genetic testing.[2]

Definition

- Pheochromocytomas are neuroendocrine tumors arising from catecholamine-producing chromaffin cells of the adrenal medulla.
- Tumors arising from extra-adrenal chromaffin tissue (sympathetic or parasympathetic ganglia) are paragangliomas.[3]

Classification

- Pheochromocytoma is more common than paraganglioma, with extra-adrenal tumors comprising only 15% to 20% of cases.[1]
- Adrenal tumors are usually benign and secrete both epinephrine and norepinephrine in at least half of all cases. Extra-adrenal paragangliomas can be either sympathetic or parasympathetic in origin. Sympathetic paragangliomas mostly secrete catecholamines. They are located in the chest, abdomen, and pelvis—often at the junction of inferior vena cava and left renal vein or at the organ of Zuckerkandl. Parasympathetic paragangliomas are usually found in the base of the skull and neck, near the carotids and are mostly nonsecretory.[4,5]
- Tumors can also be classified as sporadic (solitary, unilateral, and intra-adrenal) or familial (also typically intra-adrenal, but often multicentric and bilateral).

Epidemiology

- The prevalence of pheochromocytoma in patients with hypertension is 0.1% to 0.6%.[6]
- Approximately 5% of all asymptomatic adrenal incidentalomas >1 cm in size are pheochromocytomas.[7]
- Most pheochromocytomas are sporadic, but up to 40% have germline susceptibility mutations.[1]
- Prevalence of pheochromocytoma is approximately 40% in multiple endocrine neoplasia (MEN)2A, 10% in von Hippel–Lindau (VHL), and 5% in neurofibromatosis type 1 (NF1).[8]
- Prevalence of metastases ranges from 2% to 13% in pheochromocytoma and 2% to 50% for paraganglioma.[9]

Etiology

- Pheochromocytomas can occur in the context of autosomal dominant hereditary syndromes with 40% of cases now thought to have hereditary basis.[10]
- Germline mutations in various genes are responsible for familial pheochromocytomas: the *RET* proto-oncogene in MEN2 and tumor suppressor genes *VHL* in von Hippel–Lindau syndrome and *NF1* in neurofibromatosis. Genes encoding the A, B, C, and D subunits of mitochondrial succinate dehydrogenase (*SDHA, SDHB, SDHC,* and *SDHD*) and a gene involved in flavination of SDHA (*SDHAF2*) are implicated in familial nonsyndromic paragangliomas and pheochromocytomas.[11,12]
- More recently, germline mutation of *FP/TMEM127*, the *MAX* tumor suppressor gene, and an isocitrate dehydrogenase mutation have been associated with pheochromocytoma and paraganglioma.[13]

Pathophysiology

- Most of the norepinephrine produced and released by sympathetic nerves is metabolized within the nerves by monoamine oxidase (MAO) to dihydroxyphenylglycol (DHPG).
- Vanillylmandelic acid (VMA), the major end product of norepinephrine and epinephrine metabolism, is produced almost exclusively from metabolism by the liver of circulating catecholamines and their metabolites. The majority of VMA is derived from circulating DHPG and 3-methoxy-4-hydroxyphenylglycol (MHPG), most of which is derived from neuronal norepinephrine metabolism, which explains why VMA is a relatively insensitive marker for pheochromocytoma.
- Approximately 90% of metanephrines and up to 40% of normetanephrines are formed from metabolism of epinephrine and norepinephrine within the adrenals before release into the circulation, making it the single largest source in the body.[14]
- Over 94% of elevated plasma normetanephrines and metanephrines are derived from metabolism of catecholamines by catechol-0-methyltransferase (COMT) within the tumor cells independent of catecholamine release, which supports measuring metanephrines and normetanephrines in diagnosing pheochromocytoma.[15]

DIAGNOSIS

Clinical Presentation

History

- Patients with pheochromocytoma often experience characteristic paroxysms or crises caused by the release of catecholamines.
- The classic symptomatic triad includes episodes of headache (60% to 90%), sweating (55% to 75%), and palpitations (50% to 70%).[6]
- Hypertension is the most common feature and occurs in up to 90% of patients and is paroxysmal in 30%.[6]
- Other less frequent symptoms include pallor (40% to 45%), nausea (20% to 40%), fatigue (25% to 40%), panic attacks (20% to 40%), weight loss (20% to 40%), hyperglycemia (40%), and orthostatic hypotension (10% to 50%).[6]
- Patients with pheochromocytoma may also be completely asymptomatic. Retrospective case series from large centers document incidental discovery on imaging in 10% to 58% of cases.[16–18] Therefore, the diagnosis of pheochromocytoma requires a high index of suspicion, especially in patients with one or more of the following:
  - Refractory hypertension and/or onset of hypertension before 20 years of age;
  - Nonexertional palpitations, spells, diaphoresis, headache, or tremor;
  - Familial syndrome (e.g., MEN2, NF1, VHL) or a family history of pheochromocytoma;

○ Incidental adrenal mass with imaging characteristics consistent with pheochromocytoma (marked enhancement on contrast CT or high-signal intensity on T2-weighted MRI);

○ Hypertensive response during anesthesia and surgery;

○ Idiopathic dilated cardiomyopathy;

○ A history of gastrointestinal stromal tumor or pulmonary chondromas (Carney triad).

- Paroxysms associated with pheochromocytoma may be precipitated by displacement of abdominal contents (e.g., lifting or palpation). Typically, paroxysms last **30 to 40 minutes** and occur **every 1 to 2 days**. Paroxysms tend to increase in frequency and severity over time. Blood pressure can be extremely elevated when measured during a paroxysm.

- Several classes of medications may precipitate a hypertensive crisis in the setting of pheochromocytoma: dopamine (D_2) antagonists, β-adrenergic receptor blockers, sympathomimetics, opioid analgesics, tricyclic antidepressants, selective serotonin reuptake inhibitors, MAO inhibitors, corticosteroids, adrenocorticotropic hormone (ACTH), glucagon, and neuromuscular blockers. These drugs should be avoided until pheochromocytoma has been excluded or resected or the patient has been premedicated with an α-adrenergic antagonist.[2]

Physical Examination

- Hypertension is the most common physical examination finding in pheochromocytoma. It is usually severe, refractory to conventional therapy, and associated with signs of end-organ damage such as proteinuria or retinopathy; however, it may also resemble essential hypertension in the absence of paroxysms.

- Rare presentations include episodic hypotension (when the tumor secretes only epinephrine) or rapid cyclic fluctuations of blood pressure.

Diagnostic Criteria

Definitive diagnosis of pheochromocytoma is made by a biochemical evaluation followed by anatomical and functional imaging to localize the tumor.

Differential Diagnosis[6]

- Endocrine: hyperthyroidism, carcinoid, hypoglycemia, medullary thyroid carcinoma, mastocytosis or mast cell activation syndrome, menopausal symptoms

- Cardiovascular: heart failure, arrhythmias, ischemic heart disease, baroreflex failure

- Neurologic: migraine, stroke, meningioma, postural orthostatic tachycardia syndrome (POTS)

- Miscellaneous: porphyria, panic disorder or anxiety, use of sympathomimetic drugs, MAO inhibitors, clonidine withdrawal, illicit drugs (i.e., cocaine)

Diagnostic Testing

There are two essential components to the diagnosis of pheochromocytoma: (a) **biochemical confirmation**, and subsequently (b) **anatomic localization of the tumor**.

Laboratories

- Diagnosis of pheochromocytoma requires biochemical evidence of excessive catecholamine production by the tumor, which is achieved by measurements of catecholamines and certain catecholamine metabolites in plasma or urine (Table 16-1).[19-21]

- The potentially fatal consequences of a missed diagnosis necessitate the need for a laboratory test with high degree of sensitivity. Plasma-free metanephrines and urinary fractionated metanephrines have been shown to offer the highest sensitivity for diagnosis of pheochromocytoma, and are recommended as the initial test.[2,3]

| TABLE 16-1 | PERFORMANCE CHARACTERISTICS OF BIOCHEMICAL ASSAYS FOR PHEOCHROMOCYTOMA | |

Test	Sensitivity (%)	Specificity (%)
NIH series[19]		
Plasma		
Free metanephrines	99	89
Catecholamines	84	81
24-hr urine		
Fractionated metanephrines	97	69
Total metanephrines	77	93
Catecholamines	86	88
Vanillylmandelic acid	64	95
Mayo series[20]		
Plasma-free metanephrines	97	85
24-hr urine total metanephrines and catecholamines	90	98
Perry et al.[21]	97	91
24-hr urine fractionated metanephrines		

Lenders JW, Pacak K, Walther MM, et al. Biochemical diagnosis of pheochromocytoma: which test is best? *JAMA* 2002;287(11):1427–1434. Sawka AM, Jaeschke R, Singh RJ, et al. A comparison of biochemical tests for pheochromocytoma: measurement of fractionated plasma metanephrines compared with the combination of 24-hour urinary metanephrines and catecholamines. *J Clin Endocrinol Metab* 2003;88(2):553–558; and Perry CG, Sawka AM, Singh R, et al. The diagnostic efficacy of urinary fractionated metanephrines measured by tandem mass spectrometry in detection of pheochromocytoma. *Clin Endocrinol (Oxf)* 2007;66(5):703–708.

- Dietary factors, drugs, or inappropriate sampling conditions can interfere with biochemical testing (Table 16-2).[6] These confounders can be avoided by fasting and abstaining from beverages containing caffeine overnight before blood draws. Patients should also be placed supine for at least 30 minutes before sampling to avoid false-positive results.[22]
- Tricyclic antidepressants and phenoxybenzamine are major causes of false-positive results on urinary and plasma normetanephrine and norepinephrine (see Table 16-2).[23]
- Measurement of fractionated metanephrines using liquid chromatography with mass spectrometric or electrochemical detection methods is preferred over enzyme immunoassay.[2]
- The high sensitivity of these biochemical tests means that negative test results essentially rule out pheochromocytoma; however, a positive test does not always reliably indicate disease. Most true-positive results can be distinguished from false positives by the magnitude of increases in test results above the reference range. Biochemical parameters are typically elevated more than twofold to threefold above normal when a pheochromocytoma is present.
- Positive test results that are not twofold to threefold above normal should be evaluated with clinical judgment, based on pre-test probability for disease.[23]
- Before further investigation, careful consideration of the various causes of false-positive results from medications and other factors is warranted.
- The clonidine suppression test may be useful when plasma catecholamines are elevated but nondiagnostic. In one series, using persistent elevation of normetanephrine and lack of suppression of normetanephrine by >40% after clonidine yielded the best sensitivity

TABLE 16-2 FACTORS INTERFERING WITH BIOCHEMICAL TESTING[2]

Stimulation of endogenous catecholamines	Exogenous catecholamines	Drugs that alter catecholamine metabolism	Drugs that interfere with biochemical assays
• Emotional and physical stress (surgery, trauma) • Drug withdrawal (alcohol, clonidine) • Drugs (vasodilators, caffeine, nicotine, theophylline, ephedrine, amphetamines) • Hypoglycemia • Obstructive sleep apnea • Myocardial ischemia • Stroke	• Bronchodilators • Appetite suppressants • Decongestants	• β-Blockers (falsely increases urine catecholamines and metanephrines) • Phenoxybenzamine (falsely increases plasma and urine norepinephrine and normetanephrine) • Tricyclic antidepressants (falsely increases plasma and urine norepinephrine and normetanephrine) • Levodopa • Theophylline • MAO inhibitors	• Labetalol, sotalol[a] • Acetaminophen[b] • Clofibrate • Quinidine

[a]Interference only with the spectrophotometric assay for metanephrines; catecholamines measured by HPLC and metanephrines by mass spectrometry are not affected.
[b]Plasma-free metanephrines measured by HPLC are not affected.
Diuretics, ACE inhibitors, and SSRIs generally do not interfere with the biochemical tests.
ACE, angiotensin-converting enzyme; HPLC, high-performance liquid chromatography; MAO, monoamine oxidase; SSRIs, selective serotonin reuptake inhibitors.
Lenders JW, Duh QY, Eisenhofer G, et al. Pheochromocytoma and paraganglioma: an endocrine society clinical practice guideline. *J Clin Endocrinol Metab* 2014;99(6):1915–1942.

(96%) and specificity (100%).[23] Combination measurement of chromogranin A and urinary fractionated metanephrine can also be used as a follow-up test for elevated plasma metanephrine levels.[24]

Electrocardiography
Signs of left ventricular hypertrophy can be seen in ECG due to persistent hypertension.

Imaging
• Radiologic evaluation should be initiated only after catecholamine excess has been confirmed biochemically. However, in situations of a high pre-test probability even with less compelling biochemical evidence or when paragangliomas are suspected to be nonsecretory (e.g., skull base and neck paragangliomas, paragangliomas in patients with SDHx mutation), imaging studies are recommended.[2]
• Because 95% of pheochromocytomas are intra-abdominal, an abdominal CT or MRI scan is usually obtained first.
• The most recent Endocrine Society Guidelines recommend CT with contrast for first imaging because of good spatial resolution in the thorax, abdomen, and pelvis.[2]

- CT has a high sensitivity of 85% to 94% for detecting adrenal pheochromocytoma (90% for extra-adrenal, metastatic, or recurrent pheochromocytoma) but a specificity of only 29% to 50%. Following an unenhanced CT with contrast-enhanced and delayed contrast-enhanced CT imaging for adrenal lesions improves sensitivity to 98% and specificity to 92%.[25]
- Pheochromocytomas usually appear round or oval, with clear margins, usually >3 cm in diameter with heterogeneous texture punctuated by cystic areas on imaging studies. Their unenhanced CT density is >10 Hounsfield units (HU) and the contrast washout is <50% at 10 minutes because of their low lipid content (however 30% of pheochromocytomas have washout >50%).[26]
- If the CT is negative in a biochemically positive pheochromocytoma, chemical shift MRI is used to differentiate adrenal masses based on presence/absence of fat similar to the CT. The hypervascularity of pheochromocytoma makes them appear characteristically bright, with high-signal intensity on T2 sequences and no signal loss on opposed phase images. Using different techniques for assessing signal intensity, MRI achieves a sensitivity of 81% to 83% and specificity of 88% to 93%.[27,28] MRI is favored over CT in following patient populations: patients with metastatic disease, skull base and neck paragangliomas, patients with surgical clip artifacts, those needing limitation of radiation exposure, like children and pregnant women, and patients with germline mutations.[2]
- Functional imaging is indicated in patients with or at risk for metastatic disease (large primary tumor, extra-adrenal, multifocal, recurrent).
  - ^{123}I-MIBG SPECT may be useful if ^{131}I-MIBG is considered for therapy and has much better sensitivity for adrenal pheochromocytoma than extra-adrenal paraganglioma.[29]
  - ^{68}Ga-DOTATATE PET/CT has excellent sensitivity for head and neck paragangliomas, metastatic disease, and SDHB/SDHD-related tumors.[30–32] ^{18}F-FDOPA PET has good sensitivity for skull base and neck paragangliomas and nonmetastatic disease, and ^{18}F-FDG PET has the good sensitivity for metastatic SDHB-related paragangliomas.[33,34]

Diagnostic Procedures
- About 40% of patients with pheochromocytoma and paraganglioma have germline mutations.[1] Genetic testing should be considered in all patients with pheochromocytoma and paraganglioma.
- Mutations in the following genes have been implicated: *NF1*, *RET* gene in multiple endocrine neoplasia type 2 (MEN2a, MEN2b), VHL, transmembrane domain protein 127 (FP/TMEM127), MYC-associated factor X (MAX), fumarate hydratase (FH), malate dehydrogenase 2 (MDH2), hypoxia-inducible factor 2α (EPAS1), SDHA, SDHB, SDHC, SDHD, and SDHAF2.[2,8]
- Mutation of *SDHB* gene is associated with an increased risk of development of metastatic disease (40% to 60%). Mutation for this gene should be tested especially in patients with paragangliomas, large tumors, and tumors producing methoxytyramine.[1]
- Mutation of *SDHD* and *SDHAF2* are inherited in autosomal dominant fashion with only paternally inherited mutations causing disease.[8]
- Selection of genes to be tested should be prioritized according to syndromic features, metastatic presentation, young age at presentation, tumor location, and catecholamine biochemical phenotype. Pre-test and post-test genetic counseling should be provided. See Table 16-3.[2,8]

TREATMENT

- Surgical resection is the definitive therapy for pheochromocytoma.
- Removing a pheochromocytoma is a high-risk surgical procedure, and an experienced surgeon–anesthesiologist team is required. In addition, patients must undergo

TABLE 16-3 GENETIC MUTATIONS AND ASSOCIATED CLINICAL PRESENTATION

Gene	Syndrome or other associated features	Metastasis risk	Location	Biochemical profile
RET	MEN2A, MEN2B	Low	Adrenal; possibly bilateral	Adrenergic
VHL	von Hippel–Lindau	High	Adrenal; possibly bilateral Extra-adrenal	Noradrenergic
NF1	Neurofibromatosis type 1	Moderate	Adrenal	
SDHB	Renal cell carcinoma GI stromal tumors Rare pituitary adenomas	Highest	SBHN Adrenal, Extra-adrenal	Dopaminergic, Noradrenergic, Adrenergic
SDHD	Renal cell carcinoma GI stromal tumors Rare pituitary adenomas	Low–moderate	SBHN-multifocal Adrenal, Extra-adrenal	Dopaminergic, Noradrenergic, Adrenergic
SDHC	Rare renal cell carcinoma GI stromal tumors Rare pituitary adenomas	Low–moderate	SBHN Adrenal, Extra-adrenal (thoracic)	Dopaminergic, Noradrenergic, Adrenergic
SDHA	GI stromal tumors	Low		
SDHAF2		Low	SBHN-multifocal	
MAX	None defined	Moderate	Adrenal, Extra-adrenal	Adrenergic, Noradrenergic
TMEM127	Rare renal cell carcinoma	Low	Adrenal, extra-adrenal, SBHN	Adrenergic
FH	Leiomyomatosis, Renal cell carcinoma	Possibly high		
EPAS1	Polycythemia, somatostatinoma	Not defined		
MDH2	None defined	Not defined		

MEN, multiple endocrine neoplasia; SBHN, skull base head and neck.
von Hippel–Lindau: hemangioblastomas of the central nervous system, endolymphatic sac tumors, epididymal cystadenomas, renal cell carcinomas, renal cysts, pancreatic neuroendocrine tumors, pancreatic cyst, pheochromocytoma, or paraganglioma.
Neurofibromatosis type 1: cutaneous neurofibromas, plexiform neurofibromas, café au lait spots, Lisch nodules (iris hamartoma), inguinal or axillary freckling, long bone dysplasia, optic gliomas, pheochromocytoma. Lenders JW, Duh QY, Eisenhofer G, et al. Pheochromocytoma and paraganglioma: an endocrine society clinical practice guideline. *J Clin Endocrinol Metab* 2014;99(6):1915–1942; Fishbein L. Pheochromocytoma and paraganglioma: genetics, diagnosis, and treatment. *Hematol Oncol Clin North Am* 2016;30(1):135–150.

appropriate medical preparation to control the effects of excessive adrenergic stimulation and prevent intraoperative hypertensive crisis. An endocrinologist or other physician experienced in the management of pheochromocytoma should supervise preoperative therapy.

- Pheochromocytomas have traditionally been resected through an open transabdominal approach. However, several studies have shown that laparoscopic adrenalectomy results in less pain, less blood loss, fewer hospital days, and less surgical morbidity compared to open adrenalectomy and is preferred to open adrenalectomy for most adrenal pheochromocytoma.[35,36]
- Laparoscopic adrenalectomy can be done safely even with large tumors (≥ 6 cm).[37] Paragangliomas usually require open surgeries as they are often malignant and are found in places where resection through laparoscopic approach can be difficult.[2]
- For intra-adrenal sporadic pheochromocytoma, the entire gland should be removed.
- Patients with familial pheochromocytomas (MEN2 or VHL disease) have a high incidence of bilateral disease and usually require bilateral adrenalectomies. For some patients with hereditary pheochromocytoma who have had previous contralateral adrenalectomy, partial adrenalectomy can be considered (for small tumors) to prevent permanent hypocortisolism and lifelong steroid dependence. Recent series indicate <5% 10-year recurrence rate with preservation of glucocorticoid function in at least 50%.[38]
- However, risks of recurrence of the tumor should be weighed against risks associated with chronic steroid use. When bilateral adrenalectomy is planned, the patient should receive perioperative "stress-dose" glucocorticoid coverage and appropriate postoperative glucocorticoid management.
- Preoperative management
  - The main goal of preoperative management of a pheochromocytoma is to normalize blood pressure, heart rate, and function of organs by restoring volume and preventing surgery-induced catecholamine storm.
  - Without adequate preparation for surgery, perioperative mortality has been found to be 30% to 45%. With preparation, mortality drops to <1%.[39]
  - α-Adrenergic antagonists or calcium channel blockers are recommended medications.[39]
  - No consensus exists regarding the exact time of preoperative adrenergic blockade. In most medical centers, adrenergic blockade is usually started 7 to 14 days preoperatively to have adequate time to normalize blood pressure and heart rate and to expand the contracted blood volume.
- α-Adrenergic blockade
  - Selective or nonselective α-blockade is the cornerstone of preoperative therapy, ideally started 10 to 14 days prior to surgery
    - Nonselective α-blocker: phenoxybenzamine
      - Start 10 mg bid-tid (up to 100 mg total daily dose)
      - Longer acting, irreversible, more expensive
      - Increased-risk orthostatic hypotension, reflex tachycardia, nasal congestion, syncope
  - Selective α_1-blockers: doxazosin, prazosin, terazosin
    - Doxazosin: 2 to 4 mg bid-tid; prazosin: 1 to 2 mg bid; terazosin: 1 to 4 mg qday
    - Shorter acting, less expensive
    - Increased-risk intraoperative hypertension[39]
- There are no prospective randomized controlled studies, but retrospective chart reviews at Mayo and Cleveland clinics demonstrated selective α-blockade resulted in more intraoperative hypertension without differences in outcomes. A prospective study comparing phenoxybenzamine to prazosin in India found that prazosin use also resulted in more intraoperative hypertension.[40,41]
- α-Adrenergic blockade improves surgical outcome with fewer perioperative complications.[42]
- Volume expansion (e.g., with oral salt supplements or intravenous fluids) helps minimize orthostatic hypotension associated with α-adrenergic blockade.

- Tachycardia may develop during α-blockade and require treatment with a β-blocker. However, β-blockers should not be started until after adequate α-adrenergic blockade is achieved (usually 2 to 3 days later) to prevent a paradoxical rise in blood pressure due to unopposed α-adrenergic receptor stimulation. There is not enough evidence to support β_1-selective adrenergic receptor blockers over nonselective β-adrenergic receptor blockers. Labetalol, with more potent β- than α-blocking property should not be used as initial therapy as it can cause paradoxical hypertension.
  - Nonselective β-blocker: propranolol (10 to 40 mg bid-tid)
  - Selective β-blocker: metoprolol (25 to 100 mg bid)
- Start low dose to control tachycardia and watch for signs of acute pulmonary edema related to underlying cardiomyopathy.
- Preoperative target blood pressure of <130/80 mm Hg while seated and >90 mm Hg systolic while standing and target heart rate 60 to 70 bpm seated and 70 to 80 bpm standing is recommended, but can be modified based on age and cardiovascular risk.[2]
- Intraoperative hypertension and cardiac arrhythmias usually occur during anesthesia induction, intubation, or tumor manipulation.
- Acute hypertensive crises should be treated intravenously with sodium nitroprusside, phentolamine, or nicardipine. Lidocaine or esmolol can be used for cardiac arrhythmias.
- After tumor resection, patients may experience mild hypotension, but severe hypotension can be avoided with aggressive fluid replacement. Approximately 10% to 15% of patients may experience postoperative hypoglycemia that can be managed by short-term infusion of glucose.[43]
- Other agents
  - Dihydropyridine calcium channel blockers: nicardipine, amlodipine
    - Nicardipine: 30 mg bid; amlodipine 5 to 10 mg qday
    - May be adjunct or alternative to α- and β-blockade[2]
  - Tyrosine hydroxylase inhibitor: metyrosine
    - 250 to 500 mg qid
    - Inhibits catecholamine biosynthesis
    - May be adjunct or alternative to traditional α- and β-blockade
- Risk factors for perioperative complications such as hypertension include high norepinephrine production, large tumor size (>4 cm), high blood pressure at presentation and after α-adrenergic blockade, and a more pronounced postural drop in blood pressure after preoperative treatment.[44]

SPECIAL CONSIDERATIONS

- **Malignant pheochromocytoma**
  - Other than local invasion or distant metastases, there are no distinctive histologic or biochemical characteristics that differentiate benign from malignant pheochromocytomas/paragangliomas.[6] However, recent studies have shown that mutations in *SDHB* lead to metastatic disease in 40% or more of the patients.[2] Other risk factors for malignant disease include tumor size >5 cm or tumors in an extra-adrenal location.[45]
  - The most common sites of metastases are the bones, lungs, liver, and lymph nodes.
  - There remains no effective treatment for malignant pheochromocytoma. Surgery to reduce tumor burden can help with subsequent radiation therapy, which may be useful for treatment of symptomatic bone metastases, though no survival advantage is demonstrated. ^{131}I-MIBG therapy can be used as a therapeutic option if the tumor is shown to have 123I-MIBG uptake.[46] If there is no radionuclide uptake, then combination chemotherapy with cyclophosphamide, vincristine, and dacarbazine may result in tumor regression and symptom relief in up to 50% of patients, but the responses are

short lived.[11,47] A recent study has raised the possibility for use of the tyrosine kinase inhibitor sunitinib in metastatic paraganglioma.[48]

- **Pregnancy**
  - Pheochromocytoma is a rare but potentially lethal cause of hypertension during pregnancy, with similar features to the general population. However, if hypertension and proteinuria occur, pheochromocytoma may be difficult to distinguish from preeclampsia.
  - Diagnosis is still made with elevated plasma and/or urinary fractionated metanephrines and anatomic localization by MRI. Nuclear scintigraphy and stimulation tests are not safe during pregnancy.
  - Women should be prepared for surgery with phenoxybenzamine followed by β-blockade as necessary for tachycardia. Although phenoxybenzamine is safe for the fetus, it does cross the placenta and can cause perinatal depression and transient hypotension.
  - If the diagnosis of pheochromocytoma is made before 24 weeks of gestation, surgical resection is usually performed. Second trimester is usually preferred for surgery.[49] After 24 weeks of gestation, medical management is continued until fetal maturation (as close to term as possible), at which time combined cesarean delivery and tumor resection are performed.[50]

MONITORING/FOLLOW-UP

- Long-term follow-up is indicated in all patients. Plasma and urine metanephrines should be checked 2 to 6 weeks after surgery to assess the adequacy of tumor resection. If levels are elevated, additional imaging studies should be considered.
- Even after complete resection of the tumor, there is about 5% risk of local, metastatic or new tumor formation. Risk of recurrence is higher in younger patients, age <20 years, patients with syndromic presentation, large tumor size, and in those with paragangliomas.
- Annual follow-up is recommended for all operated patients for at least 10 years and for those at high risk of recurrent disease; follow-up should be continued lifelong.[51] History, blood pressure measurements, and urine or plasma metanephrine levels should be included in the annual examination.

OUTCOME/PROGNOSIS

- Hypertension-free survival in patients without recurrence was 74% at 5 years and 45% at 10 years. Survival does not appear to be affected by the site of the tumor.[52]
- Patients with malignant tumors have a 5-year survival of <85% (79% for pheochromocytoma and 89% for paraganglioma), 10-year overall survival of 73%, and 15-year overall survival of 65%.[9]

REFERENCES

1. Lenders JWM, Eisenhofer G. Update on modern management of pheochromocytoma and paraganglioma. *Endocrinol Metab (Seoul)* 2017;32(2):152–161.
2. Lenders JW, Duh QY, Eisenhofer G, et al. Pheochromocytoma and paraganglioma: an endocrine society clinical practice guideline. *J Clin Endocrinol Metab* 2014;99(6):1915–1942.
3. Pacak K, Eisenhofer G, Ahlman H, et al. Pheochromocytoma: recommendations for clinical practice from the First International Symposium. October 2005. *Nat Clin Pract Endocrinol Metab* 2007;3(2):92–102.
4. Welander J, Soderkvist P, Gimm O. Genetics and clinical characteristics of hereditary pheochromocytomas and paragangliomas. *Endocr Relat Cancer* 2011;18(6):R253–R276.
5. Lee JA, Duh QY. Sporadic paraganglioma. *World J Surg* 2008;32(5):683–687.
6. Lenders JW, Eisenhofer G, Mannelli M, et al. Phaeochromocytoma. *Lancet* 2005;366(9486):665–675.

7. Young WF Jr. Management approaches to adrenal incidentalomas. A view from Rochester, Minnesota. *Endocrinol Metab Clin North Am* 2000;29(1):159–185.

8. Fishbein L. Pheochromocytoma and paraganglioma: genetics, diagnosis, and treatment. *Hematol Oncol Clin North Am* 2016;30(1):135–150.

9. Hamidi O, Young WF, Jr., Iniguez-Ariza NM, et al. Malignant pheochromocytoma and paraganglioma: 272 patients over 55 years. *J Clin Endocrinol Metab* 2017;102(9):3296–3305.

10. Buffet A, Venisse A, Nau V, et al. A decade (2001-2010) of genetic testing for pheochromocytoma and paraganglioma. *Horm Metab Res* 2012;44(5):359–366.

11. Karagiannis A, Mikhailidis DP, Athyros VG, Harsoulis F. Pheochromocytoma: an update on genetics and management. *Endocr Relat Cancer* 2007;14(4):935–956.

12. Yao L, Schiavi F, Cascon A, et al. Spectrum and prevalence of FP/TMEM127 gene mutations in pheochromocytomas and paragangliomas. *JAMA* 2010;304(23):2611–2619.

13. Brito JP, Asi N, Bancos I, et al. Testing for germline mutations in sporadic pheochromocytoma/paraganglioma: a systematic review. *Clin Endocrinol (Oxf)* 2015;82(3):338–345.

14. Eisenhofer G, Friberg P, Pacak K, et al. Plasma metadrenalines: do they provide useful information about sympatho-adrenal function and catecholamine metabolism? *Clin Sci* 1995;88(5):533–542.

15. Eisenhofer G, Keiser H, Friberg P, et al. Plasma metanephrines are markers of pheochromocytoma produced by catechol-O-methyltransferase within tumors. *J Clin Endocrinol Metab* 1998;83(6):2175–2185.

16. Motta-Ramirez GA, Remer EM, Herts BR, Gill IS, Hamrahian AH. Comparison of CT findings in symptomatic and incidentally discovered pheochromocytomas. *AJR Am J Roentgenol* 2005;185(3):684–688.

17. Kudva Y, Young W, Thompson G. Adrenal incidentaloma: An important component of the clinical presentation spectrum of benign sporadic adrenal pheochromocytoma. *The Endocrinologist* 1999;9(77).

18. Baguet JP, Hammer L, Mazzuco TL, et al. Circumstances of discovery of phaeochromocytoma: a retrospective study of 41 consecutive patients. *Eur J Endocrinol* 2004;150(5):681–686.

19. Lenders JW, Pacak K, Walther MM, et al. Biochemical diagnosis of pheochromocytoma: which test is best? *JAMA* 2002;287(11):1427–1434.

20. Sawka AM, Jaeschke R, Singh RJ, Young WF Jr. A comparison of biochemical tests for pheochromocytoma: measurement of fractionated plasma metanephrines compared with the combination of 24-hour urinary metanephrines and catecholamines. *J Clin Endocrinol Metab* 2003;88(2):553–558.

21. Perry CG, Sawka AM, Singh R, Thabane L, Bajnarek J, Young WF Jr. The diagnostic efficacy of urinary fractionated metanephrines measured by tandem mass spectrometry in detection of pheochromocytoma. *Clin Endocrinol (Oxf)* 2007;66(5):703–708.

22. Darr R, Pamporaki C, Peitzsch M, et al. Biochemical diagnosis of phaeochromocytoma using plasma-free normetanephrine, metanephrine and methoxytyramine: importance of supine sampling under fasting conditions. *Clin Endocrinol (Oxf)* 2014;80(4):478–486.

23. Eisenhofer G, Goldstein DS, Walther MM, et al. Biochemical diagnosis of pheochromocytoma: how to distinguish true- from false-positive test results. *J Clin Endocrinol Metab* 2003;88(6):2656–2666.

24. Algeciras-Schimnich A, Preissner CM, Young WF Jr, Singh RJ, Grebe SK. Plasma chromogranin A or urine fractionated metanephrines follow-up testing improves the diagnostic accuracy of plasma fractionated metanephrines for pheochromocytoma. *J Clin Endocrinol Metab* 2008;93(1):91–95.

25. Ilias I, Pacak K. Current approaches and recommended algorithm for the diagnostic localization of pheochromocytoma. *J Clin Endocrinol Metab* 2004;89(2):479–491.

26. Young WF Jr. Clinical practice. The incidentally discovered adrenal mass. *N Engl J Med* 2007;356(6):601–610.

27. Schieda N, Alrashed A, Flood TA, Samji K, Shabana W, McInnes MD. Comparison of quantitative MRI and CT washout analysis for differentiation of adrenal pheochromocytoma from adrenal adenoma. *Am J Roentgenol* 2016;206(6):1141–1148.

28. Borhani AA, Hosseinzadeh K. Quantitative versus qualitative methods in evaluation of T2 signal intensity to improve accuracy in diagnosis of pheochromocytoma. *Am J Roentgenol* 2015;205(2):302–310.

29. Wiseman GA, Pacak K, O'Dorisio MS, et al. Usefulness of 123I-MIBG scintigraphy in the evaluation of patients with known or suspected primary or metastatic pheochromocytoma or paraganglioma: results from a prospective multicenter trial. *J Nucl Med* 2009;50(9):1448–1454.

30. Archier A, Varoquaux A, Garrigue P, et al. Prospective comparison of (68)Ga-DOTATATE and (18)F-FDOPA PET/CT in patients with various pheochromocytomas and paragangliomas with emphasis on sporadic cases. *Eur J Nucl Med Mol Imaging* 2016;43(7):1248–1257.

31. Janssen I, Blanchet EM, Adams K, et al. Superiority of [68Ga]-DOTATATE PET/CT to other functional imaging modalities in the localization of SDHB-associated metastatic pheochromocytoma and paraganglioma. *Clin Cancer Res* 2015;21(17):3888–3895.

32. Janssen I, Chen CC, Taieb D, et al. 68Ga-DOTATATE PET/CT in the localization of head and neck paragangliomas compared with other functional imaging modalities and CT/MRI. *J Nucl Med* 2016;57(2):186–191.

33. Timmers HJ, Kozupa A, Chen CC, et al. Superiority of fluorodeoxyglucose positron emission tomography to other functional imaging techniques in the evaluation of metastatic SDHB-associated pheochromocytoma and paraganglioma. *J Clin Oncol* 2007;25(16):2262–2269.

34. Timmers HJ, Taieb D, Pacak K. Current and future anatomical and functional imaging approaches to pheochromocytoma and paraganglioma. *Horm Metab Res* 2012;44(5):367–372.

35. Agarwal G, Sadacharan D, Aggarwal V, et al. Surgical management of organ-contained unilateral pheochromocytoma: comparative outcomes of laparoscopic and conventional open surgical procedures in a large single-institution series. *Langenbecks Arch Surg* 2012;397(7):1109–1116.

36. Shen WT, Grogan R, Vriens M, Clark OH, Duh QY. One hundred two patients with pheochromocytoma treated at a single institution since the introduction of laparoscopic adrenalectomy. *Arch Surg* 2010;145(9):893–897.

37. Wang W, Li P, Wang Y, et al. Effectiveness and safety of laparoscopic adrenalectomy of large pheochromocytoma: a prospective, nonrandomized, controlled study. *Am J Surg* 2015;210(2):230–235.

38. Castinetti F, Taieb D, Henry JF, et al. Management of endocrine disease: Outcome of adrenal sparing surgery in heritable pheochromocytoma. *Eur J Endocrinol* 2016;174(1):R9–R18.

39. Naranjo J, Dodd S, Martin YN. Perioperative management of pheochromocytoma. *J Cardiothorac Vasc Anesth* 2017;31(4):1427–1439.

40. Weingarten TN, Cata JP, O'Hara JF, et al. Comparison of two preoperative medical management strategies for laparoscopic resection of pheochromocytoma. *Urology* 2010;76(2):508 e6–e11.

41. Agrawal R, Mishra SK, Bhatia E, et al. Prospective study to compare peri-operative hemodynamic alterations following preparation for pheochromocytoma surgery by phenoxybenzamine or prazosin. *World J Surg* 2014;38(3):716–723.

42. Goldstein RE, O'Neill JA Jr, Holcomb GW 3rd, et al. Clinical experience over 48 years with pheochromocytoma. *Ann Surg* 1999;229(6):755–764; discussion 64–66.

43. Akiba M, Kodama T, Ito Y, Obara T, Fujimoto Y. Hypoglycemia induced by excessive rebound secretion of insulin after removal of pheochromocytoma. *World J Surg* 1990;14(3):317–324.

44. Bruynzeel H, Feelders RA, Groenland TH, et al. Risk factors for hemodynamic instability during surgery for pheochromocytoma. *J Clin Endocrinol Metab* 2010;95(2):678–685.

45. Bravo EL, Tagle R. Pheochromocytoma: state-of-the-art and future prospects. *Endocr Rev* 2003;24(4):539–553.

46. van Hulsteijn LT, Niemeijer ND, Dekkers OM, Corssmit EP. (131)I-MIBG therapy for malignant paraganglioma and phaeochromocytoma: systematic review and meta-analysis. *Clin Endocrinol (Oxf)* 2014;80(4):487–501.

47. Niemeijer ND, Alblas G, van Hulsteijn LT, Dekkers OM, Corssmit EP. Chemotherapy with cyclophosphamide, vincristine and dacarbazine for malignant paraganglioma and pheochromocytoma: systematic review and meta-analysis. *Clin Endocrinol (Oxf)* 2014;81(5):642–651.

48. Joshua AM, Ezzat S, Asa SL, et al. Rationale and evidence for sunitinib in the treatment of malignant paraganglioma/pheochromocytoma. *J Clin Endocrinol Metab* 2009;94(1):5–9.

49. Pearl J, Price R, Richardson W, et al. Guidelines for diagnosis, treatment, and use of laparoscopy for surgical problems during pregnancy. *Surg Endosc* 2011;25(11):3479–3492.

50. Lenders JW. Pheochromocytoma and pregnancy: a deceptive connection. *Eur J Endocrinol* 2012;166(2):143–150.

51. Plouin PF, Amar L, Dekkers OM, et al. European Society of Endocrinology Clinical Practice Guideline for long-term follow-up of patients operated on for a phaeochromocytoma or a paraganglioma. *Eur J Endocrinol* 2016;174(5):G1–G10.

52. Plouin PF, Chatellier G, Fofol I, Corvol P. Tumor recurrence and hypertension persistence after successful pheochromocytoma operation. *Hypertension* 1997;29(5):1133–1139.

Amenorrhea

17

Lauren D. Reschke and Emily S. Jungheim

GENERAL PRINCIPLES

- Regular, cyclic menstruation is defined as nine or more menstrual cycles per year and typically occurs every 28 to 35 days.
- Regular menses are the result of complex interactions within the hypothalamic–pituitary–ovarian (HPO) axis and require a functional endometrium and an intact genital outflow tract.
- Pathology affecting any of the structures involved may lead to menstrual irregularity which warrants investigation.[1,2]

Definition

Amenorrhea is the absence of menses. It is physiologic prior to puberty, during pregnancy, during lactation, in menopause, and with certain medications.[3]

Classification

- Primary versus secondary amenorrhea:
  - **Primary amenorrhea:**
    - No menses by age 13 in the absence of secondary sexual development
    - No menses by age 15 in the presence of secondary sexual development
  - **Secondary amenorrhea:**
    - No menses for three menstrual cycles with a history of regular menses
    - No menses for 6 months with a history of irregular menses
- World Health Organization (WHO) classification:
  - **Group I (hypogonadotropic hypoestrogenic):** normal or low follicle-stimulating hormone (FSH) levels, absent estrogen production, normal prolactin (PRL) levels, no hypothalamic or pituitary lesion
  - **Group II (normogonadotropic normoestrogenic):** estrogen production present, normal FSH and PRL levels
  - **Group III (hypergonadotropic hypoestrogenic):** elevated FSH levels, absent estrogen production[3]

Epidemiology

Prevalence of pathologic amenorrhea ranges from 3% to 4% in reproductive-aged populations.[3]

Etiology

- HPO axis and menstrual physiology
  - The hypothalamus secretes gonadotropin-releasing hormone (GnRH) into the pituitary portal venous circulation in a pulsatile fashion.
  - Pulsatile GnRH stimulates gonadotrope cells of the anterior pituitary, and regulates synthesis, storage, and systemic release of FSH and luteinizing hormone (LH).

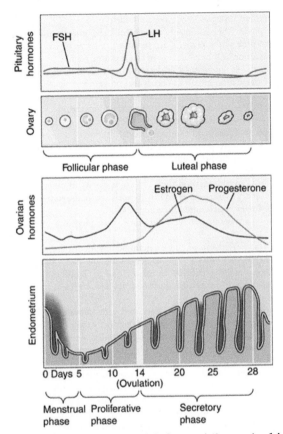

FIGURE 17-1 The menstrual cycle. (**Top**) Before ovulation on day 14, the follicle is ripening in the ovary; after ovulation, the follicle becomes the corpus luteum. (**Bottom**) Changes in the uterine endometrium during the menstrual cycle. Cyclic hormone production in relation to follicle maturation and ovulation, and to proliferative and secretory phases of the uterine lining. FSH, follicle-stimulating hormone; LH, luteinizing hormone. Reprinted from Cohen B. *Memmler's The Human Body in Health and Disease*. 12th ed. Philadelphia, PA: Wolters Kluwer; 2013, with permission.

- LH and FSH stimulate ovarian steroid synthesis according to the **two-cell theory involving crosstalk between the theca and granulosa cells of the ovarian follicle:**
  - LH stimulates androgen production by theca cells. Androgen diffuses across the basement membrane to neighboring granulosa cells.
  - FSH stimulates estradiol production by granulosa cells via aromatase which converts androgens to estradiol.[1,4,5]
- Events of the menstrual cycle can be conceptualized from the perspective of the ovary or endometrium as follows (see Fig. 17-1)[6]:

- Follicular and luteal phases of the ovarian follicle
  - Follicular phase: FSH stimulates ovarian follicular growth and estrogen production. Once peak estrogen levels are sustained, a surge of LH from the pituitary induces ovulation and luteinization of the ruptured follicle.
  - Luteal phase: The luteinized follicle/corpus luteum secretes progesterone. In the absence of pregnancy, luteolysis occurs and progesterone levels fall. Normal luteal phase length is typically 12 to 14 days.
- Proliferative and decidual phases of the uterine endometrium
  - Proliferative phase: Estrogen drives growth of the endometrium.
  - Decidual phase: Progesterone induces decidualization of the endometrium making the endometrium receptive to an embryo. In the absence of pregnancy, progesterone levels fall and menses begin.

- **Etiologies of amenorrhea**
  - Many conditions can cause amenorrhea, but the **majority of cases are accounted for by polycystic ovary syndrome (PCOS), hypothalamic amenorrhea, hyperprolactinemia, or primary ovarian insufficiency (POI).**[3]
  - If patients are of a menopausal age (>40 years), then physiologic menopause should be considered.
  - The cause of amenorrhea can often be determined by identifying the anatomic origin of the defect in the HPO axis and/or the genital outflow tract (Table 17-1).
  - Various etiologies are grouped below as anatomic or by WHO classification.
  - **Anatomic disorders of the genital outflow tract and uterus.**
    - **Congenital disorders:**
      - Lower outflow tract obstruction is associated with **imperforate hymen, complete transverse vaginal septum**, and **isolated vaginal atresia**. Patients will have age-appropriate secondary sexual characteristics with normal ovarian function. They typically present after puberty with acute cyclic pelvic or abdominal pain due to retrograde menstruation.
      - In **müllerian agenesis**, also known as **Mayer–Rokitansky–Küster–Hauser syndrome (MRKH)**, patients have a 46,XX karyotype with normal ovarian function, but lack müllerian structures. Physical examination shows a vaginal dimple. In partial müllerian agenesis, patients may have rudimentary müllerian structures with functioning endometrium resulting in cyclic pelvic pain. MRI can assist with classifying anomalies. One-third of women with müllerian agenesis have associated renal anomalies including horseshoe kidney, pelvic kidney, and unilateral renal agenesis.
      - **Complete androgen insensitivity syndrome** is an X-linked recessive disorder characterized by 46,XY karyotype. It is caused by a defect in the androgen receptor thus preventing normal testosterone binding. Anti-müllerian hormone (AMH) secreted by the testes induces regression of müllerian structures, thus the uterus, fallopian tubes, and the upper third of the vagina are absent. Breast development occurs during puberty from peripheral conversion of testosterone to estradiol. Testosterone levels are within or above the normal male range. Testes can often be palpated in the labia or inguinal region and should be surgically removed after puberty due to an increased risk of malignancy.
    - **Acquired disorders:**
      - **Cervical stenosis** can be acquired following surgical trauma or radiation, or with certain conditions like vaginal atrophy, or neoplasia. Patients may present with hematometra. Management requires dilation of the cervix.
      - **Intrauterine synechiae (Asherman syndrome)** results from damage of the basal endometrium, thus impeding menstrual flow or preventing response to ovarian steroids. It may follow vigorous uterine curettage, or uterine infection.[1,3,4]
  - **Hypogonadotropic hypoestrogenic amenorrhea**

TABLE 17-1 ETIOLOGIES OF AMENORRHEA

Disorders of genital outflow tract and uterus
Müllerian agenesis (Mayer–Rokitansky–Küster–Hauser syndrome)
Androgen insensitivity syndrome
Imperforate hymen
Transverse vaginal septum
Intrauterine synechiae (Asherman syndrome)
Cervical stenosis
Isolated cervical/vaginal agenesis

Ovarian causes
Gonadal dysgenesis: Turner syndrome (45,X), Mosaic Turner syndrome (45,X/46,XX), Swyer syndrome (46,XY), 46,XX gonadal dysgenesis/agenesis
Primary ovarian insufficiency: idiopathic, chemotherapy, radiation, mumps oophoritis, fragile X mutations, structural and numerical chromosomal abnormalities, autoimmune
Enzymatic deficiencies: galactosemia, 17α-hydroxylase deficiency, aromatase deficiency, 17,20-lyase deficiency

Pituitary causes
Prolactinoma
Other pituitary tumors
Empty sella syndrome
Pituitary infarction (Sheehan syndrome)
Infiltrative diseases: lymphocytic hypophysitis, hemochromatosis
Radiation
Surgery
FSH or LH receptor mutations
Panhypopituitarism

Hypothalamic causes
Functional hypothalamic amenorrhea (exercise, anorexia nervosa, weight loss, stress, chronic disease, depression)
Congenital GnRH deficiency: idiopathic hypogonadotropic hypogonadism, Kallmann syndrome
Infiltrative diseases: sarcoidosis, lymphoma, Langerhans cell histiocytosis, hemochromatosis
Infection: tuberculosis, syphilis, encephalitis/meningitis
Tumors (craniopharyngioma, germinoma, hamartoma, etc.)
GnRH receptor mutations

Other endocrine causes
Adrenal disease: late-onset adrenal hyperplasia, Cushing syndrome
Thyroid disorders
Cushing syndrome
Polycystic ovary syndrome
Ovarian tumors: granulosa–theca cell tumors, Brenner tumors, teratomas, cystadenomas, metastatic carcinoma

Physiologic causes
Pregnancy
Lactation
Menopause
Constitutional delay of puberty

- In hypogonadotropic hypogonadism, the primary pathology lies in the hypothalamus and/or pituitary gland. Impaired GnRH and/or gonadotropin secretion leads to diminished ovarian stimulation and estrogen production.
- Congenital disorders:
  - **Kallmann syndrome** is an X-linked disorder caused by failure of GnRH and olfactory neuronal migration. Patients are anosmic, and present with primary amenorrhea and absent breast development.
  - **Isolated GnRH deficiency, GnRH receptor mutations, and isolated gonadotropin deficiency** are rare. Patients have a broad range of phenotypes based on the mutation.
- Acquired disorders:
  - **Functional hypothalamic amenorrhea** may be associated with **psychological stress, eating disorders, or excessive exercise**. The term **female athlete triad** is used to describe women with low energy availability with or without disordered eating, menstrual dysfunction, and low bone mineral density. Other causes of amenorrhea must be excluded prior to making this diagnosis.
  - **Chronic diseases** such as end-stage kidney disease, liver disease, malignancies, malabsorption, and acquired immunodeficiency syndrome, as well as **conditions impacting the central nervous system (CNS)** (i.e., tumors, trauma, radiation, infections, or infiltrative diseases) may be associated with amenorrhea.
  - **Lesions affecting the anterior pituitary gland** such as **prolactinomas, adenomas**, or **empty sella syndrome** may negatively impact gonadotropin secretion. **Sheehan syndrome** is a condition of pituitary necrosis and panhypopituitarism following postpartum hemorrhage and hypotension.
  - **Hyperprolactinemia** caused by medications, hypothyroidism, or prolactinomas impairs GnRH secretion.[1,3,4,7]
- ○ **Normogonadotropic normoestrogenic amenorrhea**
  - In normogonadotropic normoestrogenic amenorrhea, gonadotropin and estrogen production is usually normal, however ovarian follicular recruitment and ovulation are disturbed.
  - **PCOS** is the most common cause of amenorrhea due to anovulation. There are a number of different criteria used to diagnose PCOS. The most recent outlined by the Androgen Excess Society include clinical and/or biochemical signs of hyperandrogenism in the presence of oligo- or anovulation, or polycystic-appearing ovaries on ultrasound. Other causes of amenorrhea and hyperandrogenism need to be excluded to make this diagnosis. PCOS is further discussed in Chapter 21.
  - **Late-onset congenital adrenal hyperplasia (CAH)** is typically due to a mutation in the *CYP21A2* gene which encodes the 21-hydroxylase enzyme. It presents similarly to PCOS. Patients with CAH are unable to convert an adequate amount of progesterone to cortisol and aldosterone, resulting in disrupted follicular maturation.[1,4,8]
- ○ **Hypergonadotropic hypoestrogenic amenorrhea**
  - In hypergonadotropic hypogonadism, the ovary fails to respond to gonadotropin. This is physiologic at menopause, but prior to 40 years of age it is referred to as POI.
  - Congenital disorders:
    - In **gonadal dysgenesis**, oocytes undergo accelerated atresia and the ovary is replaced with fibrous streaks. This is classically seen in patients with **Tuner syndrome** (45,X), **chromosomal mosaicism** (45,X/46,XX), and in individuals with **pure gonadal dysgenesis** resulting from genetic, environmental, or infectious insults during early embryonic development.
    - Two percent of women with sporadic POI have a premutation in the *FMR1* gene.
    - Several genetic mutations have been linked to POI including mutations of genes encoding for galactose-1-phosphate uridyltransferase, the FSH receptor, and autoimmune regulator gene.
  - Acquired disorders

- POI has been associated with autoimmune disorders including systemic lupus erythematous, myasthenia gravis, idiopathic thrombocytopenic purpura, rheumatoid arthritis, vitiligo, and autoimmune hemolytic anemia.
- POI can be acquired from infection, or medical exposures like radiation or certain chemotherapeutic agents which result in premature depletion of ovarian follicles.[1,3,4,9]

DIAGNOSIS

Clinical Presentation

Diagnostic testing and evaluation of amenorrhea are guided by history and physical examination and may be organized by testing the functional components of the menstrual cycle including those of the HPO axis and the genital outflow tract.

History
- Age of menarche and thelarche, cycle frequency, and duration of previous menstrual cycles
- Cyclic symptoms including breast changes, pelvic or lower abdominal pain indicative of obstructed menstrual flow (cryptomenorrhea)
- Past medical history with particular consideration for chronic illnesses
- Sexual activity, history of pelvic infections, number of pregnancies including outcomes and complications (hemorrhage, inability to breastfeed, retained products of conceptions), and lactation history
- Lifestyle changes including changes in diet or exercise, weight changes, and physical or emotional stress
- Prescription medications
- Alcohol and substance abuse
- Surgical history focusing on prior abdominal, pelvic, or uterine surgery
- History of chemotherapy or radiation exposure
- Symptoms of estrogen deficiency (e.g., hot flashes, vaginal dryness, decreased libido)
- Symptoms of endocrine diseases (e.g., weight change, fatigue, galactorrhea)
- Symptoms of CNS disorder (e.g., headache, seizures, visual disturbance, anosmia)
- Family history of abnormal pubertal development, mental retardation[1,4]

Physical Examination
- Body weight and physical habitus should be noted
- Skin findings including signs of acne, hirsutism, and striae
- In the setting of primary amenorrhea, specific attention should be given to height, identification of normal urogenital anatomy, and to the presence of breast development
- In women with secondary amenorrhea, thyroid gland should be evaluated for size, shape, and nodules[1,4]

Diagnostic Testing

- Laboratory and radiologic examination should be guided by history and physical examination. All reproductive-aged women should receive a urinary pregnancy test to rule out pregnancy.
- Figure 17-2 provides a general diagnostic algorithm of amenorrhea, listing the most common causes of amenorrhea.
- Imaging with pelvic ultrasound, uterine saline sonohysterogram, hysterosalpingogram, hysteroscopy, and/or MRI may be necessary to evaluate uterine anatomy. Absence of müllerian structures should prompt further evaluation with a karyotype analysis and serum testosterone level.

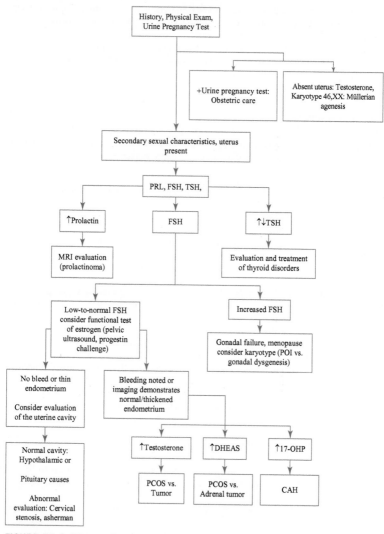

FIGURE 17-2 Diagnostic algorithm to evaluate amenorrhea.

- Primary laboratory tests should include thyroid-stimulating hormone (TSH), PRL, and FSH.
- **Elevated prolactin:** Further evaluation and management for women with hyperprolactinemia are discussed in Chapter 2.
- **Abnormal TSH:** Evaluation and treatment for patients with thyroid disorders are covered in Chapters 8 and 9.
- **FSH levels:**
  ○ **Low-to-normal FSH levels:** Normoestrogenic and hypoestrogenic causes of amenorrhea need to be distinguished from one another. Low serum estradiol levels should

be interpreted with caution and functional tests of estrogen production may be more helpful. Functional tests of estrogen production include pelvic ultrasound evaluating for the presence of thickened endometrium or the progestin challenge test (see below).

- In the absence of bleeding after a progestin challenge or visualization of a thin endometrium on pelvic ultrasound: Consider a central etiology (hypothalamic or pituitary pathology). Cranial MRI is indicated in most cases to rule out a hypothalamic or pituitary lesion before other etiologies are considered.
- In secondary amenorrhea, uterine scarring (Asherman syndrome, cervical stenosis) should be ruled out with examination and possible imaging.
- In the presence of bleeding after a progestin challenge or visualization of a normal/thick endometrium on pelvic ultrasound:
  □ PCOS is the most common cause. Other causes should be ruled out prior to confirming the diagnosis (see Chapter 21).
  □ In the presence of hirsutism, 17-hydroxyprogesterone (17-OHP) should be checked to rule out nonclassic CAH (see Chapter 13), and total testosterone to assess for an androgen-secreting tumor. IGF-1 and dehydroepiandrosterone sulfate (DHEAS) should be considered, particularly if there is virilization.
  □ Cushing syndrome can be ruled out with a 1-mg overnight dexamethasone suppression test or 24-hour urine-free cortisol (see Chapter 15).
- ○ **Elevated FSH levels** (hypergonadotropic amenorrhea) suggest an ovarian etiology and gonadal failure.[7]
  - In primary amenorrhea with the absence of secondary sexual characteristics, a karyotype analysis should be performed to rule out a chromosomal abnormality such as Turner syndrome (45,XO), POI (46,XX), or to assess for the presence of a Y chromosome.
  - In women under age 40 years with POI, a karyotype analysis should also be performed to assess for mosaic Turner syndrome and other various chromosomal abnormalities.[3]
  - Other causes for ovarian failure such as ovarian tumors, prior trauma, pelvic radiation, and chemotherapy should be evaluated.
- **Further testing:**
  ○ One standard approach for a **progestin challenge test** is the administration of medroxyprogesterone, typically 10 mg orally daily for 10 days. Subsequent bleeding rules out an outflow tract obstruction, and the woman is assumed to produce estrogen. Test results may be difficult to interpret though, as 20% of women who are normoestrogenic will have no bleeding and 40% to 50% of women with hypoestrogenism will have withdrawal bleeding.
  ○ AMH, a growth factor, is expressed by granulosa cells of small preantral follicles. AMH is often elevated in PCOS, but this application is not established.
  ○ Antral follicle count (AFC) on transvaginal sonography reflects the resting follicular pool. Antral follicles between 2 and 10 mm are counted in both ovaries. The total AFC usually ranges between 10 and 20 in reproductive-aged women and is often increased in women with PCOS, although 20% of normal women also have increased AFC. The utility of this test in the setting of amenorrhea is not established.[1,3,4]

TREATMENT

- Treatment depends on etiology and patient goals. Patients should be counseled about long-term implications of their condition and prevention of sequelae.
- Anatomic abnormalities may require surgical correction. Patients with a Y chromosome are at increased risk for germ cell tumors and postpubertal removal of the gonads should be considered.[1]
- With primary amenorrhea, potential for achieving sexual maturation and reproduction should be discussed. If indicated, estrogen may be used to induce puberty with special consideration for optimization of adult height and normal breast development.

- Hypothyroidism is treated with thyroid replacement. Hyperprolactinemia is often treated with a dopamine agonist or an ergoline derivative. Women with macroadenomas may require surgery.
- Correcting precipitating factors may restore cycles for women with functional hypothalamic amenorrhea. In women with eating disorders or excessive exercise, a collaborative team approach that addresses mental health is imperative.[7]
- Patients with hypogonadism require estrogen treatment to prevent osteoporosis. Women with a uterus also require continuous or intermittent progesterone treatment to protect against endometrial hyperplasia associated with use of unopposed estrogen use. Hormone therapy should be continued until menopause, at which time continuation of hormone therapy is often symptom based.[2,7]
- Ovulation and fertility may be achieved in some patients under the direction of a reproductive endocrinologist. Initial treatment with oral ovulation induction agents like clomiphene citrate or aromatase inhibitors, exogenous gonadotropins, and/or assisted reproductive technologies depends on etiology and patient preference. Donor oocytes are an option for women with POI.[1,3,10]
- Specific therapy for PCOS is discussed in Chapter 21, and is aimed at controlling hirsutism, resuming menstruation, achieving fertility, and avoiding long-term sequelae of PCOS including glucose intolerance, endometrial hyperplasia, and cardiovascular complications.

REFERENCES

1. Hoffman BL, Schorge JO, Bradshaw KD, Halvorson LM, Schaffer JI, Corton MM. *Williams Gynecology*. 3rd ed. New York: McGraw-Hill Education; 2016:369–385.
2. American College of Obstetricians and Gynecologists. ACOG Committee Opinion No. 651: Menstruation in girls and adolescents: using the menstrual cycle as a vital sign. *Obstet Gynecol* 2015;126(6):e143–e146.
3. Practice Committee of American Society for Reproductive Medicine. Current evaluation of amenorrhea. *Fertil Steril* 2008;90(5 Suppl):S219–S225.
4. Fritz MA, Speroff L. Amenorrhea. *Clinical Gynecologic Endocrinology and Infertility*. 8th ed. Philadelphia, PA: Lippincott Williams & Wilkins; 2011:435–493.
5. Hall JE. Neuroendocrine control of the menstrual cycle. In: Strauss JF, Barbieri RL, eds. *Yen and Jaffe's Reproductive Endocrinology: Physiology, Pathophysiology, and Clinical Management*. 7th ed. Philadelphia, PA: Saunders/Elsevier; 2014:141–156.
6. Cohen B. *Medical Terminology*. 7th ed. Philadelphia, PA: Lippincott Williams & Wilkins; 2013.
7. American College of Obstetricians and Gynecologists. Committee Opinion No. 702: Female athlete triad. *Obstet Gynecol* 2017;129(6):e160–e167.
8. American College of Obstetricians and Gynecologists. ACOG Practice Bulletin No. 108: Polycystic ovary syndrome. *Obstet Gynecol* 2009;114(4):936–949.
9. American College of Obstetricians and Gynecologists. Committee Opinion No. 605: Primary ovarian insufficiency in adolescents and young women. *Obstet Gynecol* 2014;123:193–197.
10. Sullivan SD, Sarrel PM, Nelson LM. Hormone replacement therapy in young women with primary ovarian insufficiency and early menopause. *Fertil Steril* 2016;106(7):1588–1599.

Gynecomastia

Maamoun Salam and Marina Litvin

GENERAL PRINCIPLES

Definition

Gynecomastia is a benign glandular enlargement (≥ 0.5 cm) of the male breast that is often asymmetrical or unilateral, and may be tender.[1-3]

Classification

- Gynecomastia can be divided into two main categories: **physiologic** or **pathologic**.
  - **Physiologic gynecomastia** occurs from normal fluctuations in hormonal levels (estrogen/androgen ratio) observed at different ages. Treatment is typically not necessary due to spontaneous resolution.
    - Transient gynecomastia occurs in **60% to 90% of newborns** due to high levels of circulating estrogen during pregnancy, and typically regresses within 2 to 3 weeks after birth.[1]
    - **Pubertal gynecomastia** occurs in early adolescence, regresses within 18 months, and is uncommon after 17 years of age. Gynecomastia results from transient imbalance of estrogen/androgen, as estradiol concentrations rise to adult levels before testosterone does.[1,3]
    - **Gynecomastia of aging** occurs in otherwise healthy men aged 50 to 80, and is due to decreased testosterone synthesis and a relative increase in the estrogen-to-androgen ratio. Age-associated increased aromatase activity and increased body fat composition also contributes to gynecomastia via aromatization of testosterone to estradiol.[3]
  - **Pathologic gynecomastia** is due to a congenital or acquired imbalance of estrogen to androgen. Gynecomastia results from an increase in the estrogen-to-androgen ratio, excessive estrogen production, deficient androgen production, increased estrogen precursors available for peripheral conversion, blockade of androgen receptors, and/or increased binding of androgen to sex-hormone binding globulin (SHBG).
- Types of gynecomastia[1,3]:
  - **Florid gynecomastia:** Acute presentation with breast enlargement and tenderness. Can last up to **6 months**. May reverse spontaneously, with resolution of offending etiology, or with treatment.
  - **Quiescent gynecomastia:** Present for **more than a year**, usually asymptomatic and **may not reverse** with treatment
  - **Intermediate phase:** Contains features of both types and is seen in gynecomastia 4 to 12 months in duration.

Pathophysiology

- Hormones affecting breast development[1]:
  - **Estrogen:** stimulates the growth and differentiation of breast epithelium into ducts (ductal hyperplasia)
  - **Progesterone:** promotes acinar development and formation of glandular bud (glandular formation). Since progesterone levels are not high enough in men, galactorrhea is rarely seen in gynecomastia even in the presence of hyperprolactinemia.

- ○ Growth hormone, IGF-1, insulin, cortisol, and thyroid hormone all facilitate breast development.
- ○ **Non-aromatized androgens**, such as testosterone, inhibit growth and differentiation of breast tissue.
- ○ **Prolactin** stimulates differentiated breast acinar cells to produce milk.
- Serum androgens[4]:
  - ○ Testes secrete most testosterone and 15% of estradiol.
  - ○ Both bind to SHBG while small amount circulates unbound.
  - ○ Bioavailable fraction is the free and albumin-bound steroids.
  - ○ Aromatase enzyme in extragonadal tissues converts testosterone to estradiol and adrenal androstenedione to estrone, which can be converted further to estradiol (a more potent estrogen) by 17β-hydroxysteroid dehydrogenase.

Etiology

Common causes of gynecomastia are summarized in Table 18-1.

Associated Conditions

- Conditions affecting the production and effect **of androgens[5]**:
  - ○ In **primary hypogonadism**, deficiency in testosterone leads to a compensatory increase in LH, enhancing aromatization of testosterone to estradiol, resulting in relative estrogen excess and gynecomastia.
  - ○ Less commonly, **secondary hypogonadism** can also be associated with gynecomastia. In secondary hypogonadism, the pituitary fails to produce LH, leading to decreased testosterone secretion, but the adrenal cortex continues to produce estrogen precursors that are aromatized in extraglandular tissues. The net effect is an estrogen–androgen imbalance, which leads to breast tissue growth.
  - ○ **Elevated prolactin** does not cause gynecomastia, unless inhibition of the endogenous gonadotropin and testosterone production lead to loss of the inhibitory influence of androgens on the breast. This is seen in both prolactinomas, and with medications that increase prolactin, such as antipsychotics, antidepressants, and sedatives.[1]
  - ○ In **androgen insensitivity syndrome**, ineffective testosterone action due to defects in, or absence of intracellular androgen receptors in target tissues, results in genotypic males appearing as phenotypic females, with gynecomastia.
- Conditions that **increase estrogen** production[1,5]:
  - ○ Tumors may secrete estrogen leading to gynecomastia.
    - ▪ **Leydig** and **Sertoli cell** tumors are usually small and benign.
    - ▪ Feminizing Sertoli tumors are associated with a family history of gynecomastia in association with autosomal dominant conditions like Peutz–Jeghers (GI polyps, mucocutaneous pigmentation, increased risks of GI and non-GI malignancy) or Carney complex (cardiac or cutaneous myxomas, pigmented skin lesions, adrenal or testicular tumors).
    - ▪ **Feminizing adrenocortical carcinomas** may manifest with a palpable abdominal mass and are usually large and malignant.
    - ▪ **Germ cell tumors** of the testes or bronchogenic carcinomas can secrete human chorionic gonadotropin (hCG), stimulating Leydig cell aromatase, leading to increased conversion of androgen precursors to estrone and estradiol, resulting in gynecomastia.
    - ▪ Patients with **true hermaphroditism** may have gynecomastia due to increased estrogen production from the ovarian component of their gonads.
- **Drugs** can cause gynecomastia via several mechanisms (please see Table 18-2)[3,4,6]:
  - ○ Analogs of estrogen and gonadotropins increase estrogenic activity.

TABLE 18-1   CAUSES OF GYNECOMASTIA

Physiologic causes	
Maternal estrogens	Neonatal
Increase in estrogen/androgen ratio	Pubertal
Increased aromatase activity	Aging, obesity
Pathologic causes	
Estrogen excess	
Increased aromatization	
Tumors	Sertoli cell, leydig cell, sex cord, adrenocortical, germ cell
Glandular	Primary aromatase excess, hermaphroditism, obesity, hyperthyroidism, testicular feminization, refeeding after starvation, liver disease
Decreased estrogen metabolism	Cirrhosis
Exogenous sources	Embalming fluid, topical estrogen creams, oils, lotions
Eutopic hCG production	Choriocarcinoma
Ectopic hCG production	Lung, liver, kidney, gastric carcinoma
hCG treatment	
Drugs	Testosterone, other androgens, estrogens, digoxin, marijuana
Androgen deficiency	
Primary gonadal disorders	
Inherited	Klinefelter, anorchia, hermaphroditism, hereditary defects in testosterone synthesis
Acquired	Viral orchitis, granulomatous disease, castration, androgen deprivation therapy
Secondary	Hypogonadotrophic hypogonadism, hemochromatosis, hyperprolactinemia, acromegaly, Cushing syndrome, chronic kidney disease
Androgen resistance disorders	Congenital and acquired androgen resistance
Drugs that interfere with androgen action	Spironolactone, 5α-reductase inhibitors, marijuana, histamine-2 receptorantagonist, androgen receptor antagonists, insulin, HIV therapy with HAART, anti-tuberculous therapy, GH
Other	
Direct stimulation of breast tissue	
Idiopathic	Persistent prepubertal macromastia

GH, growth hormone; HIV, human immunodeficiency virus; HAART, highly active antiretroviral treatment.

TABLE 18-2	MEDICATIONS ASSOCIATED WITH GYNECOMASTIA
Hormones	Androgens, anabolic steroids, estrogens, growth hormone, HCG, glucocorticoids, phytoestrogens
Anti-androgens	Cyproterone acetate, finasteride, flutamide, dutasteride, tea tree oil
Inhibitors of androgen synthesis	Ketoconazole, bicalutamide, nilutamide, lavender oil
Antibiotics	Ethionamide, isoniazid, ketoconazole, metronidazole
Anti-ulcer agents	Cimetidine, ranitidine, omeprazole
Cancer chemotherapeutic agents	Alkylating agents, vince alkaloids, methotrexate, imatinib, combination chemotherapy
Cardiovascular drugs	Amiodarone, spironolactone, methyodopa, reserpine, captopril, enalapril, verapamil, diltiazem, nifedipine
Psychoactie agents	Diazepam, phenothiazines, haloperidol, tricyclic antidepressants, atypical anti-psychotics
Drugs of abuse	Alcohol, opioids, methadone, marijuana, heroin, amphetamines
Other	Auranofin, etretinate, sulindac, diethylpropion, metoclopramide, theophylline, domperidone, phenytoin, HAART, penicillamine

These associations are based on case reports, and therefore may not represent a true cause-and-effect relationship.[4]

○ Anti-androgens, such as spironolactone, block androgen receptors, increasing the estrogen-to-androgen ratio.
○ Some drugs displace more estrogen than testosterone from SHBG, leading to relative increase in bioavailable estrogen.
○ Alkylating agents and ketoconazole suppress testosterone biosynthesis.
○ Lavender and tea tree oil have weak estrogenic and anti-androgenic properties that may cause imbalance in estrogen and androgen ratio leading to gynecomastia. Use of products containing these oils should be suspected when cause of gynecomastia is not identified, specifically in prepubertal boys.[7,8]
• Systemic illnesses associated with gynecomastia[1,5]:
○ Cirrhosis and liver disease cause gynecomastia via multiple mechanisms:
  ▪ Increased androstenedione levels (decreased catabolism by liver and increased production by the adrenals)
  ▪ Enhanced aromatization of androgens/androstenedione to estrone and estradiol
  ▪ Increased SHBG, which binds testosterone with greater affinity than estradiol
  ▪ Associated primary or secondary hypogonadism

- **End-stage renal disease (ESRD)** causes gynecomastia due to Leydig cell dysfunction, leading to decreased testosterone levels. Patients with ESRD may also exhibit primary and secondary hypogonadism.
- **Hyperthyroidism** elevates estradiol levels by increasing SHBG and LH, stimulating more estradiol secretion than testosterone by Leydig cells.

DIAGNOSIS

Clinical Presentation

- True gynecomastia presents as a symmetric ridge of glandular tissue, rubbery-firm in consistency, freely mobile, and is located under the areola.[1]
- History should include a **detailed medication list**, onset, presence of breast pain, and symptoms of systemic illnesses such as liver disease, renal disease, or thyrotoxicosis.
- **Physical examination** should focus on breast and testicular examinations, as well as an assessment for virilization.

Differential Diagnosis

- **Pseudogynecomastia** occurs in obese men, and is characterized by soft, nondiscrete, and irregularly lobular adipose tissue deposition without glandular proliferation.[1,9]
- **Male breast cancer** is rare and is generally unilateral, hard or firm, eccentric in location, and may be associated with skin changes, bloody nipple discharge, and lymphadenopathy.[1,10]

Diagnostic Testing

Laboratories
- Mild, asymptomatic, isolated gynecomastia does not warrant evaluation.
- Indication for laboratory evaluation include[1,11]:
  - Rapid and recent onset
  - Size of >5 cm in obese men and >2 cm in lean men
  - Symptomatic
  - Asymmetric
  - Suspicious for malignancy
- **Laboratory workup** includes testosterone, estradiol, LH, FSH, TSH, prolactin, β-hCG, renal and liver function studies.
- Figure 18-1 summarizes gynecomastia evaluation and workup, including the interpretation of hormone levels and recommendations for further evaluation.

Imaging

Imaging is used to rule out malignancy and is not cost effective if physical examination does not provide signs of other illness.[12] While mammography is sensitive for malignancy, ultrasound (US) is specific. However, due to low incidence of male breast cancer, both have low positive predictive value (55% mammogram and 17% US).[12]

TREATMENT

When an underlying cause for gynecomastia is identified during the florid phase, treatment of that condition typically leads to resolution of gynecomastia.[1] Medication-induced gynecomastia starts to regress within 1 month after discontinuation of the drug as long as gynecomastia has not been present for more than 1 year or progressed to the fibrotic quiescent phase.[3]

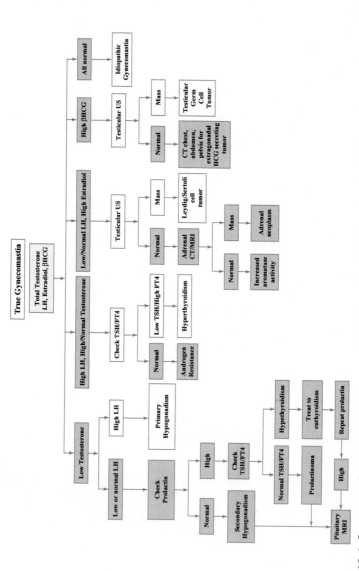

FIGURE 18-1 Gynecomastia workup flow. CT, computed tomography; FT4, free thyroxine; HCG, human chorionic gonadotropin; LH, luteinizing hormone; MRI, magnetic resonance imaging; TSH, thyroid stimulating hormone; US, ultrasound.

Medications

- Medical therapy is most effective during the first phase of gynecomastia and is usually reserved for men with severe painful gynecomastia while surgery is being contemplated.
- Several classes of medications have been studied, but none are currently approved by the FDA for treatment of gynecomastia.
  - **Selective estrogen receptor modulators (SERMs)**, such as **tamoxifen** or **raloxifene**, are effective in treating painful gynecomastia.[11,13] Decrease in pain and tenderness might be noticed within 1 month of therapy initiation. However, these medications do not always result in complete regression of breast tissue. Additionally, use of these agents is associated with adverse side effects such as headache, nausea, impotence, and loss of libido, increased risk of thromboembolism, and patients tend to relapse after the medication has been discontinued. **Testosterone** replacement is only useful in hypogonadal men. It has no utility in eugonadal men and, in some cases, could actually worsen gynecomastia due to aromatization of the additional testosterone to estradiol.
  - **Aromatase inhibitors**, such as anastrozole, are not effective.[14]
  - In men with prostate cancer on androgen deprivation, or when surgical orchiectomy is planned, gynecomastia may be prevented by treatment with ER antagonists (tamoxifen or raloxifene) or by a prophylactic low-dose breast irradiation.

Surgical Management

- Surgery is indicated if there is continued growth, tenderness, malignancy, cosmetic issues, or severe psychological problems, or if the underlying cause cannot be corrected.[15]
- Approaches include subcutaneous mastectomy, US-assisted liposuction, and suction-assisted lipectomy.[16,17]

REFERENCES

1. Matsuomoto AM, Bremer WJ. Testicular disorder. In: Melmed S, Polonsky K, Larsen PR, Kronenberg H, eds. *Williams Textbook of Endocrinology*. 12th ed. Philadelphia, PA: Elsevier/Saunders; 2011:688–774.
2. Johnson RE, Murad MH. Gynecomastia: Pathophysiology, evaluation and management. *Mayo Clin Proc* 2009;84(11):1010–1015.
3. Braunstein GD. Clinical practice. Gynecomastia. *N Engl J Med* 2007;357(12):1229–1237.
4. Mathur R, Braunstein GD. Gynecomastia: pathomechanisms and treatment strategies. *Horm Res* 1997;48(3):95–102.
5. Wilson JD, Aiman J, MacDonald PC. The pathogenesis of gynecomastia. *Adv Intern Med* 1980;25:1–32.
6. Thompson DF, Carter JR. Drug-induced gynecomastia. *Pharmacotherapy* 1993;13(1):37–45.
7. Diaz A, Luque L, Badar Z, Kornic S, Danon M. Prepubertal gynecomastia and chronic lavender exposure: report of three cases. *J Pediatr Endocrinol Metab* 2016;29(1):103–107.
8. Henley DV, Lipson N, Korach KS, Bloch CA. Prepubertal gynecomastia linked to lavender and tea tree oils. *N Engl J Med* 2007;356(5):479–485.
9. Yazici M, Sahin M, Bolu E, et al. Evaluation of breast enlargement in young males and factors associated with gynecomastia and pseudogynecomastia. *Ir J Med Sci* 2010;179(4):575–583.
10. Volpe CM, Raffetto JD, Collure DW, Hoover EL, Doerr RJ. Unilateral male breast masses: Cancer risk and their evaluation and management. *Am Surg* 1999;65(3):250–253.
11. Gikas P, Mokbel K. Management of gynecomastia: An update. *Int J Clin Pract* 2007;61(7):1209–1215.
12. Hines SL, Tan WW, Yasrebi M, DePeri ER, Perez EA. The role of mammography in male patients with breast symptoms. *Mayo Clin Proc* 2007;82(3):297–300.
13. Lawrence SE, Faught KA, Vethamuthu J, Lawson ML. Beneficial effects of raloxifene and tamoxifen in the treatment of pubertal gynecomastia. *J Pediatr* 2004;145(1):71–76.

14. Plourde PV, Reiter EO, Jou HC, et al. Safety and efficacy of anastrozole for the treatment of pubertal gynecomastia: a randomized, double-blind, placebo-controlled trial. *J Clin Endocrinol Metab* 2004;89(9):4428–4433.
15. Cordova A, Moschella F. Algorithm for clinical evaluation and surgical treatment of gynaecomastia. *J Plast Reconstr Aesthet Surg* 2008;61(1):41–49.
16. Tashkandi M, Al-Qattan MM, Hassanain JM, Hawary MB, Sultan M. The surgical management of high-grade gynecomastia. *Ann Plast Surg* 2004;53(1):17–20; discussion 21.
17. Rohrich RJ, Ha RY, Kenkel JM, Adams WP Jr. Classification and management of gynecomastia: defining the role of ultrasound-assisted liposuction. *Plast Reconstr Surg* 2003;111(2):909–923; discussion 924–925.

Hirsutism and Virilization

19

Ritika Puri and Kim Carmichael

GENERAL PRINCIPLES

Definition

- **Hirsutism** is the development of excessive androgen-dependent terminal body hair in a male distribution pattern in a woman.
- True hirsutism needs to be differentiated from **hypertrichosis**, a condition in which there is an increase in androgen-independent total body hair.

Epidemiology

Hirsutism affects 5% of women of reproductive age and is commonly accompanied by other cutaneous manifestations such as acne and temporal hair loss.[1]

Etiology

- Hirsutism is caused by increased androgen production by the ovaries or adrenal glands or increased target-organ responsiveness to androgen.
- Among androgen excess disorders, polycystic ovary syndrome (PCOS) (72.1%) is the most common, followed by idiopathic hyperandrogenism (15.8%), idiopathic hirsutism (7.6%), 21-hydroxylase-deficient nonclassic congenital adrenal hyperplasia (NCCAH) (4.3%), and androgen-secreting tumors (0.2%).[2]
- Causes of hirsutism are listed in Table 19-1 and fall into the following general categories[3]:
  - **PCOS** is the most common cause of hyperandrogenism in women of reproductive age. The criteria for diagnosis are menstrual irregularity and clinical or biochemical evidence of hyperandrogenism. Hirsutism usually develops within the first several years after menarche. Insulin resistance is thought to play a role in this disorder by promoting ovarian hyperandrogenism. Insulin and androgens also decrease the sex hormone–binding globulin (SHBG) concentration, thereby increasing the free testosterone level. The clinical features, diagnosis, and management of PCOS are discussed in Chapter 21.
  - **Idiopathic hyperandrogenism:** women have clinical and biochemical evidence of hyperandrogenism with normal menstrual cycles and ovarian morphology.[2]
  - **Idiopathic hirsutism:** women present with hirsutism with regular menses, normal serum androgen levels without an underlying identifiable disorder. It is proposed that these women may have increased cutaneous 5α-reductase activity.[3]
  - **NCCAH:** NCCAH presents at puberty with hirsutism and menstrual irregularity. It is usually due to 21-hydroxylase deficiency and results in excessive production of 17-hydroxyprogesterone and androstenedione.
  - **Ovarian neoplasms:** androgen-secreting tumors of the ovary, such as Sertoli–Leydig cell tumors, hilus cell tumors, and granulosa–theca cell tumors, usually occur later in life and progress rapidly.
  - **Adrenal neoplasms** can secrete dehydroepiandrosterone sulfate (DHEA-S), dehydroepiandrosterone (DHEA), androstenedione, cortisol (Cushing syndrome), and in rare instances, testosterone.

TABLE 19-1	CAUSES OF HIRSUTISM

Ovarian
PCOS
Hyperthecosis (a severe PCOS variant)
Ovarian tumor (e.g., Sertoli–Leydig cell tumor)

Adrenal
Nonclassic adrenal hyperplasia
Cushing syndrome
Glucocorticoid resistance
Adrenal tumor (e.g., adenoma, carcinoma)

Specific conditions of pregnancy
Luteoma of pregnancy
Hyperreactio luteinalis
Aromatase deficiency of fetus

Other causes
Hyperprolactinemia, hypothyroidism
Medications (danazol, testosterone, anabolic agents)
Idiopathic hirsutism (normal serum testosterone in an ovulatory woman)
Idiopathic hyperandrogenism (patients who do not fall into any of the other
  categories listed)

PCOS, polycystic ovarian syndrome.
Adapted from Bulun SE. Chapter 17: Physiology and pathology of the female reproductive axis. In: Melmed S, Polonsky KS, Larsen PR, Kronenberg HM, eds. *Williams Textbook of Endocrinology.* 13th ed. Philadelphia, PA: Saunders/Elsevier; 2011.

- ○ **Other causes:** certain medications, conditions associated with pregnancy, and other endocrinopathies are rare causes of hirsutism (see Table 19-1). Certain medications such as minoxidil may cause non–androgen-dependent hair growth.

Pathophysiology

- Testosterone is the major circulating androgen with one third released by the ovaries and the remainder as a byproduct of other prohormones. Testosterone is locally converted to biologically active form, dihydrotestosterone (DHT) by 5α-reductase within the target cells.[4]
- Androgens are necessary for the growth of sexual hair and transform vellus hair into terminal hair in sex-specific areas. Vellus hairs are fine, soft, and nonpigmented. Terminal hairs are thick, coarse, and pigmented.
- The growth cycles of terminal hairs are nonsynchronous and last approximately 4 months. Results of hormonal therapy for hirsutism may not be apparent for 6 months due to the long duration of the growth cycle.
- The levels of circulating androgens do not always correlate with the extent of hirsutism. Local conversion of testosterone to the more potent DHT and variability in sensitivity of the hair follicle to androgen also effect hair growth.

DIAGNOSIS

The following goals should be kept in mind while approaching a patient with hirsutism:

- Determine the underlying etiology.
- Assess the degree of hirsutism objectively and hirsutism-related patient distress.

- Assess reproductive goals, since hormonal treatment cannot be used in patients seeking pregnancy.

Clinical Presentation

History

- Most women with hirsutism have either the idiopathic form or PCOS. However, it is very important to exclude rare but serious causes such as androgen-secreting neoplasms or other endocrinopathies.
- **Clinical features suggestive of ovarian or adrenal neoplasm are:**
  - Virilization (voice deepening, increased muscle mass, clitoromegaly, breast atrophy),
  - Late onset of symptoms (during or after the third decade of life),
  - Rapid progression of hirsutism.
- Hirsutism can be associated with Cushing syndrome, thyroid dysfunction, hyperprolactinemia, severe insulin-resistance syndromes, or acromegaly. However, these disorders usually present with other typical disease-specific manifestations.
- It is important to know age of onset, distribution of hair growth, rapidity of progression, and associated features such as acne or hairline recession.
- A **menstrual history** helps distinguish PCOS from idiopathic hirsutism. Irregular menses due to PCOS usually present at menarche while onset after menarche suggests otherwise.
- A **weight history** should also be elicited since gradual weight gain over time is more consistent with and can worsen hirsutism due to PCOS, whereas rapid weight gain may suggest Cushing syndrome.
- Certain **medications** can cause hirsutism, including oral contraceptives containing androgenic progestins, danazol, anabolic or androgenic steroids, and valproic acid.
- **Ethnic background** and **family history** can be helpful in diagnosis of NCCAH.
- Clinicians should always **assess the degree to which patients are distressed** by their hirsutism, since idiopathic hirsutism that does not cause patient distress does not require treatment.
- **Reproductive goals** should be discussed prior to initiating treatment.

Physical Examination

- **Height, weight, BMI**, and **blood pressure** should be measured.
- **Objective assessment of hair distribution and quality of hair** should be documented. A scoring scale such as the modified Ferriman–Gallwey scale can be used to objectively assess degree of hirsutism (Fig. 19-1).[5]
- **Skin** should be examined for acne, seborrhea, temporal balding, acanthosis nigricans, striae, abnormal thickness, or bruising.
- **Signs of virilization** such as deepening of the voice, increased muscle mass, and clitoromegaly should be carefully sought.
- **Gynecologic examination** for palpable ovarian masses should be done.

Diagnostic Criteria

- A Ferriman–Gallwey score ≥8 has traditionally defined hirsutism, since 95% of white and black women of reproductive age have a score <8 (see Fig. 19-1).[3]
- The Ferriman–Gallwey score has several limitations, the most important of which are:
  - "Normal" hair growth varies by ethnic group. Women of Mediterranean origin tend to have more hair, whereas Asian women have less hair in androgen-dependent areas.
  - Previous cosmetic treatments may not allow for accurate assessment of hair growth.
  - The scale does not reflect the degree of distress the hirsutism causes an individual patient.

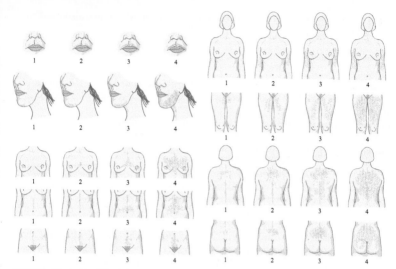

FIGURE 19-1 Modified Ferriman–Gallwey scale for assessing hirsutism. (Modified from *Hatch R, Rosenfield RL, Kim MH, Tredway D*. Hirsutism: Implications, etiology, and management. *Am J Obstet Gynecol* 1981; 140(7):815–830.) A score of 0 to 4 is given for each of the nine androgen-dependent sites. A score ≥8 is suggestive of hirsutism.

- Therefore, clinicians should not be dogmatic in their approach and should instead focus their effort on uncovering and treating serious disorders that cause hirsutism. Once an underlying condition has been excluded, the clinician can focus on the cosmetic concerns of the individual patient.

Differential Diagnosis

- Hypertrichosis is excessive vellus hair in a non-androgen pattern. It is usually due to hereditary factors or drugs such as phenytoin, minoxidil, cyclosporine, etc. It may be associated with metabolic disorders such as thyroid disorders, anorexia nervosa, and porphyria.
- Hypertrichosis lanuginose is a condition with excessive lanugo hair. It may be congenital or acquired. It is often associated with advanced or metastatic cancers.

Diagnostic Testing

- Patients with isolated mild hirsutism do not require testing for elevated androgen levels.
- Patients with moderate or severe hirsutism, or hirsutism of any degree associated with symptoms compatible with PCOS or an androgen-secreting neoplasm, should be evaluated for androgen excess. These symptoms include:
  ○ Signs of virilization
  ○ Rapid progression of hirsutism
  ○ Menstrual irregularity
  ○ Acanthosis nigricans
  ○ Central obesity
- Patients with features of an underlying endocrine disorder should be evaluated for that disorder.

Laboratories

- **Serum testosterone** can be measured either as total or free testosterone and provides the best overall estimate of androgen production in hirsute women. Free testosterone, the biologically active form, is typically elevated in women with androgen excess even when total levels are within the normal range. Therefore, free testosterone is the most sensitive test for androgen excess, but reliability of the assay (particularly radioimmunoassays) is variable. Testing for total testosterone is widely available and better standardized. Serum total testosterone >200 ng/dL is suggestive of androgen-secreting tumors.[1] Patients with PCOS or idiopathic hirsutism typically have normal or slightly elevated levels of testosterone.
- **Serum DHEA-S:** Measuring DHEA-S is indicated to rule out adrenal androgen excess when signs of virilization are present or symptoms are abrupt in onset and rapidly progressive. Women with androgen-secreting adrenal tumors typically have DHEA-S levels >700 mcg/dL.[1]
- **Serum prolactin** can be measured in women with hirsutism and irregular menstrual cycles to rule out hyperprolactinemia.
- **Serum thyroid-stimulating hormone (TSH)** can be measured in women with hirsutism and irregular menstrual cycles to rule out hypothyroidism.
- **Serum 17-hydroxyprogesterone:** Measurement of 17-hydroxyprogesterone is useful to differentiate between NCCAH and PCOS. Testing in women of Hispanic or Eastern European Jewish origin may have a higher yield due to increased prevalence. Because oral contraceptives and/or antiandrogens are the first-line treatments for hirsutism due to NCCAH and PCOS,[6] formal diagnosis of NCCAH may not be necessary unless pregnancy is desired.
- **Screening tests for Cushing syndrome:** Cushing syndrome and PCOS can present in a similar fashion with hirsutism, irregular menses, and weight gain. Screening tests for Cushing syndrome include the low-dose dexamethasone suppression test, 24-hour urine collection for free cortisol, or measurement of late-night salivary cortisol. For a full description of these tests, see Chapter 15.
- **Other tests** to rule out insulin-resistance syndromes or acromegaly may also be warranted in the appropriate clinical setting.

Imaging

Radiologic studies, such as pelvic ultrasound and abdominal CT and MRI, are indicated only if a tumor is suspected.

TREATMENT

- Treatment for hirsutism should focus first on identification of treatable underlying disorders.
- Diet and weight loss may result in lower androgen levels.
- Patients may be treated systemically with medications and/or locally with direct hair removal according to patient preference.
- The response to pharmacologic therapy is slow, and a trial of at least 6 months should be given before doses are changed or new medications are added.
- None of the pharmacologic treatments for hirsutism result in permanent hair removal, and hirsutism generally recurs with discontinuation of therapy.

Medications

- **Drug treatment should be limited to patients who are not seeking immediate pregnancy.**
- Oral contraceptives are the first-line medical therapy for hirsutism in most cases. If response is inadequate after 6 months of treatment with oral contraceptives, an antiandrogen can be

added.[5] **Because of their teratogenic potential, antiandrogens should never be used in premenopausal women unless adequate contraceptive measures are used.**

- **Oral contraceptives**
  - Combination estrogen–progestin oral contraceptives are the first-line agents in patients who do not desire pregnancy.
  - A preparation that contains ethinyl estradiol in conjunction with a progestin with minimal androgenic activity (desogestrel or norgestimate) or antiandrogenic activity (drospirenone) should be selected.
  - Oral contraceptives act to reduce hirsutism through a variety of mechanisms. They cause a suppression of luteinizing hormone release, leading to decreased ovarian androgen production; an increase in SHBG levels, thereby lowering the free testosterone level; and a mild reduction in adrenal androgen production, with some inhibition of the binding of androgen to its receptor.

- **Antiandrogens**
  - **Spironolactone** (100 to 200 mg orally daily) can decrease the effect of androgens by blocking the androgen receptor. When used in combination with an oral contraceptive, both androgen levels and action are decreased. Spironolactone can cause hyperkalemia, and potassium level should be checked after initiation of therapy and with dose titration. Menstrual irregularity can be prevented by concomitant use of oral contraceptives.[7]
  - **Finasteride** (5 to 7.5 mg orally daily) competitively inhibits 5α-reductase and can also be used to treat hirsutism by reducing DHT levels.[7]
  - **Flutamide** is not FDA approved for treatment of hirsutism, and its use is limited as it can cause hepatotoxicity.[4,6,7]
  - **Cyproterone acetate** is an antiandrogen widely available worldwide but not currently available in the United States.
  - Topical antiandrogens are not currently recommended due to inconclusive data regarding their efficacy.

- **Gonadotropin-releasing hormone (GnRH) agonists**
  - GnRH agonists inhibit ovarian androgen production by inhibiting gonadotropins. The ensuing estrogen deficiency can be treated with a combination estrogen–progestin pill. The GnRH agonist–oral contraceptive combination is more cumbersome, more expensive, and has not been shown to be more efficacious than the antiandrogen–contraceptive combination.[3,6]
  - However, GnRH agonists may be considered in patients with severe hirsutism secondary to androgen-secreting ovarian tumor or ovarian hyperthecosis.[6,8]
  - Bone density should be monitored during treatment.

- **Glucocorticoids**
  - Glucocorticoids, which suppress adrenal androgen production, are no longer considered a first-line treatment option for hirsutism due to NCCAH, as oral contraceptive pills and antiandrogens may be more efficacious and have a better side effect profile.[6]
  - Glucocorticoids can be used as a second-line treatment for hirsutism in CAH patients with a poor response to, intolerance of, or contraindication to oral contraceptives and/or antiandrogens.[6]
  - Dexamethasone (0.2 to 0.5 mg) or prednisone (5 to 10 mg) should be taken at bedtime to suppress the nocturnal surge of ACTH.

- **Insulin-lowering drugs**: The benefits of the insulin-sensitizing drugs (metformin and the thiazolidinediones) in treating hirsutism are not well established and as such cannot be recommended for treatment of idiopathic hirsutism.[4,6,9] However, metformin is often prescribed to treat the metabolic derangements of PCOS.

- **Other**: **Topical eflornithine** (13.9%) is approved for facial hirsutism. It irreversibly inhibits L-ornithine decarboxylase which is critical for regulation of cell growth and differentiation of hair cycle.[3,10]

Other Nonpharmacologic Therapies

- Nonpharmacologic treatment should be considered in all patients, either as the sole treatment or as an adjunct to drug therapy.
- Weight loss should be encouraged in overweight or obese women, as it can lower androgen levels and improve hirsutism.[7]
- Bleaching, waxing, shaving, depilatories, electrolysis, and laser treatment are all ways of removing undesired hair. Electrolysis and laser treatment can be expensive, time consuming, and painful but can have long-lasting effects.

PATIENT EDUCATION

Pharmacologic treatment for hirsutism can be expected to reduce, not eliminate, terminal hair growth. Realistic goals of treatment should be explained to patients beginning treatment for hirsutism.

REFERENCES

1. Rosenfield RL. Clinical practice. Hirsutism. *N Engl J Med* 2005;353(24):2578–2588.
2. Carmina E, Rosato F, Janni A, Rizzo M, Longo RA. Extensive clinical experience: relative prevalence of different androgen excess disorders in 950 women referred because of clinical hyperandrogenism. *J Clin Endocrinol Metab* 2006;91(1):2–6.
3. Escobar-Morreale HF, Carmina E, Dewailly D, et al. Epidemiology, diagnosis and management of hirsutism: a consensus statement by the Androgen Excess and Polycystic Ovary Syndrome Society. *Hum Reprod Update* 2012;18(2):146–170.
4. Bulun SE. Chapter 17: Physiology and pathology of the female reproductive axis. In: Melmed S, Polonsky KS, Larsen PR, Kronenberg HM, eds. Williams Textbook of Endocrinology. 13th ed. Philadelphia, PA: Saunders/Elsevier; 2011.
5. Hatch R, Rosenfield RL, Kim MH, Tredway D. Hirsutism: Implications, etiology, and management. *Am J Obstet Gynecol* 1981;140(7):815–830.
6. Martin KA, Chang RJ, Ehrmann DA, et al. Evaluation and treatment of hirsutism in premenopausal women: An endocrine society clinical practice guideline. *J Clin Endocrinol Metab* 2008;93(4):1105–1120.
7. Goodman NF, Bledsoe MB, Futterweit W, et al. American Association of Clinical Endocrinologists medical guidelines for clinical practice for the diagnosis and treatment of hyperandrogenic disorders. *Endocr Pract* 2001;7:120–134.
8. Franks S. The investigation and management of hirsutism. *J Fam Plann Reprod Health Care* 2012;38(3):182–186.
9. Van Zuuren EJ, Fedorowicz Z, Carter B, Pandis N. Interventions for hirsutism (excluding laser and photoepilation therapy alone). *Cochrane Database Syst Rev* 2015;(4):CD010334.
10. Koulouri O, Conway GS. Management of hirsutism. *BMJ* 2009;338:b847.

Male Hypogonadism

20

Maamoun Salam and Charles A. Harris

GENERAL PRINCIPLES

Hypogonadism is the most common disorder of testes function in clinical practice.[1] Symptoms of male hypogonadism depend on the age of the patient at the onset of disease. The production of an adequate amount of testosterone is necessary for the development of external genitalia and secondary sexual characteristics in children and adolescents. In adults, androgen production is necessary for the maintenance of lean body mass, bone mass, libido, sexual function, and spermatogenesis.[2,3] Men with a total testosterone level less than about 300 ng/dL often develop symptoms and signs of hypogonadism that can have long-term clinical effects.

Definition

Male hypogonadism is defined as the **failure of the testes to produce testosterone, sperm, or both**.

Classification

- Hypogonadism is classified as primary, secondary, and combined primary and secondary hypogonadism.
- **Primary hypogonadism** is caused by failure of the testis (hypergonadotropic hypogonadism).
- **Secondary hypogonadism** is caused by defects at the hypothalamic–pituitary level (hypogonadotropic hypogonadism).
- **Combined hypogonadism form**, manifested by both testicular and hypothalamic–pituitary defects.
- **Late onset of hypogonadism** is a distinct clinical syndrome manifested by testosterone deficiency and three sexual symptoms (decreased sexual interest, decreased morning erections, and erectile dysfunction) in aging men.[4,5]

Epidemiology

- Four to 5 million men in the United States have hypogonadism.
- Prevalence of symptomatic androgen deficiency in men between 30 and 79 years of age is 5.6%.[6]
- In longitudinal studies, as men advance in age, total testosterone declines. Serum testosterone declines at <1% to 2% a year after age 30. It is estimated that 30% to 40% of men older than 65 years of age, and 49% to 80% of men older than age 80 have hypogonadism.[7,8]

Etiology

- **Primary hypogonadism**
  - **Developmental defects:**
    - **Klinefelter syndrome** is the most common congenital defect causing male hypogonadism (1 in 1,000 males). Clinical features include small, firm testis; varying degrees of impaired sexual development; azoospermia; gynecomastia; and elevated

gonadotropins. The underlying defect is the presence of an extra X chromosome, 47,XXY being the most common. Diagnosis is confirmed by karyotype analysis.[9] It is associated with the development of diabetes mellitus (DM), systemic lupus erythematosus (SLE), and cancer-like germ cell tumor and breast cancer and possibly non-Hodgkin lymphoma later in life.[10–14] There is a higher mortality from breast cancer but a lower mortality from prostate cancer.[14]

- **The 46,XY/XO karyotype** (mosaic for loss of Y chromosome) clinically presents with a broad spectrum from Turner syndrome to mixed gonadal dysgenesis (MGD), male pseudohermaphroditism (MPH), or phenotypically normal male. The gonads vary from streak to normal testes. If both a streak gonad and a dysgenetic testis ("MGD") are found, there is at least a 20% risk of developing gonadoblastoma. Therefore, gonadectomy should be performed.[15,16]
- **Mutations in genes encoding testosterone synthesis and secretion** can lead to a decrease or absence of testosterone secretion leading to incomplete virilization.
- **Cryptorchidism** may affect one or both testes which will be reflected in the sperm count, serum FSH, and testosterone levels. It is associated with increased risk of testicular cancer.[17]
- **Others defects** include mutation in the follicle-stimulating hormone (FSH) and luteinizing hormone (LH) receptor genes,[1,18,19] myotonic dystrophy,[1,20] congenital anorchia,[1,21] varicocele.[1]

○ **Acquired diseases:**
- **Mumps** is the most common infection affecting the testes usually with adulthood onset and may lead to infertility and reduced testosterone levels.[1] Radiation affects both spermatogenesis and testosterone production.[1]
- **Drugs** such as ketoconazole, spironolactone, cyproterone, and suramin[22] interfere with testosterone synthesis. P450 enzyme-inducing drugs, such as phenytoin and carbamazepine, can lower bioavailable testosterone, raise sex hormone–binding globulin (SHBG) and LH levels, and decrease metabolic clearance. Alkylating agents, such as cyclophosphamide, chlorambucil, cisplatin, and busulfan can damage the seminiferous tubules and to a lesser degree impair testosterone secretion.[1] Spironolactone, cyproterone, cimetidine, and omeprazole compete for the androgen receptor causing gynecomastia and impotence.[23]
- **Other** causes include environmental toxins, testicular trauma, testicular torsion, and bilateral orchiectomy.[1]

- **Secondary hypogonadism**
  ○ **Congenital disorders:**
  - **Isolated hypogonadotropic hypogonadism (IHH)**[1,24] or congenital gonadotropin-releasing hormone (GnRH) deficiency is primarily a disease of males. It is broadly broken down to the anosmic and normosmic subtypes.
  - IHH can present at any age.
  - Affected individuals at birth may have impaired phallic development characterized by micropenis and/or cryptorchidism owing to lack of testosterone production in the final trimester.
  - During childhood, a diagnosis is suspected only by the nonreproductive phenotypes (e.g., the lack of sense of smell in some patients [anosmia] or skeletal abnormalities, such as cleft lip/cleft palate or syndactyly).
  - Presentation in teenage years is characterized by deficient sexual maturation. These individuals have a normal male phenotype at birth because maternal human chorionic gonadotropin (hCG) stimulates normal sexual differentiation in the first trimester.
  - Other clinical features include delayed bone age (typically not beyond 11 to 12 years in males), osteopenia, eunuchoid body proportions, gynecomastia, and delayed puberty.

- Male patients with testes ≥4 cm have incomplete IHH, but those with testes <4 cm have complete IHH. Gonadotropin and testosterone values cannot differentiate between the two disorders.
- IHH must be differentiated from delay of puberty, and the diagnosis cannot be made until patients are >18 years of age. Pulsatile GnRH treatment induces full pubertal development.
- Kallmann syndrome is the anosmic form of IHH. It is characterized by hypogonadotropic hypogonadism and anosmia with or without other nongonadal anomalies. Patients may have midfacial clefting, renal agenesis, and neurologic abnormalities (deafness, cerebellar dysfunction, mental retardation, eye abnormalities).
- A number of genes have been implicated in the etiology of congenital IHH: *ANOS1* (formerly *KAL1*) gene, *FGF8* and *FGFR1* (*KAL2* gene), prokineticin 2 (*PROK2*) and prokineticin receptor 2 (*PROKR2*) mutations (*KAL3* and *KAL4*), kisspeptin and *KISS1* receptor (formerly *GPR54* gene), *GNRH1* and GnRH receptor mutations, tachykinin 3 (*TAC3*) and tachykinin 3 receptor (*TAC3R*) mutations, and *CHD7* and semaphorin 3A.
- Karyotype analysis is not recommended unless multiple congenital anomalies are present.
- Secondary hypogonadism can also occur in **leptin and leptin receptor mutations** (presenting with morbid obesity),[1,25] **LH and FSH β-subunit mutations,**[1] **Laurence–Moon syndrome, and Bardet–Biedl syndrome**.
- **Androgen receptor dysfunction** causes incomplete virilization in 46,XY males, who have bilateral testes and normal testosterone production. The diagnosis should be considered in girls with inguinal or labial masses, women with primary amenorrhea, adolescent girls who become virilized and develop clitoromegaly, adolescent boys who have persistent gynecomastia and fail to undergo puberty, and adult males with undervirilization or infertility associated with azoospermia or severe oligospermia.
- **Impaired development of the pituitary gland** leads to hypogonadism. Mutations in the *PROP1* gene result in absence of several pituitary hormones; *HESX1* gene mutations result in septo-optic dysplasia, which may include poor development of the pituitary.[26]

○ **Acquired disorders**
- Any disease that affects the hypothalamus, pituitary stalk, and the pituitary gland can lead to hypogonadotropic hypogonadism by either suppression of the gonadotropin secretion or direct damage to gonadotropes.
- **Mass lesions** of the pituitary or hypothalamus (sellar or suprasellar lesions) can destroy the pituitary gland or interrupt the nerve fibers that bring GnRH to the hypophyseal circulation. Patients present with headaches, visual disturbances, and variable manifestations of hypopituitarism.
- **Adrenocorticotropic hormone (ACTH)–producing tumors** can cause impotence, decreased libido, and infertility. Testosterone levels are low, and GnRH-stimulated LH concentrations are suppressed.
- **Prolactinoma** affects pulsatile GnRH secretion. Men have low testosterone levels and attenuated pulsatile LH secretion. Treatment with dopamine agonists can normalize prolactin levels and restore sexual function.
- **Infiltrative diseases** such as Langerhans cell histiocytosis and sarcoidosis may involve the hypothalamus and pituitary gland, thereby causing hypogonadism.
- **Infections**—Meningitis is a rare cause of hypogonadism in the United States. Tuberculous meningitis can lead to hypopituitarism more often seen in countries where tuberculosis is common.
- **Leydig cell tumors** and **adrenal tumors** produce estradiol, leading to gynecomastia and gonadotropin deficiency. hCG secreted by **choriocarcinoma** can increase estradiol levels and suppress gonadotropins.

- **Excessive exercise** can cause hypothalamic hypogonadism in men similar to exercise-induced hypothalamic amenorrhea in women. Serial measurement of testosterone levels has been proposed as one means of screening for overtraining syndromes in elite male athletes.
- **Primary hypothyroidism** can cause hyperprolactinemia and hypogonadism (due to elevated thyrotropin-releasing hormone [TRH]).
- **Trauma** severing the pituitary stalk, **postinfectious lesions** of the central nervous system (CNS), **vascular abnormalities** of the CNS, **critical illness**, **brain irradiation**, and **pituitary apoplexy** are some other causes of secondary hypogonadism. Traumatic brain injury may cause temporary or persistent pituitary hypofunction of one or several axes (up to 68.5%).[27,28] The most commonly affected is the pituitary gonadal axis (up to 22.7% in some series). This is followed in frequency by growth hormone deficiency (<18.2%) and ACTH and thyroid-stimulating hormone (TSH) (both 5% or less).[29]
- **Chronic glucocorticoid use** can decrease the action of GnRH by unclear mechanism. There might also be a direct effect on testicular production of testosterone.[30]
- **Drugs** can suppress GnRH, LH, and FSH secretion. GnRH analogs used in treatment of prostate cancer lead to loss of the pulsatility of GnRH secretion. Gonadal steroids like androgen, estrogen, progestin, and megestrol, used as appetite stimulants can cause secondary hypogonadism. Chronic opiates use can suppress the hypothalamic-pituitary-gonadal axis.
- **Other** conditions associated with secondary hypogonadism include anorexia nervosa, DM, and obstructive sleep apnea.[1]
- When all causes of hypogonadotropic hypogonadism have been excluded a diagnosis of acquired idiopathic hypogonadotropic hypogonadism can be made.[31]
- **Combined (primary and secondary) hypogonadism:**
  - **Congenital adrenal hyperplasia** (CAH) can lead to primary hypogonadism if testicular adrenal rest tumor is present. Excessive adrenal androgen production due to untreated or inadequate glucocorticoid therapy for 21-hydroxylase deficiency **suppresses** gonadotropin secretion by sex steroid negative feedback regulation and causes secondary hypogonadism.[1]
  - **Systemic illnesses**, such as renal failure (testicular failure, **hyperprolactinemia**), liver failure (testicular failure and inhibition of the hypothalamic–pituitary axis), sickle cell disease, thalassemia, chronic illness, thyrotoxicosis, human immunodeficiency virus (HIV), and acquired immunodeficiency syndrome (AIDS).
  - **Hemochromatosis** can cause selective gonadotropin deficiency owing to deposition of iron in the pituitary cells, but can also cause primary **hypogonadism** via iron deposition in testes.
  - **Obesity** can cause low testosterone not only by increased aromatization of estrogen in fat tissue and decreased SHBG but also by a combined effect of hormonal, metabolic, and inflammatory mediators at different levels of the hypothalamic–pituitary–testicular axis.[1,32]
  - **Ethanol ingestion** reduces testosterone levels by inhibiting the synthesis of testosterone and impairing the hypothalamic–pituitary axis.[33]

Pathophysiology

- The testes function as part of the hypothalamic–pituitary–gonadal axis.
- A hypothalamic pulse generator resides in the arcuate nucleus, which releases GnRH into the hypothalamic–pituitary portal system.
- In response to these pulses of GnRH, the anterior pituitary secretes the gonadotropins—FSH and LH—which in turn stimulate gonadal activity.

- LH stimulates Leydig cells in pulsatile manner to produce testosterone. An adult testis produces approximately 7 mg of testosterone daily.
- FSH controls spermatogenesis and stimulates synthesis of androgen-binding protein (ABP) by Sertoli cells in the seminiferous tubules. LH helps with sperm production through local secretion of testosterone. Both FSH and testosterone are required to stimulate spermatogenesis quantitatively.
- GnRH secretion is negatively regulated by testosterone.
- LH secretion is negatively regulated by testosterone, estradiol, and dihydrotestosterone (DHT).
- FSH is under the negative influence of inhibin B and testosterone. Sixty percent of testosterone is transported in plasma bound to SHBG, 1% to 3% is free, and the remainder is bound to albumin. Both free testosterone and albumin-bound testosterone are bioavailable.[34]
- Circulating SHBG levels (and, therefore, total testosterone) can be increased in chronic hepatitis, hepatic cirrhosis, hyperthyroidism, HIV infection, estrogen use, anticonvulsant use, and aging.[1] Reduction in SHBG level is associated with obesity, type 2 DM, low-protein states (nephrotic syndrome), hypothyroidism, acromegaly, familial SHBG deficiency, hyperinsulinism, glucocorticoids, progestins, and androgens use.[1]
- Approximately 6% to 8% of testosterone is converted to more potent DHT by 5α-reductase in prostate, testes, liver, kidney, and skin. A small proportion (0.2%) of testosterone is converted to estradiol by aromatase.
- The actions of testosterone are the combined effects of testosterone, plus its active androgenic (DHT) and estrogenic (estradiol) metabolites.
- Testosterone is converted to DHT by 5α-reductase. Both metabolites bind to the same androgen receptor, but DHT is more potent. Testosterone is sufficient for gonadotropin regulation, stimulation of spermatogenesis, and virilization of the Wolffian ducts, whereas DHT is required to mediate virilization of the external genitalia during embryogenesis and to fully complete the virilization that occurs at male puberty. Estradiol inhibits gonadotropin secretion and promotes epiphyseal maturation in the adolescent male.
- Primary hypogonadism results if the testes do not produce the amount of sex steroid sufficient to suppress secretion of LH and FSH to normal levels.
- Secondary hypogonadism may result from failure of the hypothalamic GnRH pulse generator or from inability of the pituitary to respond with secretion of LH and/or FSH.

DIAGNOSIS

- Diagnosis is based on a thorough history, physical examination, and laboratory data. The general scheme for assessment of hypogonadism is outlined in Figure 20-1.
- Testosterone levels are high in the morning and reach nadir in the afternoon. The magnitude of this diurnal rhythm decreases with age. This diurnal variation need to be considered when interpreting results.[35]
- Total testosterone levels should be checked in the morning, fasting, ideally between 8 and 10 AM. A man with total testosterone levels below 300 ng/dL is likely hypogonadal, but levels need to be repeated. Levels between 200 and 400 ng/dL should be repeated with measurement of free testosterone.
- Measurement of free testosterone might be helpful if an abnormality in testosterone binding to SHBG is suspected. Free testosterone should be performed by equilibrium dialysis and not the analog method as the latter test may give misleading information.[36]
- Food, especially glucose ingestion, decreases testosterone level, so the blood should be drawn fasting.[37]

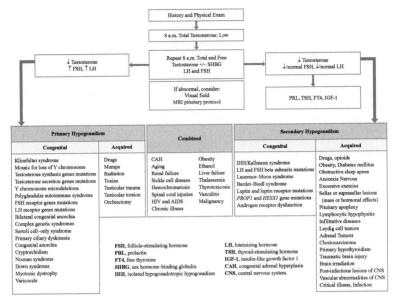

FIGURE 20-1 Algorithm for assessment of type and etiology of hypogonadism.

Clinical Presentation

- Clinical features depend on whether the impairment involves spermatogenesis or testosterone secretion, or both. It also depends on the time of onset of the defect.
- Impaired spermatogenesis typically leads to reduced sperm count and testicular size.
- Reduced testosterone production during the first trimester of pregnancy leads to partial virilization—ranging from severe deficiency causing posterior labial fusion to mild deficiency resulting in hypospadias. Complete lack of testosterone during this period results in female external genitalia (both clitoris and labia).
- If testosterone deficit occurs during the third trimester, it leads to micropenis and cryptorchidism.
- If testosterone production is inhibited before puberty, males will fail to initiate (average age 14) or complete puberty (completed in 3 to 4 years).
- Postpubertal testosterone deficit leads to decreased libido, muscle mass, hair growth, energy, mood, concentration, hematocrit, and bone mass. Decreased libido and fatigue develop early on, whereas other symptoms take years to manifest. Long-standing hypogonadism in males manifests with decreased facial hair growth (female hair distribution) and development of fine wrinkles at the corners of the mouth and eyes. Adults may be infertile as well.
- Hypogonadal men are still able to have some nocturnal erection activity. However, the penile rigidity is not sufficient to permit vaginal penetration.[38]
- Primary hypogonadism is more likely to be associated with gynecomastia. Supernormal serum FSH and LH levels stimulate testicular aromatase to increase the conversion of testosterone to estradiol, resulting in elevated levels of estradiol relative to testosterone.

History

- History should include developmental milestones, with emphasis on sexual development, current symptoms, and information pertaining to possible causes. History of ambiguous genitalia; micropenis; cryptorchidism; failed or delayed puberty; or decrease in libido, sexual function, and/or energy gives clues regarding time of onset of the hypogonadism.
- Inquiry should be made about the rapidity of onset and progression of the symptoms, presence or absence of early morning erections, headaches, anosmia, and changes in voice, vision, muscle strength, or hair growth.
- Questions about culprit systemic illness, trauma, and potential drugs and medications should be asked.
- Patients should be screened for sleep apnea symptoms.
- Inquire about history of other comorbid diseases such as metabolic syndrome, diabetes, osteoporosis, bone fracture, and coronary artery disease. A history of opioid use should be taken.

Physical Examination

- A complete physical examination should be done to look for developmental anomalies, visual problems, abnormal hair distribution, and the presence of eunuchoid proportions (a lower body segment [floor to pubis] that is more than 2 cm longer than upper body segment [pubis to crown], and an arm span that is more than 5 cm longer than height). These proportions occur due to increased length of long bones and delayed epiphyseal closure mediated by the presence of growth hormone and the absence of the estrogenic (estradiol) metabolites of testosterone.[1]
- Examination of the external genitalia should include measuring testicular size (normal, 4 to 7 cm) and volume (normal, 15 to 30 mL) and Tanner stage for adolescents. Decreased testicular size is more pronounced in prepubertal than postpubertal hypogonadism. Consistency of the testicle should also be noted. Typically, firm testes are associated with Klinefelter syndrome owing to hyalinization or fibrosis. Small, rubbery testes are characteristically found in males with prepubertal onset, whereas postpubertal testicular atrophy results in a soft or mushy consistency.
- Gynecomastia may be present, as may increased body fat and reduced muscle mass.
- Physical findings are not always present in adults, since some secondary sexual characteristics, such as reduced muscle mass, may take years to develop. In such instances, appropriate laboratory evaluation may be helpful.

Diagnostic Criteria

The history and physical examination will suggest hypogonadism and laboratory data will reveal an unequivocal lower level of testosterone, usually <300 ng/dL. Further categorization into a diagnosis of primary, secondary, or combined hypogonadism is necessary. The diagnosis of late onset of hypogonadism is made in a similar manner.

Differential Diagnosis

Patients with other diseases may present with similar signs and symptoms. Patients with headaches, visual problems, galactorrhea, papilledema, or optic disc pallor should raise concern for a pituitary tumor. Malaise, fatigue, anorexia, and weight loss are very nonspecific, and can be seen in hypopituitarism and a wide variety of other medical conditions.

Diagnostic Testing

Laboratories

- **Initial laboratory evaluation** should include **testosterone, FSH, LH, and prolactin levels**. Presence of low testosterone with elevated FSH and LH denotes primary hypogonadism, whereas low testosterone and low or normal FSH and LH levels indicate secondary hypogonadism.

- **Semen analysis** is the best means of analyzing sperm count and is typically ordered for men who desire fertility. It should be performed after 1 to 3 days of sexual abstinence and examined within 2 hours of specimen collection. Sperm are analyzed for number, motility, and morphology. Typically, normal semen analysis parameters are $>15 \times 10^6$ sperm per mL, >32% progressive motility, and >4% normal morphology (lower limits are permissible for patients desiring artificial reproductive technology).[39] Abnormal results might be caused by recent fever, trauma, or drug exposure that can transiently impair spermatogenesis.
- Subnormal sperm count and supranormal serum FSH in the setting of normal serum testosterone concentration and normal LH concentration indicate damage to seminiferous tubules (resulting in loss of inhibin feedback on FSH secretion), whereas testosterone production by Leydig cells remains normal.
- If secondary hypogonadism is suspected, **prolactin, TSH, free thyroxine (T_4), insulin-like growth factor-1 ([IGF-1] as a surrogate for GH), and cortisol** (8 AM level or cosyntropin stimulation testing) should be tested.
- Other laboratory tests may be indicated if HIV, end-stage renal disease (ESRD), hemochromatosis, Langerhans cell histiocytosis, or sarcoidosis is suggested.

Imaging
- **Magnetic resonance imaging (MRI)** is indicated if a low testosterone level and low LH or elevated prolactin level is found, if other pituitary hormones are abnormal, and if visual field abnormalities or other neurologic abnormalities are present. If an MRI is contraindicated, although of inferior quality, a head computed tomography (CT) scan with and without contrast could be performed to visualize larger lesions.
- **Assessment of bone density** at 2-year intervals is advised in hypogonadal men and serum testosterone measurements should be obtained in all men with less than normal bone mineral density.

TREATMENT

Medications
- **Testosterone** should be administered only to men who are hypogonadal, as evidenced by symptoms and signs consistent with androgen deficiency and a distinctly subnormal serum testosterone concentration. Increasing the serum testosterone in a man who has symptoms suggestive of hypogonadism but has normal testosterone concentrations will typically not relieve those symptoms.
- Treatment for both primary and secondary hypogonadism consists of replacing testosterone. The following are initial dose and preparation recommendations.[40]
  - Testosterone enanthate/cypionate intramuscular injections, 75 to 100 mg weekly or 150 to 200 mg every 2 weeks.
  - Testosterone gel 1% (AndroGel or Testim), 5 to 10 g applied daily and topically over a covered area of nongenital skin, usually to upper arm.
  - Transdermal testosterone patches (Androderm), one or two 5-mg patch daily applied nightly over the skin of the back, thigh, or upper arm, away from pressure areas.
  - Scrotal patch, 6-mg patch daily (hair needs to be shaved and adhesive may not last 24 hours).
  - Bioadhesive buccal tablet (Striant), 30 mg every 12 hours applied to buccal mucosa.
  - Testosterone pellets implanted subcutaneously at intervals of 3 to 6 months; the dose and regimen vary with the formulation used.
  - Oral testosterone undecanoate, injectable testosterone undecanoate, testosterone-in-adhesive matrix patch, and testosterone pellets where available.

- Generally, the gels are the most costly, whereas patches and injectable esters are the least expensive. The possibility of skin transfer of the gel to a female partner or children in close contact is possible and needs to be avoided by washing thoroughly before close contact.
- Transdermal testosterone patches can be associated with skin rash and itching and may require application of corticosteroid cream.
- Men treated with testosterone injections will have wide swings of plasma testosterone levels and can develop emotional and physiologic effects. These include breast tenderness, hyperactivity at peak levels, and at the nadir fatigue, depression, or anger. Thus, it is advisable to start at lower doses, especially in older men, and then titrate upward to reduce mood fluctuations.
- Other pharmacologic therapies used when fertility is desired include hCG, hCG in combination with FSH, and pulsatile GnRH administration.[41,42] These methods stimulate testicular production of both testosterone and sperm.
- Clomiphene citrate, an estrogen antagonist, decreases the estrogen-induced inhibition of gonadotropin secretions at the hypothalamic level leading to increased secretions of testosterone. Hence, it can be used to treat hypogonadotropic hypogonadism with a dose between 25 mg three times per week and 50 mg daily.[43–45] Clomiphene is currently only FDA-approved for induction of spermatogenesis, but is used off-label to treat hypogonadism. Bone density is a theoretical concern with clomiphene given it is an estrogen antagonist, but studies have not been performed.

Other Nonpharmacologic Therapies

- Therapeutic lifestyle changes are also indicated in treating male hypogonadism. It is still controversial if physical inactivity, alcohol, and smoking decrease testosterone levels.
- **Urgent surgical correction is needed if cryptorchidism is found.**
- A pituitary or hypothalamic mass might need surgical or radiation therapy or medical therapy for prolactinoma.
- If opioid-induced hypogonadism is suspected, cessation of opioids may restore normal gonadal function.

SPECIAL CONSIDERATIONS

- Use of gonadotropins in conjunction with artificial reproductive technologies is a consideration.
- Offering testosterone therapy to older hypogonadal men should be individualized and done only after explicit discussion of the uncertainty about the risks and benefits of testosterone therapy.[40]
- A short-term testosterone therapy may be considered as an adjunctive therapy in HIV-infected men with low testosterone levels and weight loss to promote weight maintenance and gains in lean body mass and muscle strength, or for hypogonadal men receiving high doses of glucocorticoids to promote preservation of lean body mass and bone mineral density.[40]

MONITORING/FOLLOW-UP[40]

- Serum testosterone levels should be checked 3 to 6 months after initiating treatment. They should be measured midway between injections in patients receiving injectable testosterone. The dosage should be adjusted to maintain total testosterone levels in the mid-normal range (400 to 700 ng/dL). In patients treated with a testosterone patch, levels should be checked 3 to 12 hours after application. With use of the gel or buccal tablets, serum levels of testosterone can be measured at any time and should be in the mid-normal range.
- In postpubertal men, it is reasonable to treat with the minimum amount of testosterone that alleviates symptoms of decreased libido, impaired sexual function, and energy levels.

- In primary hypogonadism, normalization of serum LH can be used as a surrogate marker to determine the adequacy of therapy.
- Patients receiving testosterone should be monitored for potential side effects, including erythrocytosis, benign prostatic hyperplasia, prostate cancer, and the development or worsening of sleep apnea. Other minor effects are acne/oily skin and reduced sperm production/infertility.
- **Hemoglobin and hematocrit** should be checked at baseline and monitored at 3 to 6 months and then yearly to screen for the development of erythrocytosis. If the hematocrit increases to above 54%, testosterone replacement needs to be held until the hematocrit decreases to a safe level then testosterone can be restarted at a lower dose. The patient may need to be further evaluated for hypoxia and sleep apnea.
- **Obstructive sleep apnea** may worsen while on testosterone replacement. Symptoms of obstructive sleep apnea such as daytime drowsiness or witnessed apnea should be evaluated at each visit.
- **Bone density scan** should be done after 1 to 2 years of testosterone therapy if osteoporosis or low trauma fractures are present.
- **Digital rectal examination (DRE) and prostate-specific antigen (PSA)** should be performed in all men 40 years or older with PSA of 0.6 ng/mL or higher before initiation of testosterone therapy and at 3 to 6 months, and then according to the evidence-based guidelines for prostate cancer screening. The use of PSA as a screening and following up for prostate cancer is still very controversial. The benefits and risks should be thoroughly discussed with patients.
- Testosterone therapy should be avoided in patients with breast cancer, prostate cancer, hematocrit above 50%, untreated severe OSA, severe lower urinary tract symptoms and poorly controlled heart failure and those desiring fertility.
- Testosterone therapy should be avoided and urologic consultation is warranted in patients with palpable prostate nodule, PSA ≥4 ng/mL or PSA ≥3 ng/mL with risk factors for prostate cancer such as African Americans and those with first-degree relatives with prostate cancer before age 65.[40,46]

OUTCOME/PROGNOSIS

- Normalizing testosterone levels typically leads to improvement in symptoms and normal virilization in men in 3 to 6 months.[3]
- Increases in lean body mass, prostate volume, erythropoiesis, energy, and sexual function occur within the first 3 to 6 months.[3]
- Bone mineral density reaches maximum values by 24 months.[3]
- Ten percent of patients with IHH (including Kallmann syndrome), previously thought to require lifelong therapy, were found to have sustained remission of IHH after discontinuation of hormonal therapy. Therefore, it is reasonable to try brief discontinuation of hormonal therapy to assess reversibility of hypogonadotropic hypogonadism after full virilization is achieved.[47]
- Administration of hCG/human menopausal gonadotropin (hMG) in IHH can increase sperm production in 71% of the large testes subjects (testis volume >4 mL), but only in 36% of the small testes subjects (testis volume <4 mL).[48]

REFERENCES

1. Matsuomoto AM, Bremer WJ. Testicular disorder. In: Melmed S, Polonsky K, Larsen PR, Kronenberg H, eds. *Williams Textbook of Endocrinology*. 12th ed. Philadelphia, PA: Elsevier/ Saunders; 2011:688–777.

2. Bhasin S, Storer TW, Berman N, et al. Testosterone replacement increases fat-free mass and muscle size in hypogonadal men. *J Clin Endocrinol Metab* 1997;82(2):407–413.

3. Snyder PJ, Peachey H, Berlin JA, et al. Effects of testosterone replacement in hypogonadal men. *J Clin Endocrinol Metab* 2000;85(8):2670–2677.

4. Morales A, Schulman CC, Tostain J, C W Wu F. Testosterone deficiency syndrome (TDS) needs to be named appropriately–the importance of accurate terminology. *Eur Urol* 2006;50(3):407–409.

5. Wu FC, Tajar A, Beynon JM, et al. Identification of late-onset hypogonadism in middle-aged and elderly men. *N Engl J Med* 2010;363(2):123–135.

6. Araujo A, Esche G, Kupelian V, et al. Prevalence of symptomatic androgen deficiency in men. *J Clin Endocrinol Metab* 2007;92(11):4241–4247.

7. Feldman HA, Longcope C, Derby CA, et al. Age trends in the level of serum testosterone and other hormones in middle-aged men: Longitudinal results from the Massachusetts male aging study. *J Clin Endocrinol Metab* 2002;87(2):589–598.

8. Harman SM, Metter EJ, Tobin JD, Pearson J, Blackman MR. Longitudinal effects of aging on serum total and free testosterone levels in healthy men. Baltimore Longitudinal Study of Aging. *J Clin Endocrinol Metab* 2001;86(2):724–731.

9. Giltay JC, Maiburg MC. Klinefelter syndrome: Clinical and molecular aspects. *Expert Rev Mol Diagn* 2010;10(6):765–776.

10. Geffner ME, Kaplan SA, Bersche N, et al. Insulin resistance in Klinefelter syndrome. *J Pediatr Endocrinol* 1987;2:173.

11. Scofield RH, Bruner GR, Namjou B, et al. Klinefelter's syndrome (47,XXY) in male systemic lupus erythematosus patients: support for the notion of a gene-dose effect from the X chromosome. *Arthritis Rheum* 2008;58(8):2511–2517.

12. Völkl TM, Langer T, Aigner T, et al. Klinefelter syndrome and mediastinal germ cell tumors. *Am J Med Genet A* 2006;140(5):471–481.

13. Weiss JR, Moysich KB, Swede H. Epidemiology of male breast cancer. *Cancer Epidemiol Biomarkers Prev* 2005;14(1):20–26.

14. Swerdlow AJ, Schoemaker MJ, Higgins CD, Wright AF, Jacobs PA. Cancer incidence and mortality in men with Klinefelter syndrome: a cohort study. *J Natl Cancer Inst* 2005;97(16):1204–1210.

15. Telvi L, Lebbar A, Del Pino O, Barbet JP, Chaussain JL. 45,X/46,XY mosaicism: Report of 27 cases. *Pediatrics* 1999;104(2):304–308.

16. Bianco B, Lipay M, Guedes A, Oliveira K, Verreschi IT. SRY gene increases the risk of developing gonadoblastoma and/or nontumoral gonadal lesions in Turner syndrome. *Int J Gynecol Pathol* 2009;28(2):197–202.

17. van Brakel J, Kranse R, de Muinck Keizer-Schrama SM, et al. Fertility potential in a cohort of 65 men with previously acquired undescended testes. *J Pediatr Surg* 2014;49(4):599–605.

18. Simoni M, Gromoll J, Höppner W, et al. Mutational analysis of the follicle-stimulating hormone (FSH) receptor in normal and infertile men: identification and characterization of two discrete FSH receptor isoforms. *J Clin Endocrinol Metab* 1999;84(2):751–755.

19. Latronico A, Anasti J, Arnhold IJ, et al. Brief report: testicular and ovarian resistance to luteinizing hormone caused by inactivating mutations of the luteinizing hormone-receptor gene. *N Engl J Med* 1996;334(8):507–512.

20. Harper P, Penny R, Foley TP Jr, Migeon CJ, Blizzard RM. Gonadal function in males with myotonic dystrophy. *J Clin Endocrinol Metab* 1972;35(6):852–856.

21. Rousso I, Iliopoulos D, Athanasiadou F, Zavopoulou L, Vassiliou G, Voyiatzis N. Congenital bilateral anorchia: hormonal, molecular and imaging study of a case. *Genet Mol Res* 2006;5(4):638–642.

22. Danesi R, La Rocca RV, Cooper MR, et al. Clinical and experimental evidence of inhibition of testosterone production by suramin. *J Clin Endocrinol Metab* 1996;81(6):2238–2246.

23. Eckman A, Dobs A. Drug-induced gynecomastia. *Expert Opin Drug Saf* 2008;7(6):691–702.

24. Quinton R, Duke VM, Robertson A, et al. Idiopathic gonadotrophin deficiency: genetic questions addressed through phenotypic characterization. *Clin Endocrinol (Oxf)* 2001;55(2):163–174.

25. Strobel A, Issad T, Camoin L, Ozata M, Strosberg AD. A leptin missense mutation associated with hypogonadism and morbid obesity. *Nat Genet* 1998;18(3):213–215.

26. Davis SW, Castinetti F, Carvalho LR, et al. Molecular mechanisms of pituitary organogenesis: In search of novel regulatory genes. *Mol Cell Endocrinol* 2010;323(1):4–19.

27. Hohl A, Mazzuco TL, Coral MH, Schwarzbold M, Walz R. Hypogonadism after traumatic brain injury. *Arq Bras Endocrinol Metabol* 2009;53(8):908–914.

28. Agha A, Thompson CJ. Anterior pituitary dysfunction following traumatic brain injury (TBI). *Clin Endocrinol (Oxf)* 2006;64(5):481–488.

29. Kelly DF, Gonzalo IT, Cohan P, Berman N, Swerdloff R, Wang C. Hypopituitarism following traumatic brain injury and aneurysmal subarachnoid hemorrhage: A preliminary report. *J Neurosurg* 2000;93(5):743–752.

30. Odell WD. Testosterone treatment of men treated with glucocorticoids. *Arch Intern Med* 1996;156(11):1133–1134.

31. Nachtigall LB, Boepple PA, Pralong FP, Crowley WF Jr. Adult-onset idiopathic hypogonadotropic hypogonadism–a treatable form of male infertility. *N Engl J Med* 1997;336(6):410–415.

32. Wang C, Jackson G, Jones TH, et al. Low testosterone associated with obesity and the metabolic syndrome contributes to sexual dysfunction and cardiovascular disease risk in men with type 2 diabetes. *Diabetes Care* 2011;34(7):1669–1675.

33. Emanuele MA, Emanuele N. Alcohol and the male reproductive system. *Alcohol Res Health* 2001;25(4):282–287.

34. Carruthers M, Trinick TR, Wheeler MJ. The validity of androgen assays. *Aging Male* 2007;10(3):165–172.

35. Brambilla DJ, Matsumoto AM, Araujo AB, McKinlay JB. The effect of diurnal variation on clinical measurement of serum testosterone and other sex hormone levels in men. *J Clin Endocrinol Metab* 2009;94(3):907–913.

36. Vermeulen A, Verdonck L, Kaufman JM. A critical evaluation of simple methods for the estimation of free testosterone in serum. *J Clin Endocrinol Metab* 1999;84(10):3666–3672.

37. Caronia LM, Dwyer AA, Hayden D, Amati F, Pitteloud N, Hayes FJ. Abrupt decrease in serum testosterone levels after an oral glucose load in men: implications for screening for hypogonadism. *Clin Endocrinol (Oxf)* 2013;78(2):291–296.

38. Kwan M, Greenleaf WJ, Mann J, Crapo L, Davidson JM. The nature of androgen action on male sexuality: a combined laboratory-self-report study on hypogonadal men. *J Clin Endocrinol Metab* 1983;57(3):557–562.

39. Cooper TG, Noonan E, von Eckardstein S, et al. World Health Organization reference values for human semen characteristics. *Hum Reprod Update* 2010;16(3):231–245.

40. Bhasin S, Cunningham GR, Hayes FJ, et al. Testosterone therapy in men with androgen deficiency syndromes: An Endocrine Society clinical practice guideline. *J Clin Endocrinol Metab* 2010;95(6):2536–2559.

41. Han TS, Bouloux PM. What is the optimal therapy for young males with hypogonadotropic hypogonadism. *Clin Endocrinol (Oxf)* 2010;72(6):731–737.

42. Silveira LF, Latronico AC. Approach to the patient with hypogonadotropic hypogonadism. *J Clin Endocrinol Metab* 2013;98(5):1781–1788.

43. Liel Y. Clomiphene citrate in the treatment of idiopathic or functional hypogonadotropic hypogonadism in men: a case series and review of the literature. *Endocr Pract* 2017;23(3):279–287.

44. Bardin CW, Ross GT, Lipsett MB. Site of action of clomiphene citrate in men: a study of the pituitary-Leydig cell axis. *J Clin Endocrinol Metab* 1967;27(11):1558–1564.

45. Ioannidou-Kadis S, Wright PJ, Neely RD, Quinton R. Complete reversal of adult-onset isolated hypogonadotropic hypogonadism with clomiphene citrate. *Fertil Steril* 2006;86(5):1513.e5–e9.

46. Wolf AM, Wender RC, Etzioni RB, et al. American Cancer Society Prostate Cancer Advisory Committee. American Cancer Society guideline for the early detection of prostate cancer: update 2010. *CA Cancer J Clin* 2010;60(2):70–98.

47. Raivio T, Falardeau J, Dwyer A, et al. Reversal of idiopathic hypogonadotropic hypogonadism. *N Engl J Med* 2007;357(9):863–873.

48. Miyagawa Y, Tsujimura A, Matsumiya K, et al. Outcome of gonadotropin therapy for male hypogonadotropic hypogonadism at university affiliated male infertility centers: A 30-year retrospective study. *J Urol* 2005;173(6):2072–2075.

Polycystic Ovary Syndrome

21

Rong Mei Zhang and Marina Litvin

GENERAL PRINCIPLES

- Polycystic ovary syndrome (PCOS), first described in 1935, presents with amenorrhea, hirsutism, enlarged ovaries, and obesity.[1] It is also associated with hyperinsulinemia, glucose intolerance, and dyslipidemia.
- PCOS impacts fertility, and has been linked to insulin resistance and increased risk of endometrial cancer and cardiovascular disease.[2,3] Its multifactorial etiology has not been clearly established.

Epidemiology

PCOS is the most common endocrine disorder in women of reproductive age, affecting 8% to 20% of women, depending on the population studied and the diagnostic criteria used.[4] In women with type 2 diabetes, prevalence can reach 27%.[5]

Pathophysiology

- Hallmark of PCOS is the coexistence of varying degrees of reproductive (hyperandrogenism, anovulation) and metabolic (insulin resistance, obesity) disturbances. In PCOS, luteinizing hormone (LH) pulse frequency and amplitude are increased, likely due to accelerated GnRH pulse. Increased LH pulse frequency favors earlier differentiation of granulosa cells, disordered follicular development, and increased androgen production by the ovary, exacerbated by hyperinsulinemia.[6] Hyperandrogenism is worsened by upregulation of adrenal androgen enzymes.[6]
- Elevated androgens and low progestin, due to multiple anovulatory cycles, feedback to the hypothalamus, accelerating GnRH pulse frequency, and creating a vicious cycle.[6]
- Risk of developing PCOS is compounded by environmental exposures (endocrine disrupters) and intrauterine growth restriction. In addition, inflammatory conditions may affect ovarian remodeling.[7]

DIAGNOSIS

PCOS has multiple manifestations that vary between individuals, and vary over time in the same individual.

Clinical Presentation

- Features of PCOS develop during puberty, and range in severity from mild hirsutism to amenorrhea and infertility.
- Most patients are overweight or obese, with the degree of weight gain influenced by ethnicity.

History
- **Menstrual history** is critical in evaluation of PCOS. Onset of menarche, menstrual regularity, and history of abnormal bleeding should be documented. Patients should be asked about contraception and prior pregnancies.

- **Irregular menses** are due to chronic oligo- or anovulation, and can result in endometrial hyperplasia and dysfunctional uterine bleeding. Oligomenorrhea is defined as menstrual cycle >35 days, while cycle length of 32 to 36 days may require further evaluation with a mid-luteal phase progesterone (levels >2.5 ng/mL indicating ovulation).[8]
- The onset and severity of **hirsutism** and acne should be recorded. Hirsutism involves terminal hair growth in androgen sensitive areas, and can be graded by the Ferriman–Gallwey score. Hirsutism is challenging to follow over time, and the score has not been validated in certain ethnicities or adolescents.
- Androgen excess can result in **androgenic alopecia** (male pattern baldness) and may be exacerbated by weight gain. Frank alopecia is rare.
- **Central obesity** is present in 40% to 60% of patients, and up to 69% of U.S. women with PCOS are obese.[9]
- **Hyperinsulinemia** and **insulin resistance** can exist in lean patients, but are exacerbated by obesity.
- **Sleep apnea** may be present.
- Family members may exhibit conditions of insulin resistance (diabetes, hypertension).

Physical Examination
- Assess the degree of **acne, alopecia**, and **hirsutism**.
- **Acanthosis nigricans**, a marker of insulin resistance, is a velvety hyperpigmented plaque that can be seen on posterior neck, axilla and groin.
- To assess cardiovascular risk, measure **blood pressure, weight**, and **waist/hip circumference**.

Diagnostic Criteria

- Criteria for diagnosing PCOS have evolved with better ultrasound techniques. The NIH working group criteria, Rotterdam PCOS Consensus, and the Androgen Excess and PCOS Society guidelines are compared in Table 21-1.[10] Each requires a combination of specific findings, including **hyperandrogenism, oligomenorrhea**, and **polycystic ovaries** on ultrasound for diagnosis.
- **Hyperandrogenism** is the primary defect in PCOS, since its absence, regardless of menstrual irregularities, makes PCOS less likely.[11]
- Exclusion of other etiologies of hyperandrogenism is essential to the diagnosis PCOS.
- PCOS is **challenging to diagnose in adolescents**, who often have menstrual cycle irregularities,[8] and for whom criteria for ovarian ultrasound findings are lacking.

Differential Diagnosis[12]

- **Late-onset congenital adrenal hyperplasia (CAH)** is more common in the Ashkenazi Jewish population; patients present with more virilization than typical PCOS and have a family history of infertility and/or hirsutism (see Chapter 13, CAH).
- In **androgen-secreting neoplasms**, symptoms occur later, and are more severe (clitoromegaly, voice deepening). Although dehydroepiandrosterone sulfate (DHEAS) levels may be elevated in PCOS, levels >700 mcg/dL should prompt imaging.
- **Cushing syndrome** may present at any age, progress slowly, and have overlapping features with PCOS (see Chapter 15).
- **Hyperprolactinemia** and **hypothyroidism** are not usually associated with hyperandrogenemia, but a **serum prolactin** and **TSH** should be checked in all women with menstrual irregularities.
- Consider **acromegaly** if pathognomonic features are present (see Chapter 3).
- **Drugs** (androgens, valproate, cyclosporine) can cause hyperandrogenism and menstrual irregularities. Cross-contamination from household members using topical testosterone should also be considered.

TABLE 21-1 DIAGNOSTIC CRITERIA FOR PCOS[a,b]

Criteria	NIH 1990 "Classic"	Rotterdam 2003 (Any 2 of 3)	AE-PCOS 2005
Clinical or biochemical hyperandrogenism[d]	+	+/–	+
Oligomenorrhea[c]	+	+/–	+/–
Polycystic ovaries on ultrasound[e]	Criteria not used	+/–	+/–

[a]NIH: presence of both oligomenorrhea and clinical/biochemical hyperandrogenism; Rotterdam: any two of the above criteria; AE-PCOS: presence of clinical/biochemical hyperandrogenism and one other criterion.

[b]All guidelines require exclusion of other causes of androgen excess or ovulatory disorders (Cushing syndrome, nonclassical CAH, virilizing tumors).

[c]Eight or fewer menses per year.

[d]Acne or hirsutism or androgenic alopecia.

[e]Ovarian volume >10 mL and/or ≥25 follicles 2–9 mm in size in at least one ovary (follicular number changed due to improved technology).

AE-PCOS, androgen excess-polycystic ovary syndrome society; NIH, National Institutes of Health.

From Wild RA, Carmina E, Diamanti-Kandarakis E, et al. Assessment of cardiovascular risk and prevention of cardiovascular disease in women with the polycystic ovary syndrome: A consensus statement by the Androgen Excess and Polycystic Ovary Syndrome (AE-PCOS) Society. *J Clin Endocrinol Metab* 2010;95:2038–2049. Reprinted with permission.

Diagnostic Testing

- PCOS is a diagnosis of exclusion, and laboratory work up is aimed at ruling out other disorders. There are no universally accepted hormonal cutoffs for PCOS, making it a clinical diagnosis.
- Normal testosterone levels do not exclude PCOS.

Laboratories

- Free testosterone measurement by equilibrium dialysis is recommended.[8] Up to 80% of patients with PCOS have total and free testosterone levels in the upper normal or above the normal range. Decreased production of hepatic sex hormone–binding globulin (SHBG) leads to elevated free testosterone levels, while total testosterone levels may be normal. DHEA-S may be mildly elevated.
- Additional laboratory abnormalities in PCOS
  - **Elevated LH** and normal FSH result in an **elevated LH/FSH** ratio. Due to pulsatile gonadotropin secretion and day-to-day variability, gonadotropin levels are too insensitive for diagnosis. LH levels can be useful, especially in lean women with amenorrhea.
  - Serum estrone may be increased, while serum estradiol is usually normal.
  - **Impaired glucose tolerance** and **diabetes** are present in up to 40% of women with PCOS when challenged with a 75 g, 2-hour oral glucose tolerance test (OGTT).[13] Guidelines suggest screening all women with PCOS with an OGTT every 1 to 2 years.[14]
  - Atherogenic lipid profiles (high very-low–density lipoprotein (VLDL), high LDL, and low HDL) are common in women with PCOS, even after adjusting for BMI. Low HDL levels are associated with obesity, while high LDL levels with hyperandrogenemia.

Imaging[15]
- Criteria
  - Follicle number per ovary (FNPO) ≥25 is suggestive of PCOS **OR**
  - Ovarian volume of ≥10 mL per ovary
- FNPO is recommended over use of ovarian volume due to higher predictive power and less variability.
- If ultrasound is not available, anti-mullerian hormone (AMH), secreted by granulosa cells, can be used as a marker of ovarian reserve.[16]

TREATMENT

- Most manifestations of PCOS can be reversed by improving insulin resistance, either by weight loss and/or medications.
- Clinical response to therapy is slow, lagging behind biochemical improvement.

Contraindications to treatment, and **pregnancy** should be excluded before starting medications.

Medications

Oral Contraceptives (OCPs)
- OCPs are standard therapy for patients not desiring pregnancy. Oral formulation is recommended, since first pass liver metabolism increases SHBG, decreasing androgen levels. Nonoral formulations bypass first pass metabolism and may not be as effective.
- OCPs restore normal menses and prevent unopposed, estrogenic stimulation of the endometrium.
- Preparations containing ethinyl estradiol with low androgenic activity progestin, such as norgestimate or desogestrel should be used.[17]
- Drospirenone, a progestin with antimineralocorticoid and antiandrogenic activity, can be used in combination with ethinyl estradiol.
- The use and choice of OCP should be individualized based on manifestations of PCOS (degree of insulin resistance, androgenicity, etc). Insulin resistance can be worsened by OCP use.[17]
- Contraindications for OCP must be considered, including age, smoking, and prior venous thromboembolism.
- In women who are not candidates for OCP, intermittent oral progestin with a 7- to 10-day course of medroxyprogesterone acetate every 1 to 3 months can be considered. This offers endometrial protection, but does not improve hyperandrogenism.

Insulin Sensitizers
Improving insulin sensitivity through weight loss or medications improves hyperandrogenemia and induces ovulation. Although not approved by the Food and Drug Administration (FDA) for treatment of PCOS, metformin effectively decreases testosterone, fasting insulin, and glucose levels. It improves ovulation, but without overall increase in live birth rate when compared to placebo.[18] Metformin is pregnancy category B.

Antiandrogens
- Antiandrogens can be used with OCPs to further improve hirsutism, but the effect may not be seen for up to 6 months. Patients taking antiandrogens must use effective contraception due to teratogenicity of these drugs.
- **Spironolactone** inhibits androgen biosynthesis and 5α-reductase, and blocks the androgen receptor. When used alone, it has minimal effects on free testosterone. Used in combination with OCP, both androgen levels and androgen action are decreased.

- **Finasteride** and **flutamide** can also be used to treat hirsutism. Flutamide may cause hepatotoxicity.
- **Eflornithine hydrochloride** cream, which slows hair growth, can be used to treat facial hirsutism. Topical **minoxidil** can be used for alopecia.

Other Pharmacologic Interventions
- Liraglutide (a glucagon-like peptide (GLP)-1 receptor agonist) can be an effective treatment for weight loss in women with PCOS, and can improve insulin resistance, compared to placebo and metformin, without affecting menstrual frequency or androgen levels.[19]
- Use of agents for weight loss, such as Orlistat may reduce testosterone levels in addition to weight loss.[20]
- Statins used with or without an OCP improved testosterone levels, hirsutism, and lipid profiles.[21,22]
- More research is needed to determine the safety and efficacy of these drugs.

Nonpharmacologic Therapies
- Weight reduction, through caloric restriction and exercise, should be a central feature in treatment of PCOS.
- An effective weight loss plan includes supervised weight loss and maintenance phases by using diet, exercise, and behavioral therapy.[23]

COMPLICATIONS

- **Infertility** is an important concern for women with PCOS.
- An infertility evaluation of the couple, including semen analysis, should be completed.
- Weight loss and insulin sensitizers may induce ovulatory cycles, leading to conception.
- **Clomiphene citrate** is a nonsteroidal agent that may restore gonadotropin secretion. It is superior to metformin in achieving conception, but has a relatively high rate of multiple pregnancies. Combination of clomiphene and metformin may increase pregnancy rates.
- **Letrozole**, an aromatase inhibitor, can improve live birth rates compared to clomiphene, without a difference in increasing congenital anomalies.[24] If pregnancy is not achieved after 6 to 9 months of clomiphene with or without metformin, a fertility specialist should be consulted.
- Increased incidence of spontaneous miscarriages is associated with PCOS, and may be reduced by metformin.
- In patients able to conceive, there is an increased risk of pregnancy-induced hypertension, preeclampsia, gestational diabetes, pregnancy loss, and preterm labor.
- The prevalence of **impaired glucose tolerance** and **type 2 diabetes** is increased in women with PCOS, who have a three to seven times greater risk of developing diabetes. This association is present in both obese and lean women with PCOS.[25]
- **Hypertension** is not common in young women with PCOS, can be proportional to menstrual cycle length, and dramatically increases in prevalence by perimenopause.
- Women with PCOS also have an increased risk for **dyslipidemia** and may have abnormal vascular function, higher rates of coagulopathy, and increased inflammatory markers. There is likely an increased cardiovascular risk, but this research is still ongoing.[26]
- Unopposed estrogenic stimulation of the uterus increases the risk of **endometrial hyperplasia** and **carcinoma**.
- There is an increased incidence of **nonalcoholic fatty liver disease** (NAFLD) in patients with PCOS, and 71% of females with NAFLD have PCOS. Insulin resistance contributes to both conditions.[27]

- PCOS increases risk of **obstructive sleep apnea** (OSA), and treatment improves blood pressure and insulin resistance with effects dependent on the duration of continuous positive airway pressure (CPAP) use.[28]
- Decreased bone mineral density has been linked to PCOS, with increased inflammation associated with decreased bone strength.[29]

MONITORING/FOLLOW-UP

- A **multidisciplinary** approach encompassing several specialties including endocrinology, nutrition, dermatology, psychiatry, and exercise physiology is required to provide optimal care to PCOS patients.
- The long-term metabolic and cardiovascular risks associated with PCOS heighten the importance of proper follow-up.
- OGTT, as described above, is recommended for those with obesity, advanced age, personal history of gestational diabetes, or family history of type 2 diabetes.
- Other risk factors for cardiovascular disease, including tobacco use, sleep apnea, and hyperlipidemia, should be assessed annually.
- In PCOS, relative hyperandrogenemia and increased risk for glucose intolerance and dyslipidemia persist after menopause, and ongoing screening is warranted.[30]

REFERENCES

1. Stein IF, Leventhal ML. Amenorrhea associated with bilateral polycystic ovaries. *Am J Obstet Gynecol* 1935;29:181–191.
2. Haoula Z, Salman M, Atiomo W. Evaluating the association between endometrial cancer and polycystic ovary syndrome. *Human Reprod* 2012;27:1327–1331.
3. De Groot PC, Dekkers OM, Romijn JA, Dieben SW, Helmerhorst FM. PCOS, coronary heart disease, stroke and influence of obesity: A systematic review and meta-analysis. *Human Reproduction Update* 2011;17:495–500.
4. Sirmans SM, Pate KA. Epidemiology, diagnosis, and management of polycystic ovary syndrome. *Clinical Epidemiology* 2014;6:1–13.
5. Peppard HR, Marfori J, Iuorno MJ, Nestler JE. Prevalence of polycystic ovary syndrome among premenopausal women with type 2 diabetes. *Diabetes Care* 2001;24:1050–1052.
6. Baskin NE, Balen AH. Hypothalamic-pituitary, ovarian and adrenal contributions to polycystic ovary syndrome. *Best Pract Res Clin Obstet Gynaecol* 2016;37:80–97.
7. Akcali A, Bostanci N, Özçaka Ö, et al. Gingival inflammation and salivary or serum granulocyte secreted enzymes n patients with polycystic ovary syndrome. *J Periodontol* 2017;88:1145–1152.
8. Goodman NF, Cobin RH, Futterweit W, Glueck JS, Legro RS, Carmina E. AACE, American College of Endocrinology, and Androgen Excess and PCOS Society Disease State Clinical Review: Guide to the best practices in the evaluation and treatment of polycystic ovary syndrome–part 1. *Endocr Pract* 2015;21:1291–1300.
9. Moran LJ, Pasquali R, Teede HJ, Hoeger KM, Norman RJ. Treatment of obesity in polycystic ovary syndrome: A position statement of the Androgen Excess and Polycystic Ovary Syndrome Society. *Fertil Steril* 2009;92:1966–1982.
10. Wild RA, Carmina E, Diamanti-Kandarakis E, et al. Assessment of cardiovascular risk and prevention of cardiovascular disease in women with the polycystic ovary syndrome: A consensus statement by the Androgen Excess and Polycystic Ovary Syndrome (AE-PCOS) Society. *J Clin Endocrinol Metab* 2010;95:2038–2049.
11. Azziz R, Carmina E, Dewailly D, et al. Criteria for defining polycystic ovary syndrome as a predominantly hyperandrogenic syndrome: An Androgen Excess Society guideline. *J Clin Endocrinol Metab* 2006;91:4237–4245.
12. Legro RS, Arslanian SA, Ehrmann DA, et al. Diagnosis and treatment of polycystic ovary syndrome: An endocrine society clinical practice guideline. *J Clin Endocrinol Metab* 2013;98:455–492.

13. Legro RS, Kunselman AR, Dodson WC, Dunaif A. Prevalence and predictors of risk for type 2 diabetes mellitus and impaired glucose tolerance in polycystic ovary syndrome: A prospective, controlled study in 254 affected women. *J Clin Endocrinol Metab* 1999;84:165–169.

14. Salley KE, Wickham EP, Cheang KI, Essah PA, Karjane NW, Nestler JE. Position statement: Glucose intolerance in polycystic ovary syndrome—a position statement of the androgen excess society. *J Clin Endocrinol Metab* 2007;92;4546–4556.

15. Dewailly D, Lujan ME, Carmina E, et al. Definition and significance of polycystic ovarian morphology: A task force report from the androgen excess and polycystic ovary syndrome society. *Hum Reprod Update* 2014;29:334–332.

16. Falbo A, Rocca M, Russo T, et al. Serum and follicular anti-mullerian hormone levels in women with polycystic ovary syndrome (PCOS) under metformin. *J Ovarian Res* 2010;3;16.

17. Diamanti-Kandarakis E, Baillargeon JP, Iuorno MJ, Jakubowicz DJ, Nestler JE. A modern medical quandary: Polycystic ovary syndrome, insulin resistance, and oral contraceptive pills. *J Clin Endocrinol Metab* 2003;88;1927–1932.

18. Tang T, Lord JM, Norman RJ, Yasmin E, Balen AH. Insulin-sensitizing drugs (metformin, rosiglitazone, pioglitazone, D-chiro-inositol) for women with polycystic ovary syndrome, oligo amenorrhoea and subfertility. *Cochrane Database Syst Rev* 2010;20(1).

19. Jensterle M, Salamun V, Kocjan T, Vrtacnik Bokal E, Janez A. Short term monotherapy with glp-1 receptor agonist liraglutide or pde 4 inhibitor roflumilast is superior to metformin in weight loss in obese pcos women: A pilot randomized study. *J Ovarian Res* 2015;8:32.

20. Cho LW, Kilpatrick ES, Keevil BG, Coady AM, Atkin SL. Effect of metformin, orlistat and pioglitazone treatment on mean insulin resistance and its biological variability in polycystic ovary syndrome. *Clin Endocrinol (Oxf)* 2009;70:233–237.

21. Banaszewska B, Pawelczyk L, Spaczynski RZ, Dziura J, Duleba AJ. Effects of simvastatin and oral contraceptive agent on polycystic ovary syndrome: Prospective, randomized, crossover trial. *J Clin Endocrinol Metab* 2007;92:456–461.

22. Stamets K, Taylor DS, Kunselman A, Demers LM, Pelkman CL, Legro RS. A randomized trial of the effects of two types of short-term hypocaloric diets on weight loss in women with polycystic ovary syndrome. *Fertil Steril* 2004;81:630–637.

23. Brennan L, Teede H, Skouteris H, Linardon J, Hill B, Moran L. Lifestyle and behavioral management of polycystic ovary syndrome. *J Womens Health (Larchmt)* 2017;26(8):836–848.

24. Legro RS, Brzyski RG, Diamond MP, et al. Letrozole versus clomiphene for infertility in the polycystic ovary syndrome. *N Engl J Med* 2014;371:119–129.

25. Moran LJ, Misso ML, Wild RA, Norman RJ. Impaired glucose tolerance, type 2 diabetes and metabolic syndrome in polycystic ovary syndrome: A systematic review and meta-analysis. *Hum Reprod Update* 2010;16:347–363.

26. Carmina E. Cardiovascular risk and events in polycystic ovary syndrome. *Climateric* 2009;12:22–25.

27. Kelley CE, Brown AJ, Diehl AM, Seti TL. Review of nonalcoholic fatty liver disease in women with polycystic ovary syndrome. *World J Gastroenterol* 2014;20:14172–14184.

28. Tasali E, Chapotot F, Leproult R, Whitmore H, Ehrmann DA. Treatment of obstructive sleep apnea improves cardiometabolic function in young obese women with polycystic ovary syndrome. *J Clin Endocrinol Metab* 2011;96:365–374.

29. Kaylan S, Patel MS, Kingwell E, Côté HCF, Liu D, Prior JC. Competing factors link to bone health in polycystic ovary syndrome: Chronic low-grade inflammation takes a toll. *Sci Rep* 2017;7:3432–3439.

30. Puurunen J, Piltonen T, Morin-Papunen L, et al. Unfavorable hormonal, metabolic, and inflammatory alterations persist after menopause in women with PCOS. *J Clin Endocrinol Metab* 2011;96:1827–1834.

Gender Dysphoria and Transgender Medicine

22

Brian D. Muegge, Christopher Lewis, and
Thomas J. Baranski

GENERAL PRINCIPLES

- Transgender people increasingly seek out hormonal and/or surgical treatments that allow them to live with a body that matches their gender identity.
- Gender affirming therapy has consistently been shown to improve mental and physical health for transgender people.[1]
- Endocrinologists are part of a multidisciplinary team, including primary care providers, gynecologists, surgeons, social workers, and mental health professionals, that provide integrated medical care to transgender people. At all levels of medical education, more training is needed to adequately prepare for this responsibility. Surveys show that while 80% of practicing endocrinologists have provided care for a transgender patient, only 19% of those physicians had received formal training in transgender medicine and the majority of respondents desired more opportunities for education.[2]
- There are almost no high-quality randomized trials to guide treatment decisions in transgender medicine. Expert recommendations from the Endocrine Society and the World Professional Association for Transgender Health (WPATH) form the backbone of most treatment protocols.[3,4] Providers caring for transgender patients should familiarize themselves with the most recent guidelines from these societies.
- Understanding the basic terminology of gender and self-expression improves compassionate and respectful patient care for transgender patients.[5,6] Commonly used definitions are summarized in Table 22-1.[5,6]

Epidemiology

- Data from The Netherlands, which have had a longstanding centralized referral center to serve all transgender patients, estimates that 1 in 11,900 biologic males and 1 in 30,400 biologic females seek treatment for transgender-related care.[7] The roughly threefold excess of identified transgender women compared to transgender men is found in many other countries among adults, though children present for medical attention of gender nonconformity at roughly equal ratios.
- A meta-analysis including studies from multiple countries estimates that between 6.8 and 9.2 people per 100,000 are transgender, as measured by diagnostic codes or provision of medical therapy.[8]
- More recent studies estimate that 0.4% of the United States population identifies as transgender.[9]
- There are significant differences in prevalence and experience of transgender people around the world.[10] Reasons are multiple, but include different cultural norms of gender identity, patterns of discrimination, and possibly genetic factors.
- Transgender populations face significant social and health disparities, including higher rates of depression, substance abuse, HIV infection, suicide, and a greater likelihood to be homeless, unemployed or a victim of physical or sexual violence.[11,12]
- Transgender patients report significant negative experiences when seeking health care such as having to teach the provider about transgender health (50%), refusal of care (19%), and harassment in the health care setting (28%).[13]

TABLE 22-1	**DEFINITIONS OF SELECTED TERMS USED IN THIS CHAPTER**[5,6]
Sex	Sex assigned at birth based on external genitalia, chromosomes, and/or gonads
Gender identity	An individual's sense of being a man, a woman or of indeterminate gender
Transgender	When someone's gender identity differs from the sex assigned at birth
Transgender man	A person with a male gender identity and a female birth assigned sex, also known as female-to-male (FTM)
Transgender woman	A person with a female gender identity and a male birth assigned sex, also known as male-to-female (MTF)
Gender dysphoria	DSM-V diagnosis for the clinically significant distress experienced if gender identity and sex are not congruent
Transsexual	A clinical term used to describe transgender people who seek medical intervention (hormones, surgery) for gender affirmation
Cisgender	A person whose gender identity does not differ from the sex that was assigned at birth

DIAGNOSIS

Diagnosis in Children

- Gender nonconforming behaviour is relatively common in children of all ages, with a wide spectrum of presentation.[14]
- Most children who display gender nonconformity will "desist" during puberty and identify with their biologic sex. For those children whose gender dysphoria "persists" or intensifies during puberty, that gender identity will almost certainly continue for life.
- There are no reliable methods to predict which children will go on to "desist" or "persist." Psychologists are actively studying these populations to gain deeper understanding.[15]
- DSM (Diagnostic and Statistical Manual) and International Statistical Classification of Diseases and Related Health Problems (ICD) use different criteria for the diagnosis of gender dysphoria in children. Diagnosis should be performed by mental health providers with specific training in child developmental psychology.

Diagnostic Criteria in Adolescents and Adults

- Providers are encouraged to use the DSM 5th edition (DSM-V) diagnostic criteria for "gender dysphoria" summarized in Table 22-2.[16] "Gender dysphoria" replaces the DSM-IV and ICD diagnostic codes for "gender identity disorder" to deemphasize pathology and remove stigmatization of transgender identity.
- The diagnosis should be established by a mental health care professional with training and competence in the assessment of gender dysphoria.
- There is significant controversy around these diagnoses. Many advocates still argue that label of gender dysphoria stigmatizes gender identity as a mental illness, as does the requirement for mental health evaluation prior to hormone therapy.
- Some clinics and advocates instead use an "informed consent" model, which does not require a specific mental health or medical diagnosis.[17] In this model, a provider can

TABLE 22-2	DSM-V DIAGNOSTIC CRITERIA FOR GENDER DYSPHORIA IN ADOLESCENTS AND ADULTS*

A. A marked incongruence between one's experienced/expressed gender and assigned gender, of at least 6 months' duration, as manifested by at least two of the following:
- A marked incongruence between one's experienced/expressed gender and primary and/or secondary sex characteristics (or in young adolescents, the anticipated sex characteristics)
- A strong desire to be rid of one's primary and/or secondary sex characteristics because of a marked incongruence with one's experienced/expressed gender (or in young adolescents, a desire to prevent the development of the anticipated secondary sex characteristics)
- A strong desire for the primary and/or secondary sex characteristics of the other gender
- A strong desire to be of the other gender (or some alternative gender different from one's assigned gender)
- A strong desire to be treated as the other gender (or some alternative gender different from one's assigned gender)
- A strong conviction that one has the typical feelings and reactions of the other gender (or some alternative gender different from one's assigned gender)

B. The condition is associated with clinically significant distress or impairment in social, occupational, or other important areas of functioning

*Reproduced with permission from American Psychiatric Association. Gender Dysphoria. In: Diagnostic and Statistical Manual of Mental Disorders. 5th ed. Washington, DC: American Psychiatric Association; 2013.

initiate hormonal therapy after discussing and documenting a conversation of risks, benefits, and reasonable alternatives with patients seeking hormonal therapy.

TREATMENT

- Before initiating hormone therapy, the provider should confirm and document the diagnosis of gender dysphoria (via referring provider or direct assessment).
- It is the responsibility of the performing physician to ensure that the patient (or the parents of adolescent patients) has full medical decision-making capacity and consents to therapy. Any significant mental or medical conditions that would impact treatment have been appropriately addressed before starting therapy.
- All patients should be counseled on possible impacts of hormonal therapy or surgery on future fertility. If fertility preservation is desired, patients should be referred to reproductive specialists for further evaluation and planning.
- Absolute contraindications to hormonal therapy include active sex hormone sensitive malignancies (e.g., estrogen-sensitive breast cancer or androgen-sensitive prostate cancer). Patients with prior history of such tumors should complete oncologic evaluation.

Female to Male Hormonal Therapy

- Transgender men are treated with testosterone to: (a) suppress endogenous estrogen production via negative feedback on pituitary gonadotropin release; and (b) induce male secondary sexual characteristics.[18]

- Typical doses and formulations are presented in Table 22-3.[3,19] Doses are similar to those used for testosterone replacement in hypogonadal men (Chapter 21).
- Clinical evaluation along with laboratory measurement of testosterone and estradiol levels should occur every 3 to 6 months during the 1st year of therapy. Expected physical changes include:
  - Almost all patients experience **improved quality of life, decreased gender dysphoria**, and **reduction in depression and anxiety** (if present).
  - **Voice deepening** begins immediately and reaches peak in 1 to 2 years. Due to structural changes in the larynx, this effect is irreversible.
  - **Facial and body hair** emerge within months. In some patients, **androgenic alopecia** emerges as a result of long term androgen therapy.

TABLE 22-3	MEDICATIONS FOR TRANSGENDER HORMONE THERAPY	
Class[a]	Typical dosage	Considerations
Testosterone		
Transdermal: testosterone gel, 1%	2.5–10 g/day	
Testosterone patch	2.5–7.5 mg/day	
Parenteral: enanthate	100–200 mg IM every 2 weeks	
Cypionate	50–100 mg IM or SC weekly	
Estrogen		
Oral: 17β-estradiol	2–6 mg/day	Avoid conjugated estrogens
Transdermal: estradiol patch	0.1–0.4 mg daily dose	
Parenteral: estradiol valerate	5–20 mg IM every 2 weeks	
Estradiol cypionate	2–10 mg IM weekly	
Antiandrogens		
Spironolactone	100–400 mg/day	Contraindicated in renal failure
Cyproterone acetate	50–100 mg/day	Not approved in U.S. Depression, hepatotoxicity
Gonadotropin-releasing hormone agonist		
Goserelin[b]	3.6 mg SC monthly	All expensive
Leuprolide[b]	3.75–7.5 mg IM monthly	
Histrelin	50 mg SC implant yearly	

[a]All medications for transgender hormone therapy used off-label in U.S.
[b]Three month formulations also available.
IM, intra-muscular; SC, subcutaneous.

TABLE 22-4   MONITORING TRANSGENDER HORMONE THERAPY

	Male-to-female	Female-to-male
Evaluation, measurement of sex hormone levels	First year of treatment: every 3 to 6 months After 1st year: once or twice per year	
Total testosterone target	<55 ng/dL	Normal range for biologic males
Estradiol target	Normal range for premenopausal women, roughly 100–200 pg/mL	<50 pg/nL
Metabolic measures (annual)	Fasting triglycerides Electrolytes (spironolactone) Liver enzymes (cyproterone)	Hematocrit Fasting lipid panel
Bone density	Consider bone mineral density test prior to hormone therapy if risk factors for osteoporosis Otherwise, screen per population guidelines Consider earlier testing if: (a) noncompliance with hormonal therapy; or (b) persistently low sex hormone levels	
Cancer screening	Colon, breast, prostate (if present) per population guidelines	Colon; breast and cervical if present

- **Acne** is almost universal after several months. Face and back are typically involved.
- **Menses cease** in >90% of patients receiving appropriate doses of intramuscular or subcutaneous testosterone within 6 months.[20]
- **Clitoral enlargement** begins immediately and reaches peak effect in 6 to 12 months. **Increased libido** is commonly reported.
- **Lean muscle mass is modestly increased**, which is matched by a **decrease in adiposity**.
- **Breast tissue** becomes less glandular and more fibrotic.
- Testosterone doses should be adjusted until serum levels are in the male normal range, and symptoms of dysphoria and secondary sex characteristics are adequately addressed; see Table 22-4.
- Some transgender men have high total testosterone levels with normal free testosterone levels over the first 6 to 9 months of therapy. This is attributed to higher baseline levels of sex hormone–binding globulin, and resolves over time.
- If persistent menstrual bleeding continues despite adequate testosterone dosing, gonadotropin-releasing hormone (GnRH) agonists or progestins can be added to further reduce estrogen levels. Endometrial ablation is also an option.

Male to Female Hormonal Therapy

- Transgender women are treated with estradiol to: (a) suppress endogenous testosterone production via negative feedback on pituitary gonadotropin release; and (b) induce female secondary sexual characteristics.[21] Estradiol monotherapy is usually insufficient to drive testosterone levels to the normal range of biologic women, so androgen receptor antagonists or GnRH agonists are usually required to achieve full testosterone suppression.
- Typical doses and formulations are presented in Table 22-3. Doses of estradiol necessary to achieve target serum estradiol and testosterone levels are typically much higher than

doses used in postmenopausal women. Antiandrogen therapy or GnRH agonists are often started concurrently with estrogen.

- Clinical evaluation along with laboratory measurement of estradiol and testosterone levels should occur every 3 to 6 months during the 1st year of therapy; see Table 22-4.
- Expected physical changes include:
  - Almost all patients experience **improved quality of life, decreased gender dysphoria**, and **reduction in depression and anxiety** (if present).
  - **Decreased frequency of erections** and **decreased libido** are noted in most patients within the first months of treatment. Over time, **testicular and prostate volumes** are reduced.
  - **Skin is softened** and acne is often reduced.
  - **Terminal hair growth is decreased**, resulting in decreased body hair. Facial hair is relatively resistant and often requires cosmetic removal.
  - **Breast tissue develops** over time in a pattern that roughly recapitulates thelarche in pubertal girls. Full development will be completed within 2 to 3 years for most patients.
  - **Lean mass is decreased** and most patients note **redistribution of adipose tissue**, with less abdominal fat and increased adiposity at hips.
  - Estrogen therapy has no impact on voice pitch.
- If estrogen levels are not in the normal range for females at follow-up visits, the dose of estrogen should be increased until serum levels are at target.
- Progesterone can be added to augment breast development, although there are no placebo-controlled studies to support efficacy. Some transgender women report increased breast, areola development, and improved mood.
- Antiandrogen therapy or GnRH agonists are initiated or increased if testosterone levels remain above normal female range despite adequate estrogen treatment, or if the development of secondary female sexual characteristics is insufficient.
- Choices for antiandrogren therapy include spironolactone and cyproterone.
- In addition to well-recognized mineralocorticoid receptor antagonism, spironolactone is a weak androgen receptor antagonist and also a mixed agonist/antagonist at the estrogen receptor.[22] Serum electrolytes, especially potassium, must be monitored.
- Cyproterone acetate is probably a more potent androgen receptor antagonist than spironolactone. It is used extensively in Europe but is not approved for use in the United States. Adverse effects include depression and hepatotoxicity.

Gonadal Blockade

- GnRH agonists disrupt the pulsatile activation of GnRH receptors thereby causing receptor desensitization and decreased production of luteinizing hormone (LH) and follicle stimulating hormone (FSH) production in the pituitary. The net effect is decreased sex hormone production in the gonads.
- The effects of GnRH agonists are fully reversible with discontinuation of the medication.
- GnRH agonists are extensively used in adolescent medicine for pubertal delay (see below), and are an option in adult medicine instead of antiandrogens if endogenous sex hormone production is not adequately suppressed by hormonal therapy.[19]
- The side effect profile is very favorable, but high cost is a major limitation to widespread use.
- The main concern with GnRH agonists revolves around unknown long-term effects on bone health and mineralization.

Adolescents

- Because there is a significant desistance of gender nonconformity during puberty, hormonal therapy is never indicated prior to puberty.
- For children who have persistent transgender identity after the onset of puberty, dysphoria is typically intensified. Further, the physical changes of puberty like breast development

or voice deepening can exacerbate the incongruence of outward appearance and personal identity.[23]

- For these reasons, reversible pubertal delay with GnRH agonist is recommended at the early stages of puberty in transgender children experiencing intensifying dysphoria during early puberty (Tanner 2 or 3). Reversible gonadal blockade will prevent the further development of secondary sexual characteristics, while maintaining the body in a primed state for future sex hormone–mediated development when the child is prepared to commit to gender affirming therapy.[24]

- Current Endocrine Society guidelines recommend that hormonal therapy of the affirmed gender be added to the GnRH blockade by age 16 in those children who have persistent transgender identity, and that no surgical intervention be performed before age 18. Many pediatric transgender health experts advocate initiation of gender affirming hormones as young as 14 years of age.

- In the event that GnRH agonists are unavailable or prohibitively expensive, high doses of progestins and antiandrogens can also inhibit pubertal progression. They are associated with numerous side effects at high doses and require close monitoring.

Surgical Management

- Some transgender patients pursue gender confirming surgeries that change outward physical appearance, genitalia, or internal sex organs to match the expressed gender identity. Examples include contour shaping, mastectomy or breast augmentation, orchiectomy or hysterectomy and oophorectomy, and phalloplasty, metoidioplasty or vaginoplasty.

- As with all other areas of transgender health, surgical care should be integrated into a multidisciplinary care team. Each surgical procedure is associated with specific recommendations for prerequisite mental health evaluation, duration of hormonal treatment, or social transition.[25]

- If preoperative testosterone and estrogen levels were appropriate, no dose change is necessary after gonadectomy. Some patients may choose to lower their dose, since high-dose suppression of gonadotropins is no longer necessary. Adequate doses should maintain secondary sex characteristics and relieve gender dysphoria, while maintaining bone health.

- After orchiectomy, testosterone levels become negligible with only minimal residual production from the adrenal glands. Antiandrogens or GnRH agonists can be discontinued.

- It is sometimes recommended that estrogen therapy be suspended prior to surgery to minimize the chance of venous thromboembolism (VTE). There is no high-quality evidence to guide these treatment decisions, and complete cessation of estrogen therapy can lead to significant distress. Decisions should ideally be personalized to the individual, considering other risk factors for blood clots and the expected risk of the surgical procedure.

- For many patients, the cost of gender confirming surgery is not covered by insurance, and access to qualified surgeons may be limited.

SPECIAL CONSIDERATIONS

Considerations in older patients:

- There is no high-quality evidence to guide approaches to hormonal therapy in older transgender patients.
- Testosterone therapy should be continued in transgender men, targeting patient relief from dysphoric symptoms and normal serum levels.[26]
- Treatment decisions in transgender women are more nuanced.[27] Since estrogen levels fall at menopause in women, dose reduction in transgender women should be considered at about age 50. Estrogen can be completely withdrawn without loss of secondary sexual

characteristics in transgender women who have had an orchiectomy, but full withdrawal in a transgender woman with functioning testes could result in virilization.

- Withdrawal of estrogen can result in typical symptoms of menopause, for example, hot flashes.

MONITORING/FOLLOW-UP

- Recommended sex hormone level targets and other considerations are summarized in Table 22-4.
- Long-term outcome studies are significantly limited by small numbers and absence of prospective data.

Venous Thromboembolism

- Early literature from transgender clinics identified significantly increased frequency of VTE among transgender women treated with estrogen.
- Several studies have suggested that most of this increase was due to conjugated or synthetic estrogens. VTE rates are not clearly elevated in transgender patients treated with oral or transdermal estradiol.[21]
- In transgender women with personal history of VTE or risk factors for VTE, such as smoking or advancing age, providers should emphasize risks versus benefits of estrogen treatment. Use of the lowest effective dose and/or transdermal preparations have theoretical appeal in these cases.

Cardiovascular Health

- Numerous studies have shown that transgender men do not have significantly increased risk of cardiovascular disease.
- Several studies in transgender women treated with estrogen have suggested an increased risk of cardiovascular mortality.[28,29] These studies did not account for mode of estrogen delivery or other cardiovascular risk factors.
- One study reported that transgender women had a significantly increased risk of myocardial infarction (MI) compared to age-matched cisgender women, but not an increased risk compared to age-matched cisgender men.[30] The majority of those who suffered an MI were older, had been on hormone therapy for a shorter duration of time, and had other risk factors such as smoking.
- Estrogen therapy in transgender women is associated with increased triglyceride levels and LDL, while testosterone therapy in transgender men is a risk factor for higher triglycerides and lower HDL. It is unclear if there is any clinical significance to these altered lipid levels. Decision to initiate lipid-lowering drugs should depend on associated risk factors and cardiovascular risk prediction. For transgender patients, there is no evidence to guide if calculations should be performed with respect to biologic or affirmed gender.
  - While overall lifespan among transgender patients is roughly the same as population controls, suicide rates are significantly greater than the general population.[28,31]
  - Hyperprolactinemia was detected in 21% of transgender women treated with ethinyl estradiol in one series.[32] This is most noticeable in the 1st year of treatment, and there is no evidence estrogen treatment causes an increased risk of pituitary adenoma. Transgender women with known macroprolactinomas prior to the initiation of estrogen therapy should have careful risk/benefit conversations and close monitoring.[3] It is possible that estrogen treatment might promote symptoms from a previously silent macroprolactinoma. Current guidelines suggest periodic measurement of serum prolactin levels.
  - Pre-existing polycythemia might be exacerbated by testosterone therapy. If polycythemia is identified prior to treatment, the cause should be identified if possible and closely monitored during treatment. If polycythemia is identified on treatment,

testosterone dose should be reduced until the hematocrit is in the normal reference range for males.

○ Severe migraine headaches might be exacerbated by estrogen therapy. Use of the lowest effective dose and transdermal preparations may be helpful.

○ Estrogen therapy can lower seizure threshold and thereby worsen seizure frequency and/or severity in patients with a seizure disorder.

○ Breast cancer has been rarely reported in transgender women, and also in transgender men with intact breasts. Prostate cancer has been reported in transgender women, and gynecologic cancers in transgender men. There is insufficient evidence to determine the precise risk or benefit of hormonal therapy in these populations. Thus, mammography is recommended in all transgender women and transgender men with intact breasts, using population guidelines for women as the reference for initiation and frequency. Prostate and cervical cancer screens should be performed if those organs are present, along with general colon cancer screening.

REFERENCES

1. Murad MH, Elamin MB, Garcia MZ, et al. Hormonal therapy and sex reassignment: A systematic review and meta-analysis of quality of life and psychosocial outcomes. *Clin Endocrinol (Oxf)* 2010;72(2):214–231.

2. Davidge-Pitts C, Nippoldt TB, Danoff A, Radziejewski L, Natt N. Transgender health in endocrinology: Current status of endocrinology fellowship programs and practicing clinicians. *J Clin Endocrinol Metab* 2017;102(4):1286–1290.

3. Hembree WC, Cohen-Kettenis PT, Gooren L, et al. Endocrine treatment of gender-dysphoric/gender-incongruent persons: An Endocrine Society clinical practice guideline. *J Clin Endocrinol Metab* 2017;102(11):3869–3903.

4. World Professional Association for Transgender Health. *Standards of Care for the Health of Transsexual, Transgender, and Gender Nonconforming People.* 7th ed. Minneapolis, MN: World Professional Association for Transgender Health; 2011. Retrieved August, 17, 2017, from http://www.wpath.org.

5. James SE, et al. *The Report of the 2015 U.S. Transgender Survey.* Washington: DC: National Center for Transgender Equality; 2016. Retrieved August 16, 2017, from http://www.ustranssurvey.org/report/.

6. Deutsch MB, ed. *Guidelines for the Primary and Gender-Affirming Care of Transgender and Gender Nonbinary People.* 2nd ed. San Francisco: Center of Excellence for Transgender Health, Department of Family and Community Medicine, University of California San Francisco; 2016. Retrieved August 17, 2017, from http://www.transhealth.ucsf.edu/guidelines.

7. Van Kesteren PJ, Gooren LJ, Megens JA. An epidemiological and demographic study of transsexuals in The Netherlands. *Arch Sex Behav* 1996;25(6):589–600.

8. Collin L, Reisner SL, Tangpricha V, Goodman M. Prevalence of transgender depends on the "case" definition: A systematic review. *J Sex Med* 2016;13(4):613–626.

9. Meerwijk EL, Sevelius JM. Transgender population size in the United States: A meta-regression of population-based probability samples. *Am J Public Health* 2017;107(2):e1–e8.

10. de Cuypere G, Van Hemelrijck M, Michel A, et al. Prevalence and demography of transsexualism in Belgium. *Eur Psychiatry* 2007;22(3):137–141.

11. Bradford J, Reisner SL, Honnold JA, Xavier J. Experiences of transgender-related discrimination and implications for health: Results from the Virginia Transgender Health Initiative Study. *Am J Public Health* 2013;103(10):1820–1829.

12. Safer JD, Coleman E, Feldman J, et al. Barriers to healthcare for transgender individuals. *Curr Opin Endocrinol Diabetes Obes* 2016;23(2):168–171.

13. Grant JM, et al. *Injustice at Every Turn: A Report of the National Transgender Discrimination Survey.* Washington, DC: National Center for Transgender Equality and National Gay and Lesbian Task Force; 2011. Retrieved September 25, 2017, from http://www.thetaskforce.org/static_html/downloads/reports/reports/ntds_full.pdf.

14. Rosenthal SM. Transgender youth: Current concepts. *Ann Pediatr Endocrinol Metab* 2016;21(4):185–192.

15. Steensma TD, McGuire JK, Kreukels BP, Beekman AJ, Cohen-Kettenis PT. Factors associated with desistence and persistence of childhood gender dysphoria: A quantitative follow-up study. *J Am Acad Child Adolesc Psychiatry* 2013;52(6):582–590.

16. American Psychiatric Association. Gender dysphoria. In: *Diagnostic and Statistical Manual of Mental Disorders*. 5th ed. Washington, DC: American Psychiatric Association; 2013.

17. Cavanaugh T, Hopwood R, Lambert C. Informed consent in the medical care of transgender and gender-nonconforming patients. *AMA J Ethics* 2016;18(11):1147–1155.

18. Irwig MS. Testosterone therapy for transgender men. *Lancet Diabetes Endocrinol* 2017;5(4): 301–311.

19. Garthwaite SM, McMahon EG. The evolution of aldosterone antagonists. *Mol Cell Endorinol* 2004;217(1-2):27–31.

20. Nakamura A, Watanabe M, Sugimoto M, et al. Dose-response analysis of testosterone replacement therapy in patients with female to male gender identity disorder. *Endocr J* 2013;60(3): 275–281.

21. Tangpricha V, der Heijer M. Oestrogen and anti-androgen therapy for transgender women. *Lancet Diabetes Endocrinol* 2017;5(4):291–300.

22. Spack NP. Management of transgenderism. *JAMA* 2013;309(5):478–484.

23. de Vries AL, McGuire JK, Steensma TD, Wagenaar EC, Doreleijers TA, Cohen-Kettenis PT. Young adult psychological outcome after puberty suppression and gender reassignment. *Pediatrics* 2014;134(4):696–704.

24. Rosenthal SM. Approach to the patient: transgender youth: Endocrine considerations. *J Clin Endocrinol Metab* 2014;99(12):4379–4389.

25. Berli JU, Knudson G, Fraser L, et al. What surgeons need to know about gender confirmation surgery when providing care for transgender individuals: A review. *JAMA Surg* 2017;152(4):394–400.

26. Travison TG, Vesper HW, Orwoll E, et al. Harmonized reference ranges for circulating testosterone levels in men of four cohort studies in the United States and Europe. *J Clin Endocrinol Metab* 2017;102(4):1161–1173.

27. Gooren L, Lips P. Conjectures concerning cross-sex hormone treatment of aging transsexual persons. *J Sex Med* 2014;11(8):2012–2019.

28. Dhejne C, Lichtenstein P, Boman M, Johansson AL, Långström N, Landén M. Long-term follow-up of transsexual persons undergoing sex reassignment surgery: Cohort study in Sweden. *PloS One* 2011;6(2):e16885.

29. Asscheman H, Giltay EJ, Megens JA, de Ronde WP, van Trotsenburg MA, Gooren LJ. A long-term follow-up study of mortality in transsexuals receiving treatment with cross-sex hormones. *Eur J Endocrinol* 2011;164(4):635–642.

30. Wierckx K, Elaut E, Declercq E, et al. Prevalence of cardiovascular disease and cancer during cross-sex hormone therapy in a large cohort of trans persons: A case-control study. *Eur J Endocrinol* 2013;169(4):471–478.

31. Van Kesteren PJ, Asscheman H, Megens JA, Gooren LJ. Mortality and morbidity in transsexual subjects treated with cross-sex hormones. *Clin Endocrinol (Oxf)* 1997;47(3):337–342.

32. Asscheman H, Gooren LJ, Assies J, Smits JP, de Slegte R. Prolactin levels and pituitary enlargement in hormone-treated male-to-female transsexuals. *Clin Endocrinol (Oxf)* 1988;28(6): 583–588.

Hypercalcemia and Hyperparathyroidism

23

Naga Yalla and Karin Hickey

GENERAL PRINCIPLES

- Calcium homeostasis maintains serum calcium levels by balancing dietary intake with urinary excretion and formation of new bone. Daily calcium intake is about 1 g, with 150 mg of that being absorbed. Effective calcium absorption is dependent on vitamin D. Absorbed calcium is incorporated into bone or excreted by the kidneys.
- Calcium circulates both free (<50%) or bound to protein or anion. The free, ionized portion is sensed and regulated. Parathyroid hormone (PTH) is released when calcium is low. It causes bone resorption, calcium reabsorption in the kidney, and increased production of activated vitamin D in the kidney, all leading to a rise in calcium. PTH-mediated bone resorption is mediated by the RANK–RANK ligand–OPG system.

Definition

Hypercalcemia is an elevation of free, ionized calcium in the serum. Elevated total serum calcium can occur without increased ionized calcium if calcium-binding proteins are elevated, but this does not constitute true hypercalcemia.

Epidemiology

- Depending on the population being studied, hypercalcemia affects up to 0.1% to 2.6% of hospitalized patients.[1]
- The two most common causes of hypercalcemia are **primary hyperparathyroidism** (pHPT) and **malignancy-associated hypercalcemia** (MAH). pHPT accounts for 50% to 60% of outpatient hypercalcemia, while MAH is the most common cause of inpatient hypercalcemia, occurring in 20% to 30% of malignancies.[2]

Etiology

Causes of hyperglycemia are described in Table 23-1.

Pathophysiology

- PTH causes hypercalcemia through three mechanisms:
  - In the kidney, PTH acts to increase calcium reabsorption on the distal convoluted tubule and decrease phosphate reabsorption in the proximal tubule.
  - PTH acts to increase the activity of 1α-hydroxylase in proximal tubular cells, increasing the level of 1,25-dihydroxy vitamin D over several hours, and ultimately leading to increased absorption of calcium and phosphate by the small intestine.
  - Over time, prolonged secretion of PTH increases bone resorption and decreases bone mass.
- **Primary hyperparathyroidism** occurs when one or more of the parathyroid glands produce an excessive amount of PTH for the amount of calcium present in the blood. A **single benign parathyroid adenoma** is found in 80% to 90% of cases and **four-gland hyperplasia** is seen in approximately 6% of cases.
- **Secondary hyperparathyroidism** (sHPT) is a physiologic elevation in PTH in response to a derangement in calcium homeostasis that causes, or would otherwise lead to, frank

TABLE 23-1 CAUSES OF HYPERCALCEMIA

Parathyroid mediated
Primary hyperparathyroidism
Tertiary hyperparathyroidism (renal failure)
Inherited variants
Multiple endocrine neoplasia(MEN) syndromes
Familial isolated hyperparathyroidism
Hyperparathyroidism jaw syndrome
Parathyroid carcinoma
Familial hypocalciuric hypercalcemia
Lithium therapy

Nonparathyroid mediated
Hypercalcemia of malignancy
Vitamin D intoxication
Chronic granulomatous disorders

Medications
Thiazide diuretics
Lithium
Excessive vitamin A
Theophylline toxicity

Endocrine causes
Hyperthyroidism
Adrenal insufficiency
Pheochromocytoma
Acromegaly

Miscellaneous
Milk–alkali syndrome
Parenteral nutrition
Immobilization

hypocalcemia (e.g., renal failure, hyperphosphatemia, or vitamin D deficiency). In contrast with primary hyperparathyroidism, it does not result in hypercalcemia.
- **Tertiary hyperparathyroidism** develops in the setting of long-standing severe sHPT with parathyroid hyperplasia in patients with end-stage renal disease. The increased mass of the parathyroid gland produces a constitutive excess of PTH resulting in hypercalcemia.
- **Familial hyperparathyroidism** is rare and is most commonly associated with multiple endocrine neoplasia (MEN) 1 and MEN 2A (See Chapter 37).
  ○ **MEN1** is caused by a defect in gene encoding the tumor suppressor menin and is inherited in an autosomal-dominant fashion. It is most commonly associated with parathyroid hyperplasia, pancreatic tumors, and pituitary adenomas, although it may also be associated with other tumors. Hypercalcemia can be found in approximately 95% of those with MEN1, typically developing around age 25 years as the earliest manifestation of the syndrome. Although it may be associated with a single parathyroid adenoma at presentation, it almost always involves multiglandular hyperplasia.
  ○ **MEN2A** is inherited in an autosomal-dominant fashion and it is associated with defects in the RET proto-oncogene. It is characterized by medullary thyroid cancer,

which occurs with complete penetrance, pheochromocytoma, and asymmetric parathyroid hyperplasia that occurs in 25% to 35% of patients.

- **Familial isolated hyperparathyroidism** and **hyperparathyroidism–jaw tumor syndrome** are less common causes of pHPT. These are important to consider since the risk for developing parathyroid carcinoma is greatly increased to approximately 10%.
- **Parathyroid carcinoma** is reported to occur in 0.5% to 1% of cases, but is probably in the lower half of this range. Carcinomas may have characteristic pathologic findings, but are often only distinguished from adenomas by the degree of vascular/local invasion or the presence of lymph node metastases.
- **Familial hypocalciuric hypercalcemia** (FHH) is an autosomal-dominant disorder that is caused by a heterogeneous spectrum of mutations of the calcium sensing receptor (CaSR) that shift the set point for serum calcium to a higher level. FHH is typically asymptomatic and is thought to be a rare disorder. Nevertheless, since the biochemical abnormalities in FHH overlap with those of pHPT, the diagnosis must be considered; otherwise, a patient may undergo an unnecessary parathyroidectomy that is rarely curative in this disorder.[3,4]
- **Lithium therapy** may also lead to hypercalcemia in 15% to 60% of patients by an unknown mechanism that shifts the set point for calcium sensing at the parathyroid gland.
- **Hypercalcemia of malignancy.** Malignancy can lead to hypercalcemia via four mechanisms, three of which are directly related to increased bone resorption.[5]
    - Systemic secretion of PTH-related peptide (PTHrP), termed humoral hypercalcemia of malignancy (HHM), is seen primarily in squamous cell carcinomas. It can also be seen in cancers of the kidney, ovary, and bladder. It is a frequent complication in patients with lymphomas associated with human T-cell lymphoma/leukemia virus 1 (HTLV-1).
    - Osteolytic hypercalcemia occurs in cancers with extensive skeletal metastases (e.g., multiple myeloma, breast cancer). Local release of cytokines leads to osteoclast differentiation and inhibition of osteoblasts, resulting in bone destruction.[6]
    - Ectopic PTH secretion from carcinomas of the lung, thymus, ovary, and undifferentiated neuroendocrine tumors can cause hypercalcemia.
    - Elevated 1,25-hydroxy vitamin D levels rarely found in lymphoma and some ovarian dysgerminomas can cause hypercalcemia by increasing calcium absorption.
- **Vitamin D–mediated hypercalcemia.** Elevated vitamin D levels lead to hypercalcemia by increasing intestinal calcium absorption. Chronic ingestion of more than 50,000 to 100,000 IU/day of ergocalciferol (vitamin D_2) or cholecalciferol (vitamin D_3) can produce significant hypercalcemia in normal individuals. Because vitamin D is highly fat soluble, intoxication may persist for weeks. Excessive or accidental ingestion of 1,25-dihydroxy vitamin D (calcitriol) can also lead to hypercalcemia, but should resolve within days after discontinuation.[7]
- **Granulomatous diseases** may cause hypercalcemia through increased conversion of 25-hydroxy vitamin D to 1,25-dihydroxy vitamin D by macrophages, which is insensitive to feedback regulation by calcium or PTH. Hypercalcemia develops in 10% to 20% of patients with sarcoidosis and has also been associated with lymphomas, berylliosis, Crohn disease, Bacille Calmette–Guérin (BCG) therapy, and lipoid pneumonia. It is seen in various granulomatous processes including Wegener granulomatosis, eosinophilic granuloma, acute granulomatous pneumonia, and granulomatosis of the liver, and due to talc and silicone. Several infectious causes, including tuberculosis, histoplasmosis, candidiasis, coccidioidomycosis, and cat scratch fever have also been implicated.[8]
- **Medications that can cause hypercalcemia:**
    - **Thiazide diuretics**, in particular, are frequently implicated as a cause of hypercalcemia. However, hypercalcemia due to thiazides is typically mild and transient (1 to 2 weeks) unless some other high bone turnover state is present, such as pHPT.

- ○ **Excessive intake of vitamin A** (>50,000 to 100,000 IU daily) rarely causes hypercalcemia. This can be seen with supplement ingestion or in the use of retinoic acid derivates in treatment of some malignancies. This process is likely mediated through elevated interleukin-6 levels.[9]
- ○ **Additional medications** that have been reported to cause hypercalcemia include estrogens used in the treatment of breast cancer with bony metastases, growth hormones in intensive care unit patients, ganciclovir in renal transplantation, omeprazole in acute interstitial nephritis, 8-Cl-cAMP chemotherapy, manganese toxicity, foscarnet, hepatitis B vaccination, theophylline and lithium.[8]
- **Endocrine causes of hypercalcemia:**
  - ○ **Thyrotoxicosis** leads to hypercalcemia due to increased bone turnover (with greater proportional osteolysis) in 15% to 20% of patients with hyperthyroidism.[10]
  - ○ **Adrenal insufficiency** has been associated with hypercalcemia. Primary adrenal failure has been implicated more commonly, but there are case reports in secondary adrenal failure as well. The exact pathophysiology is not known, but hypercalcemia is thought to be caused by a decrease in intravascular volume and relative hemoconcentration of serum albumin and bound calcium.
  - ○ **Pheochromocytoma** may be associated with pHPT as part of MEN2A. In addition, **PTHrP-mediated hypercalcemia** is implicated in pheochromocytoma.
  - ○ **Islet cell tumors of the pancreas** can rarely lead to hypercalcemia. This is either in association with MEN, through PTHrP, or through secretion of vasoactive intestinal peptide (VIP), leading to a syndrome of hypercalcemia with watery diarrhea, hypokalemia, and achlorhydria.[11]
- **Miscellaneous causes of hypercalcemia:**
  - ○ **Milk–alkali syndrome** results from ingestion of large amounts of milk or calcium carbonate, as in the treatment of dyspepsia or osteoporosis. The hypercalcemia is associated with metabolic alkalosis and renal insufficiency. Typically, more than 5 g of calcium per day is required to produce the syndrome, but this is dependent on individual patient susceptibility (intestinal absorption and renal clearance of calcium).[12]
  - ○ **Prolonged immobilization** typically causes bone resorption with hypercalciuria that, in rare cases, may also cause hypercalcemia. Hypercalcemia due to immobilization is more common in children and adolescents, but has also been described in burn patients, patients with spinal cord injuries, or other severe neurologic deficits, and patients with underlying high bone turnover states (e.g., Paget disease).[13] The mechanism by which this occurs is not entirely known, but is thought to be due to an uncoupling of bone turnover with increased osteoclast and decreased osteoblast activity.

DIAGNOSIS

Clinical Presentation

- Hypercalcemia can have a variable clinical presentation with the majority of cases being asymptomatic.
- The symptoms and signs of hypercalcemia often correlate with the age of the patient, the underlying disease process, concurrent comorbidities and the degree, duration, and rate of development of hypercalcemia. Patients who are older or who have significant comorbidities are more likely to be sensitive to the effects of hypercalcemia. Likewise, hypercalcemia associated with malignancies or infectious disorders may present with symptoms of the underlying disease, which may overlap with mild symptoms of hypercalcemia.
- **In general, levels <12 mg/dL are asymptomatic; levels >15 mg/dL may cause severe** symptoms such as coma and cardiac arrest. However, long-standing or slowly developing hypercalcemia may be well tolerated, whereas **rapidly progressing hypercalcemia is more likely to be symptomatic.**

- Hypercalcemia affects multiple organ systems. The saying "stones, bones, (psychiatric) moans, and (abdominal) groans" is a useful tool for remembering the most common symptoms.
- **Neuropsychiatric symptoms** are common but are usually subtle. Patients with chronic, mild hypercalcemia complain of fatigue, difficulty concentrating, depression, and anxiety. Some may complain of headaches, emotional lability, and irritability. With more severe hypercalcemia, especially with a rapid rise or in elderly patients, alterations in the sensorium, including coma, weakness, personality changes, hallucinations, and psychosis can occur.
- Hypercalcemia may be associated with hypertension and, rarely, with bradyarrhythmias.[14] Ventricular arrhythmias have also been reported, but without proven causality. Chronic hypercalcemia can cause calcified myocardial fibers, heart valves, and coronary arteries.
- **Constipation** is the most common gastrointestinal complaint associated with hypercalcemia. Other symptoms include nausea, vomiting, and anorexia. Due to increased gastric acid and pancreatic enzyme secretion, severe and recurrent peptic ulcer disease and pancreatitis can occur, but this is most commonly seen in association with MEN, type 1.
- **Polyuria and polydipsia** may develop as chronically elevated calcium levels cause nephrogenic diabetes insipidus. **Nephrolithiasis** is associated with long-standing hypercalcemia, most commonly in the setting of pHPT. Renal insufficiency secondary to chronic hypercalcemic nephropathy may be irreversible. Type 1 renal tubular acidosis infrequently occurs. Acute hypercalcemia can cause acute kidney injury due to direct renal vasoconstriction and volume depletion.
- **Skeletal manifestations** of hypercalcemia depend on the underlying pathophysiology. Patients with hyperparathyroidism may develop osteoporosis or osteitis fibrosa cystica. Patients with an underlying malignancy may present with bone pain due to metastases or pathologic fractures.

Physical Examination
- Physical examination findings in hypercalcemia are scant. Rarely, corneal examination will show band keratopathy—visible as a horizontal band across the cornea in the area exposed between the eyelids on slit lamp examination.
- Some nonspecific findings may be present: confusion, mental status changes, possible findings of arthritis, slow pulse, proximal muscle weakness (e.g., difficulty in rising from a squatting position) and decreased bowel sounds with history of constipation.
- A palpable neck mass should raise concerns of malignancy (thyroid/MEN, metastasis; up to 50% of parathyroid carcinomas may exhibit a palpable neck mass).

Diagnostic Testing
- The work-up of hypercalcemia is primarily based on laboratory examination. This is guided by a comprehensive history including symptoms of other endocrine disorders, prescribed and over-the-counter medications, and occupational exposures; please see Figure 23-1.
- One must first **identify true hypercalcemia**. Hypercalcemia without elevated ionized calcium can occur in hyperalbuminemia, severe dehydration, or multiple myeloma with a calcium-binding paraprotein. Elevated ionized calcium with normal serum calcium may be seen in hypoalbuminema due to malnutrition or chronic liver disease.

Laboratories
- **Serum calcium** needs to be adjusted for changes in albumin and pH. Acidosis decreases and alkalosis increases ionized calcium. Calcium should be changed by 0.8 mg/dL for every 1 g/dL change in albumin outside of the normal range.
- Start with measurement of **intact PTH**. If this elevated, it is most likely pHPT. To differentiate pHPT from FHH, measure 24-hour urine calcium and creatinine (usually <100 mg/day in FHH and >4 mg/kg/24 hours in pHPT). Vitamin D insufficiency must be

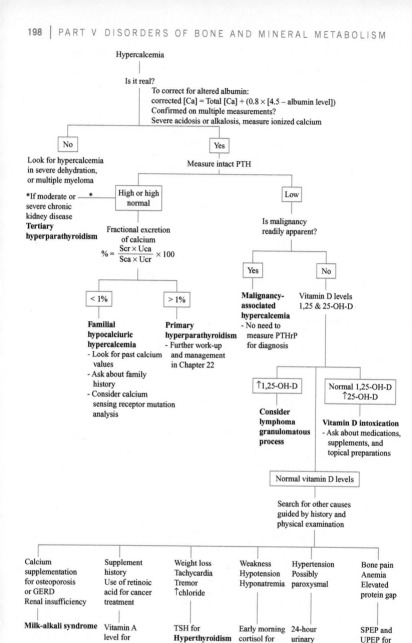

FIGURE 23-1 Algorithm for Hypercalcemia.

excluded. Calculate a fractional excretion of calcium. A value of <0.01 is highly suggestive of FHH, and a value >0.02 essentially rules out the condition, but overlap between urine calcium excretion in pHPT and FHH does occur. An elevated calcium and PTH can also be seen in lithium use.

- **If PTH is suppressed (<20 pg/mL), look for other causes of hypercalcemia.**
  - Malignancy leading to hypercalcemia is usually readily evident and therefore measurement of PTHrP is typically not needed.
  - Measure **1,25-dihydroxy vitamin D** next. If this is elevated, consider chest x-ray and complete blood count (CBC) to evaluate for lymphoma or other granulomatous diseases such as sarcoidosis.
  - If 25-hydroxy Vitamin D but not 1,25-dihydroxy vitamin D is elevated, consider exogenous vitamin D intoxication.
- Other laboratory work-up of hypercalcemia should be guided by history and could include thyroid-stimulating hormone (there may be a concomitant elevation of chloride) or cortisol (in the setting of weakness, hypotension, and hyponatremia). Other tests include vitamin A levels, urinary catecholamines for pheochromocytoma, and evaluation for multiple myeloma.

Electrocardiography
Electrocardiographic findings may include a shortened QT interval and mild prolongations of the PR and QRS intervals. With severe hypercalcemia, there may be alterations in the T-wave configuration, as well.[15]

Imaging
- Bone mineral density measurement by **dual electron X-ray absorptiometry** (DXA) should be obtained as part of the initial workup and surveillance of patients with pHPT. It is an indicator of disease severity. Multiple sites should be measured including distal one-third radius, spine, and hip.
- The following imaging modalities can be used in the preoperative workup of pHPT.
  - **Neck ultrasonography** (US) has been reported to have a sensitivity of 72% to 89% in detecting solitary adenomas, but has poor sensitivity for detecting multigland disease. An advantage of US is the ability to fully image the thyroid gland and help characterize any thyroid nodules that also may require surgical management.
  - **99mTc-sestamibi scanning** exhibits sensitivity similar to ultrasound and is reported to be 68% to 95% in detecting single adenomas, but like ultrasound has poor sensitivity for detecting multigland disease. Because 99mTc-sestamibi is also taken up by thyroid tissue, false positives may occur. An advantage of scintigraphy, however, is that it can detect ectopic glands outside the neck, identifying adenomas missed by ultrasound.
  - Therefore, some favor a combined approach to preoperative evaluation. High-resolution neck US and 99mTc-sestamibi scanning—planar, single photon emission computed tomography (SPECT), or SPECT coupled with anatomic x-ray CT overlay (SPECT/CT)—have emerged as the two most useful imaging techniques for locating a single parathyroid adenoma versus multigland disease prior to surgery in patients with pHPT.[16] The combination of preoperative US followed by SPECT/CT as needed localizes 95% of solitary adenomas, and prospectively guides the selection of patients as candidates for minimally invasive surgery.

TREATMENT

- Determining when to treat hypercalcemia depends on its chronicity and the degree of elevation.
- Mild chronic elevations in calcium (<12 mg/dL) with minimum to no symptoms do not require emergent treatment.

- Moderate hypercalcemia (12 to 14 mg/dL) may not require active treatment if it is chronic and mildly symptomatic. However, if the rise to this level is acute and patients are symptomatic they require emergent treatment.
- Severe hypercalcemia (>14 mg/dL) requires immediate treatment.

Medications

- The **primary focus of treating acute hypercalcemia is to increase urinary calcium excretion**. Patients should be **aggressively hydrated** with normal saline over 24 to 48 hours to lower the serum calcium concentration by as much as 3 to 9 mg/dL, depending on the initial degree of hypercalcemia. Close monitoring is needed, as fluid overload can develop, especially if there is underlying cardiac or renal insufficiency. The traditional use of loop diuresis with saline hydration has recently been questioned.[17] **Loop diuresis should be reserved for the setting of fluid overload.** Aggressive diuresis in a volume-depleted patient may worsen the hypercalcemia by exacerbating the volume loss. In addition, precautions should be taken to prevent potassium and magnesium depletion.
- **Bisphosphonates**
  - **Intravenous bisphosphonate** treatment provides a longer-term solution to hypercalcemia when a cause has been identified and reversible causes have been fixed. Bisphosphonates are analogs of pyrophosphate that are concentrated in areas of high bone turnover and inhibit both calcification and osteoclastic bone resorption.
  - These agents have maximum effect at 2 to 4 days and last 3 to 4 weeks. Two agents are FDA approved—**pamidronate** and **zoledronic acid**. While zoledronic acid has been found to be slightly more potent in head-to-head studies and has a shorter infusion time, pamidronate is less expensive and nearly as efficacious.[18] In HHM pamidronate has been found to be less effective.[19]
  - The recommended dose of zoledronic acid 4 mg IV over 30 to 60 minutes and pamidronate doses of 60 to 90 mg given over 2 to 4 hours can also be administered.
  - Both agents are well tolerated, and side effects are usually mild and transient. Fever is the most common reaction to intravenous administration. Renal toxicity is the most common serious side effect—doses should be given over a longer period of time or possibly reduced if renal insufficiency is present. Osteonecrosis of the jaw is a rare complication of bisphosphonate therapy, but should be considered when treating patients who have had a recent dental procedure or who are planning for major dental surgery.
- **Denusomab**
  - Denusomab is indicated for the management of hypercalcemia of malignancy. The recommended dose is 120 mg subcutaneously every 4 weeks.
  - It can be used in treatment of hypercalcemia refractory to bisphosphonates or in patients with renal impairment where bisphosphonates are contraindicated.[20]
- **Calcitonin:** Until the time when bisphosphonates reach potency, salmon calcitonin administered subcutaneously or intramuscularly (4 U/kg every 12 hours, increased up to 6 to 8 U/kg every 6 hours) can be used as a temporizing measure. It acts quickly—within 6 to 8 hours—and has few side effects. Unfortunately, it is a relatively weak agent, only lowering serum calcium concentrations by 1 to 2 mg/dL, and acquired resistance often develops within the first 48 hours, limiting its use. Nasal calcitonin is not effective in the treatment of hypercalcemia.
- **Other Treatments**
  - **Dialysis** against a no- or low-calcium bath may be needed in the setting of acute symptomatic hypercalcemia and renal or cardiac insufficiency leading to volume overload.
  - Hypercalcemia in hematologic malignancies and granulomatous diseases associated with increased production of 1,25-dihydroxy vitamin D may be treated effectively with moderately high-dose **glucocorticoids** (e.g., prednisone 40 to 60 mg daily). Glucocorticoids increase urinary calcium excretion and decrease intestinal calcium absorption,

but may also have direct antitumor effects. Calcium levels usually fall within 48 hours, with a peak response in 7 to 10 days.[2] Corticosteroids are also effective therapy for hypercalcemia related to adrenal insufficiency and excessive vitamin A or D ingestion.

○ **Cinacalcet** is a calcimemetic that increases the sensitivity of the CaSR, leading to reduced PTH levels. It is currently approved for treatment of pHPT (in patients who are poor surgical candidates or have persistent hypercalcemia after surgery), sHPT, chronic kidney disease and parathyroid carcinoma where it reduces adverse outcomes from hypercalcemia.[21,22]

○ **Ketoconazole** and hydroxychloroquine inhibit hydroxylation of 25-hydroxy vitamin D to 1,25-dihydroxy vitamin D, and may also be effective in treating hypercalcemia caused by elevated 1,25-dihydroxy vitamin D levels.[23,24]

Surgical Management

- **Parathyroidectomy** by an experienced surgeon is the mainstay of therapy for symptomatic pHPT.
- Surgery is indicated if a patient meets one of the following criteria:
  ○ Symptomatic hypercalcemia
  ○ Age <50 years
  ○ Serum calcium 1 mg/dL above the upper limit of normal
  ○ Osteoporosis (T score <−2.5 on DXA scan)
  ○ Presence of vertebral compression fracture by x-ray, CT, MRI or vertebral fracture analysis
  ○ Creatinine clearance <60 cc/min
  ○ 24-hour urine calcium >400 mg/day and increased stone risk by biochemical stone risk analysis
  ○ Presence of nephrolithiasis or nephrocalcinosis by x-ray, ultrasound or CT
- Patients that do not meet surgical criteria should be monitored annually with measurement of serum calcium, creatinine, and glomerular filtration rate. DXA scans should be performed every 1 to 2 years. X-ray or vertebral fracture assessment (VFA) of the spine should be done if patients are experiencing neck pain or height loss. If the patient demonstrates a progressive reduction in bone mineral density that exceeds the least significant change at any site and T-score falls between −2.0 and −2.5, the physician may opt to recommend surgery.[25]

Lifestyle/Risk Modification

- Patients with mild and moderate hypercalcemia should be instructed to avoid factors that exacerbate hypercalcemia. These include lithium, thiazide diuretics, volume depletion, prolonged bed rest, and a diet high in calcium (>1 g/day).
- Patients should be instructed to maintain adequate hydration (about 3 L/day) to prevent nephrolithiasis.

REFERENCES

1. Dent DM, Miller JL, Klaff L, Barron J. The incidence and causes of hypercalcaemia. *Postgrad Med J* 1987;63(743):745–750.
2. Lafferty FW. Differential diagnosis of hypercalcemia. *J Bone Miner Res* 1991;6(Suppl 2):S51–S59; discussion S61.
3. Hinnie J, Bell E, McKillop E, Gallacher S. The prevalence of familial hypocalciuric hypercalcemia. *Calcif Tissue Int* 2001;68(4):216–218.
4. Gunn IR, Gaffney D. Clinical and laboratory features of calcium-sensing receptor disorders: A systematic review. *Ann Clin Biochem* 2004;41(Pt 6):441–458.
5. Stewart AF. Clinical practice. Hypercalcemia associated with cancer. *N Engl J Med* 2005;352(4):373–379.

6. Tian E, Zhan F, Walker R, et al. The role of the Wnt-signaling antagonist DKK1 in the development of osteolytic lesions in multiple myeloma. *N Engl J Med* 2003;349(26):2483–2494.

7. Nordt SP, Williams SR, Clark RF. Pharmacologic misadventure resulting in hypercalcemia from vitamin D intoxication. *J Emerg Med* 2002;22(3):302–303.

8. Jacobs TP, Bilezikian JP. Clinical review: Rare causes of hypercalcemia. *J Clin Endocrinol Metab* 2005;90(11):6316–6322.

9. Niesvizky R, Siegel DS, Busquets X, et al. Hypercalcaemia and increased serum interleukin-6 levels induced by all-trans retinoic acid in patients with multiple myeloma. *Br J Haematol* 1995;89(1):217–218.

10. Iqbal AA, Burgess EH, Gallina DL, Nanes MS, Cook CB. Hypercalcemia in hyperthyroidism: Patterns of serum calcium, parathyroid hormone, and 1,25-dihydroxyvitamin D3 levels during management of thyrotoxicosis. *Endocr Pract* 2003;9(6):517–521.

11. Mao C, Carter P, Schaefer P, et al. Malignant islet cell tumor associated with hypercalcemia. *Surgery* 1995;117(1):37–40.

12. Abreo K, Adlakha A, Kilpatrick S, Flanagan R, Webb R, Shakamuri S. The milk-alkali syndrome. A reversible form of acute renal failure. *Arch Intern Med* 1993;153(8):1005–1010.

13. Sam R, Vaseemuddin M, Siddique A, et al. Hypercalcemia in patients in the burn intensive care unit. *J Burn Care Res* 2007;28(5):742–746.

14. Ziegler R. Hypercalcemic crisis. *J Am Soc Nephrol* 2001;12(Suppl 17):S3–S9.

15. Douglas PS, Carmichael KA, Palevsky PM. Extreme hypercalcemia and electrocardiographic changes. *Am J Cardiol* 1984;54(6):674–675.

16. Johnson NA, Tublin ME, Ogilvie JB. Parathyroid imaging: Technique and role in the preoperative evaluation of primary hyperparathyroidism. *AJR Am J Roentgenol* 2007;188(6):1706–1715.

17. LeGrand SB, Leskuski D, Zama I. Narrative review: Furosemide for hypercalcemia: An unproven yet common practice. *Ann Intern Med* 2008;149(4):259–263.

18. Lumachi F, Brunello A, Roma A, Basso U. Cancer-induced hypercalcemia. *Anticancer Res* 2009;29(5):1551–1555.

19. Major P, Lortholary A, Hon J, et al. Zoledronic acid is superior to pamidronate in the treatment of hypercalcemia of malignancy: A pooled analysis of two randomized, controlled clinical trials. *J Clin Oncol* 2001;19(2):558–567.

20. Dietzek A, Connelly K, Cotugno M, Bartel S, McDonnell AM. Denosumab in hypercalcemia of malignancy: A case series. *J Oncol Pharm Pract* 2015;21(2):143–147.

21. Peacock M, Bilezikian JP, Klassen PS, Guo MD, Turner SA, Shoback D. Cinacalcet hydrochloride maintains long-term normocalcemia in patients with primary hyperparathyroidism. *J Clin Endocrinol Metab* 2005;90(1):135–141.

22. *Sensipar (Cinacalcet) Prescribing Information.* Thousand Oaks, CA: Amgen Inc; March 2017.

23. Sayers J, Hynes AM, Srivastava S, et al. Successful treatment of hypercalcemia associated with a CYP24A1 mutation with fluconazole. *Clin Kidney J* 2015;8(4):453–455.

24. Barre PE, Gascon-Barre M, Meakins JL, Goltzman D. Hydroxychloroquine treatment of hypercalcemia in a patient with sarcoidosis undergoing hemodialysis. *Am J Med* 1978;82(6):1259–1262.

25. Bilezikian JP, Brandi ML, Eastell R, et al. Guidelines for the management of asymptomatic primary hyperparathyroidism: Summary statement from the Fourth International Workshop. *J Clin Endocrinol Metab* 2014;99(10):3561–3569.

Hypocalcemia

24

Marjorie Ann Malbas and Naga Yalla

GENERAL PRINCIPLES

Calcium homeostasis is vital for normal cellular function, neurotransmission, membrane stability, bone health, blood coagulation, muscle contraction, and intracellular signaling. Unrecognized or poorly treated hypocalcemic emergencies can lead to significant morbidity or mortality.

Definition

- Hypocalcemia is defined as serum ionized calcium <4.5 mg/dL or serum albumin–corrected total calcium <8.6 mg/dL.
- Normal reference range for serum total calcium is 8.6 to 10.4 mg/dL (2.15 to 2.58 mmol/L) and for ionized calcium is 4.5 to 5.1 mg/dL (1.13 to 1.28 mmol/L).[1]
- Hypocalcemia can be classified into acute and chronic.

Epidemiology

Hypocalcemia is estimated to occur in up to 85% of patients in an intensive care unit (ICU) and 15% of those admitted to a non-ICU facility.[2,3]

Etiology

Causes for hypocalcemia can be broadly classified (see Table 24-1) into:
- Inadequate parathyroid hormone (PTH) production (hypoparathyroidism)
- PTH resistance
- Vitamin D deficiency
- Vitamin D resistance
- Miscellaneous causes

Pathophysiology

- 99% of total body calcium is sequestered in the skeleton. Of the remaining 1%, ~50% exists in free biologically active or ionized form, 40% is albumin bound, and ~10% is complexed with anions (e.g., citrate or PO_4).[1]
- Serum calcium levels vary with changes in serum pH, protein and anion levels, and calcium-regulating hormone function.
- The average skeletal turnover of calcium is approximately 250 mg/day. Gastrointestinal calcium absorption is matched by urinary excretion in healthy individuals. Serum levels of ionized calcium are tightly regulated by an integrated hormonal system that includes PTH, vitamin D, and their receptors, and the calcium-sensing receptors (CaSRs).[1]
- **CaSR**
  - CaSR is a G-protein cell membrane receptor expressed in parathyroid and renal tubular cells that senses changes in extracellular ionized calcium level.
  - In the parathyroid gland, CaSR activates phospholipase C and in turn reduces PTH gene transcription, synthesis, and ultimately, secretion.
  - CaSR in the renal tubular system has an inhibitory effect on the reabsorption of calcium.
- **Parathyroid hormone**
  - Parathyroid gland chief cells secrete PTH in response to decreases in ionized calcium.

TABLE 24-1 CAUSES OF HYPOCALCEMIA

Inadequate PTH production (Hypoparathyroidism)	• Surgical/postoperative • Autoimmune destruction • Genetic (DiGeorge syndrome) • Postradiation therapy, infiltrative processes • CaSR receptor defect • Idiopathic
PTH resistance	• Pseudohypoparathyroidism • Magnesium deficiency
Inadequate vitamin D	• Nutritional deficiency • Lack of sunlight exposure • Malabsorption syndrome • End-stage liver disease and cirrhosis • Chronic kidney disease
Resistance to vitamin D	• Pseudovitamin D deficiency rickets (vitamin D–dependent rickets type 1) • Vitamin D–resistant rickets (vitamin D–dependent rickets type 2)
Miscellaneous	• Hyperphosphatemia • Drugs (e.g., foscarnet, IV bisphosphonate therapy in patients with vitamin D deficiency) • Rapid transfusion with citrate-containing blood • "Hungry bone syndrome" or recalcification tetany • Postthyroidectomy for Graves' disease • Postparathyroidectomy • Acute pancreatitis • Rhabdomyolysis or tumor lysis syndrome • Acute critical illness

- ○ It acts to maintain normocalcemia by directly stimulating bone resorption and decreasing renal calcium excretion (also increasing phosphate excretion), and indirectly increasing intestinal calcium absorption by stimulating renal production of $1,25(OH)_2D$ or also calcitriol.
- **Vitamin D**
  - ○ Vitamin D is derived from dietary sources or from UV light–medicated conversion of cholesterol precursors in the dermis. It is then converted to $25(OH)D$ by the liver and then to the active form $1,25(OH)_2D$ by PTH-regulated 1α-hydroxylase in the proximal renal tubule.
  - ○ Active vitamin D (calcitriol) stimulates intestinal absorption of calcium and phosphorus and regulates PTH release.

DIAGNOSIS

Clinical Presentation

- Manifestations depend on severity and chronicity of hypocalcemia, and can range from asymptomatic laboratory abnormality to life-threatening seizure and laryngospasm.
- Low extracellular fluid ionized calcium enhances neuromuscular excitability, an effect accentuated by hyperkalemia or hypomagnesemia.[1]
- Please see Table 24-2.[5]

TABLE 24-2 SYMPTOMS AND SIGNS OF HYPOCALCEMIA

Neuromuscular excitability
  Circumoral paresthesia
  Acral numbness and tingling
  Carpopedal spasm
  Muscle weakness and cramps
  Laryngospasm or bronchospasm
  Chvostek sign
  Trousseau sign
CNS
  Seizures
  Confusion
  Memory impairment
  Basal ganglia calcification may result in movement disorders
Cardiac
  Syncope
  Arrhythmia
  Angina (acute)
  Cardiomyopathy (chronic)
  Prolonged QT interval on EKG
Gastrointestinal
  Abdominal pain
  Biliary or intestinal colic
  Dysphagia
Others
  Eyes—Cataract, pseudopapilledema
  Skin—Dry skin, coarse hair, brittle nails, psoriasis, chronic pruritus

History
- **Pertinent medical history** includes pancreatitis, renal or liver failure, gastrointestinal disorders, hyperthyroidism or hyperparathyroidism, other autoimmune diseases.
- **Pertinent surgical history** includes thyroid, parathyroid, or bowel surgeries, or recent neck trauma.
- Exposure to radiocontrast media, estrogen, loop diuretics, bisphosphonates, denosumab, calcium supplements, antibiotics, and antiepileptics should be investigated.
- Family history of hypocalcemia may aid in the diagnosis of inherited conditions.

Physical Examination
- The two classic physical examination findings are **Chvostek sign** and **Trousseau sign**.
- Chvostek sign is elicited by tapping facial nerve 2-cm anterior to tragus and observing for ipsilateral contraction of facial muscles. This is neither sensitive nor specific and may be seen in normocalcemic individuals.
- Trousseau sign is elicited by inflating a blood pressure cuff to 20 mm Hg above the systolic blood pressure for 3 minutes and observing for carpopedal spasm. It can be uncomfortable and even painful. It is reported to have a better sensitivity and lower false-positive rate compared to Chvostek sign. Features of Albright hereditary osteodystrophy (AHO) may be seen (please see Pseudohypoparathyroidism section for details).

Differential Diagnosis

- **Inadequate PTH production (hypoparathyroidism)**
  - ○ Hypoparathyroidism is defined as an **inappropriately low or normal secretion of PTH for subnormal ionized or albumin-corrected calcium**. Characteristic laboratory findings include **hypocalcemia and hyperphosphatemia, with inappropriately low or normal PTH levels.**[6] Twenty-four-hour urinary excretion of calcium is low, as is 1,25(OH)$_2$D and bone turnover marker levels.
  - ○ **Postoperative hypoparathyroidism**
    - ■ It is the most common cause of hypoparathyroidism and can be a complication of anterior neck surgery (thyroid, parathyroid, laryngeal, spine or lymph node dissection). It results from destruction of parathyroid glands or disruption of its tenuous vascular supply.
    - ■ It can be classified as transient (≤12 months) or permanent (>12 months). Risk factors include neck surgery for malignancy, presence of autoimmune thyroid disease, bilaterality, repeat operation, and surgeon experience.[7]
    - ■ Incidence of permanent hypoparathyroidism varies from 0.12% to 5%, with a lower incidence in high-volume surgical centers.[7]
    - ■ Intraoperative PTH value during total thyroidectomy has been useful in predicting risk for developing symptomatic postoperative hypocalcemia, where levels less than 12 pg/mL was found to be 71% sensitive and 95% specific.[8]
    - ■ Other causes of postoperative hypocalcemia include:
      - □ "Hungry bone syndrome" after surgery for hyperparathyroidism can cause hypocalcemia due to rapid bone mineralization with sudden withdrawal of PTH action. Unlike hypoparathyroidism, phosphorus is low and PTH is appropriately elevated.
      - □ Multiple blood transfusions due to calcium chelation by citrate preservative in the blood.
  - ○ **Hypoparathyroidism associated with autoimmune disease**
    - ■ Autoimmune parathyroid gland destruction occurs either in isolation or as part of autoimmune polyglandular syndrome type 1 (APS-1) (see Chapter 39).
    - ■ APS-1 can be sporadic or autosomal recessive, caused by mutations in the autoimmune regulator (AIRE) gene located on chromosome 21q22.3. It includes the classic triad of *hypoparathyroidism, adrenal insufficiency*, and *chronic mucocutaneous candidiasis*, two of which (diagnostic dyad) are required for diagnosis. The typical presentation is childhood candidiasis, followed by hypoparathyroidism, and then adrenal insufficiency during late childhood. Associated conditions may include hypogonadism, hepatitis, pernicious anemia, type 1 diabetes mellitus, autoimmune thyroid disease, alopecia, and vitiligo.[9] Antibodies against a parathyroid autoantigen, NACHT leucine-rich-repeat protein 5 (NALP5), have been identified in 49% of APS-1 with hypoparathyroidism.[10] Activating antibodies against the CaSR have also been described.[11]
    - ■ In patients with isolated hypoparathyroidism, activating antibodies against CaSR have also been identified.[9]
  - ○ **Defect in CaSR receptor**
    - ■ Autosomal dominant hypocalcemic hypercalciuria results from activating mutation of CaSR gene leading to inappropriate suppression of PTH secretion at subnormal calcium level.
    - ■ Similarly, calcimimetic agents such as cinacalcet, bind to CaSR and lower the threshold for its activation by extracellular calcium. Consequently, PTH release from parathyroid cells decreases. Hypocalcemia has been described in up to 5% of these patients.
  - ○ **Hypoparathyroidism secondary to developmental disorders**
    - ■ DiGeorge syndrome is associated with parathyroid glands defect caused by malformation of the third and fourth branchial pouches from microdeletion in chromosome 22q11. Features of patients with DiGeorge syndrome include cardiac anomalies, abnormal facies, thymic hypoplasia, cleft palate, and hypocalcemia (in 50% to 60%).[6]

- Mutations in pre-proPTH gene and transcription factors (GCMB, GCM2, GATA3) that control parathyroid development have been identified. These are rare causes of hypoparathyroidism and include familial isolated hypoparathyroidism; x-linked hypoparathyroidism; hypoparathyroidism, deafness, and renal dysplasia (HDR) syndrome; and hypoparathyroidism, growth/mental retardation, and dysmorphism (HRD) syndrome.[6]
  - **Radiation therapy and infiltration:** Rarely, hypoparathyroidism can be caused by infiltration of parathyroid gland by iron (hemochromatosis or transfusion dependent), copper (Wilson disease), metastatic cancer, granulomatous disease, or amyloidosis. Extensive neck radiation has been described as a cause of hypoparathyroidism.
- **PTH resistance**
  - **Pseudohypoparathyroidism:**[12]
    - Is a cluster of inherited disorders caused by end-organ resistance to PTH. Laboratory findings include hypocalcemia, hyperphosphatemia, and low $1,25(OH)_2D$, however, unlike hypoparathyroidism, PTH levels are elevated.
    - Pseudohypoparathyroidism is classified into types 1 and 2. Type 1 is further subdivided into types 1a, 1b, and 1c.
      - Pseudohypoparathyroidism type 1 is caused by mutations in GNAS gene on chromosome 20, which encodes for Gsα subunit of the PTH receptor, rendering it unresponsive to PTH. The defect in Gsα may also affect other hormonal systems that use cAMP as a second messenger (e.g., resistance to TSH, gonadotropins, and GHRH).
      - Pseudohypoparathyroidism type 1a, the most common variant, presents with proximal tubule PTH resistance and physical features of AHO, which include brachydactyly, shortening of the 4th and 5th metacarpals, short stature, rounded facies, obesity, mental retardation, and heterotopic ossification. The defect is due to mutation of maternal-derived GNAS gene. If the mutated allele is inherited from the father, there is the physical appearance of AHO, but serum calcium homeostasis is maintained. This latter disorder is termed pseudopseudohypoparathyroidism.
      - Pseudohypoparathyroidism type 1b is characterized by selective defect in renal PTH signaling without features of AHO. Imprinting defects in GNAS have been identified as a cause.
      - Pseudohypoparathyroidism type 1c, considered a variant of type 1a, presents with AHO, biochemical features of PTH resistance and multiple other hormones resistance. A normal Gsα protein expression distinguishes this condition from pseudohypoparathyroidism type 1a.[14]
      - Pseudohypoparathyroidism type 2 is caused by a mutation in protein kinase cAMP-dependent type 1 regulatory subunit alpha (PRKAR1A) downstream to Gsα and is characterized by biochemical features of PTH resistance. Pseudohypoparathyroidism type 2 is quite rare.
  - **Magnesium deficiency or excess:**[6]
    - Serum magnesium has a paradoxical effect on PTH secretion.
    - Magnesium deficiency impairs PTH secretion and causes PTH resistance (at levels <0.8 mEq/L or 1 mg/dL or 0.4 mmol/L), leading to hypocalcemia with low or inappropriately normal PTH level. Malabsorption, diuretics, parenteral fluid administration, chronic alcoholism, and cisplatin therapy are the most common causes of hypomagnesemia. Hypocalcemia secondary to hypomagnesemia is resistant to administration of calcium and vitamin D, and restoration of the calcium levels can occur only after the magnesium deficiency is corrected.
    - On the other hand, very high levels of magnesium (>5 mEq/L or 6 mg/dL or 2.5 mmol/L) can suppress PTH release via activation of CaSR and lead to hypocalcemia. This occurs in the setting of intravenous magnesium infusion for tocolysis.
- **Vitamin D deficiency**
  - Vitamin D deficiency leads to hypocalcemia by decreasing absorption of dietary calcium.

○ In vitamin D deficiency and hypocalcemia, the compensatory increase in PTH results in mild increases in serum calcium. However, this comes at the expense of serum phosphate, since PTH increases phosphaturia. The combined effects lead to bone demineralization and, if uncorrected, cause syndromes of rickets and osteomalacia.

■ Rickets occurs in growing bone of children, and results from diminished calcification of cartilage at the epiphysis. The typical presentation involves bowing of the limbs and cupping of the costochondral junctions (the rachitic rosary).

■ Osteomalacia occurs after growth plates close and has a clinical appearance that may be difficult to distinguish from osteoporosis.

○ Vitamin D deficiency can result from inadequate sun exposure, dietary insufficiency, intestinal malabsorption (gastrojejunostomy, gastric resection, or celiac disease), chronic liver disease (impaired 25-hydroxylation, decreased bile salts, decreased vitamin D–binding protein synthesis), chronic pancreatitis and chronic renal disease (impaired 1-alpha hydroxylation of vitamin D).

- **Vitamin D resistance**
  ○ Patients with vitamin D–dependent rickets type 1, also known as pseudovitamin D deficiency, have a genetic deficiency of 1α-hydroxylase. This condition is rare and is inherited in an autosomal recessive fashion typically manifesting prior to 2 years of age with hypocalcemia, hypophosphatemia, elevated PTH, elevated alkaline phosphatase and low 1,25(OH)$_2$D. 25(OH)D level is variable. Calcitriol administration can correct the defect.
  ○ Vitamin D–dependent rickets type 2, also known as hereditary calcitriol–resistant rickets, involves typical symptoms of rickets as well as alopecia. It is inherited as an autosomal recessive disease and is the result of a mutation in the vitamin D receptor gene. These patients have high serum levels of 1,25(OH)$_2$D, which are ineffective due to end-organ resistance. Treatment involves high doses of calcium and calcitriol, and calcium infusions may be required if the resistance is complete.

- **Miscellaneous causes of acute hypocalcemia**
  ○ **Acute hyperphosphatemia**, as seen in rhabdomyolysis or tumor lysis syndrome, can acutely lower calcium level since the rapid release of phosphorous from cell lysis quickly forms complexes with calcium.
  ○ Widespread **osteoblastic malignancy**, typically from breast or prostate cancer, can cause hypocalcemia. Osteoblast activation in this case results in deposition of calcium in metastatic lesions.
  ○ **Chelation of calcium** by citrate (anticoagulant in banked blood or plasma), lactate, gadolinium-based contrast material used in magnetic resonance imaging (MRI, gadodiamide and gadoversetamide), and ethylenediaminetetraacetic acid (EDTA) reduce serum ionized calcium concentrations, but not serum total calcium concentrations. Calcium is also chelated in acute pancreatitis, most likely due to the release of free fatty acids. The degree of hypocalcemia seen with pancreatitis can be a prognosticator, with lower levels predicting a worse prognosis.
  ○ Hypocalcemia in the ICU setting is common and often associated with sepsis.
  ○ Multiple **medications** cause hypocalcemia. Those that inhibit bone resorption include calcitonin, plicamycin, gallium nitrate, and estrogens. Cimetidine decreases gastric pH, slowing fat breakdown, which is necessary to complex calcium for gut absorption. Anticonvulsants may stimulate microsomal enzymes with resultant abnormal metabolism of vitamin D. Reports also show that phenytoin interferes with the intestinal absorption of vitamin D. Patients on anticonvulsant therapy may present with hypocalcemia, normal calcitriol levels, and increased PTH levels.
  ○ Treatment with intravenous bisphosphonates and denosumab has been associated with hypocalcemia and in the setting of severe vitamin D deficiency, these patients can develop symptomatic hypocalcemia. Use of intravenous bisphosphonates is contraindicated in the setting of vitamin D deficiency; therefore, prior to use, serum 25(OH)D level should be obtained.

Diagnostic Testing

Laboratories[3,4]

- **Total serum calcium** should be corrected in the setting of hypoalbuminemia using the following equation: corrected calcium = measured calcium (mg/dL) + [0.8 × (4 – measured albumin in g/dL)].
- **Serum ionized calcium** can measured directly. It can be falsely elevated with prolonged ischemia of the arm during blood draw, and is sensitive to sample handling.
- Other tests should include measurement of **serum phosphorus, intact PTH, magnesium, creatinine, vitamin D metabolites, and alkaline phosphatase**.
- A low 25(OH)D level suggests vitamin D deficiency. Low levels of 1,25(OH)$_2$D in association with high PTH suggest PTH resistance or failure to induce the 1α-hydroxylase, as observed in patients with chronic renal failure, vitamin D–dependent rickets type 1, and pseudohypoparathyroidism.
- Additional test as clinically indicated: 24-hour urinary calcium and creatinine; urinary cAMP response to PTH may help to differentiate hypoparathyroidism from pseudohypoparathyroidism types 1 and 2; DNA sequence analysis.

Electrocardiography

The ECG finding of hypocalcemia includes prolongation of the QTc interval and shortening of RR interval, proportional to the degree of hypocalcemia.

Imaging

- Imaging study results varies with etiology of hypocalcemia.
- Skeletal x-rays may show rickets or osteomalacia with pathognomonic "Looser zones" best observed in the pubic ramus, the upper femur, and the ribs.
- In chronic hypoparathyroidism, bone mineral density by DXA is usually above average, more so in the lumbar spine. High-resolution peripheral quantitative computed tomography (HRpQCT) shows increased cortical and trabecular volume.[13]
- In a retrospective analysis, renal sonogram was better than CT scan in assessing nephrocalcinosis and is preferred given its low cost, lack of radiation, and portability.[14]

TREATMENT

- Treatment depends on the severity and rapidity of development of hypocalcemia and associated symptoms.
- Goals of treatment include alleviation of symptoms, correction of serum calcium to acceptable level, and avoidance complications like hypercalciuria or hypercalcemia.
- The indications for emergent correction of hypocalcemia include severe symptomatic tetany, stridor due to laryngospasm and bronchospasm, arrhythmia-altered mental status or seizures.

Medications

- **Acute hypocalcemia:**[4,14]
  - This emergent condition is **treated by replacing calcium intravenously with either calcium gluconate or calcium chloride**. A 10 mL solution of 10% calcium gluconate (1 ampule = 1 g = 90 mg elemental calcium) in 50 to 100 mL D5W or normal saline can be infused over 10 minutes (rule of 10s) and can be repeated once or twice; calcium chloride, if used, is equally effective although less preferred due to risk of tissue necrosis with extravasation. The effect of this bolus is transient and raises serum calcium for 2 to 3 hours only, so prolonged intravenous therapy should follow.
  - A 1 mg/mL infusion can be prepared using 11 g of calcium gluconate (11 amps = 990 mg elemental calcium) in D5W or NS to provide final volume of 1,000 mL. This can be infused at a rate of 0.5 to 1.5 mg/kg/hr.[15]

○ Rapid infusion should be avoided due to risk of arrhythmia, cardiac dysfunction, and cardiac arrest. Patients should be monitored using telemetry to detect cardiac arrhythmias during IV calcium treatment.

○ Intravenous calcium administration should be considered in patients with marked hypocalcemia (<7.0 mg/dL or <1.75 mmol/L) since life-threatening symptoms can develop suddenly.

○ Bicarbonate- and phosphate-containing solutions cause calcium to precipitate and should not be run simultaneously. **Serum calcium should be measured every 4 to 6 hours during intravenous infusion** and the rate adjusted to maintain a serum calcium level in the low normal range and control symptoms.

○ Oral calcium salts and vitamin D should be started as soon as able and infusion tapered over a 24 to 48 hour period while oral therapy is adjusted.

○ Hypomagnesemia should be corrected concurrently, preferably with magnesium sulfate infusion in the acute setting.

• **Chronic hypocalcemia:**[4,14]

○ Chronic management of hypocalcemia is accomplished using oral calcium salts, vitamin D metabolites, and less commonly thiazide diuretics.

○ **The goal of chronic calcium replacement therapy is to keep the calcium in the low range of normal, especially in hypoparathyroid states to avoid hypercalciuria.** Approximately 1 to 3 g of elemental calcium daily should be given in divided doses to facilitate absorption and minimize rapid rise in serum calcium, which increases complications related to hypercalcemia. There are multiple different preparations of oral calcium; in general, calcium carbonate is the cheapest, although absorption may be less than with other products (see Table 24-3).

○ Vitamin D supplementation is typically given as ergocalciferol (vitamin D_2) or cholecalciferol (vitamin D3). Please see Table 24-4. This preparation is the least expensive and has the longest biological half-life. The typical dose range varies depending on etiology of hypocalcemia and vitamin D deficiency, and may be in the order of 50,000 IU orally daily for patients with hypoparathyoidism (1.25 to 2.5 mg/day). Serum 25(OH) D levels can be measured along with serum calcium levels to assess for adequacy of treatment. Vitamin D is extremely lipophilic and may require several weeks to reach a steady state with a new dose. Calcitriol (1,25[OH]D), which has rapid onset of action and a shorter half-life, may also be given with at a dose of 0.25 to 1 mcg orally once or twice daily. This may be preferred during initial treatment of hypocalcemia due to its rapid onset of action, and requires closer monitoring of calcium, typically every 1 to 3 days. Please see Table 24-4.

○ Thiazide diuretic may be added in patients who develop hypercalciuria, in combination with low salt diet to promote calcium retention. Effective dose of hydrochlorothiazide is 25 to 100 mg daily or chlorthalidone 25 to 100 mg daily.[16]

○ Serum calcium, phosphorus, creatinine, and vitamin D should be monitored regularly.

• **Hypocalcemia secondary to hypoparathyroidism and pseudohypoparathyroidism**

○ Goals of treatment are:[16]
  ▪ Symptom relief
  ▪ Maintaining serum total calcium slightly below normal (up to 0.5 mg/dL below lower limit of normal) to low normal range
  ▪ Maintaining serum phosphorus within normal to slightly elevated range
  ▪ Avoiding hypercalciuria (24-hour urine calcium should be <300 mg/day)
  ▪ Keep calcium-phosphate product <55 mg^2/dL^2 or 4.4 $mmol^2/L^2$
  ▪ Prevention of extraskeletal or renal (stones and nephrocalcinosis) ectopic calcification.

○ Initial management is accomplished with oral calcium supplements. Calcitriol is usually required due to lack of PTH-mediated conversion of inactive vitamin D (25[OH] D) to active vitamin D (1,25[OH]2D).

TABLE 24-3 CALCIUM SALT PREPARATIONS

	Elemental calcium	Comments
Calcium Carbonate (Os-cal, Tums, Caltrate, Titralac)	40%	Best absorbed with food and presence of stomach acid; constipation is a common side effect; least expensive
Calcium Citrate (Citracal)	21%	Does not require stomach acid for absorption, so preferred formulation in patients with achlordyria or taking proton-pump inhibitors; higher pill burden

○ Recombinant human PTH (1-84) (Natpara ®) is identical to endogenous PTH, has been shown to be effective in reducing oral calcium and active vitamin D treatment while maintaining target serum calcium with similar adverse events compared to placebo.[17] Treatment for 6 years revealed similar efficacy and safety profile, as well as lower urinary calcium excretion.[18] Natpara ® is FDA approved for management of hypoparathyroidism as an adjunct to calcium and vitamin D in patients who are not well-controlled on conventional therapy. It carries a black box warning for osteosarcoma risk and is contraindicated in patients with increased risk for osteosarcoma (Paget disease, young patients with open epiphysis, radiation exposure involving the skeleton, and unexplained elevation of alkaline phosphatase). It can only be prescribed under the Risk Evaluation and Mitigation Strategies (REMS) program. The starting dose is 50 mcg once daily SC injection which can be increased by 25 mcg every 4 weeks to maximum dose of 100 mcg daily. Careful monitoring and titration of oral calcium, calcitriol, and recombinant PTH is required to achieve desired serum calcium levels.[16]

Other Nonpharmacologic Therapies

In patients with a higher risk of developing permanent hypoparathyroidism, parathyroid tissue may be autotransplanted into the brachioradialis or sternocleidomastoid muscle at the time of parathyroidectomy.

TABLE 24-4 VITAMIN D METABOLITE PREPARATIONS

	Dose	Onset of action	Offset of action	Comments
Vitamin D2 (ergocalciferol) or Vitamin D3 (cholecalciferol)	5,000–50,000 IU daily (depending on etiology)	10–14 days	14–75 days	Longer half-life, therefore dose adjustment and serum levels must be checked every 4–6 weeks
1,25(OH) D3 (calcitriol)	0.25–1 mcg once or twice daily	1–2 days	2–3 days	Most active metabolite; more expensive

COMPLICATIONS

- Complications of treatment with calcium salts and vitamin D include hypercalcemia, nephrolithiasis, calciphylaxis, and basal ganglia calcification.
- If hypercalcemia develops, vitamin D and calcium supplementation should be withheld until levels return to normal. The doses should then be decreased. The effects of calcitriol typically last 1 week, but ergocalciferol can last more than 1 month.

PROGNOSIS

The prognosis for correcting hypocalcemia is good but is dependent upon the etiology. Most symptoms can be alleviated. However, cataract or mental retardation from long-standing hypocalcemia cannot be reversed.

REFERENCES

1. Peacock M. Calcium metabolism in health and disease. *Clin J Am Soc Nephrol* 2010;5 (Suppl 1): S23–S30.
2. Zivin JR, Gooley T, Zager RA, Ryan MJ. Hypocalcemia: A pervasive metabolic abnormality in the critically ill. *Am J Kidney Dis* 2001;37(4):689–698.
3. Hannan FM, Thakker RV. Investigating hypocalcemia. *BMJ* 2013;346:f2213.
4. Schafer AL, Shoback D. Hypocalcemia: Definition, etiology, pathogenesis, diagnosis and management. Primer on metabolic bone disease and disorders of mineral metabolism. *ASBMR* 2013:572–578.
5. Shonback DM, Bilezikian JP, Costa AG, et al. Presentation of hypoparathyroidism: Etiologies and clinical features. *J Clin Endocrinol Metab* 2016;101(6):2300–2312.
6. Shoback D. Clinical practice. Hypoparathyroidism. *N Eng J Med* 2008;359(4):391–403.
7. Stack BD, Bimston DN, Bodenner DL, et al. American Association of Clinical Endocrinologist and America College of Endocrinology disease state clinical review: Postoperative hypoparathyroidism—definitions and management. *Endocr Pract* 2015;21(6):674–685.
8. Mcleod IK, Arciero C, Noordzij JP, et al. The use of rapid parathyroid hormone assay in predicting postoperative hypocalcemia after total or completion thyroidectomy. *Thyroid* 2006;16(3):259–265.
9. Perheentupa J. Autoimmune polyendocrinopathy-candidiasis-ectodermal dystrophy. *J Clin Endocrinol Metab* 2006;91:2843–2850.
10. Alimohammadi M, Bjorklund P, Hallgren A, et al. Autoimmune polyendocrine syndrome type 1 and NALP5, a parathyroid autoantigen. *New Engl J Med* 2008;358(10):1018–1028.
11. Kemp EH, Gavalas NG, Krohn KJ, Brown EM, Watson PF, Weetman AP. Activating Autoantibodies against the calcium-sensing receptor detected in two patients with autoimmune polyendocrine syndrome type 1. *J Clin Endocrinol Metab* 2009;94(12):4749–4756.
12. Juppner H, Bastepe M. Pseudohypoparathyroidism. Primer on metabolic bone disease and disorders of mineral metabolism. *ASBMR* 2013:590–600.
13. Silva BC, Rubin MR, Cusano NE, Bilezekian JP. Bone imaging in hypopapathyroidism. *Osteoporosis Int* 2017;28(2):463–471.
14. Boyce AM, Shawker TH, Hill SC, et al. Ultrasound is superior to computed tomography for assessment of medullary nephrocalcinosis in hypoparathyroidism. *J Clin Endocrinol Metab* 2013;98(3):989–994.
15. Cooper MS, Gittoes NJ. Diagnosis and management of hypocalcemia. *BMJ* 2008;336(7656): 1298–1302.
16. Bilezikian JP, Brandi ML, Cusano NE, et al. Management of hypoparathyroidism: Present and future. *J Clin Endocrinol Metab* 2016;101(6):2213–2324.
17. Mannstadt M, Clarke BL, Brandi ML, et al. Efficacy and safety of recombinant human parathyroid hormone (1-84) in hypoparathyroidism (REPLACE): A double-blinded, placebo-controlled, randomized, phase 3 study. *Lancet Diabetes Endocrinol* 2013;1(4):275–283.
18. Rubin MR, Cusano NE, Fan WW, et al. Therapy of hypoparathyroidism with PTH (1-84): A prospective six year investigation of efficacy and safety. *J Clin Endocrinol Metab* 2016;101(7): 2742–2750.

Vitamin D Deficiency

25

Amy E. Riek, Ana Maria Arbelaez, and Carlos Bernal-Mizrachi

GENERAL PRINCIPLES[1-3]

- Vitamin D is a prohormone that exists in two forms: D_3 (cholecalciferol), which is generated in the skin of animals, and D_2 (ergocalciferol), which is derived from plants.
- Humans largely obtain vitamin D in two ways:
  - **Sunlight exposure** causes photolysis of provitamin D_3 in skin to form previtamin D_3, which isomerizes into vitamin D_3, the main source of vitamin D in humans.
  - **Dietary vitamin D** is fat soluble and principally absorbed in the proximal small intestine. Absorption of dietary vitamin D requires bile salts and an intact absorptive surface.
- Once vitamin D enters the circulation, it is stored in fat or metabolized in the liver.
- D_2 and D_3 are biologically inert. To become physiologically active, vitamin D requires two hydroxylation steps.
  - Initial hydroxylation to produce 25(OH)D occurs primarily in the **liver** via CYP2R1. **25(OH)D is the major circulating form** of vitamin D and has a half-life of 10 days to 3 weeks. Hepatic 25-hydroxylation is poorly regulated. **Serum levels of 25(OH) D increase in proportion to cutaneous synthesis and dietary intake of vitamin D, and thus are the best indicator of vitamin D status.**
  - Secondary hydroxylation of 25(OH)D to form **active vitamin D, or 1,25(OH)₂D,** via 1α-hydroxylation occurs mainly in the **kidney**. The half-life of 1,25(OH)₂D is approximately 4 to 6 hours. Renal 1α-hydroxylase activity is highly regulated to maintain normal calcium levels. Hypocalcemia induces parathyroid hormone (PTH) expression, enhancing renal production of 1,25(OH)₂D directly by induction of 1α-hydroxylase expression and indirectly by renal phosphate wasting. **1,25(OH)₂D levels remain normal and nearly constant regardless of 25(OH)D levels.**
- Numerous cells and tissues express 1α-hydroxylase and can produce local 1,25(OH)2D to serve as an autocrine–paracrine factor, which is fundamental for cell-specific functions. The contribution of these extrarenal sources to circulating 1,25(OH)2D levels is minimal.
- 1,25(OH)2D binds to vitamin D receptor (VDR) with 100-fold affinity compared to 25(OH)D. VDR is expressed in almost all human tissues and acts as a ligand-activated transcription factor to regulate the expression of vitamin D–responsive genes.
- Catabolism of both 25(OH)D and 1,25(OH)2D is carried out by 24-hydroxylase in the kidney, which is stimulated by 1,25(OH)2D. 25(OH)D deficiency decreases intestinal absorption of calcium and phosphorus. Serum ionized calcium levels drop, triggering a compensatory synthesis and secretion of PTH. Increased plasma PTH levels maintain serum calcium levels by enhancing renal production of 1,25(OH)2D, promoting tubular calcium reabsorption and phosphate excretion, and increasing bone turnover. Increased 1,25(OH)2D induces intestinal absorption of calcium and phosphorus and stimulates osteoclast activity, which increases the availability of calcium and phosphorus in the blood.

Definition[3]

- **Vitamin D deficiency**—25(OH)D levels ≤20 ng/mL
- **Vitamin D insufficiency**—25(OH)D levels 21 to 29 ng/mL
- **Vitamin D adequacy**—25(OH)D levels 30 to 50 ng/mL

Epidemiology[4]

Data from The National Health Nutrition and Examination Survey (NHANES) 2007–2010 demonstrated **deficient 25(OH)D levels** in 5.9% of those sampled: 2.3% of non-Hispanic whites, 24% of non-Hispanic blacks, and 6.4% of Hispanics. **Insufficient levels** were present in 24% overall: 13% of non-Hispanic whites, 62% of non-Hispanic blacks, and 36% of Hispanics.

Etiology[3,5]

- **Decreased bioavailability:** malabsorption resulting from cystic fibrosis, celiac disease, Whipple disease, Crohn disease, gastric bypass surgery, biliary atresia, or medications that reduce cholesterol absorption; obesity.
- **Increased catabolism:** anticonvulsants, glucocorticoids, highly active antiretroviral therapy, and transplant antirejection medications.
- **Decreased synthesis of 25(OH)D:** liver cirrhosis.
- **Increased urinary loss of 25(OH)D:** nephrotic syndrome.
- **Decreased synthesis of 1,25(OH)$_2$D:** chronic kidney disease.
- **Rickets:** heritable disorders (vitamin D–dependent rickets types I, II, III; X-linked hypophosphatemic rickets; autosomal-dominant hypophosphatemic rickets; autosomal-recessive hypophosphatemic rickets); acquired disorders (tumor-induced osteomalacia).
- **Increased conversion of 25(OH)D to 1,25(OH)$_2$D:** primary hyperparathyroidism (PTH-induced 1α-hydroxylase activation); granulomatous disorders (via cytokine induction of macrophage 1α-hydroxylase, converting 25(OH)D to 1,25(OH)$_2$D).
- **Accelerated metabolism:** hyperthyroidism.

Risk Factors[3,5]

- Premature birth
- Pigmented skin
- Low sunshine exposure
- Breast feeding
- Use of sunscreen
- Indoor activities
- Obesity
- Advanced age
- Seasons
- Latitudes further from the equator

DIAGNOSIS[2,3,5]

Clinical Presentation

Vitamin D deficiency is **largely asymptomatic and physical examination is typically unremarkable** unless severe enough to lead to rickets in children or osteomalacia in adults. These are characterized by generalized bone pain, muscle weakness, waddling gait, and pseudofractures. Clinical suspicion should be high in any patient with risk factors.

Diagnostic Testing

- Vitamin D status is usually estimated by measuring serum 25(OH)D levels (see section Definition). Testing for free 25(OH)D is available but requires further clinical correlation. **Of note, most patients with suboptimal vitamin D levels are not hypocalcemic.**
- **Osteomalcia and rickets** are characterized by low serum and urinary calcium, low serum phosphorous, and high serum alkaline phosphatase and PTH. Radiologic features include reduced bone density and thinning of the cortex. More advanced features include

concavity of the vertebral bodies and pseudofractures, radiolucent lines with surrounding sclerosis in the long bones.

TREATMENT

Indications

We suggest vitamin D adequacy in all children and adults to maintain nutrition and prevent rickets and osteomalacia. Several conditions with proven benefit of vitamin D treatment require special mention:

- Community-dwelling and institutionalized 65 or older adults: reduces hip fractures and decreases mortality.[6]
- Chronic corticosteroids: reduces fractures.[7]
- Asthma: reduces asthma exacerbations requiring systemic corticosteroids, emergency department visit, and hospitalization.[8]
- Pregnancy: reduces maternal preeclampsia and low birth weight infants (less than 2,500 g).[9]

Prevention[4,6,10]

- Current recommendations to maintain vitamin D levels are 400 international units (IU) per day for infants, 600 IU per day for children and adults up to age 70 years, and 800 IU per day for those older than 70 years. However, many studies suggest these are insufficient.
- Sun exposure to the arms and legs for 5 to 10 minutes in summer provides 3,000 IU vitamin D for a light-skinned adult.
- One serving of fortified milk, orange juice, yogurt, or breakfast cereal provides 100 IU vitamin D_3, while a serving of oily fish provides at most 1,000 IU.

Medications[3,10]

- The ideal serum 25(OH)D level is controversial. While the Institute of Medicine recommends a target of 20 ng/mL, we support the Endocrine Society clinical practice guideline that suggests levels of at least 30 ng/mL, while 25(OH)D levels >50 ng/mL may increase the risk of toxicity.
- Vitamin D is available in two forms for supplementation:
  - **Ergocalciferol** (vitamin D_2) is available as prescription or over the counter in capsules or tablets ranging from 400 to 50,000 IU or solution of 8,000 IU/mL.
  - **Cholecalciferol** (vitamin D_3) is available over the counter in capsules or tablets ranging from 400 to 50,000 IU or solution ranging from 400 to 12,000 IU/mL.
- Cholecalciferol is not regulated by the FDA but is slightly more efficient and predictable than ergocalciferol at raising 25(OH)D levels, so its use is typically favored when available. We recommended a dose of 4,000 IU daily for 8 to 12 weeks. If the 25(OH)D levels are >30 ng/mL, maintenance therapy of 1,000 to 2,000 IU daily can be used.
- Ergocalciferol can also be used weekly, at a dose of 50,000 IU for 8 weeks, to treat vitamin D deficiency. If the patient does not achieve 25(OH)D levels >30 ng/mL, another 8 weeks of therapy is recommended. If the 25(OH)D levels are >30 ng/mL, levels can typically be maintained with 50,000 IU once or twice per month.
- Patients that do not achieve >30 ng/dL, those with morbid obesity, nephrotic syndrome, or malabsorption, or those taking cholestyramine, colestipol, mineral oil, orlistat, olestra, ketoconazole, anticonvulsants, glucocorticoids, highly active anti-retroviral treatment (HAART), or transplant antirejection medications may need higher doses. We suggest ergocalciferol 50,000 IU three times per week for 4 to 6 weeks followed by maintenance of 50,000 IU per week or cholecalciferol 6,000 to 10,000 IU daily for 8 to 12 weeks, followed by maintenance therapy of at least 3,000 to 6,000 IU daily.

COMPLICATIONS[3,5]

- Toxicity is extremely rare and is typically only reported with ingestion of more than 40,000 IU daily and 25(OH)D levels >150 ng/mL. Serum $1,25(OH)_2D$ levels are usually normal. The main criterion for vitamin D–induced toxicity is **hypercalcemia**, which can result in metastatic calcification of soft tissues (kidney, vasculature, heart, lungs) and increased risk for nephrolithiasis.
- **Treatment for vitamin D toxicity** is to decrease the hypercalcemia by forcing a negative calcium balance. Intravenous saline, glucocorticoids, furosemide, calcitonin, and/or bisphosphonates have been used. Because vitamin D is stored in fat, vitamin D intoxication may persist for weeks after cessation of vitamin D ingestion. The half-life of vitamin D is about 3 weeks to 1 month. Persistent treatment with corticosteroid or an oral bisphosphonate for this period may be required.

MONITORING/FOLLOW-UP

An elevated morning **calcium-to-creatinine ratio** (normal <0.20 mg/mg) increases the risk for nephrolithiasis, and increased caution in replacement dosing, hydration, and monitoring should be exercised. If the patient is at risk of nephrolithiasis we suggest an assessment of this ratio 2 to 4 weeks after starting vitamin D replacement therapy.

REFERENCES

1. Dusso AS, Brown AJ, Slatopolsky E. Vitamin D. *Am J Physiol Renal Physiol* 2005;289(1):F8–F28.
2. Bikle D, Adams JS, Christakos S. Vitamin D: Production, metabolism, mechanism of action, and clinical requirements. In: Rosen C, ed. *Primer on the Metabolic Bone Diseases and Disorders of Mineral Metabolism*. 8th ed. Ames: John Wiley & Sons, 2013:235–248.
3. Holick MF, Binkley NC, Bischoff-Ferrari HA, et al. Evaluation, treatment and prevention of vitamin D deficiency: An Endocrine Society clinical practice guideline. *J Clin Endocrinol Metab* 2011;96(7):1911–1930.
4. Schleicher RL, Sternberg MR, Looker AC, et al. National estimates of serum total 25-hydroxyvitamin D and metabolite concentrations by liquid chromatography-tandem mass spectrometry in the US population during 2007–2010. *J Nutr* 2016;146(5):1051–1061.
5. Lips P, van Schoor NM, Bravenboer N. Vitamin D–related disorders. In: Rosen C, ed. *Primer on the Metabolic Bone Diseases and Disorders of Mineral Metabolism*. 8th ed. Ames: John Wiley & Sons, 2013:613–623.
6. Avenell A, Mak JC, O'Connell D. Vitamin D and vitamin D analogues for preventing fractures in post-menopausal women and older men. *Cochrane Database Syst Rev* 2014;(4):CD000227.
7. Homik J, Suarez-Almazor ME, Shea B, Cranney A, Wells G, Tugwell P. Calcium and vitamin D for corticosteroid-induced osteoporosis. *Cochrane Database Syst Rev* 1998;(2):CD000952.
8. Martineau AR, Cates CJ, Urashima M, et al. Vitamin D for the management of asthma. *Cochrane Database Syst Rev* 2016;9:CD011511.
9. De-Regil LM, Palacios C, Lombardo LK, Pena-Rosas JP. Vitamin D supplementation for women during pregnancy. *Cochrane Database Syst Rev* 2016;(1):CD008873.
10. Ross AC, Taylor CL, Yaktine AL, Del Valle HB, eds. *Dietary Reference Intakes for Calcium and Vitamin D*. Washington, DC: National Academy of Sciences; 2011:10.

Osteoporosis

26

Marjorie Ann Malbas, Naga Yalla, Kathryn Diemer, and Roberto Civitelli

GENERAL PRINCIPLES

Definition

Osteoporosis is a common skeletal disorder characterized by decreased bone mineral density (BMD) and bone quality, leading to impairment in bone strength. Bone density is a measure of the amount of minerals per given area or volume, and is a function of peak bone mass and degree of bone loss over time. Bone quality is contributed to by bone macro- and microarchitecture, mineralization, remodeling rate, and accumulation of microdamage. Processes that result in low bone mass and architectural deterioration lead to enhanced bone fragility, and a consequent increase in the risk of fractures.[1]

Epidemiology

- Osteoporosis is the most common metabolic bone disorder. The spectrum of osteoporosis and low bone mass affects more than 53 million people (8 million women and 2 million men have osteoporosis, and an additional 43 million have low bone mass) in the United States and 200 million worldwide.[2] Progression from low bone mass to osteoporosis increases with age.[3]
- There are racial/ethnic differences in prevalence as reported on older women from recent NHANES 2005–2010 data, with low bone mass and osteoporosis reported in 52% and 15%, respectively, of non-Hispanic white older women, 36% and 7% of non-Hispanic black women, and 47% and 20% of Mexican American women.[2]
- Osteoporotic fractures, in particular hip fractures, are associated with significant short-term and long-term disability and mortality, with economic costs projected to reach $25 billion by 2025 consequent to aging population.[4]
- To reduce the burden of osteoporotic fractures, early identification and appropriate intervention in patients at high risk of fractures is needed. Advances in diagnostic testing have made osteoporosis relatively easy to diagnose. Multiple pharmacotherapeutic agents are now available that enhance bone density and decrease the rates of fracture at various clinical sites. Unfortunately, a significant percentage of patients with osteoporosis, including those who have experienced fractures, remain undiagnosed and untreated.

Pathophysiology

- Total bone mineral content in adults is dependent on peak bone mass achieved during early adulthood (age 25 to 30) and bone loss related to aging and estrogen deficiency, in women. Peak bone mass is primarily determined by genetic factors, race/ethnicity and gender, with contribution from environmental and metabolic conditions (nutritional status, calcium intake, physical activity, tobacco use, alcohol intake, hormonal deficiencies, and other medical comorbidities). Black men and women have higher peak bone mass, which may explain lower rates of osteoporosis and fractures in these groups.[5]

217

- Osteoporosis can result from failure to achieve expected peak bone mass in the first two to three decades of life, increase bone remodeling (bone resorption exceeding formation), and bone loss with age.[5]
- Age-related bone loss occurs at 0.5% to 1%/year. Gonadal sex steroid deficiency appears to be the dominant factor contributing to bone loss in older adults. Accelerated bone loss occurs during menopausal transition in women due to loss of estrogen inhibition of osteoclastogenic factors. Menopause-related bone loss is most prominent in trabecular bones (spine), where rate of bone loss of 3% to 5%/year for up to 10 years can occur. Cortical bone loss (proximal femur and distal radius and ulna) is more gradual. Since men have higher peak bone mass, larger cortical cross-section, and do not have the equivalent of female menopausal transition, in the absence of secondary disorders, bone loss in men do not reach levels that increase the risk for fractures until age 65 to 70. Bone loss and fragility, aggravated by age-related decline in function leading to increased falls and poor balance, are associated with increased fracture risk.[5]

Risk Factors

- Multiple risk factors have been shown to be independently associated with low bone mass (Table 26-1). Some of these risk factors are modifiable and are important to address in a comprehensive regimen to prevent or treat osteoporosis.[6]
- Numerous chronic medical conditions and medications cause secondary osteoporosis (Table 26-2).[6]
- Osteoporotic fractures commonly result from falls. As such, risk factors for falling, independent of those for low bone mass, are important contributors to morbidity from osteoporotic fractures (Table 26-3).[6]

Associated Conditions

Osteoporotic Fractures:

- **Fragility fractures are the primary cause of morbidity and mortality in adults with osteoporosis.** The most common sites for osteoporotic fractures are the hip, spine, and distal radius. Approximately 1.5 million osteoporotic fractures occur each year in the United States (700,000 vertebral; 300,000 hip; 200,000 wrist; and 300,000 other).[5] A 50-year-old white woman has a 40% lifetime risk of experiencing an osteoporotic fracture

TABLE 26-1	RISK FACTORS FOR OSTEOPOROSIS AND FRACTURES

Female sex
White race
Advanced age
Personal history of a fracture
Family history of osteoporosis/fracture in a first-degree relative
Small body habitus/low body weight
Sedentary lifestyle/lack of physical activity
Tobacco use
Excessive alcohol intake (>2 drinks/day)
Insufficient intake of calcium or vitamin D
Excessive caffeine intake
Ovarian failure or early (medical or surgical) menopause (age <45 years)
Frequency of falls

TABLE 26-2 CAUSES OF SECONDARY OSTEOPOROSIS

Endocrine disorders
Acromegaly
Amenorrhea (primary or secondary amenorrhea of any cause)
Anorexia/bulimia
Cushing syndrome/hypercortisolism
Diabetes mellitus, type 1 and 2
Hyperparathyroidism
Hyperprolactinemia
Hyperthyroidism
Hypogonadism (primary or secondary)
Hypopituitarism

Genetic/collagen disorders
Ehlers–Danlos
Glycogen storage diseases
Homocystinuria
Hypophosphatasia
Osteogenesis imperfect porphyria

Gastrointestinal/hepatic disorders
Celiac disease
Chronic cholestatic liver disease
Chronic malabsorptive conditions
Cirrhosis
Gastric bypass/gastrectomy
Hemochromatosis
Inflammatory bowel disease

Hematologic disorders
Amyloidosis
Leukemia/lymphoma
Mastocytosis
Monoclonal gammopathies
Multiple myeloma

Infectious diseases
HIV/AIDS

Metabolic/nutritional disorders
Alcoholism
Hyperhomocysteinemia

Hypocalcemia
Malnutrition
Smoking
Vitamin D deficiency

Neurologic disorders
Epilepsy
Muscular dystrophy
Spinal cord injury

Pulmonary disorders
Chronic obstructive pulmonary disease

Renal disorders
Chronic kidney disease (of any cause)
Hypercalciuria
Renal tubular acidosis

Rheumatologic/immunologic disorders
Ankylosing spondylitis
Rheumatoid arthritis
Systemic lupus
Systemic mastocytosis

Medications
Aluminum
Anticonvulsant (Dilantin, phenobarbital)
Aromatase inhibitor
Cyclosporine
Glucocorticoids
Gonadotropin agonists (e.g., Lupron)
Heparin (prolonged use)
Methotrexate
Protease inhibitors
Tamoxifen
Thiazolidinediones
Thyroxine (excessive replacement)

(compared to the 23% in a man). With an aging of the population, osteoporotic fractures are predicted to increase several-fold worldwide by 2050.[7]

- **Hip fractures are the most devastating cause of morbidity and mortality attributable to osteoporosis.** In the 1st year following a hip fracture, mortality rate is 20%, 50% lose independent daily functioning, and only 30% regain their prefracture level of function. The cost of treating hip fractures and their complications are estimated at $14 billion in 1995 and $17 billion in 2001.[6]
- **Vertebral fractures are often asymptomatic** (only one-third present clinically) and can result from routine everyday activities. Vertebral fractures are associated with significant

TABLE 26-3	RISK FACTORS FOR FALLING

History of falls
Dementia
Impaired vision
Poor physical condition/frailty
Foot problems or inappropriate footwear
History of stroke or Parkinson disease
Environmental hazards
Use of benzodiazepines, anticonvulsants, or anticholinergic medications

---

disability leading to chronic back pain, height loss, kyphosis, restrictive lung disease, or gastrointestinal complications, which have been shown to decrease quality of life. Long-term prospective studies have shown that vertebral fractures, symptomatic or not, are associated with a 15% to 30% increased rate of overall mortality.[8]

- **Prior osteoporotic fracture represents the greatest risk factor for future fracture** with relative risk ranging from 1.4 to 4.4 depending on the site of initial fracture.[9]

DIAGNOSIS

Clinical Presentation

- **All postmenopausal women and men age 50 and above should be evaluated for osteoporosis risk.**
- Most patients with osteoporosis are asymptomatic until they develop fractures. Therefore, it is important to perform a complete assessment of the patient's history and physical findings to identify patients at high risk of osteoporosis or fragility fractures who will benefit from additional testing and treatment. Inquire about risk factors for low bone mass, fracture, and falls (Tables 26-1 through 26-3). In the physical examination, look for findings suggestive of fracture such as significant historical height loss (1.5 in or 4 cm), sequelae of prior fracture and disability or deformity contributing to fracture risk (loss of height, kyphosis, localized spinal tenderness, chest deformity, rib–pelvis overlap, respiratory difficulty, protuberant abdomen, posture, balance and muscle strength), or abnormalities suggestive of secondary causes of osteoporosis (thyrotoxicosis, Cushing).
- **Fracture Risk Assessment:** Combination of bone density and clinical risk factors predicts fracture better than either one alone. The WHO developed **FRAX (Fracture Risk Assessment Tool)**, an algorithm to estimate the 10-year probability of hip fracture or major osteoporotic fracture (includes clinical spine, hip, proximal humerus and distal forearm) using information easily obtained from clinical risk factors and femoral neck BMD or T-score (when available). FRAX is available online at www.sheffield.ac.uk/FRAX or www.nof.org, or in software of newer DXA machines. It incorporates age, gender, ethnicity, geographic locality, weight, height, personal and family fracture history, tobacco use, glucocorticoid use, diagnosis of rheumatoid arthritis, alcohol use, presence of secondary osteoporosis (type 1 diabetes, osteogenesis imperfecta, untreated hyperthyroidism, hypogonadism, premature menopause <40 years old, chronic malnutrition or malabsorption, or chronic liver disease) and femoral neck BMD or T-score to generate an estimated fracture risk. If femoral neck BMD is provided, the section for secondary osteoporosis will no longer factor into the algorithm. FRAX should be used in patients without history of fragility fracture and T-score >–2.5 but <–1.0 (osteopenia) to provide a numerical estimate of fracture risk and can identify patients that may be candidates for

treatment. However, it may underestimate or overestimate risk since it does not take into consideration dose, duration or severity of exposure (for instance, glucocorticoids), other contributory risk factors such as falls, frailty, or spine BMD. It has not been validated in currently or previously treated patients, and it cannot be used to monitor treatment response.[10] Patients may be considered "untreated" if they have been off osteoporosis medications for 1 to 2 years.[6]

Diagnostic Criteria

- The World Health Organization (WHO) established osteoporosis criteria based on BMD and T-score of the lumbar spine, femoral neck or total hip. **T-score** is used for **postmenopausal or perimenopausal women and men ≥50 years old**.[10,11]
  - **Normal:** BMD within 1 SD of the young adult reference mean (T ≥–1.0)
  - **Low bone bass ("osteopenia"):** BMD between 1 and 2.5 SDs below the young adult reference mean (–2.5< T <–1.0)
  - **Osteoporosis:** BMD ≥2.5 SDs below the young adult reference mean (T ≤–2.5)
  - **Established or severe osteoporosis:** BMD ≥2.5 SDs below the young adult reference mean (T ≤–2.5) and the presence of one or more fragility fractures
- Several professional societies have established **criteria for diagnosis of osteoporosis**. The general consensus is the presence of fragility or low trauma fractures (fall from standing height or in the absence of major trauma), T-score ≤–2.5 or combination of low bone mass (T-score between –1 and –2.5) plus elevated FRAX score is consistent with osteoporosis. **All patients diagnosed with osteoporosis should be evaluated for secondary cause** (Table 26-2 and Table 26-4).[6,12,13]
- In **premenopausal women and men <50 years**, the International Society for Clinical Densitometry (ISCD) recommends using **Z-scores**[14]
  - **"Within the expected range for age":** BMD within 2.0 SDs of the reference mean (Z >–2.0)
  - **"Below the expected range for age":** BMD ≥2.0 SDs below the reference mean (Z ≤–2.0).

TABLE 26-4 DIAGNOSIS OF OSTEOPOROSIS

National Osteoporosis Foundation	• Adulthood low trauma hip or vertebral fracture (≥50 years old) • Lumbar spine, femoral neck or total hip BMD ≥2.5 SD below young adult reference mean (T ≤–2.5)
American Association of Clinical Endocrinologist and National Bone Health Alliance	• Low trauma hip or vertebral fracture • Lumbar spine, total hip, femoral neck or 33% radius BMD ≥2.5 SD below young adult reference mean (T ≤–2.5) • Low bone mass (–1 < T <–2.5) plus fragility fracture of proximal humerus, pelvis or distal forearm • Low bone mass (–1 < T <–2.5) plus high FRAX based on country-specific threshold—for U.S.-adapted risk, ≥3% 10-year probability of hip fracture and ≥20% 10-year probability of any osteoporotic fracture

Diagnostic Testing

Laboratories

- Laboratory assessment of asymptomatic postmenopausal women and men with osteoporosis identified a secondary etiology in 32%[15] and 75%, respectively.[16]
- **Baseline analysis should include:** chemistry panel (including calcium, phosphorus, creatinine), hepatic function panel (including liver transaminases, alkaline phosphatase, total protein, albumin), 25-OH vitamin D (25[OH]D), complete blood count, and testosterone in men.[6,12]
- Additional tests to pursue as clinically indicated: intact PTH, 24-hour urine for calcium and creatinine, thyroid function tests, serum or urine protein electrophoresis, 24-hour urine for cortisol, antibodies for assessment of celiac disease.[6,12]
- **Bone turnover markers (BTMs)** are enzymes involved in bone formation or resorption, or by-products of type 1 collagen production or degradation. Bone formation markers include serum bone alkaline phosphatase, osteocalcin, and N-terminal propeptide of type 1 procollagen (P1NP). Bone resorption markers include C-telopeptide (CTX) and N-telopeptide (NTX).
- **BTMs cannot be used to diagnosis osteoporosis.** They provide dynamic information about skeletal activity and can offer insights into mechanism of bone loss. However, their high biologic and analytical variability limit their clinical utility. Recently, the International Osteoporosis Foundation (IOF) and the International Federation of Clinical Chemistry (IFCC) Bone Marker Standards Working Group have identified serum PINP and CTX as reference BTMs that may be useful in fracture risk prediction and monitoring of osteoporosis treatment.[17] The Bone Health Alliance endorsed steps to standardize sample collection and processing, and patient preparation to reduce variability, which include collection of fasting morning CTX specimen.[18]

Imaging

- **BMD testing is standard for diagnosis and evaluation of adults for osteoporosis.** Several radiologic tests are available to measure BMD, including central and peripheral dual energy X-ray absorptiometry (DXA), central and peripheral quantitative computed tomography (QCT), and quantitative ultrasonography (QUS).
  - ○ BMD correlates with bone strength, with the risk of fracture approximately doubling for each 1 SD decrease in the T-score. Low BMD at one site is associated with increased fracture risk at all sites. However, the best predictor of fracture at a specific site is the bone density at that site. This is most important at the hip, where for each 1 SD decrease in hip BMD, the risk of hip fractures increases by 2.6-fold, that of vertebral fractures by 1.8-fold, that of wrist fractures by 1.4-fold, and the risk of all fractures increases by 1.5-fold. The risk of a subsequent hip fracture associated with decreased BMD at other sites is somewhat lower.[19,20]
- **DXA** measures areal BMD and is the current **standard method for bone density testing.** It is used for diagnostic classification, fracture risk assessment, and monitoring BMD changes over time. It has a low level of radiation exposure (approximately one-tenth that of a traditional x-ray) and has good precision and reproducibility.[14]
  - ○ **Lumbar spine and the proximal femur** should be measured. The **nondominant distal radius (33%)** can be used in patients with morbid obesity, hyperparathyroidism, or if hip or spine BMD cannot be measured or interpreted. BMD reflects bone mineral content divided by the area of bone measured (g/cm^2). In the lumbar spine, measurements are made at the L1, L2, L3, and L4 vertebrae and vertebrae-specific and total L1–L4 spine BMD data are given. The femoral neck BMD, composed almost equally of cortical and trabecular bone, is an excellent predictor of fracture risk and used in FRAX; whereas the total hip BMD is used for monitoring changes.[14]

○ BMD results are reported in comparison to reference ranges and normalized to the standard deviation of the reference population. The **T-score** uses the average peak BMD of young healthy Caucasian female as reference, while the **Z-score** uses average BMD of age-, gender-, and ethnicity-matched reference. T-scores (and Z-scores) are technique specific and results obtained from different methods of assessing bone density are not comparable. DXA measurements should be performed by trained technologists using properly maintained and calibrated machines.[14]

○ Several international societies have issued guidelines for osteoporosis screening using DXA (Table 26-5). In general, **women with fragility fractures** should be tested. **Most U.S. guidelines support bone density testing on all women over age 65**, with **some supporting testing all men over age 70**, regardless of risk factors. In younger adults, testing is typically recommended in the presence of previous fractures or **risk factors for osteoporosis**. Although the majority of data on the diagnosis and treatment of osteoporosis are on white women, the recommendations for screening for osteoporosis are irrespective of race.[6,12,14,21]

- **Quantitative CT scanning (QCT) and peripheral QCT (pQCT)** measures volumetric BMD (reported as g/cm^3) of axial (hip and spine) and peripheral (radius and tibia) sites. In addition, QCT can investigate bone content of trabecular, cortical, and subcortical compartments separately. High-resolution pQCT provides insight into bone microarchitecture in vivo, such as cortical porosity and trabecular structure.[22] In postmenopausal women, femur BMD by QCT can predict hip fractures and monitor treatment-related changes. However, QCT is more expensive, has larger radiation dose, and in the case of high-resolution peripheral quantitative CT (HRpQCT), not frequently available in the clinical setting. Therefore, DXA remains the preferred method of screening.[23]

- **Trabecular bone score (TBS)** is a non-BMD index derived from lumbar spine DXA images available in some densitometers. It is associated with vertebral, hip, and major osteoporotic fractures in postmenopausal women, and hip and major osteoporotic fractures in men over the age of 50. The fracture risks are partially independent on DXA BMD and clinical risks. It is approved by the FDA and European agency as an addition to DXA and FRAX, and should not be used by itself, to guide treatment decisions.[24]

- **Peripheral (extremities excluding the proximal femurs) bone density testing** can be performed with DXA, QCT, or QUS (quantitative ultrasound). Locations measured include the forearm, finger, and heel. Benefits of peripheral bone densitometry techniques are portability and ability to be performed in a primary care office, in the case of QUS. While these modalities have been shown to be predictive of fractures, there are no universally accepted diagnostic criteria for the variety of machines available. Peripheral testing is not recommended for diagnosis of osteoporosis. If results are abnormal, this should be followed up with a central DXA to establish or confirm the diagnosis.[14,21,23]

- **Conventional radiography (plain films)** is an unreliable marker of bone mass, as 30% of bone must be lost before changes are evident on x-ray. If osteopenia is suggested by radiographs, bone densitometry should be performed to confirm low bone mass.[25]

- **Vertebral imaging using plain films or vertebral fracture assessment (VFA)** from DXA, provide accurate assessment for vertebral fracture, which can be asymptomatic. **Vertebral imaging should be considered** in the following individuals: women ≥70 years old and men ≥80 years old if BMD T-score is ≤–1.0 at lumbar spine, total hip and femoral neck; women 65 to 69 years old and men 70 to 79 years old if BMD T-score is ≤–1.5 at lumbar spine, total hip, and femoral neck; postmenopausal women and men ≥50 years old with low trauma fracture after age 50, historical height loss of 1.5 in (4 cm), prospective height loss of 0.8 in (2 cm), or recent long-term glucocorticoid use.[6,12,14]

TABLE 26-5	RECOMMENDED BMD SCREENING GUIDELINES FOR OSTEOPOROSIS	

Group	Recommendations for women	Recommendations for men
National Osteoporosis Foundation, International Society for Clinical Densitometry	• All women ≥65 years old • Younger peri- or post-menopausal women with fragility fractures after age 50 or have clinical risk factors for fracture or low bone mass • Any age adults with high-risk condition or medication associated with bone loss	• All men ≥70 years old • Men 50–69 years old with fragility fractures after age 50 or have clinical risk factors for fracture or low bone mass • Any age with high-risk condition or medication associated with bone loss
American Association of Clinical Endocrinologists	• All women ≥65 years old • All postmenopausal women with fragility fracture, osteopenia on radiographs, or on systemic glucocorticoids for ≥3 months • Peri- or postmenopausal women with risk factors for osteoporosis (weight <127 lbs or BMI <20, family history of osteoporotic fracture, early menopause <40 years old, smoker or excessive alcohol intake • Secondary osteoporosis	None
Endocrine Society	None	• All men ≥70 years old • 50–69 years old with fragility fractures after age 50 or additional risk factors for fracture or low bone mass, or have secondary osteoporosis
U.S. Preventative Services Task Force	• All women ≥65 years old • Younger women if fracture risk is equal to or greater than that of a 65 year old	None

TREATMENT

- Goal of intervention is to prevent fractures. Treatment decisions should be individualized taking into consideration patient comorbidities, clinical risk factors, and preference. Decision to proceed with treatment in the appropriate setting should be made in partnership with the patient.
- Nonpharmacologic and lifestyle recommendations (see Lifestyle/Risk Modification section) should complement pharmacologic therapy and should be recommended to all adults, including those who do not meet the criteria for specific pharmacologic therapy for osteoporosis.

Medications

Indications for pharmacologic treatment[6,12]: FDA-approved therapies should be considered in postmenopausal women or men age 50 and older with the following:

- Low trauma hip or vertebral fracture.
- DXA T-score ≤−2.5 (osteoporosis) at the lumbar spine, total hip or femoral neck.
- DXA T-score between −1.0 and −2.5 (low bone mass) with FRAX 10-year risk for hip fracture ≥3% or major osteoporotic fracture ≥20% in the United States or based on country-specific threshold.

First Line

For information about U.S. FDA-approved medications for osteoporosis, see Tables 26-6 and 26-7.

- **Aminobisphosphonates** include alendronate, risedronate, ibandronate, and zoledronic acid and are the most widely used medication to treat osteoporosis. They are now available in generic formulation. The chemical structure of bisphosphonate resembles pyrophosphate and binds to hydroxyapatite crystals at sites of active bone remodeling, thereby potently inhibiting osteoclast-mediated bone resorption. These **improve bone density** at 3 years and **decrease the rates of hip and vertebral fractures** (except ibandronate, which has only been shown to decrease vertebral fractures).[26–34]
  - ○ **Oral bisphosphonates** include alendronate, risedronate, and ibandronate. Alendronate is available with supplemental vitamin D, and risedronate is available with supplemental calcium. Oral bisphosphonate are poorly absorbed and should be **taken early in the morning after overnight fast with a glass of water followed by at least 30 minutes without recumbency, food, or other medications**. Delayed-release Atelvia must be taken after breakfast, but still requires 30 minutes without recumbency. In randomized, placebo-controlled trials there was no significant difference in gastrointestinal side effects between treatment and placebo, and more recent once-weekly and once-monthly dosing regimens have improved compliance. However, in clinical practice, about 10% of patients have gastrointestinal distress, and severe erosive esophagitis related to pill "reflux" is a rare but serious complication.
  - ○ **Intravenous bisphosphonates**, including ibandronate and zoledronic acid, are preferred in patients with malabsorption, intolerant to or cannot remember to take oral bisphosphonate. Acute phase "flu-like" reaction during infusion has been observed, and can be tempered by pretreatment with acetaminophen.[35] Renal failure has been reported with intravenous formulations, so **creatinine should be checked prior to each infusion**.[36] Atrial fibrillation was reported in one zoledronic acid trial but has not been confirmed in other trials with the same or another bisphosphonate.[27]
  - ○ **Contraindications** to use of oral or IV bisphosphonate include hypersensitivity, hypocalcemia, and impaired renal clearance (**GFR <30 mL/min for risedronate and ibandronate, or <35 mL/min for alendronate and zoledronic acid**).

TABLE 26-6	**AVAILABLE AGENTS AND DOSING FOR OSTEOPOROSIS**			
Agent	FDA approved for prevention	Dose for prevention	FDA approved for treatment	Dose for treatment
Alendronate (Fosamax)	Yes	5 mg PO daily 35 mg PO weekly	Yes (W, M, G)	10 mg PO daily 70 mg PO weekly
Risedronate (Actonel, Atelvia)	Yes	5 mg PO daily 35 mg PO weekly 75 mg PO on two consecutive days monthly	Yes (W, M, G)	5 mg PO daily 35 mg PO weekly 75 mg PO on two consecutive days monthly
Ibandronate (Boniva)	Yes	150 mg PO monthly 150 mg PO monthly	Yes (W)	150 mg PO monthly 150 mg PO monthly 4 mg IV every 3 months
Zoledronate (Reclast)	Yes	5 mg IV every 2 years	Yes (W, M, G)	5 mg IV yearly
Raloxifene (Evista)	Yes	60 mg PO daily	Yes (W)	60 mg PO daily
Bazedoxifene/conjugated estrogen (Duavee)	Yes	20 mg/0.45 mg PO daily	No	Not applicable
Estrogen +/- progesterone; multiple combinations available	Yes	Variable, typically 0.625 mg PO daily conjugated estrogen	No	Not applicable
Calcitonin (Miacalcin)	No	Not applicable	Yes (W)	200 IU intranasally daily
Teriparatide (Forteo)	No	Not applicable	Yes (W, M, G)	20 mcg SQ daily
Denosumab (Prolia)	No	Not applicable	Yes (W, M)	60 mg SQ every 6 months
Abaloparatide (Tymlos)	No	Not applicable	Yes (W)	80 mcg SQ daily

G, glucocorticoid-induced osteoporosis; M, men; W, postmenopausal women.

TABLE 26-7 AVAILABLE AGENTS FOR OSTEOPOROSIS: IMPACT ON BONE MINERAL DENSITY (BMD) AND FRACTURES

Agent	Increase in BMD of spine	Increase in BMD of hip	Decrease in rate of vertebral fractures	Decrease in rate of hip fractures	Decrease in rate of nonvertebral fractures
Alendronate (Fosamax)	6–13%	4–7%	40–55%	50–55%	20–47%
Risedronate (Actonel, Atelvia)	5–11%	2–5%	40–60%	40–60%	20–40%
Ibandronate (Boniva)	3–5%	2–5%	50–60%	Studies not powered	Studies not powered
Zoledronate (Zometa, Reclast)	4–7%	3–6%	70%	41%	25%
Raloxifene (Evista)	3%	2%	30–50%	Not significant	Not significant
Bazedoxifene/conjugated estrogen (Duavee)	1.5%	1.2%	42% (bazedoxifene alone)	Not significant	Not significant
Teriparatide (Forteo)	8–14%	3–5%	65–70%	Studies not powered	53%
Denosumab (Prolia)	9%	6%	68%	40%	20%
Abaloparatide (Tymlos)	9%	4%	86%	No hip fracture reported	46%
Estrogen/hormone replacement therapy[a]	4–7%	2–4%	35%	33%	23%
Calcitonin (Miacalcin)	1–2%	No change	33%	Not significant	Not significant
Strontium ranelate	14%	8%	40%	36%	Not studied

[a]Data for estrogen-/hormone-replacement therapy are from studies in postmenopausal women and not in women with known osteoporosis.

○ **Osteonecrosis of the jaw (ONJ)** is a rare complication of antiresorptive use, occurring in 1/10,000 to 1/100,000 patients. It is characterized by nonhealing, exposed necrotic bone in the maxillofacial region that persists for 8 weeks after recognition by a health care provider in patients with exposure to antiresorptive (bisphophonate or denosumab) and no history of jaw radiation. Risk factors include high cumulative parenteral doses of antiresorptive typically used in oncology (much less common in osteoporosis), invasive oral surgery, infection, and poor oral hygiene. In high-risk individuals, consider delaying or withholding antiresorptive treatment until after planned oral surgery and until mucosa is fully healed, or avoiding oral surgery, if possible, while on these medications. Given much lower risk in osteoporosis patients, the American Dental Association recognized that it was not necessary to discontinue oral bisphosphonate prior to dental procedures. Treatment involves use of topical antibiotic oral rinses, systemic antibiotic, and surgical debridement in rare instances.[37]

○ **Atypical femoral fractures (AFF)** have been reported with antiresorptive therapy (bisphosphonate and denosumab), and also seen in individuals with no prior exposure. These are atraumatic fractures located along the femoral diaphysis (between the lesser trochanter and supracondylar flare) and characterized by its lateral cortex origin, transverse or slightly oblique orientation, minimal or noncomminuted nature, and localized periosteal or endosteal thickening at fracture site. Other notable features are thickening of femoral diaphysis, prodromal symptoms (pain in groin or thigh), bilaterality, and delayed fracture healing. Pathogenesis remains uncertain and may be related to altered bone quality and prolonged inhibition of bone turnover. Although the relative risk is high with bisphosphonate use (OR 2.1 to 66), the absolute risk remains very low. Some epidemiologic studies suggested higher risk with longer exposure where age-adjusted incidence rate increase from 1.8/100,000 cases per year with 2-year exposure to 113/100,000 cases per year after 8 to 9 years of exposure. In contrast, osteoporotic fractures are much more common and the benefit of reduced fracture incidence after 5 years of bisphosphonate use outweighs the potential risk of AFF. Estimates show that 5 years of bisphosphonate therapy prevented 2,590/100,000 fractures (spine, hip, or forearm) for 16/100,000 AFF associated with treatment, which corresponds to 162 fractures prevented per AFF potentially caused. **If AFF occurs, antiresorptive should be discontinued and alternative therapy considered.**[38,39]

• **Selective estrogen-receptor modulators (SERM)** exhibit selective antagonist or agonist effects on different target tissues, and therefore, have the advantage of retaining beneficial and minimizing adverse effects of estrogen.

○ **Raloxifene** (Evista) has estrogenic, anti-estrogenic, and neutral effects on bone, breast, and endometrium respectively. It is FDA-approved for osteoporosis, and breast cancer risk reduction. Treatment for 3 years has been shown to **improve BMD (spine and hip)** and to **decrease the rate of new vertebral fractures** without reduction in hip or nonvertebral fractures.[40] Treatment for 5 years in postmenopausal women with coronary heart disease (CHD) or risk factors for CHD did not increase risk of primary coronary events but **increased risk of venous thromboembolism and fatal strokes** (both are included in black box warning), although total all-cause mortality was similar with placebo.[41] Adverse events reported were hot flushes, leg cramps, and peripheral edema.[40,41] Raloxifene can be considered in postmenopausal woman with predominantly low spine and preserved hip BMD and high risk for breast cancer, who cannot tolerate bisphosphonate. Raloxifene should be discontinued at least 72 hours before surgery in patients at risk for venous thromboembolism.

○ **Bazedoxifene/conjugated estrogen** (Duavee) is a tissue-selective estrogen complex (TSEC), which involves pairing of SERM with estrogen. It has estrogenic activity on bone and anti-estrogenic activity on breast and uterus, and was approved by the FDA for postmenopausal osteoporosis prevention and treatment of vasomotor symptoms. Phase 3 trials demonstrated **BMD increase at lumbar spine and hip**, reduction of

BTMs and improvement in vasomotor symptoms. Rate of endometrial hyperplasia was low, and in comparison to hormone replacement therapy (HRT), mammographic breast density and breast tenderness were less frequent. Adverse effects reported include spasms, diarrhea, nausea, and dizziness.[42,43] Since it contains estrogen, Duavee carries the same precautions and black box warnings as estrogen. Fracture data are not available for Duavee, however, bazedoxifene (Conbriza) which is approved in Europe for postmenopausal osteoporosis treatment, showed a 42% significant reduction in vertebral fracture in postmenopausal women with osteoporosis.[44]

- **Teriparatide** (Forteo) is a recombinant human 34-aminoacid N-terminus peptide of PTH that stimulates bone formation. Paradoxically, continuous exposure to PTH (primary hyperparathyroidism) increases bone resorption while intermittent exposure stimulates bone formation. It is administered as daily subcutaneous injections at a dose of 20 mcg.[45]
  - Treatment for 18 months in postmenopausal women with prevalent vertebral fracture **increased BMD (spine and hip)** and **reduced vertebral fractures and nonvertebral fractures**. However, the study was not powered to investigate hip fracture reduction.[46] Use of teriparatide is usually reserved for patients with severe osteoporosis, and those who cannot tolerate or have not responded to bisphosphonates.
  - Side effects reported were nausea, headache, dizziness, leg cramps, and transient hypercalcemia.[46] Very high doses in rats resulted in an increased rate of osteosarcoma, which has not been seen in human trials. Teriparatide thus carries a **black-box warning about osteosarcoma** and is **contraindicated in patients with pre-existing hypercalcemia, metastatic bone disease, or increased osteosarcoma risk** (Paget disease, history of bone radiation, open epiphyses, or unexplained alkaline phosphatase elevation). Treatment is not recommended for >2 years.[45]
  - Hip and spine BMD declined 6 months after teriparatide discontinuation, however vertebral and nonvertebral fracture risk reduction persisted for 18 and 30 months respectively. Use of bisphosphonate after teriparatide maintained or further increased BMD gained during teriparatide treatment.[47,48] As such, antiresorptive agents, usually bisphosphonate, is commonly started after teriparatide to maintain BMD.

- **Denosumab** (Prolia) is a human monoclonal antibody against receptor activator of nuclear factor kappa B ligand (RANKL), which is released by osteoblasts to stimulate the differentiation, activity, and survival of osteoclasts, and therefore, inhibits osteoclast-mediated bone resorption. Like bisphosphonates, denosumab also inhibits osteoblast-mediated bone formation since both processes are tightly coupled. Denosumab is approved for treatment of postmenopausal women and men with osteoporosis at high risk of fractures, as well as in high-risk patients receiving androgen-deprivation therapy for prostate cancer or aromatase inhibitor for breast cancer. Denosumab is administered by subcutaneous injection of 60 mg every 6 months.[49]
  - In postmenopausal women with osteoporosis (23% had prior vertebral fracture and average spine T-score −2.8), 3 years of denosumab **improved BMD (spine and total hip), suppressed BTMs, and reduced the risk of vertebral, hip, and nonvertebral fractures**. Fracture risk reduction was comparable to zoledronic acid and teriparatide.[48] Study extension for 10 years revealed maintenance of fracture risk reduction, persistent BTMs suppression, and continuous accrual in spine and hip BMD without plateau.[50]
  - As with other antiresorptives, hypocalcemia and drug hypersensitivity are contraindications. Adverse effects reported include skin infection, eczema, and pancreatitis.[49] Dose adjustment is not required with renal insufficiency. However, hypocalcemia incidence requiring vitamin D and calcium supplementation is higher. 10-year treatment was generally well tolerated and adverse event rates remained stable over time. However, 2 cases of AFF (on years 3 and 7) and 13 incidences of ONJ were reported (11 resolved while 2 discontinued the study and their outcomes were not reported).[50] Incidence of AFF and ONJ are thought to be related to treatment dose and duration. Optimal duration of

denosumab use is unknown. Several cases of spontaneous vertebral fractures occurring 9 to 16 months after denosumab discontinuation not followed by other therapies have been reported.[51] When denosumab was stopped after 2 years of use, BTMs increased to values above baseline and rapid bone loss was observed, wherein bone density gained in spine and hip over 2 years was lost after 12 months.[52] Therefore, drug holiday or a longer than 6 months interval between denosumab doses are not recommended and alternative agents should be considered if denosumab is stopped.

- **Abaloparatide** (Tymlos) is the most recently FDA-approved drug for the treatment of postmenopausal osteoporosis. It is a novel 34-aminoacid N-terminus analog of PTHrP that activates PTH receptor type 1 and has been shown to have potent osteoanabolic activity with decreased bone resorption.[53] It is administered by daily subcutaneous injection of 80-mcg pen.
  - In postmenopausal women with osteoporosis (24% of whom had prior vertebral fractures) comparing abaloparatide, placebo, and teriparatide, 18 months of abaloparatide **improved spine, femoral neck and total hip BMD, increased both bone formation and resorption markers, and reduced the risk of vertebral, nonvertebral, clinical, and major osteoporotic fractures.** Hip BMD improvement was greater and BTMs increase was less profound compared to teriparatide group. Adverse events reported were nausea, dizziness, headache, and palpitation. Compared to teriparatide, incidence of hypercalcemia was lower which could be explained by the smaller increase in bone resorption markers.[53]
  - Like teriparatide, abaloparatide carries a **black-box warning about osteosarcoma risk** and has similar contraindications. In doses 4 to 28 times the exposure in humans receiving the 80-µg dose, osteosarcoma was observed in rats.[54] However, risk in humans remains unknown. Cumulative use of abaloparatide and other parathyroid hormone analogs for more than 2 years is not recommended.

Second Line

- **Estrogen/HRT** improves bone density by inhibiting osteoclast activity.
  - In the Women's Health Initiative (WHI), combination of estrogen–progesterone improved BMD (spine and hip) and reduced fractures (total, vertebral, hip, and lower arm).[54,55] In the WHI, the rates of CHD, stroke, venous thromboembolism, and invasive breast cancer were increased by 29%, 41%, 111%, and 26% respectively in the HRT group. Risks exceeded the benefit of fracture reduction.[56]
  - Given the availability of agents with better efficacy and safety profile, the use of HRT for osteoporosis prevention and treatment has fallen out of favor. In women considering HRT for relief of menopausal symptoms (use lowest effective dose for the shortest duration) may gain benefit in BMD and fracture risk. However, other treatments should be strongly considered first for osteoporosis prevention in women with no other indication for HRT.
- **Calcitonin** (Miacalcin) is an endogenous peptide that inhibits osteoclast activity. The intranasal formulation is FDA-approved for osteoporosis treatment in women who are at least 5 years postmenopausal if first line agents are contraindicated or intolerable.
  - Improvements in spine BMD are much less than those seen with other agents, and were minimal at the hip. The 200 IU/day dose decreased vertebral fractures after 5 years, but there was no significant decrease in hip or nonvertebral fractures.[56,57] It can rarely cause nasal irritation and epistaxis. Intranasal calcitonin has an analgesic effect and may relieve the pain associated with acute vertebral compression fractures.[58]

Medications not FDA-Approved

- **Strontium ranelate**, a strontium salt of ranelic acid is approved in some European countries for treatment of osteoporosis. Studies showed 40% reduction in vertebral fracture and 36% reduction in hip fracture in an older subgroup of patients. Its mechanism of action remains unclear, and its incorporation into the mineral phase of bone can explain the observed increase in bone density.[58] It was generally well tolerated. However, in 2013, the European Medicines Agency (EMA) issued a warning regarding increased risk of myocardial infarction associated with strontium ranelate based on their review of initial clinical trials data. Strontium ranelate is not USA FDA-approved, but strontium citrate is available in the United States over-the-counter and this preparation has no clinical fracture data.

- **Hydrochlorothiazide (HCTZ)** is a thiazide diuretic use to treat hypertension. It is not approved for treatment of osteoporosis. In a large population cohort receiving treatment for >1 year, HCTZ treatment was associated with increased BMD and decreased hip fracture.[59,60] By inhibiting thiazide-sensitive sodium chloride co-transporter (NCC) in kidney tubules and promoting calcium reabsorption, HCTZ is an effective treatment for hypercalciuria, which can contribute to low bone mass. Thiazide was shown to stimulate osteoblast differentiation in human osteoblast expressing NCC, suggesting a direct bone-forming effect.[61] Electrolyte disturbances, including hypercalcemia, are the primary adverse effects of HCTZ and need to be monitored in the elderly.

Combination Therapy

- Different combinations of dual antiresorptive agents have been studied. Adding alendronate or risedronate to HRT has shown additive effects on bone density similar to combination of raloxifene and alendronate.[62] Combining parathyroid hormone and alendronate was less effective than teriparatide alone at improving BMD and increasing new bone formation.[63] However, sequential treatment showed BMD improvements after 1 year of PTH (1-84) therapy were maintained or improved with subsequent alendronate but lost if therapy was not followed by the bisphosphonate.[64]
- Combination of denosumab and teriparatide for 2 years in postmenopausal women resulted in much greater increase in spine and hip BMD compared to either medication alone.[65] Furthermore, combination therapy for 2 years followed by 2 years of denosumab, as well as switching from 2 years of teriparatide to 2 years of denosumab resulted in progressive increase in spine, femoral, and radius BMD. On the other hand, 2-year treatment of denosumab followed by 2 years of teriparatide displayed progressive or transient bone loss.[66] When teriparatide and denosumab were discontinued after 4 years of treatment, the improvements in bone density were rapidly lost. However, such bone loss was prevented in patients who promptly received antiresorptive therapy, which demonstrated the importance of well-timed medication transition.[67] Therefore, the typical approach currently is to immediately start a bisphosphonate following discontinuation of teriparatide or denosumab treatment to maintain the gains in bone density, and in the case of denosumab, to prevent rebound vertebral fracture. Routine use of combination therapy is not recommended.

Treatment Duration

- Duration of treatment should be individualized. FLEX Study showed lower risk of clinical vertebral fractures, but not nonvertebral fractures or morphometric vertebral fractures, after 10 years of alendronate (vs. 5 years).[68] Subgroup analysis revealed reduction in nonvertebral fractures among patients with femoral neck T-score $\leq$−2.5 and no vertebral fracture at FLEX baseline.[69] Moreover, older participants with femoral neck and total hip BMD in the lowest tertile (T-score −2.5 to −4.1, and −2.3 to −4.2 respectively) who discontinued alendronate at 5 years had increased fracture risk.[70] In HORIZON-PFT, zoledronic acid treatment for 6 years (vs. 3 years) was associated with significant reduction in new morphometric vertebral fracture, but not nonvertebral or hip fractures.[71] Further analysis showed that in participants who discontinued zoledronic acid after 3 years, femoral neck and total hip T-score $\leq$–2.5 and incident morphometric vertebral fracture predicted the occurrence of new morphometric vertebral fracture, while low total hip T-score, incident nonvertebral fracture and prevalent vertebral fracture predicted occurrence of new nonvertebral fracture. In low-risk patients (total hip T score >–2.5 and no incident fracture) who discontinued zoledronic acid after 3 years, the risk for subsequent fractures over the next 3 years remained low.[72] These data suggest residual effects from long-term retention in bone, and ongoing benefit after 5 years of alendronate and 3 years of zoledronic acid in low-risk population.

- Due to safety concerns with long-term bisphosphonate use, an American Society for Bone and Mineral Research (ASBMR) task force suggested continued use of oral bisphosphonate for 5 years and IV bisphosphonate for 3 years and reassess risk. In patients who remain at high risk of fracture (older, low hip T-score, high fracture score, prior major osteoporotic fracture, or fracture on therapy), continued treatment for an additional 5 years (oral) or 3 years (IV) with periodic evaluation should be considered. For low-risk individuals, stopping bisphosphonate treatment for 2 to 3 years with periodic reassessment can be considered.[39]

- As previously mentioned, rapid bone loss and spontaneous vertebral fractures have been observed after denosumab discontinuation. Therefore, care must be taken not to interrupt denosumab treatment, and bisphosphonate or anabolic therapy should be initiated immediately after discontinuation. PTH-based therapies have recommended cumulative treatment duration of 24 months.

- Once again, treatment decisions should be individualized, based on clinical judgment balancing risk and benefit, and made in partnership with the patient.

Lifestyle/Risk Modification

Lifestyle modifications are crucial to osteoporosis treatment and prevention. Adults with osteoporosis should be encouraged to **stop smoking** and **avoid excessive alcohol intake**.

Diet

- Adequate calcium and vitamin D intake is essential to achieve peak bone mass and to maintain bone mass throughout postmenopausal life.[73] Reduction in hip and nonvertebral fractures with calcium plus vitamin D[74] and 700 to 800 IU vitamin D alone have been reported in elderly adults.[75] Calcium and vitamin D supplementation was given in the majority of osteoporosis trials.

- **Calcium**
  - The recommended intake of elemental calcium is **1,000 mg/day in women $\leq$50 and men $\leq$70 years old**, and **1,200 mg/day in women over 50 and men over 70. Calcium-rich foods** include milk, yogurt, cheeses, sardines, and fortified juices. On average, 8 ounces of milk, 6 ounces of yogurt, or 1.5 ounces of cheese contain 300 mg of elemental calcium. The average daily adult calcium intake from nondairy sources is 250 to 300 mg/day, therefore, most need guidance optimizing intake.[5,6,12]
  - There are many formulations of over-the-counter calcium supplement and patients should read the label to discern amount of elemental calcium in each tablet or pill. **Calcium carbonate has 40% elemental, while citrate has 21% elemental calcium.** Calcium salts are best absorbed with meals, however, citrate can be taken without food and is less constipating.
  - A meta-analysis showed calcium supplementation in older adults was associated with increased risk of myocardial infarction.[76] Since then, other studies have conflicting results with some suggesting increased cardiovascular risk while others showed no or decreased risk. Given the concerning cardiovascular safety, dietary calcium intake is preferred and total intake should not exceed 1,500 mg/day.

- **Vitamin D:** The **suggested level of 25(OH)D is thought to be between 30 and 50 ng/mL.**[6,12] Within this range, mineral homeostasis is balanced with optimization of intestinal calcium absorption and mineralization. Recommended intake for adults ≥50 years old is **800 to 1,000 IU/day**. However, vitamin D deficiency or insufficiency is very common and 25(OH)D level should be measured in all patients being evaluated for bone health. If deficient, ergocalciferol (vitamin D$_2$) 50,000 IU weekly for 8 to 12 weeks or equivalent dose of cholecalciferol (vitamin D$_3$) should be given to achieve 25(OH) D level around 30 ng/mL. Thereafter, daily maintenance with cholecalciferol 1,000 to 2,000 IU or equivalent is given to maintain healthy 25(OH)D levels.[6,12]

Activity

Lifelong regular weight-bearing exercise should be encouraged and has been shown to maximize peak bone mass in young women, decrease age-related bone loss, improve BMD in some circumstances, and help maintain muscle balance and strength. The improvement in agility, posture, and balance may reduce fall risk. The Nurses' Health Study demonstrated that for every three metabolic equivalents per week of activity in postmenopausal women without osteoporosis, hip fracture was decreased by 6%.[76] Reversible causes of falls (such as overmedication, neurologic or vision problems, poor footwear, and home environment) should be evaluated and addressed.[77]

SPECIAL CONSIDERATIONS

- **Glucocorticoid-induced osteoporosis** is the most common cause of secondary osteoporosis. Bone loss occurs early and rapidly (~6% to 12% loss/year) within the 1st year and fracture risk increases by 75% within the first 3 months of use. Rate of bone loss is a function of dose and duration of glucocorticoid use. Fragility fractures occur even at bone density levels otherwise associated with low fracture risk. Glucocorticoids inhibit osteoblast function, cause osteocyte apoptosis, and prolong osteoclast lifespan, thus tipping the balance toward net bone loss and increased skeletal fragility.[78] In 2017, the American College of Rheumatology (ACR) released guidelines for glucocorticoid-induced osteoporosis prevention and management. Fracture risk assessment (comorbidities, fractures, falls, glucocorticoid dose) and BMD testing are recommended for patients upon initiation of glucocorticoid therapy equivalent to prednisone >2.5 mg/day for ≥3 months. FRAX should be adjusted for prednisone >7.5 mg/day by multiplying 10-year risk for major osteoporotic fracture and hip fracture by 1.15 and 1.2, respectively. Patients taking glucocorticoid (dose above) who have moderate-high fracture risk (prior osteoporotic fracture, hip or spine T-score ≤−2.5 or Z-score <−3, FRAX major osteoporotic risk ≥10% and hip fracture risk ≥1%, bone loss ≥10%/year, prednisone ≥7.5 mg/day for ≥6 months) should be considered for pharmacologic therapy with oral bisphosphonate. Alternatives include intravenous bisphosphonate, teriparatide, and denosumab. Women of childbearing potential with moderate-high fracture risk can receive above treatments if there is no plan to conceive and effective birth control is implemented. Adequate calcium and vitamin D and healthy lifestyle are recommended for all. Therapy may be stopped with glucocorticoid discontinuation unless patient remains at high risk for fracture. Treatment decision should be individualized and fracture risk reevaluated regularly.[79]
- **Diabetic mellitus** has been increasingly recognized as a risk factor for fragility fracture. BMD is usually decreased in type 1 diabetes, and normal or even slightly elevated in type 2 diabetes.[80] Nonetheless, both groups have increased fracture risk compared to nondiabetics. BMD measurement and FRAX underestimates fracture risk in type 2 diabetes patients, and should be recognized by clinicians.[81] Mechanisms leading to bone fragility are multifactorial and include oxidative stress, chronic inflammation, hyperglycemia, accumulation of advanced glycosylation end product that modify collagen properties, and increase marrow adiposity. Some therapies for diabetes, such as thiazolidinedione,

SGLT-2 inhibitor, and insulin, have been associated with higher fracture incidence.[80] Currently, management of diabetes bone fragility follows along the same lines as post-menopausal osteoporosis.

MONITORING/FOLLOW-UP

- Patient on pharmacologic therapy should be monitored for complications, side effects, adequacy of vitamin D and calcium intake, continued or new risk factors, and adherence and response to treatment. Frequently assess modifiable risk factors and correct those that are reversible (see Tables 26-1, 26-2, and 26-3). Measure height annually to screen for asymptomatic vertebral fractures.
- Treatment response can be monitored using BMD by DXA or BTMs. To monitor changes in spine and hip BMD, DXA should be reevaluated every 2 years at the same facility, using the same calibrated machine, and, if possible, by the same technologist. Follow-up DXA can be done sooner or later depending on individual clinical circumstance, and BMD comparisons should be done using the same instrument. Due to the inherent variability of DXA, precision analysis and the least significant change (LSC) must be computed for each facility as per ISCD recommendations.[14] Facility-specific LSC, usually set at 95% confidence interval, establishes the smallest BMD change (not T-score) that is statistically significant and should be included in DXA reports.[6,14] Confirm validity of large BMD changes by reexamining ROI, patient positioning or presence of artifacts. Stable or increasing BMD was associated with fracture risk reduction in clinical trials.
- Trends in BTMs (suppression with antiresorptive and increase with anabolic therapy) have been predictive of bone density improvement and may have some utility in treatment response evaluation. However, at the moment, BTMs are not the standard of care. Fracture on treatment does not equate to treatment failure. Fractures, though significantly reduced, still occurred in treatment groups and may have been more numerous and severe without treatment.
- BMD loss exceeding LSC, unexpected BTMs changes, and new fracture should prompt investigation of contributing risk factors (comorbidities, treatment adherence, vitamin D and calcium intake, malabsorption) and consideration for therapy modification.

REFERENCES

1. NIH Consensus Development Panel on Osteoporosis Prevention, Diagnosis, and Therapy. Osteoporosis prevention, diagnosis, and therapy. *JAMA* 2001;285(6):785–795.
2. Wright NC, Looker AC, Saag KG, et al. The recent prevalence of osteoporosis and low bone mass in the United States based on bone mineral density at the femoral neck or lumbar spine. *J Bone Miner Res* 2014;29(11):2520–2526.
3. Looker AC, Johnston CC Jr, Wahner HW, et al. Prevalence of low femoral bone density in older U.S. women from NHANES III. *J Bone Miner Res* 1995;10(5):796–802.
4. Burge R, Dawson-Hughes B, Solomon DH, Wong JB, King A, Tosteson A. Incidence and economic burden of osteoporosis-related fractures in the United States, 2005–2025. *J Bone Miner Res* 2007;22(3):465–475.
5. *Bone Health and Osteoporosis: A Report of the Surgeon General.* Rockville, MD: U.S. Department of Health and Human Services, Office of the Surgeon General; 2004.
6. Cosman F, de Beur SJ, LeBoff MS, et al. Clinician's guide to prevention and treatment of osteoporosis. National Osteoporosis Foundation. *Osteoporosis Int* 2014;25(10):2359–2381.
7. Cummings SR, Melton LJ. Epidemiology and outcomes of osteoporotic fractures. *Lancet* 2002;359(9319):1761–1767.
8. Kado DM, Browner WS, Palermo L, Nevitt MC, Genant HK, Cummings SR. Vertebral fractures and mortality in older women: A prospective study. Study of Osteoporotic Fractures Research Group. *Arch Intern Med* 1999;159(11):1215–1220.

9. Klotzbuecher CM, Ross PD, Landsman PB, Abbott TA 3rd, Berger M. Patients with prior fractures have an increased risk of future fractures: A summary of the literature and statistical synthesis. *J Bone Miner Res* 2000;15(4):721–739.

10. Kanis JA, McCloskey EV, Johansson H, Oden A, Ström O, Borgström F. Development and use of FRAX in osteoporosis. *Osteoporosis Int* 2010;21(Suppl 2):S407–S413.

11. Assessment of fracture risk and its application to screening for postmenopausal osteoporosis. Report of a WHO Study Group. *World Health Organ Tech Rep Ser* 1994;843:1–129.

12. Camacho PM, Petak SM, Binkley N, et al. American Association of Clinical Endocrinologists and American College of Endocrinology clinical practice guidelines for the diagnosis and treatment of postmenopausal osteoporosis—2016. *Endocr Pract* 2016;22(Suppl 4):1–42.

13. Siris ES, Adler R, Bilezikian J, et al. The clinical diagnosis of osteoporosis: A position statement from the National Bone Health Alliance Working Group. *Osteoporosis Int* 2014;25(5):1439–1443.

14. Schousboe JT, Shepherd JA, Bilezikian JP, Baim S. Executive summary of the 2013 International Society for Clinical Densitometry Position Development Conference on bone densitometry. *J Clin Densitom* 2013;16(4):455–466.

15. Tannenbaum C, Clark J, Schwartzman K, et al. Yield of laboratory testing to identify secondary contributors to osteoporosis in otherwise healthy women. *J Clin Endocrinol Metab* 2002;87(10):4431–4437.

16. Ryan CS, Petkov VI, Adler RA. Osteoporosis in men: The value of laboratory testing. *Osteoporos Int* 2011;22(6):1845–1853.

17. Vasikaran S. Eastell R, Bruyere O, et al. Markers of bone turnover for the prediction of fracture risk and monitoring of osteoporosis treatment: A need for international reference standards. *Osteoporosis Int* 2011;22(2):391–420.

18. Szulc P, Naylor K, Hoyle NR, Eastell R, Leary ET. Use of CTX-1 and P1NP as bone turnover markers: National Bone Health Alliance recommendations to standardize sample handling and patient preparation to reduce pre-analytical variability. *Osteoporosis Int* 2017;28(9):2541–2556.

19. Cummings SR, Black DM, Nevitt MC, et al. Bone density at various sites for prediction of hip fractures. The Study of Osteoporotic Fractures Research Group. *Lancet* 1993;341(8837):72–75.

20. Marshall D, Johnell O, Wedel H. Meta-analysis of how well measures of bone mineral density predict occurrence of osteoporotic fractures. *BMJ* 1996;312(7041):1254–1259.

21. Colange N, Bibbins-Domingo K, Cantu AG, et al. Screening for osteoporosis: A U.S. preventive service task force recommendation statement. *Ann Intern Med* 2011;155:356–364.

22. Engelke K, Libanati C, Fuerst T, Zysset P, Genant HK. Advanced CT based in vivo methods for the assessment of bone density, structure and strength. *Current Osteoporosis Reports* 2013;11(3):246–255.

23. Shepherd JA, Schousboe JT, Broy SB, Engelke K, Leslie WD. Executive summary of the 2015 ISCD position development conference on advanced measures from DXA and QCT: Fracture prediction beyond BMD. *J Clin Densitom* 2015;18(3):274–286.

24. Silva BC, Broy SB, Boutroy S, Schousboe JT, Shepherd JA, Leslie WD. Fracture risk prediction by non-BMD DXA measures: The 2015 ISCD official positions part 2: Trabecular bone score. *J Clin Densitom* 2015;18(3):309–330.

25. Haller J, Andre MP, Resnick D, et al. Detection of thoracolumbar vertebral body destruction with lateral spine radiography. Part II: Clinical investigation with computed tomography. *Invest Radiol* 1990;25(5):523–532.

26. Black DM, Cummings SR, Karpf DB, et al. Randomised trial of effect of alendronate on risk of fracture in women with existing vertebral fractures. Fracture Intervention Trial Research Group. *Lancet* 1996;348(9041):1535–1541.

27. Black DM, Delmas PD, Eastell R, et al. Once-yearly zoledronic acid for treatment of postmenopausal osteoporosis. *N Engl J Med* 2007;356(18):1809–1822.

28. Chesnut IC, Skag A, Christiansen C, et al. Effects of oral ibandronate administered daily or intermittently on fracture risk in postmenopausal osteoporosis. *J Bone Miner Res* 2004;19(8):1241–1249.

29. Cummings SR, Black DM, Thompson DE, et al. Effect of alendronate on risk of fracture in women with low bone density but without vertebral fractures: Results from the Fracture Intervention Trial. *JAMA* 1998;280(24):2077–2082.

30. Harris ST, Watts NB, Genant HK, et al. Effects of risedronate treatment on vertebral and nonvertebral fractures in women with postmenopausal osteoporosis: A randomized controlled trial.

Vertebral Efficacy with Risedronate Therapy (VERT) Study Group. *JAMA* 1999;282(14):1344–1352.

31. Liberman UA, Weiss SR, Broll J, et al. Effect of oral alendronate on bone mineral density and the incidence of fractures in postmenopausal osteoporosis. The Alendronate Phase III Osteoporosis Treatment Study Group. *N Engl J Med* 1995;333(22):1437–1443.

32. McClung MR, Geusens P, Miller PD, et al. Effect of risedronate on the risk of hip fracture in elderly women. Hip Intervention Program Study Group. *N Engl J Med* 2001;344(5):333–340.

33. Reginster J, Minne HW, Sorensen OH, et al. Randomized trial of the effects of risedronate on vertebral fractures in women with established postmenopausal osteoporosis. Vertebral Efficacy with Risedronate Therapy (VERT) Study Group. *Osteoporos Int* 2000;11(1):83–91.

34. Reid IR, Brown JP, Burckhardt P, et al. Intravenous zoledronic acid in postmenopausal women with low bone mineral density. *N Engl J Med* 2002;346(9):653–661.

35. A once-yearly IV bisphosphonate for osteoporosis. *Med Lett Drugs Ther* 2007;49(1273):89–90.

36. Perazella MA, Markowitz GS. Bisphosphonate nephrotoxicity. *Kidney Int* 2008;74(11):1385–1393.

37. Khan AA, Morrison A, Hanley D, et al. Diagnosis and management of osteonecrosis of the jaw: A systematic review and international consensus. *J Bone Miner Res* 2015;30(1):3–23.

38. Shane E, Burr D, Abrahamsen B, et al. Atypical subtrochanteric and diaphyseal femoral fractures: Second report of a task force of the American Society for Bone and Mineral Research. *J Bone Miner Res* 2014;29(1):1–23.

39. Adler RA, El-Hajj Fuleihan G, Bauer DC, et al. Managing osteoporosis in patients on long-term bisphosphonate treatment: Report of a task force of the American Society for Bone and Mineral Research. *J Bone Miner Res* 2015;31(1):16–35.

40. Ettinger B, Black DM, Mitlak BH, et al. Reduction of vertebral fracture risk in postmenopausal women with osteoporosis treated with raloxifene: Results from a 3-year randomized clinical trial. Multiple Outcomes of Raloxifene Evaluation (MORE) Investigators. *JAMA* 1999;282(7):637–645.

41. Barrett-Connor E, Mosca L, Collins P, et al. Effects of raloxifene on cardiovascular events and breast cancer in postmenopausal women. *N Engl J Med* 2006;355(2):125–137.

42. Pinkerton JV, Harvey JA, Lindsay R, et al. Effects of bazedoxifene/conjugated estrogen on the endometrium and bone: A randomized trial. *J Clin Endocrinol Metab* 2014;99(2):E189–E198.

43. Lindsay R, Gallagher JC, Kagan R, Pickar JH, Constantine G. Efficacy of tissue-selective estrogen complex bazedoxifene/conjugated estrogen for osteoporosis prevention in at-risk postmenopausal women. *Fertil steril* 2009;92(3):1045–1052.

44. Silverman SL, Christiansen C, Genant HK, et al. Efficacy of bazedoxifene in reducing new vertebral fracture risk in postmenopausal women with osteoporosis: Results from a 3-year randomized, placebo-, and active-controlled clinical trial. *J Bone Miner Res* 2008;23(12):1923–1934.

45. Teriparatide (forteo) for osteoporsis. *Med Lett Drugs Ther* 2003;45(1149):9–10.

46. Neer RM, Arnaud CD, Zanchetta JR, et al. Effect of parathyroid hormone (1-34) on fractures and bone mineral density in postmenopausal women with osteoporosis. *N Engl J Med* 2001;344(19):1434–1441.

47. Lindsay R, Scheele WH, Neer R, et al. Sustained vertebral fracture risk reduction after withdrawal of teriparatide in postmenopausal women with osteoporosis. *Arch Intern Med* 2004;164(18):2024–2030.

48. Prince R, Sipos A, Hossain A, et al. Sustained nonvertebral fragility fracture risk reduction after discontinuation of teriparatide treatment. *J Bone Miner Res* 2005;20(9):1507–1513.

49. Cummings SR, San Martin J, McClung MR, et al. Denosumab for prevention of fractures in postmenopausal women with osteoporosis. *N Engl J Med* 2009;361(8):756–765.

50. Bone HG, Wagman RB, Brandi ML, et al. 10 years of denosumab treatment in postmenopausal women with osteoporosis: Results from phase 3 randomised FREEDOM trial and open-label extension. *Lancet Diabetes Endocrinology* 2017;5(7):513–523.

51. Lamy O, Gonzalez-Rodriguez E, Stoll D, Hans D, Aubry-Rozier B. Severe rebound-associated vertebral fractures after denosumab discontinuation: 9 clinical cases report. *J Clin Endocrinol Metab* 2017;102(2):354–358.

52. Miller PD, Bolognese MA, Lewiecki E, et al. Effect of denosumab on bone density and turnover in postmenopausal women with low bone mass after long-term combined, discontinued, and restarting of therapy: A randomized blinded phase 2 clinical trial. *Bone* 2008;43(2):222–229.

53. Miller PD, Hattersley G, Riss BJ, et al. Effect of abaloparatide vs placebo on new vertebral fractures in postmenopausal women with osteoporosis a randomized clinical trial. *JAMA* 2016;316(7):722–733.

54. Jolette J, Attalla B, Valera A, et al. Comparing the incidence of bone tumors in rats chronically exposed to the selective PTH type 1 receptor agonist abaloparatide or PTH (1-34). *Regul Toxicol Pharmacol* 2017;86:356–365.

55. Cauley JA, Robbins J, Chen Z, et al. Effects of estrogen plus progestin on risk of fracture and bone mineral density: The Women's Health Initiative randomized trial. *JAMA* 2003;290(13):1729–1738.

56. Rossouw JE, Anderson GL, Prentice RL, et al. Risks and benefits of estrogen plus progestin in healthy postmenopausal women: Principal results from the Women's Health Initiative randomized controlled trial. *JAMA* 2002;288(3):321–333.

57. Chesnut CH 3rd, Silverman S, Andriano K, et al. A randomized trial of nasal spray salmon calcitonin in postmenopausal women with established osteoporosis: The prevent recurrence of osteoporotic fractures study. PROOF Study Group. *Am J Med* 2000;109(4):267–276.

58. Knopp JA, Diner BM, Blitz M, Lyritis GP, Rowe BH. Calcitonin for treating acute pain of osteoporotic vertebral compression fractures: A systematic review of randomized, controlled trials. *Osteoporos Int* 2005;16(10):1281–1290.

59. Meunier PJ, Roux C, Seeman E, et al. The effects of strontium ranelate on the risk of vertebral fracture in women with postmenopausal osteoporosis. *N Engl J Med* 2004;350(5):459–468.

60. Schoofs MW, van der Klift M, Hofman A, et al. Thiazide diuretics and the risk for hip fracture. *Ann Intern Med* 2003;139(6):476–482.

61. Dvorak MM, De Joussineau C, Carter DH, et al. Thiazide diuretics directly induce osteoblast differentiation and mineralized nodule formation by interacting with a sodium chloride co-transporter in bone. *J Am Soc Nephrol* 2007;18(9):2509–2516.

62. Binkley N, Krueger D. Combination therapy for osteoporosis: Considerations and controversy. *Curr Osteoporos Rep* 2005;3(4):150–154.

63. Black DM, Greenspan SL, Ensrud KE, et al. The effects of parathyroid hormone and alendronate alone or in combination in postmenopausal osteoporosis. *N Engl J Med* 2003;349(13):1207–1215.

64. Black DM, Bilezikian JP, Ensrud KE, et al. One year of alendronate after one year of parathyroid hormone (1-84) for osteoporosis. *N Engl J Med* 2005;353(6):555–565.

65. Leder BA, Tsai JN, Uihlein V, et al. Two years of denosumab and teriparatide administration in postmenopausal women with osteoporosis (the DATA Extension Study): A randomized controlled trial. *J Clin Endocrinol Metab* 2014;99(5):1694–1700.

66. Leder BZ, Tsai JN, Uihlein AV, et al. Denosumab and teriparatide transitions in postmenopausal osteoporosis (the DATA-Switch study): Extension of a randomized controlled trial. *Lancet* 2015;386(9999):1147–1155.

67. Leder BZ, Tsai JN, Jiang LA, Lee H. Importance of prompt antiresorptive therapy in postmenopausal women discontinuing teriparatide or denosumab: The denosumab and teriparatide follow-up study (DATA-Follow-up). *Bone* 2017;98:54–58.

68. Black DM, Schwartz AV, Ensrud KE, et al. Effects of continuing or stopping alendronate after 5 years of treatment. The fracture intervention trial long-term extension (FLEX): A randomized trial. *JAMA* 2006;296(24):2927–2938.

69. Schwartz AV, Bauer DC, Cummings SR, et al. Efficacy of continued alendronate for fractures in women with and without prevalent vertebral fracture: The FLEX trial. *J Bone Miner Res* 2010;25(5):976–982.

70. Bauer DC, Schwartz AV, Palermo L, et al. Fracture prediction after discontinuation of 4 to 5 years of alendronate therapy. The FLEX study. *JAMA* 2014;174(7):1126–1134.

71. Black DM, Reid IR, Boonen S, et al. The effect of 3 versus 6 years of zoledronic acid treatment of osteoporosis: A randomized extension to the HORIZON-Pivotal fracture trial (PFT). *J Bone Miner Res* 2012;27(2):243–254.

72. Cosman F, Cauley JA, Estell R, et al. Reassessment of fracture risk in women after 3 years of treatment with zoledronic acid: When is it reasonable to discontinue treatment? *J Clin Endocrin Metab* 2014;99(12):4546–4554.

73. Heaney RP. Calcium, dairy products and osteoporosis. *J Am Coll Nutr* 2000;19(2 Suppl):83S–99S.

74. Chapuy MC, Arlot ME, Delmas PD, Meunier PJ. Effect of calcium and cholecalciferol treatment for three years on hip fractures in elderly women. *BMJ* 1994;308(6936):1081–1082.

75. Bischoff-Ferrari HA, Willett WC, Wong JB, Giovannucci E, Dietrich T, Dawson-Hughes B. Fracture prevention with vitamin D supplementation: A meta-analysis of randomized controlled trials. *JAMA* 2005;293(18):2257–2264.

76. Bolland MJ, Avenell A, Baron JA, et al. Effect of calcium supplements on risk of myocardial infarction and cardiovascular events: Meta-analysis. *BMJ* 2010;341:c3691.

77. Todd JA, Robinson RJ. Osteoporosis and exercise. *Postgrad Med J* 2003;79(932):320–323.

78. Weinstein RS. Clinical practice. Glucocorticoid-induced bone disease. *N Engl J Med* 2011;365(1):62–70.

79. Buckley L, Guyatt G, Fink HA, et al. 2017 American College of Rheumatology guideline for the prevention and treatment of glucocorticoid-induced osteoporosis. *Arthritis Care Res (Hoboken)* 2017;69(8):1095–1110.

80. Napoli N, Chandran M, Pierroz DD, Abrahamsen B, Schwartz AV, Ferrari SL. Mechanisms of diabetes mellitus-induced bone fragility. *Nature* 2017;13(4):208–218.

81. Gianggregorio LM, Leslie WD, Lix LM, et al. FRAX underestimates fracture risk in patients with diabetes. *J Bone Miner Res* 2012;27(2):301–308.

Paget Disease and Dense Bone Disorders

27

Naga Yalla and Michael P. Whyte

GENERAL PRINCIPLES

Definition

Increased bone mass has many causes including metabolic, endocrine, hematologic, infectious, neoplastic disease and heritable osteochondrodysplasias (Table 27-1). Nevertheless there is no accepted dual-energy X-ray absorptiometry (DXA) definition for high bone mineral density (BMD). Some consider a BMD Z-score >+2.5 worthy of further clinical evaluation.

Classification

Common causes of high bone mass revealed by DXA are "artifactual" degenerative osteoarthritis and vertebral compression fractures. Focal elevations in BMD can result from extra-skeletal factors, that is, implants, kyphoplasty, contrast studies, etc., but typically are differentiated from true causes of high bone mass by the medical history. Thus, non artefactual dense bones are investigated by family history, physical examination, radiographic and other studies. Increases in bone mass can largely be divided into inherited causes and acquired causes (see Table 27-1). Paget disease of the bone (PDB) is a common acquired focal skeletal disorder that sometimes increases bone mass. "Osteosclerosis" refers to trabecular (spongy bone) thickening whereas "hyperostosis" refers to cortical (compact bone) thickening.[1]

Paget Disease

GENERAL PRINCIPLES

Definition

PDB is characterized by acquired, focal acceleration of bone turnover (remodeling) leading to skeletal expansion of weak bone that is predisposed to fracture.

Classification

PDB can be localized to one skeletal area (monostotic), or affect multiple bones (polyostotic).

Epidemiology

- PDB has been considered the second most common metabolic bone disease (after osteoporosis). Its prevalence is slightly greater in men than women.
- PDB occurs most commonly in Western Europe, North America, Australia, and New Zealand,[2] and typically presents in middle age or later, and is considered uncommon <40 years of age.[3]

Etiology

- Evidence suggests both genetic and environmental factors, though this has been debated for decades.

TABLE 27-1 INCREASED BONE MASS

Acquired causes of high bone mass
Diffuse idiopathic skeletal hyperostosis (DISH)
Fluorosis
Hypervitaminosis A, D
Heavy metal poisoning
Hepatitis C–associated osteosclerosis
Leukemia
Lymphomas
Mastocytosis
Myelofibrosis
Multiple myeloma (indolent)
Melorheostosis
Malignancies (e.g., osteoblastoma, prostate CA)
Paget Disease
Renal osteodystrophy (CKD-MBD)
Sarcoidosis
Skeletal metastasis

Dysplasias and dysostoses (Heritable Causes)
High bone mass phenotype (LRP5 activation)
Osteopetrosis
Osteopoikilosis
Progressive diaphyseal dysplasia (Camurati–Engelman disease)
Sclerosteosis/Van Buchem disease
X-linked hypophosphatemia

- **Genetic factors:** 5% to 40% of patients with PDB have an affected first-degree relative.[4] Specific predisposing gene defects have been reported.
- **Environmental influence:** Viral infection has been postulated given electron microscopy showing viral-like inclusion bodies in osteoclasts and viral-like antigens using immunohistochemical tehniques.[5] However, these observations have not always been replicated and viruses have not been isolated from Pagetic bone.

Pathophysiology

Focally increased osteoclast activity and bone resorption is followed by disorganized skeletal repair. Three clinical/radiographic phases are reported. Different bones may simultaneously be in different stages.[6]

- The initial **osteolytic phase** features intense bone resorption by large, hypernucleated osteoclasts.
- **Mixed osteolytic/osteoblastic phase** features uncoordinated bone resorption and formation by reactive osteoblasts.
- The **late sclerotic phase** features continued bone formation resulting in thickened disorganized ("mosaic") bone of poor quality.

DIAGNOSIS

Clinical Presentation

- Most PDB is symptomatic and detected incidentally on radiographs taken for unrelated reasons, or during investigation of an elevated serum alkaline phosphatase.

- Common symptoms are **bone** and **joint** pain.[7]
  - Bone pain is typically constant, deep seated, and worse at night, and frequently increases with weight bearing. Its severity does not always correlate with the radiographic findings and tends to be more prominent with advanced lytic lesions.
  - Secondary osteoarthritis with joint pain frequently develops, particularly in weight-bearing joints, especially the hip and knee. Deafness and headaches may occur with involvement of the skull.
- Physical signs can include bony deformities such as bowing of the limbs, kyphosis or scoliosis, and enlargement of the skull with cranial nerve compromise including deafness. Local skin warmth over pagetic lesions may reflect increased bony vascularity.
- The prevalence of skeletal involvement of PDB by location is shown in Table 27-2.

Diagnostic Testing

- This involves radiographic testing and biochemical markers of bone turnover.
- The **bone scan** defines the location and extent of this disease, and can suggest its activity. Bone scans are more sensitive, but less specific, than radiographs and detect 15% to 30% of lesions not recognized on plain films.[6] Radiographs are obtained of the areas that are abnormal on the bone scan to confirm the diagnosis and to assess the phase of abnormalities.[3]
- **Serum alkaline phosphatase** is the least expensive biochemical measure and correlates with the extent of PDB on bone scan.[8] However, hyperphosphatasemia can also originate from hepatobiliary disease and other skeletal disorders. Differentiation among these can come from either fractionating the alkaline phosphatase isoforms, or by assaying serum gammaglutamyltransferase (GTT). A normal GTT effectively rules out a hepatic source. Other markers of both bone formation and resorption can provide further specificity, but at higher costs and restricted availability.[9]
- Procollagen type 1 amino-terminal propeptide (P1NP) measures bone formation. **Markers of resorption** include urinary N-terminal peptide (NTX), and serum beta-crosslaps (βCTx).
- If the traditional tests above are inconclusive, additional laboratory and imaging tests may be useful:
  - Serum calcium and phosphorus are usually normal in PDB.
  - Hypercalcemia suggests a second disorder such as primary hyperparathyroidism.

TABLE 27-2	FREQUENCY OF SKELETAL SITES INVOLVED IN PAGET DISEASE

Skeletal site	Frequency of involvement (%)
Pelvis	72
Lumbosacral spine (esp. L3–L4)	58
Femur	55
Thoracic spine	45
Sacrum	43
Skull	42
Tibia	35
Humerus	31
Scapula	23
Cervical spine	14

○ Additional radiologic testing is typically unnecessary except to evaluate for complications. Computer tomography (CT) or magnetic resonance imaging (MRI) helps to evaluate possible malignant degeneration or neurologic complications, such as spinal stenosis.

○ Despite the classic histopathologic appearance of PBD, bone biopsy is usually not required for diagnosis, but is essential if there is concern for malignant transformation.

TREATMENT

- The primary goals of treatment are to decrease pain and to hopefully decrease the rate of bone turnover to prevent progression and complications.
- The following are generally accepted **indications for bone antiresorptive treatment**:[9,10]
  ○ Symptomatic disease: bone pain, deformities, or neurologic symptoms
  ○ Patients preparing for elective orthopedic surgery on involved bone (in an effort to decrease bony vascularity)
  ○ Evidence of increased bone turnover with:
    ▪ Lytic lesions in long bones at high risk for fracture
    ▪ Joints at risk for secondary osteoarthritis
    ▪ Vertebral involvement risking spinal stenosis
    ▪ Disease in the skull risking deafness or cranial nerve palsy

Medications

- **Bisphosphonates**, particularly zoledronic acid (Zometa®), are the preferred treatment for those PDB patients requiring therapy (See Table 27-3). They decrease bone turnover (as measured by the decline in serum alkaline phosphatase levels) as well as improve/relieve symptoms.[10]
- **Supplemental calcium and vitamin D** can be given to prevent vitamin D deficiency causing secondary hyperparathyroidism.
- Salmon calcitonin is an older agent that can be considered for those unable to tolerate bisphosphonates. Calcitonin is given subcutaneously or intramuscularly. Unfortunately, symptoms and increases in bone turnover usually recur soon after stopping this therapy.[10]

Surgical Management

- Surgery may be **helpful for some complications of PDB**. The most common indication is a joint replacement, usually of a hip or a knee, for secondary osteoarthritis.[11]
- Other reasons to consider surgical intervention are for a complicated nonhealing fracture, bowing deformities of long bones, spinal stenosis, and focal nerve root compression syndromes.

TABLE 27-3	PHARMACOLOGIC TREATMENT OPTIONS
Agent	**Dose**
Alendronate	40 mg PO daily for 6 months. Retreatment may need to be considered between 2 and 6 years
Risedronate	30 mg PO daily for 2 months. Retreatment may be required between 1 and 5 years
Zoledronate Retreatment is rarely required within 5 years	5 mg IV infused over 15 minutes × 1 dose
Calcitonin	50–100 IU Sub Q daily or 3×/week for 6–12 months

TABLE 27-4	POSSIBLE COMPLICATIONS IN PAGET DISEASE
Organ system	Possible complications
Long bones	Fractures, deformities, arthritis
Neurologic	Spinal stenosis
	Chronic headaches
	Cranial neuropathies (especially II, V, VII, VIII)
	Noncommunicative hydrocephalus
	Basilar impression
	Paraplegia, quadriplegia/invagination, vascular steel syndrome
Dental	Loss of teeth/malocclusion
Cardiovascular	Increased vascular disease
	High-output heart failure
	Valvular heart disease (aortic > mitral)
Metabolic	Hypercalcemia (usually with immobility)
	Hyperuricemia/gout
Tumors	Benign giant cell tumors
	Malignant sarcoma

- Bisphosphonate therapy can be initiated prior to elective surgery to decrease bone vascularity and the risk of intraoperative bleeding.

COMPLICATIONS

- Multiple complications can occur in patients with PDB (Table 27-4), although most are infrequent.
- **Fractures** are one of the most common complications and occur in 6% to 7% of patients.[11] Fractures occur most commonly in the femur, tibia, and humerus and are often associated with poor healing and nonunion.
- **Neurologic complications** can occur because of either direct nerve root compression by pagetic bone or diversion of blood flow to bone. Spinal stenosis is an important neurologic complication. Deafness occurs in 10% to 30% of patients with disease affecting the skull.
- **Cardiovascular complications** are much less common though high-output heart failure have been reported.
- **Malignant sarcomatous degeneration** is an uncommon but severe and usually life-threatening complication of PDB, occurring in <1% of patients and most commonly in those with severe polyostotic disease.[12] Malignant transformation may lead to a sudden or severe increase in pain, a palpable mass, a rise in the alkaline phosphatase, and/or a pathologic fracture.

MONITORING/FOLLOW-UP

- Follow-up of patients with PDB includes monitoring their **symptoms**, markers of bone turnover and occasionally supplemented with occasional imaging procedures. Symptoms are initially monitored every 3 months in those on therapy and every 6 to 12 months in those not on treatment.
- Serum total **alkaline phosphatase** is the most cost effective marker of bone turnover to follow and is usually the only one needed in follow-up. The alkaline phosphatase decreases

at 6 to 12 weeks posttreatment, but maximal suppression may require measurement at 6 months.[9]

- It is usually followed annually in those not on treatment. Retreatment with another course of a bisphosphonate should be considered if the alkaline phosphatase increases by >20% to 25% above the posttreatment nadir.[3,13,14]
- Serial measurements of other markers of bone turnover could be useful in those with highly active lytic disease, where there is more pressing need to assess response to treatment, for example, spinal compression or in patients in whom the alkaline phosphatase levels are unreliable.
- βCTx fall rapidly, nadir value at 10 days in response to IV bisphosphonates,[9] whereas the markers of bone formation take longer to improve, often up to 1 month.[3,10]
- Indications for subsequent radiographs at 1-year posttreatment include known osteolytic lesions, new symptoms, worsening of symptoms, trauma, concern for fracture or concern for sarcomatous degeneration.

Dysplasias and Dysostoses (Inherited): Osteopetrosis

GENERAL PRINCIPLES

- Often referred to as "marble bone disease" or Albers-Schönberg disease (ASD). Osteopetrosis (OPT) is the consequence of failed osteoclast resorption of the skeleton during growth. Defective modeling leads to dense but weak bone.
- The two major clinical forms are an autosomal recessive infantile (malignant) type typically fatal in early childhood if untreated and the autosomal dominant (AD) adult type or ASD.
- ASD is caused by a heterozygous mutation in chloride channel 7 (CLCN7). Penetrance is between 60% and 80% giving rise to a varied clinical presentation.[15]
- OPT emerges radiographically during childhood, yet some "carriers" have only biochemical findings in adult life.
- Potential complications include fractures, facial palsy, compromised vision or hearing, psychomotor delay, osteomyelitis of the mandible, deep dental decay, carpal tunnel syndrome, osteoarthritis, and bone marrow failure.[16]

DIAGNOSIS

- Increased serum acid phosphatase and the brain isoenzyme of creatine kinase (BB-CK) from defective yet excessive osteoclasts (OCs) are biomarkers for most OPTs. Several LDH isoenzymes are elevated in ASD. Mutation analysis is offered by commercial laboratories.
- Radiographic findings of alternating sclerotic and lucent bands that parallel the iliac crest and long bone physes account for the "rugger jersey" appearance in the spine. Metaphyses widen and can develop a club shape or "Erlenmeyer flask" deformity and "bone within bone appearance." Bone density Z-score ranges from +3 to +15.[17]
- **Bone biopsy:** Increased numbers of osteoclasts lacking ruffled borders, or few osteoclasts can be identified. Unresorbed calcified cartilage is characteristic.

TREATMENT

Bone marrow transplantation can be life saving and curative in some severely affected infants with malignant OPT. In ASD treatment is largely supportive. Surgical decompression of the optic, facial nerves and auditory canal may become necessary. Joint replacement and fracture repairs are challenging. Hyperbaric oxygenation may help osteomyelitis of the jaw.

Van Buchem Disease/Sclerosteosis

GENERAL PRINCIPLES

- Van Buchem disease and sclerosteosis are characterized by increased bone formation, enhanced bone strength, and resistance to factures; mainly reported in Afrikaners or others of Dutch ancestry. These conditions are secondary to decreased levels of sclerostin.[18]
- Van Buchem disease is characterized by progressive asymmetrical enlargement and marked thickening of the jaw, which occurs during puberty, recurrent facial nerve palsy, deafness, and optic atrophy from narrowing of cranial foramina. Long bones may be painful to pressure. Sclerosteosis is even more severe with in utero onset of syndactyly. In early childhood, patients become tall and heavy with skeletal overgrowth, especially of the skull causing facial disfigurement, deafness, and facial palsy. The small cranial cavity may raise intracranial pressure and cause headache with brainstem compression which can be fatal.[19]

TREATMENT

There is no specific medical therapy for both these disorders. Treatment is largely supportive. In Van Buchem disease, decompression of narrowed foramina may help cranial nerve palsies. Sclerosteosis patients may require decompressive craniotomy and cerebrospinal fluid diversion procedures may be necessary to reduce elevated intracranial pressure.

High Bone Mass Disorder

Certain mutations of the low-density lipoprotein receptor-related protein 5 and 6 gene (*LRP6*) enhance Wnt signaling, stimulate osteoblasts, and increase skeletal mass with good quality bone. These are inherited as an AD trait. Most patients have torus palatinus, and other oropharyngeal exostoses. Some have cranial nerve palsies, sensory-motor neuropathy, spinal stenosis, headaches and bone pain. They often report marked resistance to fractures. Biochemical testing is usually within normal limits. BMD range from Z-scores +3 to +8.[8,20]

Osteopoikilosis

Osteopoikilosis is typically an incidental radiographic finding, characterized by "spotted bones." Radiologic features include numerous foci of osteosclerosis. The bony lesions are asymptomatic, but if misunderstood can precipitate investigation for metastatic disease to the skeleton.[21]

Acquired Causes of High Bone Mass: Fluorosis

GENERAL PRINCIPLES

- Skeletal fluorosis results from chronic ingestion or inhalation of high amounts of fluoride, leading to excess deposition in the skeleton. It is rare in the developed world where case reports have implicated tainted wines, mineral waters, fluoridated toothpastes, and excessive tea drinking.[22]
- The osteosclerosis is generalized but most pronounced in the axial skeleton.

- Presentation ranges from asymptomatic to skeletal deformities, pain and significantly reduced mobility. Patients may develop debilitating muscle wasting and neurologic deficits caused by spinal cord compression.
- Diagnosis can be inferred on the basis of elevated serum fluoride, 24-hour urinary fluoride measurements and characteristic radiographs. Increased bone mass with Z scores of +14 (lumbar spine) and +7 (total hip) may be found on DXA.

TREATMENT

Limiting fluoride exposure can reduce symptoms, normalize urine and blood fluoride levels, and may lead to improvement in radiographs and BMD over time.[23,24]

Hepatitis C–Associated Osteosclerosis

GENERAL PRINCIPLES

- Severe generalized osteosclerosis and hyperostosis has been reported with hepatitis C virus infection.[25] Approximately 20 cases have been reported worldwide. The increased bone mass has been attributed to increased circulating levels of insulin-like growth factor (IGF)–binding protein 2 and IGF II.[26]
- Periosteal, endosteal, and trabecular bone thickening occurs throughout the skeleton sparing the cranium.
- During active disease, the forearms and legs are painful.

TREATMENT

Gradual, spontaneous remission with decreasing bone density can occur.[27] Antiviral therapy may lead to improvement in the bone disorder.

MALIGNANCIES

Osteosclerotic lesions in the bone are typically the result of metastases.

- Metastatic carcinoma, especially from the prostate, can cause dense bones. Metastases from breast gastric, cervical cancer and Hodgkin disease have been reported to occasionally manifest as osteosclerotic lesions.
- Multiple myeloma typically features generalized osteopenia and osteolytic lesions, indolent forms can manifest widespread osteosclerosis.[28]
- Increased BMD at a single vertebra have been reported in Ewing sarcoma, and osteoblastomas.

MASTOCYTOSIS

- Systemic mastocytosis is a rare disorder characterized by excessive mast cell accumulation in one or multiple tissues.
- Mastocytosis commonly presents with diffuse osteoporosis, but a small subset (5–10%) can manifest as osteosclerosis.[29]

MELORHEOSTOSIS

- Originates from Greek, meaning "flowing hyperostosis."
- The etiology and pathogenesis of this sporadic and focal skeletal disorder can involve KRAS and MAP2K1 mutations.

- Presentation is typically during childhood and has been most commonly described in the lower extremities. Cutaneous changes may overlie the skeletal lesions and include linear scleroderma-like patches and soft tissue abnormalities often precede the hyperostosis. Pain and stiffness are the main symptoms.
- Radiographic appearance "resembles wax that has dripped down a candle." Dense, irregular, and eccentric hyperostosis of periosteal and enosteal surfaces of a single bone or several adjacent bones in a dermatomal distribution is pathognomonic of this disorder.[30]

MYELOFIBROSIS

- Chronic myeloproloferative disorders which result in a hyperplastic bone marrow and extramedullary hematopoiesis can lead to marrow fibrosis. The osteosclerosisis likely due to replacement of the normal marrow cavity with fibrous tissue.[31]
- Clinical symptoms are variable and include fatigue, weight loss, easy bruising/bleedings, fever night sweats, and splenomegaly.
- Radiographs and DXA show increased bone density that is most pronounced in the axial skeleton and proximal aspects of long bones.

DIFFUSE IDIOPATHIC SKELETAL HYPEROSTOSIS

- This is a noninflammatory disorder of unclear etiology, characterized by ossification of spinal ligaments and of peripheral enthesis. Male predominance has been noted.
- Patients typically present with pain and occasionally stiffness in the region of the thoracic spine; dysphagia from cervical osteophytes and myelopathy are less common.
- Diagnosis is based on a combination of the clinical presentation and characteristic radiographic appearance, typically of thoracic plain films.
- Plain films demonstrate calcification and ossification along the anterolateral aspects of the vertebral bodies which continues across the disc space. These can account for focal increases in spinal BMD by as much as 24% to 39%.[32]

RENAL OSTEODYSTROPHY

- Renal osteodystrophy can be associated with a diffuse increase in bone radiodensity, a finding that is seen more often in the axial skeleton, that is, spine, pelvis, and the ribs.
- Despite the increased bone mass, these patients are at high risk of fractures.
- The spine often demonstrates rugger jersey appearance, due to the alternating bands of increased density along the endplates and decreased density in the central portion of the vertebral bodies.[33,34]

REFERENCES

1. Whyte MP. Sclerosing bone disorders. In: Rosen CJ ed. *Primer on the Metabolic Bone Diseases and Disorders of Mineral Metabolism.* 8th ed. Hoboken: Wiley-Blackwell; 2013:767–785
2. Altman RD, Bloch DA, Hochberg MC, Murphy WA. Prevalence of pelvic Paget's disease of bone in the United States. *J Bone Miner Res* 2000;15(3):461–465.
3. Whyte MP. Clinical practice. Paget's disease of bone. *N Engl J Med* 2006;355(6):593–600.
4. Siris ES, Ottman R, Flaster E, Kelsey JL. Familial aggregation of Paget's disease of bone. *J Bone Miner Res* 1991;6(5):495–500.
5. Roodman GD, Windle JJ. Paget disease of bone. *J Clin Invest* 2005;115(2):200–208.
6. Shoback D, Sellmeyer D, Bikle D. Metabolic bone disease. In: Gardner DG, Shoback D, eds. *Greenspan's Basic & Clinical Endocrinology.* 8th ed. New York: McGraw-Hill Companies; 2007:337–341.
7. Tiegs RD. Paget's disease of bone: Indications for treatment and goals of therapy. *Clin Ther* 1997; 19(6):1309–1329; discussion 1523–1524.

8. Rickels MR, Zhang X, Mumm S, Whyte MP. Oropharyngeal skeletal disease accompanying high bone mass and novel LRP5 mutation. *J Bone Miner Res* 2005;20(5):878–885.

9. Singer FR, Bone HG, Hosking DR, et al. Paget's disease of bone: An endocrine society clinical practice guideline. *J Clin Endocrinol Metab* 2014;99(12):4408–4422.

10. Siris ES, Lyles KW, Singer FR, Meunier PJ. Medical management of Paget's disease of bone: Indications for treatment and review of current therapies. *J Bone Miner Res* 2006;21 Suppl 2: P94–P98.

11. Parvizi J, Klein GR, Sim FH. Surgical management of Paget's disease of bone. *J Bone Miner Res* 2006;21(Suppl 2):P75–P82.

12. Mirabello L, Troisi, RJ, Savage SA. Osteosarcoma incidence and survival rates from 1973 to 2004: Data from the Surveillance, Epidemiology, and End Results Program. *Cancer* 2009;115(7): 1531–1543.

13. Alvarez L, Guañabens N, Peris P, et al. Discriminative value of biochemical markers of bone turnover in assessing the activity of Paget's disease. *J Bone Miner Res* 1995;10(3):458–465.

14. Delmas PD. Biochemical markers of bone turnover in Paget's disease of bone. *J Bone Miner* 1999;14(Suppl 2):66–69.

15. Cleiren E, Bénichou O, Van Hul E, et al. Albers-Schönberg disease (autosomal dominant osteopetrosis, type II) results from mutations in the ClCN7 chloride channel gene. *Hum Mol Genet* 2001;10(25):2861–2867.

16. Waguespack SG, Hui SL, Dimeglio LA, Econs MJ. Autosomal dominant osteopetrosis: Clinical severity and natural history of 94 subjects with a chloride channel 7 gene mutation. *J Clin Endocrinol Metab* 2007;92(3):771–778.

17. Bollerslev J, Steiniche T, Melsen F, Mosekilde L. Structural and histomorphometric studies of iliac crest trabecular and cortical bone in autosomal dominant osteopetrosis: A study of two radiological types. *Bone* 1989;10(1):19–24.

18. Delgado-Calle J, Sato AY, Bellido T. Role and mechanism of action of sclerostin in bone. *Bone* 2017;96:29–37.

19. Hamersma H, Gardner J, Beighton P. The natural history of sclerosteosis. *Clin Genet* 2003; 63(3):192–197.

20. Boyden LM, Mao J, Belsky J, et al. High bone density due to a mutation in LDL-receptor-related protein 5. *N Engl J Med* 2002;346(20):1513–1521.

21. Whyte MP, Murphy WA, Fallon MD, Hahn TJ. Mixed-sclerosing-bone-dystrophy: Report of a case and review of the literature. *Skeletal Radiol* 1981;6(2):95–102.

22. Whyte MP, Totty WG, Lim VT, Whitford GM. Skeletal fluorosis from instant tea. *J Bone Miner Res* 2008;23(5):759–769.

23. Krishnamachari KA. Skeletal fluorosis in humans: A review of recent progress in the understanding of the disease. *Prog Food Nutr Sci* 1986;10(3-4):279–314.

24. Kurland ES, Shulman RC, Zerwekh JE, Reinus WR, Dempster DW, Whyte MP. Recovery from skeletal fluorosis (an enigmatic, American case). *J Bone Miner Res* 2007;22(1): 163–170.

25. Whyte MP, Teitelbaum SL, Reinus WR. Doubling skeletal mass during adult life: The syndrome of diffuse osteosclerosis after intravenous drug abuse. *J Bone Miner Res* 1996;11(4):554–558.

26. Khosla S, Ballard FJ, Conover CA. Use of site-specific antibodies to characterize the circulating form of big insulin-like growth factor II in patients with hepatitis C-associated osteosclerosis. *J Clin Endocrinol Metab* 2002;87(8):3867–3870.

27. Serraino C, Melchio R, Silvestri A, Borretta V, Pomero F, Fenoglio L. Hepatitis C-associated osteosclerosis: A new case with long-term follow-up and a review of the literature. *Intern Med Tokyo Jpn* 2015;54(7):777–783.

28. Gregson CL, Hardcastle SA, Cooper C, Tobias JH. Friend or foe: High bone mineral density on routine bone density scanning, a review of causes and management. *Rheumatol Oxf Engl* 2013; 52(6):968–985.

29. Greene LW, Asadipooya K, Corradi PF, Akin C. Endocrine manifestations of systemic mastocytosis in bone. *Rev Endocr Metab Disord* 2016;17(3):419–431.

30. Smith GC, Pingree MJ, Freeman LA, et al. Melorheostosis: A retrospective clinical analysis of 24 patients at the Mayo Clinic. *PM R* 2017;9(3):283–288.

31. Cloran F, Banks KP. AJR teaching file: Diffuse osteosclerosis with hepatosplenomegaly. *AJR Am J Roentgenol* 2007;188(3 Suppl):S18–S20.

32. Westerveld LA, Verlaan JJ, Lam MG, et al. The influence of diffuse idiopathic skeletal hyperostosis on bone mineral density measurements of the spine. *Rheumatol Oxf Engl* 2009;48: 1133–1136.

33. Chang CY, Rosenthal DI, Mitchell DM, Handa A, Kattapuram SV, Huang AJ. Imaging Findings of Metabolic Bone Disease. *Radiographics* 2016;36(6):1871–1887.

34. Murphey MD, Sartoris DJ, Quale JL, Pathria MN, Martin NL. Musculoskeletal manifestations of chronic renal insufficiency. *Radiographics* 1993;13(2):357–379.

Standards of Care for Diabetes Mellitus

28

Maamoun Salam and Janet B. McGill

GENERAL PRINCIPLES

- Standards of care for patients with diabetes are developed by consensus committees both in the United States and abroad to facilitate the application of evidence-based medicine to all persons with diabetes or who are at risk for diabetes.
- The stated goals of these committees are to provide practical guidelines for health care providers that will reduce the risk of morbidity and mortality from acute and chronic complications of diabetes.
- Standards of care for patients with diabetes have been established by the American Diabetes Association (ADA), the American Association of Clinical Endocrinologists (AACE), and the American College of Cardiology/American Heart Association in addition to many other associations.
- Original studies and grade of evidence supporting the recommendations discussed in this chapter are referenced in the consensus documents. Diagnostic and treatment strategies for type 1 diabetes mellitus (T1DM) and type 2 diabetes mellitus (T2DM) are discussed in Chapters 29 and 30 respectively.

SCREENING FOR DIABETES MELLITUS

Type 1 Diabetes Mellitus

- **Measurement of autoantibodies** for autoimmune T1DM may be appropriate in high-risk individuals with prior history of transient hyperglycemia, those who have close relatives with T1DM, or in the context of clinical research studies. However, widespread screening is generally not recommended for low-risk populations.[1]
- The risk of developing T1DM is >70% if two autoantibodies are positive. Counseling regarding the risk of developing T1DM should be provided to those who have positive antibody titers.

Type 2 Diabetes Mellitus

- **ADA recommends screening for T2DM** at age 45 OR in adults who are overweight (BMI ≥25 kg/m^2 or ≥23 kg/m^2 in Asians) with additional risk factors (Table 28-1).[1]
- **AACE recommends screening of all individuals who are at risk for developing T2DM.** In addition to persons meeting criteria in Table 28-1, AACE recommends screening persons taking antipsychotic drugs and glucocorticoids. Screening should be done every 3 years. Annual screening may be considered for patients with two or more risk factors.[2]
- **The EASD and ECS recommend using a risk-assessment tool** such as the Finnish Diabetes Risk Score (FINDRISC) to assess the 10-year risk of T2DM, and performing laboratory testing that includes a diagnostic oral glucose tolerance test (OGTT) or a combination of Hemoglobin A1c (HbA1c) and fasting plasma glucose (FPG). In patients with cardiovascular disease (CVD), there is no need for diabetes risk-assessment tool but an OGTT is indicated if HbA1c and/or FPG are inconclusive.[3]
- The **same tests are used for screening and diagnosis of diabetes**. Diagnostic criteria are reviewed in Chapter 30.

TABLE 28-1	ADA CRITERIA FOR TESTING FOR DIABETES IN ASYMPTOMATIC ADULTS[1]

- Testing should be considered in all adults who are overweight (BMI ≥25 kg/m^2 or ≥23 kg/m^2 in Asians) and have additional risk factors:
  - Physical inactivity
  - First-degree relative with diabetes
  - Members of a high-risk ethnic population (e.g., African American, Latino, Native American, Asian American, Pacific Islander)
  - Women who were diagnosed with gestational diabetes mellitus
  - Hypertension (≥140/90 mm Hg or on therapy for hypertension)
  - HDL cholesterol <35 mg/dL (0.90 mmol/L) and/or a triglyceride level >250 mg/dL (2.82 mmol/L)
  - Women with polycystic ovary syndrome
  - HbA1c ≥5.7% (39 mmol/mol), IGT, or IFG on previous testing
  - Other clinical conditions associated with insulin resistance (e.g., severe obesity, acanthosis nigricans)
  - History of CVD
- In the absence of the above criteria, testing for diabetes should begin at age 45
- If the results are normal, testing should be repeated at least at 3-year intervals, with consideration of more frequent testing depending on initial results (e.g., those with prediabetes should be tested yearly) and risk status

[a]At risk BMI may be lower for some ethnic groups.
Adapted from American Diabetes Association. Classification and diagnosis of diabetes: Standards of medical care in diabetes—2018. *Diabetes Care* 2018;41(Suppl 1):S13–S27, with permission.

- **Hemoglobin A1c** as a screening and diagnostic test should be performed in a laboratory using a method that is National Glycohemoglobin Standardization Program (NGSP) certified and standardized to the Diabetes Control and Complication Trial (DCCT) assay (Table 28-2).[4,5]

Gestational Diabetes Mellitus

- Gestational diabetes mellitus (GDM) is defined as **any degree of glucose intolerance with onset or first recognition during pregnancy.**
- Screening for diabetes in pregnancy is important to ensure optimal maternal and fetal outcomes.
- Because the number of pregnant women with undiagnosed T2DM has increased with the ongoing epidemic of obesity, patients with preconception T2DM may be wrongly classified as gestational. Hence **ADA recommends screening women with risk factors for diabetes** (Table 28-1) **using standard diagnostic testing at the first prenatal visit.** Women who satisfy diagnostic criteria should receive a diagnosis of overt diabetes.[1]
- All pregnant women previously undiagnosed with diabetes should undergo GDM testing with a **75-g OGTT at 24 to 28 weeks of gestation**. The OGTT should be performed in the morning after an overnight fast of at least 8 hours. The diagnosis of GDM is made if any of the following criteria are met:[1,6,7]
  - Fasting plasma glucose ≥92 mg/dL (5.1 mmol/L)
  - 1-hour plasma glucose ≥180 mg/dL (10 mmol/L)
  - 2-hour plasma glucose ≥153 mg/dL (8.5 mmol/L)
- **Women with GDM should also be tested at 4 to 12 weeks postpartum using OGTT and clinically appropriate nonpregnancy diagnostic criteria** to detect persistence of diabetes and followed more closely in subsequent years.[1,8]

TABLE 28-2 CORRELATION BETWEEN HbA1c AND MEAN PLASMA GLUCOSE[5]

HbA1c	Mean plasma glucose	
% (mmol/mol)	mg/dL	mmol/L
6 (42)	126	7.0
7 (53)	154	8.6
8 (64)	183	10.2
9 (75)	212	11.8
10 (86)	240	13.4
11 (97)	269	14.9
12 (108)	298	16.5

HbA1c, hemoglobin A1c.

Prevention of Diabetes

- People with prediabetes should be monitored annually for the development of diabetes.[9]
- Randomized controlled studies have shown that diabetes can be prevented in individuals at high risk with either lifestyle modification or with medication.[10,11]
- All consensus groups recommend **counseling in lifestyle management to reduce weight in those who are overweight and to increase physical activity.**[1–3,9]
- Studies of lifestyle management that have resulted in weight loss of ≥5% through diet and exercise (150 min/wk) have demonstrated up to 58% reduction in risk of progression to diabetes.[10,11]
- Based on these clinical trials, lifestyle changes with a goal weight loss of 5% to 7% and moderate physical activity of 150 min/wk are recommended for prevention of progression from impaired fasting glucose (IFG) or impaired glucose tolerance (IGT) to diabetes.[1–3,9]
- **Medications that have proved effective in preventing diabetes** include metformin, α-glucosidase inhibitors (e.g., acarbose), orlistat, glucagon-like peptide 1 (GLP-1) receptor agonists, and thiazolidinediones. None of these drugs have been approved by the FDA in the United States for use in prediabetes to prevent progression to diabetes. The ADA considers metformin as a prevention option in those with prediabetes, especially those with BMI ≥35 kg/m², those aged <60 years, women with prior GDM, and/or those with rising HbA1c despite lifestyle intervention.[1,2,9,12]

GLYCEMIC CONTROL

- Targets for glycemic control in diabetes reflect evidence from randomized controlled trials that have demonstrated protection from microvascular complications. Reduction in macrovascular events has been demonstrated in the intensively treated arms in long-term follow-up observational studies of the DCCT and UKPDS cohorts despite lack of persistence of tight glucose control during the follow-up period.[1,5,12,13]
- No macrovascular benefit of tight glycemic control was observed in patients with long-standing T2DM in the ACCORD and VADT clinical trials, and there were more deaths in the tight control arm of the ACCORD trial.[13]
- It is, therefore, important to individualize the goal HbA1c according to the risk of hypoglycemia, presence of comorbidities, and life expectancy.[5,12]
- In pregnancy, glycemic targets are lower than in nonpregnant adults to mimic nondiabetic pregnant women, and to ensure optimal fetal outcomes.

- **Glycemic control is monitored by** self-monitored blood glucose (SMBG), continuous glucose monitoring (CGM) and HbA1c.[5]

Self-Monitoring of Blood Glucose

- The **frequency of SMBG** should range from 1 to 4 or more readings per day, depending on the intensity of therapy, the need for medication adjustments based on glucose values and the risk of hypoglycemia. In patients with T1DM and T2DM on multiple insulin injections or insulin pump therapy, as well as pregnant women taking insulin, more frequent testing (three or more times a day) is necessary to reach HbA1c targets.[5] The optimal frequency, timing, and overall utility of SMBG for noninsulin-treated patients with T2DM is unclear.
- **SMBG is generally checked before meals and at bedtime,** with periodic checks of glucose during the postprandial period and during sleep. Also, SMBG should be done prior to exercise, prior to critical tasks such as driving and when hypoglycemia is suspected.[5]
- The capillary blood glucose levels are 10% to 15% lower than plasma glucose levels. Newer blood glucose meters are calibrated to report plasma glucose values, so each patient should be informed whether his/her meter reports plasma values.[4]
- If there is a discrepancy between SMBG values reported by the patient or depicted in meter readings and the HbA1c, it may be useful to increase the frequency of SMBG or measure postprandial glucose 1 to 2 hours after meals. Persistently high HbA1c despite lower than expected blood glucose readings, or wide fluctuations in blood glucose, should prompt further investigation, which is often done best by a certified diabetes educator (CDE).

Continuous Glucose Monitoring

- CGMs use subcutaneous, real-time sensors that measure the interstitial glucose concentration. The interstitial glucose concentrations are converted by various algorithms to mimic plasma glucose levels.
- CGM systems have variable characteristics. Some of the current systems provide real-time glucose data via blue tooth connection to a receiver (Dexcom G5 and G6, Medtronic Enlite and Guardian). These systems also provide alarms for high and low glucoses. Another system (Freestyle Libre) requires that the receiver be held in proximity to the sensor to capture glucose data, consequently there are no alarms for out of range glucoses. The Medtronic CGM systems are available for use only with specified insulin pumps, and they use the pump as the receiver. The Dexcom CGMs can utilize a dedicated receiver, an insulin pump or smart cellular phone to receive glucose data. Using a cellular phone as a receiver allows the information to be shared with others, permitting another layer of safety.
- CGM is approved by Medicare for use by patients taking multiple injections of insulin or those using an insulin pump. Data on the benefits of use in patients on less intensive regimens are limited.[5]
- CGM systems with high and low glucose alarms provide a safety net for patients on intensive insulin therapy, in particular those with hypoglycemia unawareness and/or frequent hypoglycemia.
- Pregnancy outcomes were improved in one study of CGM in pregnant women.[14]
- Optimal use of CGM requires training in both the mechanics of use and dosing algorithms that incorporate directional arrows.[5]

Hemoglobin A1c

- **HbA1c reflects blood glucose levels over the previous 2 to 3 months.** HbA1c should be monitored every 3 months until a patient reaches the goal, and then every 6 months if the patient is at target and stable.[5] Point-of-care HbA1c tests enable timely decisions on therapeutic changes during office visits. Table 28-2 shows correlation between HbA1c and mean plasma glucose levels. A calculator for converting HbA1c results into estimated average is found at: https://professional.diabetes.org/diapro/glucose_calc.

- **HbA1c can be misleading in patients with certain forms of anemia and/or hemoglobinopathies.** HbA1c assays may not be accurate in the presence of abnormal hemoglobins (list of assays and impact of abnormal hemoglobin on them is available at http://www.ngsp.org/factors.asp). HbA1c is unreliable for diagnosis and management of diabetes in conditions of abnormal cell turnover as in pregnancy or anemia from hemolysis and iron deficiency.[4,5]
- Guidelines for glycemic goals established by consensus groups are listed in Table 28-3.[1,2,3,5,8]
- The **goals for glycemic control should be individualized.** HbA1c goal may be near normal (<6%) for individuals with short duration of diabetes, long life expectancy, and no significant CVD if it is possible to achieve without hypoglycemia. Less stringent targets may be appropriate for those with a history of severe hypoglycemia, limited life expectancy, extensive comorbid conditions, advanced microvascular or macrovascular complications, and difficult to manage long-standing diabetes. Targets for children are adjusted to permit scrupulous avoidance of serious hypoglycemia.[5,12]

TREATMENT RECOMMENDATIONS

Diabetes Self-Management Education

Patients with newly diagnosed as well as established diabetes should receive comprehensive diabetes self-management education (DSME) by a certified diabetes educator (CDE). This approach should be patient centered and done in collaboration with health-care professionals.

Lifestyle Therapy

- Nutrition recommendations need to be individualized with consideration of the patient's need for caloric restriction or increase, ethnicity, diabetes therapy, and food choices.

TABLE 28-3 GLYCEMIC TARGETS FOR ADULTS WITH DIABETES

Glycemic parameter	ADA[1]	AACE[2]	EASD[3]	GDM[8]	Pregnancy[6]
Hemoglobin A1c[a]	<7.0% <6.5% if attainable without hypoglycemia <8% if less stringent goal is appropriate	≤6.5%	≤7%	N/A	<6.0%
Fasting and preprandial blood glucose	80–130 mg/dL	<110 mg/dL	≤120 mg/dL	≤95 mg/dL	60–99 mg/dL
Postprandial blood glucose	<180 mg/dL	<140 mg/dL	≤160–180 mg/dL	1-hour post meal ≤140 mg/dL 2-hour post meal ≤120 mg/dL	100–129 mg/dL

[a]Using a DCCT-referenced assay.

AACE, American Association of Clinical Endocrinologists; ADA, American Diabetes Association; EASD, European Association for the Study of Diabetes.

- **Carbohydrate intake monitoring** with carbohydrate counting, exchanges, or experience-based estimation have been shown to improve glycemic control.
- **Aerobic exercise** of at least 150 minutes (50% to 70% of maximum heart rate) per week and supplemental **repetitive resistance training** are recommended for all adults with diabetes in the absence of contraindications. Prolonged sitting should be interrupted every 30 minutes particularly in T2DM.
- Physical activity is associated with reduced cardiovascular risk in both primary and secondary prevention that is equivalent to first-line pharmacologic therapy. Health-care providers should assess the level of physical activity in patients with diabetes and provide encouragement to reach activity or exercise targets. Physical limitations should be addressed and alternative exercise programs developed as needed.
- Nutrition advice specific to cardiovascular risk reduction includes avoidance of trans and saturated fats, increased intake of fiber, and intake of five or more servings of fruits and vegetables daily. Reduction of salt intake is advised in persons who are hypertensive. This advice should be provided to all patients as part of routine health care visits and included in medical nutrition therapy (MNT) instructions.
- **Smoking cessation** is critically important for persons with diabetes, and counseling regarding smoking cessation should be documented in medical records.
- **Alcohol** consumption in moderation (no more than one drink per day for adult women or two drinks per day for adult men) does not have detrimental effects on long term blood glucose control. However, there might be increased risk of hypoglycemia especially in those using insulin or insulin secretagogue therapies.
- **Nonnutritive sweeteners** are considered generally safe to use within the defined acceptable daily intake levels. They may be preferred to sugar as they may provide less carbohydrate intake.

Drug Therapy

- Multiple daily injections of basal plus prandial insulin or continuous subcutaneous insulin infusion are the cornerstone in T1DM therapy (Chapter 29).
- Medication intervention in T2DM **should normally begin with metformin**, with other agents added sequentially to achieve glycemic targets (Chapter 30).
- **Early treatment with insulin is recommended** if HbA1c is ≥10% and/or blood glucose level >250 to 300 mg/dL at presentation or any time in the course of treatment.[12]
- Individualization of treatment strategies is needed for all patients, taking into consideration age, comorbidities such as chronic kidney disease, and risk for or presence of CVD.
- **Hypoglycemia** is a limiting factor in the glycemic management of diabetes (discussed in Chapter 33). **Glucose values <70 mg/dL should be treated with 15 to 20 g of glucose (preferred) or other simple carbohydrates, and rechecked in 15 minutes.** Persons at risk for severe hypoglycemia should have a prescription for **glucagon** and instructions for use by a companion.

Obesity and Bariatric Surgery

Evaluation and management of obesity, including lifestyle, medications and bariatric surgery is discussed in Chapter 34.

PREVENTION OF COMPLICATIONS DUE TO DIABETES

Cardiovascular Disease

- CVD is the **leading cause of mortality in persons with diabetes**. Diabetes confers an increased risk of acute coronary syndrome, myocardial infarction, heart failure, atrial fibrillation, stroke, peripheral vascular disease, and sudden death that is 2 to 5 times the risk in nondiabetic comparator groups.[13,14]

- Persons with diabetes also experience greater morbidity after vascular events, and interventions such as coronary angioplasty may not be as effective at reducing morbidity and mortality in diabetic patients compared to nondiabetic comparison groups.
- Although the increased risk is not entirely explained by usual risk factors, studies have shown that aggressive management of hypertension and lipids and the use of antiplatelet agents in patients with diabetes can reduce the risk of cardiovascular events, and that the benefits of treatment of each risk factor in diabetes may exceed the benefits in lower-risk cohorts.[15,16,17]
- CVD risk should be addressed in a comprehensive manner in all patients with diabetes, with efforts to achieve lifestyle, glycemic, blood pressure, and lipid targets.[13]

Hypertension

- Hypertension is present in more than 75% of persons with T2DM, and more than 50% of persons with T1DM.[18]
- The coexistence of diabetes and hypertension increases the risk of CVD and CVD-related mortality, and may increase the risk of retinopathy and nephropathy.
- Blood pressure should be checked at every visit in patients with diabetes, and home monitoring is encouraged.
- Lifestyle therapy should be considered if the blood pressure is ≥120/80 mm Hg. Lifestyle therapy for hypertension includes weight loss, dietary approaches to stop hypertension (DASH)-style diet, moderation of alcohol intake, and increased physical activity. DASH-style diet consists of decrease in sodium and increase in potassium intake.[18]
- The American College of Cardiology/American Heart Association and AACE recommend starting therapy with antihypertensive medications if the BP is >130/80 mm Hg, and achieving BP target of <130/80 mm Hg. ADA recommends using a BP target of <140/90 mm Hg in patients with diabetes.[12,18,19] **All of the first-line classes of antihypertensive agents, including renin–angiotensin system blockers, calcium channel blockers, and thiazide diuretics are useful in the treatment of hypertension in patients with diabetes, however angiotensin-converting enzyme inhibitors (ACEIs) or angiotensin receptor blockers (ARBs) should be considered in the presence of albuminuria.[18,19]**
- β-Blockers are indicated in patients who have had a myocardial infarction, heart failure, or for rate control in atrial fibrillation. Vasodilating agents such as carvedilol or nebivolol may be particularly useful in patients with diabetes, since they do not worsen insulin resistance or symptomatic peripheral vascular disease.[19]
- ACEIs and ARBs have been associated with birth defects, so caution is advised in premenopausal women, especially those women who indicate a desire to become pregnant or who are not using adequate birth control.

Hyperlipidemia

- Diabetic patients should have a fasting lipid profile (total cholesterol, low-density lipoprotein [LDL] cholesterol, high-density lipoprotein [HDL] cholesterol, and triglycerides) checked at diagnosis and annually (AACE guidelines), every 5 years or after a change in therapy (ADA guidelines).[12,20]
- ADA recommends lifestyle therapy followed by statin therapy for all patients with diabetes, escalating statin intensity with age, risk factors, and presence of CVD.[20] AACE recommends achievement of lipid targets in patients with diabetes (Table 28-4).[3,12]
- Therapy is initially directed toward meeting the LDL cholesterol goal with lifestyle modification and statin therapy.
- For those with triglycerides ≥200 mg/dL, the National Cholesterol Education Program/Adult Treatment Panel III guidelines have established a non-HDL cholesterol target of <130 mg/dL as the secondary goal.[21]
- If the triglyceride level is >500 mg/dL, therapy should first be directed at lowering triglycerides to prevent pancreatitis.[21]

TABLE 28-4 LIPID TARGETS FOR PERSONS WITH DIABETES

	AACE, ATP III[2]	EASD/ESC[3,a]
Total cholesterol		<4.5 mmol/L (174 mg/dL)
LDL cholesterol	<100 mg/dL	<2.5 mmol/L (97 mg/dL)[b]
• DM + ASCVD or at least one additional risk factor (hypertension, family history, low HDL or smoking)	≤70 mg/dL	<1.8 mmol/L (70 mg/dL) or at least ≥50% LDL reduction if this target goal cannot be reached
HDL	>40 mg/dL in men >50 mg/dL in women	The use of drugs to increase HDL to prevent CVD in T2DM is not recommended
Triglycerides	<150 mg/dL If >500 mg/dL, lowering TG becomes a priority	>1.7 mmol/L (151 mg/dL) is a marker for increased vascular risk; begin treatment when >2.3 mmol/L (189 mg/dL) and LDL is at target
Non-HDL (TC-HDL)	<130 mg/dL (especially for those with TG >200 mg/dL) <100 mg/dL (if DM + ASCVD or at least one additional risk factor)	0.8 mmol/L (31 mg/dL) above stated LDL goal

[a]With the Third Joint European Societies Task Force on Cardiovascular Disease Prevention in Clinical Practice.

[b]Includes patients with type 1 diabetes.

AACE, American Association of Clinical Endocrinologists; ADA, American Diabetes Association; ATP, Adult Treatment Panel; CVD, cardiovascular disease; DM, diabetes mellitus; EASD, European Association for the Study of Diabetes; ESC, European Society of Cardiology; HDL, high-density lipoprotein; LDL, low-density lipoprotein; TC, total cholesterol; TG, triglycerides.

- Additional LDL lowering with ezetimibe or a bile acid sequestrant may be required to reach LDL targets not achieved with statins. PCSK9 inhibitors evolocumab and alirocumab may be considered as adjunctive therapy for patients at high risk for ASCVD who require additional lowering of LDL or who are statin intolerant.[12,20] For specific recommendations on treatment of hyperlipidemia, refer to Chapter 33.

Retinopathy

- All patients with diabetes are at risk for retinopathy. Diabetic retinopathy poses a serious threat to vision and is the leading cause of blindness in middle-aged Americans.[22]

- Optimizing glycemic control, blood pressure, and serum lipid are recommended to reduce the risk or slow the progression of diabetic retinopathy.
- Newly diagnosed T1DM patients should have an initial dilated eye examination within 5 years after onset of their disease. Persons with T2DM should have a comprehensive eye examination at the time of diagnosis and yearly thereafter. Examinations every 2 years may be considered if there is no evidence of retinopathy for one or more annual eye examinations and glycemic control is good. However, at least annual examination is recommended when any level of retinopathy is present.[22]
- Women who are planning a pregnancy, or who present early in pregnancy, should have a comprehensive eye examination due to the risk of development or progression of retinopathy during pregnancy. An eye examination should be performed in the first trimester with close follow-up and monitoring throughout the pregnancy and for 1 year postpartum.[22]
- Eye examinations more frequently than once a year should be done in patients with active retinopathy and in patients receiving active treatment for retinopathy.
- Laser photocoagulation therapy has been the mainstay treatment for preservation of vision in diabetic retinopathy, but it does not restore lost vision. Close ophthalmologic follow-up is recommended to determine the timing and extent of laser or other therapies.
- Intravitreal injections of antivascular endothelial growth factor are indicated for center-involved macular edema.[22]
- Aspirin therapy for cardio protection does not increase the risk of retinal hemorrhage and it is not contraindicated in the presence of retinopathy.

Nephropathy

- Diabetic nephropathy (DN) accounts for nearly 50% of end-stage renal disease in the United States and is a leading cause of diabetes-related morbidity and mortality.[22]
- Screening for DN includes annual measurement of serum creatinine and urine albumin excretion, which is typically done on a spot random urine sample. In patients with T1DM, screening should be performed within 5 years of diagnosis, but in persons with T2DM, screening should start at the time of diagnosis. Calculation of estimated glomerular filtration rate (eGFR) should be done using the CKD-EPI equation.[22]
- **Microalbuminuria** is defined as a albumin:creatinine ratio of 30 to 300 mcg/mg, and **macroalbuminuria** is defined as albumin:creatinine ratio of ≥300 mcg/mg. Positive tests should be confirmed.
- DN may manifest as declining kidney function in the presence or absence of albuminuria. The presence of macroalbuminuria is associated with more rapid decline in kidney function. **Treatment with either an ACEI or an ARB** is appropriate when albuminuria is present, otherwise meeting glycemic and blood pressure goals are the most important interventions.
- Decline of kidney function should be assessed by annual assessment of eGFR. Rapid progression is defined as decline of eGFR of >3 mL/min/1.73m^2.
- When the eGFR is <60 mL/minute/1.73 m^2 testing for anemia, vitamin D, and parathyroid hormone should be undertaken and abnormal values treated. Referral to a nephrologist is recommended for patients with rapid progression, difficult to treat hypertension, electrolyte abnormalities or for assistance with management of renal complications and renal replacement planning.

Neuropathy

- Neuropathy is considered a microvascular complication of diabetes, which can present in several forms, generally categorized as focal or diffuse and involving peripheral sensory, autonomic, or sensory plus motor pathways.[22,23]
- The **most common forms are distal symmetric sensorimotor diabetic polyneuropathy (DPN) and autonomic neuropathy** involving gastrointestinal (gastroparesis, constipation, diarrhea, fecal incontinence), genitourinary (erectile dysfunction, neurogenic bladder), and

cardiovascular (resting tachycardia, orthostatic hypotension) systems, as well as contributing to hypoglycemic unawareness and sudomotor dysfunction with either increased or decreased sweating. Focal neuropathy is less common and typically presents acutely.[23]

- Evaluation of possible neuropathy should begin with a thorough history of symptoms such as pain, numbness, paresthesias, weakness in the feet or hands, early satiety, or erectile dysfunction. A neurologic examination should be performed annually and should evaluate deep tendon reflexes and various sensory modalities (pain/temperature, vibration, light touch, and joint position sense).[22]

- Individuals with diabetes should undergo annual screening for DPN using tests such as pinprick sensation, vibration perception (using a 128-Hz tuning fork), and 10-g monofilament sensory testing. Sensitivity of detecting DPN increases to >87% with combination of these tests.[23]

- Sensory testing with a 10-g monofilament detects the presence or absence of "protective sensation." Loss of monofilament sensation and vibration is predictive of foot ulcers.[23]

- Treatment of neuropathy is aimed at preventing progression and symptom relief including pain control.
  - **Strict control of blood glucose**, with attention to reducing glucose fluctuation, may prevent progression.
  - **Symptomatic pain relief** can be attained, through the use of some anticonvulsant medications, tricyclic antidepressants, and serotonin/norepinephrine reuptake inhibitors. Either pregabalin or duloxetine are recommended as initial pharmacologic therapy for neuropathic pain.
  - Large-fiber neuropathies are managed with strength, gait, and balance training; pain management; orthotics to treat and prevent foot deformities; and surgical reconstruction in some cases. Small-fiber neuropathies are managed by foot protection, supportive shoes with orthotics, regular foot and shoe inspection, prevention of heat injury, and use of emollient creams.
  - The antioxidant, α-lipoic acid was tested in a 4-year trial, was shown to be safe and effective on the Neuropathy Impairment Scale, but did not meet a composite primary endpoint of improved physiology and symptom scores.[24]
  - **Gastroparesis symptoms** respond to dietary changes and prokinetics like metoclopramide or erythromycin.
  - Erectile dysfunction is treated with phosphodiesterase type 5 inhibitors, intracorporeal or intraurethral prostaglandins, vacuum devices, or penile prosthesis.
  - A multidisciplinary approach should be adopted to manage patients with foot ulcers or at high risk for foot ulcers due to conditions such as Charcot deformity.

Lower Extremity Complications

- Patients with diabetes are at risk for several types of extremity problems, including foot infections and ulcerations, Charcot foot deformities and ischemia leading to poor wound healing.[22,23]

- Diabetes is the leading cause of nontraumatic lower extremity amputation in the United States.

- Annual foot examinations should include evaluation of touch and vibration sense (Semmes-Weinstein 10-g monofilament and 128-mHz tuning fork), deep tendon reflexes, and pedal pulses. At every visit, the feet should be visually inspected for skin breakdown, callus, discoloration, or signs of vascular or neurologic disease.

- Individuals with foot ulcers or at high risk for foot ulcers should be managed by a multidisciplinary team to ensure healing and prevent recurrence.

- Use of "diabetic shoes," which are individually fitted or crafted by orthotic specialists may help prevent skin breakdown.[22]

Antiplatelet Therapy

- Treatment with **low-dose (75 to 162 mg/day) aspirin** has been shown to reduce recurrence of cardiovascular events, including myocardial infarction and stroke in persons with diabetes.[20]
- Low-dose aspirin is recommended as primary prevention measure for individuals with T1DM and T2DM at increased cardiovascular risk (10-year risk >10%). The evidence is, however, insufficient to recommend aspirin in lower-risk individuals. Aspirin should be used as a secondary prevention strategy in those patients with CVD with diabetes.[20]
- Other antiplatelet agents such as clopidogrel are a reasonable alternative to aspirin when the patient is intolerant to aspirin.

Screening for Cardiovascular Disease

- Routine screening of asymptomatic patients for coronary artery disease is not recommended by the ADA due to evidence that shows no difference in outcome measures with screening stress electrocardiograms.[25]
- No difference was shown in intensive medical therapy versus invasive revascularization.[20]
- Individuals with typical or atypical cardiac symptoms, carotid bruits, transient ischemic attack, claudication, peripheral arterial disease, and an abnormal resting ECG should undergo exercise stress cardiac testing.[20]

Immunizations

- **Influenza vaccine should be administered annually** to all diabetic patients ≥6 months of age, beginning each October.
- The **pneumococcal polysaccharide vaccine (PPSV23)** should be administered once the diagnosis of diabetes is established to all patients 2 through 64 years of age. All adults 65 years of age or older should receive a dose of pneumococcal conjugate vaccine (PCV13) at least 1 year after PPSV23, followed by another dose of PPSV23 at least 1 year after PCV 13 and at least 5 years after the last dose of PPSV23.[26,27]
- Hepatitis B vaccine is recommended for adults with diabetes.[26]
- Other specific vaccines are left to clinical judgment.

OUTCOMES

Optimum care of patients with diabetes prevents acute complications and reduces the risk of development of long-term complications of this disease. This can be accomplished through patient education, regular health screening, medical care, laboratory evaluation, and timely referral to specialists.

SPECIAL CONSIDERATIONS

Diabetes and the fasting month of Ramadan:

- Fasting during the month of Ramadan is compulsory for all healthy Muslims from puberty onward. It includes abstinence from food and drinks starting from sunrise till sunset. This leads to a shift in meal times to two meals per day (Suhoor/predawn meal and Iftar/sunset meal) and a shift in sleeping patterns.[28]
- Ramadan timing changes from one year to another leading to variation in fasting duration, with summer fasting periods lasting up to 20 hours per day in some parts of the world. Climate conditions may vary as well, causing fasting in very dry and hot weather some years.
- Patients with diabetes who fast during Ramadan may be at increased risk for hypoglycemia, hyperglycemia, diabetic ketoacidosis, and dehydration. Patients with diabetes may be eligible for religious exemption, yet a large number will participate, often against medical

advice. Fasting in Ramadan for patients with diabetes is a personal decision that should be respected. Ensuring the optimal care of diabetic patients during Ramadan is crucial to ensure success. The International Diabetes Federation (IDF) and Diabetes and Ramadan (DAR) International Alliance have delivered comprehensive guidelines on this subject.[29] https://www.idf.org/e-library/guidelines/87-diabetes-and-ramadan-practical-25. Ramadan-focused diabetes education may reduce the incidence of possible complications. Blood glucose should be checked frequently (predawn meal, morning, midday, mid-afternoon, presunset meal, 2 hours after sunset meal, and when feeling unwell).

- IDF-DAR practical guidelines propose three categories of risk. Decisions to advise not to fast or allow fasting could be based on these categories which were approved by the Mofty of Egypt, the highest religious regulatory authority in Egypt.[29]
- All patients should break their fast if blood glucose is less than 70mg/dL or more than 300 mg/dL, if patient has symptoms of hypoglycemia or an acute illness occurs.
- Following are recommendations pharmacologic therapy adjustment during Ramadan:
  - No dose modifications are recommended for **metformin, acarbose, thiazolidinedione, DDP4 inhibitors** or **GLP-1 agonists** (after appropriate dose titration has been achieved). Timing may be changed so that medications are taken with sunset meal.
  - **Meglitinides:** TID dosing may be reduced to BID dosing with predawn and sunset meals. When using a **sulfonylurea**, switching to newer agents (gliclazide, glimepiride) when possible, reducing the dose in patients with good glycemic control and changing timing to sunset meal with once a day dosing are recommended steps to reduce the risk of hypoglycemia.
  - **SGLT-2 inhibitors** should be taken with the sunset meal. Attention should be made to stay well hydrated during nonfasting periods. No dose modification is needed.
  - **Insulin therapy** should be continuously modified based on duration of fasting and every three days assessment of glycemic control. **Basal insulin** (NPH, detemir, glargine, degludec) doses may be decreased by 15% to 30%. **Premixed insulin** doses may stay the same if given at sunset meal but decreased by 25% to 50% if given at predawn meal. **Meal time rapid or short acting insulin** doses may stay the same for the sunset meal but decreased by 25% to 50% for predawn meals. Dose titration can be done by 2 to 4 unit increments based on glycemic control with no changes in doses if blood glucose is between 90 and 126 mg/dL (5 to 7 mmol/L).

REFERENCES

1. American Diabetes Association. Classification and diagnosis of diabetes: Standards of medical care in diabetes—2018. *Diabetes Care* 2018;41(Suppl 1):S13–S27.
2. Handelsman Y, Bloomgarden ZT, Grunberger G, et al. American Association of Clinical Endocrinologists and American College of Endocrinology—Clinical practice guidelines for developing a diabetes mellitus comprehensive care plan. *Endocr Pract* 2015;21(Suppl 1):1–87.
3. Rydén L, Grant PJ, Anker SD, et al. The Task Force on Diabetes, Pre-diabetes and Cardiovascular Diseases of the European Society of Cardiology (ESC) and developed in collaboration with the European Association for the Study of Diabetes (EASD). Guidelines on diabetes, pre-diabetes, and cardiovascular diseases. *Eur Heart J* 2013;34(39):3035–3087.
4. Sacks DB, Arnold M, Bakris GL, et al. Position Statement Executive Summary: Guidelines and recommendations for laboratory analysis in the diagnosis and management of diabetes mellitus. *Diabetes Care* 2011;34(6):1419–1423.
5. American Diabetes Association. Glycemic targets: Standards of medical care in diabetes—2018. *Diabetes Care* 2018;41(Suppl 1):S55–S64.
6. Kitzmiller JL, Block JM, Brown FM, et al. Managing preexisting diabetes for pregnancy: Summary of evidence and consensus recommendations for care. *Diabetes Care* 2008;31(5);1060–1079.
7. International Association of Diabetes and Pregnancy Study Groups Consensus Panel, Metzger BE, Gabbe SG, et al. International association of diabetes and pregnancy study groups recommendations on the diagnosis and classification of hyperglycemia in pregnancy. *Diabetes Care* 2010;33(3):676–682.

8. Committee on Practice Bulletins—Obstetrics. Practice Bulletin No. 180: Gestational diabetes mellitus. *Obstet Gynecol* 2017;130(1):e17–e37.

9. American Diabetes Association. Prevention or delay of type 2 diabetes: Standards of medical care in diabetes—2018. *Diabetes Care* 2018;41(Suppl 1):S28–S37.

10. Knowler WC, Barrett-Connor E, Fowler SE, et al; Diabetes Prevention Program Research Group. Reduction in the incidence of type 2 diabetes with lifestyle intervention or metformin. *N Engl J Med* 2002;346(6):393–403.

11. Tuomilehto J, Lindström J, Eriksson JG, et al. Prevention of type 2 diabetes mellitus by changes in lifestyle among subjects with impaired glucose tolerance. *N Engl J Med* 2001;344(18):1343–1350.

12. Garber AJ, Abrahamson MJ, Barzilay JI, et al. Consensus statement by the American Association of Clinical Endocrinologists and American College of Endocrinology on the comprehensive type 2 diabetes management algorithm—2018 executive summary. *Endocrine Practice* 2018;24(1):91–120.

13. Cefalu WT, Kaul S, Gerstein HC, et al. Cardiovascular outcomes trials in type 2 diabetes: Where do we go from here? Reflections from a Diabetes Care editors' expert forum. *Diabetes Care* 2018;41(1):14–31.

14. Feig DS, Donovan LF, Corcoy R, et al. Continuous glucose monitoring in pregnant women with type 1 diabetes (CONCEPTT): A multicentre international randomised controlled trial. *Lancet* 2017;390(10110):2347–2359.

15. Ali MK, Bullard KM, Saaddine JB, Cowie CC, Imperatore G, Gregg EW. Achievement of goals in U.S. diabetes care, 1999–2010. *N Engl J Med* 2013;368(17):1613–1624.

16. Rawshani A, Rawshani A, Franzen S et al. Mortality and cardiovascular disease in type 1 and type 2 diabetes. *N Engl J Med* 2017;376(15):1407–1418.

17. Gregg EW, Li Y, Wang J, et al. Changes in diabetes-related complications in the United States, 1990–2010. *N Engl J Med* 2014;370(16):1514–1523.

18. de Boer IH, Bangalore S, Benetos A, et al. Diabetes and hypertension: A position statement by the American Diabetes Association. *Diabetes Care* 2017;40(9):1273–1284.

19. Carey RM, Whelton PK; 2017 ACC/AHA Hypertension Guideline Writing Committee. Prevention, detection, evaluation, and management of high blood pressure in adults: Synopsis of the 2017 American College of Cardiology/American Heart Association Hypertension Guideline. *Ann Int Med* 2018;168(5):351–358.

20. American Diabetes Association. Cardiovascular disease and risk management: Standards of medical care in diabetes—2018. *Diabetes Care* 2018;41(Suppl 1):S86–S104.

21. Expert Panel on Detection, Evaluation, and Treatment of High Blood Cholesterol in Adults. Executive summary of the third report of the National Cholesterol Education Program (NCEP) expert panel on detection, evaluation, and treatment of high blood cholesterol in adults (Adult Treatment Panel III). *JAMA* 2001;285(19):2486–2497.

22. American Diabetes Association. Microvascular complications and foot care: Standards of medical care in diabetes—2018. *Diabetes Care* 2018;41(Suppl 1):S105–S118.

23. Pop-Busui R, Boulton AJM, Feldman EL, et al. Diabetic neuropathy: A position statement by the American Diabetes Association. *Diabetes Care* 2017;40(1):136–154.

24. Ziegler D, Low PA, Litchy WJ, et al. Efficacy and safety of antioxidant treatment with α-lipoic acid over four years in diabetic polyneuropathy: The NATHAN 1 trial. *Diabetes Care* 2011;34(9):2054–2060.

25. Young LH, Wackers FJT, Chyun DA, et al; DIAD Investigators. Cardiac outcomes after screening for asymptomatic coronary artery disease in patients with type 2 diabetes: The DIAD study: A randomized controlled trial. *JAMA* 2009;301(15):1547–1555.

26. American Diabetes Association. Comprehensive medical evaluation and assessment of comorbidities: Standards of medical care in diabetes—2018. *Diabetes Care* 2018;41(Suppl 1):S29–S37.

27. Tomczyk S, Bennett NM, Stoecker C, et al., Use of 13-valent pneumococcal conjugate vaccine and 23-valent pneumococcal polysaccharide vaccine among adults aged ≥65 years: Recommendations of the Advisory Committee on Immunization Practices (ACIP). *MMWR Morb Mortal Wkly Rep* 2014;63(37):822–825.

28. Al-Arouj M, Assaad-Khalil S, Buse J, et al. Recommendations for management of diabetes during Ramadan: Update 2010. *Diabetes Care* 2010;33(8):1895–1902.

29. Hassanein M, Al-Arouj M, Hamdy O, et al. Diabetes and Ramadan: Practical guidelines. *Diabetes Res Clin Pract* 2017;126:303–316.

Type 1 Diabetes Mellitus

Jing W. Hughes and Janet B. McGill

GENERAL PRINCIPLES

- Type 1 diabetes mellitus (T1DM) is an illness in which autoimmune destruction of pancreatic β cells causes **insulin deficiency** and **hyperglycemia**.
- Insulin deficiency can lead to acute metabolic decompensation known as **diabetic ketoacidosis (DKA)**; however, exogenous insulin taken in excess of immediate needs can produce life-threatening hypoglycemia.
- Chronic hyperglycemia is the root cause of disabling microvascular complications and contributes to macrovascular disease.
- The treatment goal of T1DM is normalization of blood glucose (BG) by physiologically based insulin replacement therapy.

Epidemiology

- The overall prevalence of the disease is 0.25% to 0.5% of the population, or 1 in 400 children and 1 in 200 adults in the United States.
- The incidence of T1DM is increasing in developed countries, and it is appearing at younger ages.[1,2]
- The peak onset occurs at age 10 to 14 years, but it can be diagnosed from a few months of age into the ninth decade of life.
- Males and females are equally affected.
- T1DM accounts for 10% of all cases of diabetes and needs to be accurately diagnosed so that insulin therapy is not delayed or withheld inappropriately.

Etiology

- The **autoimmune process that selectively destroys pancreatic β cells** is T-cell mediated with an unknown antigenic stimulus in genetically susceptible individuals.[3,4]
  - Environmental factors, including coxsackie and rubella viruses, and dietary factors such as early exposure to cow's milk, have been implicated.
  - Insulitis (lymphocytic infiltration of pancreatic islets) is an early finding, followed by immune destruction of β cells, which leads to their virtual absence later in the disease course.
  - Antibodies to β-cell antigens can be found in the majority of patients before diagnosis and for some time after the onset of clinical diabetes.
  - These disease markers are antibodies to **glutamic acid decarboxylase (GAD65)**, to **tyrosine phosphatases IA-2** and **IA-2 beta**, **insulin (IAA)**, and **zinc transporter (ZnT8)**.
  - Of these markers, GAD65 is positive in 80% of children and adults near the time of diagnosis, whereas IA-2 and IAA are positive in ~50% of children and are less likely to be present in adults.
  - The presence of two antibodies has high sensitivity and specificity for rapid progression to insulin dependency and may help clarify the diagnosis in some patients.
- In cases of T1DM in which no evidence of autoimmunity can be detected, the classification is *idiopathic T1DM*.

- Several organ-specific and systemic **autoimmune diseases occur with increased frequency in patients with T1DM**, including autoimmune thyroiditis (Hashimoto or Graves' diseases), Addison disease, pernicious anemia, celiac sprue, vitiligo, alopecia, and autoimmune hepatitis.[5,6]
  - In a study of 265 adults with T1DM, the risk of thyroid disease was 32% for the proband, 25% for siblings, and 42% for parents, with females more commonly affected than males.
  - The risk of developing autoimmune thyroid disease and pernicious anemia increases with age, so periodic screening should continue throughout adulthood in patients with T1DM and their family members.
- The **genetic susceptibility** to T1DM is manifested by linkage with several gene loci and association with HLA-DR and DQ.[7]
  - Genome-wide association studies identified additional-risk loci BACH2, C1QTNF6, CTSH, and PRKCQ.[7]
  - The *IDDM1* gene located in the HLA region of chromosome 6p21.3, and the *IDDM2* gene in the region 5' upstream of the insulin gene on chromosome 11p15.5 contribute 42% and 10%, respectively, to the observed familial clustering.
  - In the family of a patient with T1DM, the risk of an identical twin developing T1DM is 50%, an offspring is 6%, and a sibling is 5%.
- The striking familial discordance supports the importance of environmental factors.

Pathophysiology

- Patients with both T1DM and type 2 diabetes mellitus (T2DM) are susceptible to organ dysfunction that is caused by long-term exposure to hyperglycemia and which leads to devastating morbidity and mortality.[8]
- The **microvascular complications** of diabetes are retinopathy, nephropathy, and neuropathy.
- Although they share some pathogenic features, they may not appear at the same time or with the same severity in all individuals with diabetes. The pathogenesis of these complications includes increased oxidative stress, abnormal activation of signaling cascades, and stimulation of hemodynamic regulation systems.
  - **Advanced glycation end-products** are formed by processes of glycation and/or oxidation of proteins, nucleotides, and lipids, and have intrinsic cellular toxicity.
  - High levels of glucose and reactive oxygen species have been shown to increase diacylglycerol and stimulate protein kinase C activity, causing alterations in intracellular signal transduction and production of cytokines and growth factors.[9]
- Glucose enters peripheral nerves by mass action, is converted first to sorbitol by aldose reductase, and is then converted to fructose by sorbitol dehydrogenase. These saccharides produce osmotic stress, increase glycation, and cause alterations in the NADH/NAD ratio, which collectively contribute to nerve fiber damage and symptoms of **peripheral neuropathy**.
- **Diabetic retinopathy** is associated with abnormal remodeling of the vascular endothelium due to hyperglycemia and increased cytokines such as vascular endothelial growth factor.
- In **diabetic nephropathy**, hyperglycemia induces transforming growth factor β, which stimulates matrix synthesis and inhibits matrix degradation in renal mesangial cells. Investigational agents that target these processes are currently in clinical development.

DIAGNOSIS

Clinical Presentation

- T1DM develops most commonly in childhood but can present at any age.
- Because 80% of cases occur without a positive family history, symptoms may be overlooked until hyperglycemia reaches critical levels.

- The **prodromal symptoms are related to hyperglycemia** and include weight loss, polyuria, polydipsia, polyphagia, and blurred vision.
- If DKA is present, the patient might complain of abdominal pain, nausea, vomiting, myalgia, shortness of breath, and exhibit changes in mental and hemodynamic status.

History
- In previously diagnosed patients, the **history of present illness** should document the duration of the illness, frequency of hyper- and hypoglycemia, results of self-monitored BG (SMBG) testing, dietary habits, and the status of any microvascular or macrovascular complications.
- The history of present illness or medication history should **record the insulin regimen in detail** and provide an assessment of adequacy of, or problems with, the regimen.
- In female adolescents and adult women, menstrual, sexual, and gestational histories should be elicited and the method of birth control should be documented.
- Smoking behavior, alcohol and drug use, socioeconomic status, and social support are all important factors in the care of a patient with T1DM.

Physical Examination
- If the patient presents in **DKA**, signs of dehydration and acidosis, such as tachycardia, orthostatic hypotension, and dry mucus membranes, might be evident.
- Fruity odor to the breath reflects the presence of ketones.
- Routine follow-up physical examinations should document height, weight, and Tanner staging in children to determine that growth and development are advancing normally.
- Blood pressure and heart rate are important measures for all patients with T1DM.
- At least annually, the physical examination should include skin, funduscopic, oral, thyroid, and cardiovascular examinations, as well as sensory testing and foot screening.
- Dilated eye examination by an ophthalmologist is recommended at 3 to 5 years of T1DM duration, with scheduling of repeat examinations based on clinical findings.

Diagnostic Testing
- The diagnosis of diabetes mellitus, based upon the guidelines of the American Diabetes Association (ADA) can be made based on one of these four abnormalities of glucose metabolism:[10]
  - Hyperglycemia symptoms and a random venous plasma glucose ≥200 mg/dL.
  - Fasting plasma glucose ≥126 mg/dL, confirmed on a second sample if <200 mg/dL.
  - Glycated hemoglobin (HbA1c) ≥6.5% (using an assay that is certified by the National Glycohemoglobin Standardization Program).
  - Abnormal oral glucose tolerance test (OGTT). Two-hour plasma glucose level of ≥200 mg/dL after ingestion of a 75-g glucose drink. However, OGTT is rarely needed to diagnose T1DM.
  - Typically, people with T1DM present with symptoms of hyperglycemia, possibly in DKA, and markedly elevated BG, **random plasma glucose ≥200 mg/dL.**
- After the diagnosis of diabetes mellitus is made, T1DM must be differentiated from other types of diabetes.
  - This is based upon clinical presentation (body habitus, age, signs of insulin resistance, history [family history], and if necessary, laboratory studies).
  - If patient has not had DKA and the diagnosis of T1DM is unclear, testing for islet-specific pancreatic autoantibodies, GAD65, or the 40K fragment of tyrosine phosphatase IA-2B (also known as *ICA*), or IAA, or C-peptide level can be useful.[10]
  - C-peptide levels are typically low or undetectable in patients with T1DM.
  - Of note, the absence of pancreatic autoantibodies does not rule out T1DM. Also, antibodies may be present in up to 30 percent of individuals with other forms of diabetes.

- **Hemoglobin A1c** (HbA1c) should be measured 2 to 4 times per year, and a lipid profile, serum creatinine and electrolytes, and urine microalbumin-to-creatinine ratio should be checked at least annually in adolescents and adults. Screening for thyroid antibodies is recommended, and thyroid-stimulating hormone (TSH) should be checked annually if the patient is antibody positive or has a goiter.[10]

TREATMENT

- **Goals of treatment**
  - The goal of diabetes treatment is to **maintain the BG as close to normal as possible** and to **avoid hypoglycemia**.
  - All patients with T1DM require insulin therapy, and early achievement of a near-normal HbA1c has been shown to preserve residual beta-cell function and to reduce long-term complications.[11]
  - The Diabetes Control and Complications Trial (DCCT) and its follow-up study have shown that every 1% reduction in HbA1c reduces retinopathy by 33%,[11,12] microalbuminuria by 22%,[13] and neuropathy by 38%.[14]
  - Tight control early on, during the first 5 to 10 years of diabetes before the manifestation of complications, confers long-term risk reduction, supporting the hypothesis that hyperglycemia induces organ toxicity that can be self-perpetuating (glycemic memory).
  - In children, the therapeutic goals include ensuring normal growth and development and the scrupulous avoidance of severe hypoglycemia at young ages.
  - In the postpubertal adolescent and adult patient, maintenance of normal blood pressure, achievement of target lipid levels, smoking cessation, aspirin use in patients older than age 40, and preconception counseling are important treatment goals. (Please refer to Chapter 28 for detailed recommendations.)
- **Glucose monitoring**
  - Patients with T1DM should be encouraged to do **SMBG** at least 4 times daily so that appropriate insulin adjustments can be made based on ambient glucose levels.
  - These recommendations may be modified for children with school considerations.
  - Increased monitoring is required during acute illnesses, for intense exercise, and before and during pregnancy.
    - Alternate site testing; rapid readings; and meters with averaging, graphing, and download functions have helped patients with the challenging task of SMBG.
    - Periodic monitoring during the nighttime is recommended for all patients to check for nocturnal hypoglycemia.
  - **Continuous glucose monitoring systems** (CGM) are available to assist with diabetes management. The accuracy has improved over the years, and some devices are approved for insulin dosing, which is called nonadjunctive use. Medicare and most insurers approve these devices for patients with T1DM who meet certain criteria, such as monitoring frequently and taking four injections of insulin per day. Some of the systems have alarms that can be set for high and low glucoses. This supplemental tool is especially useful for those with hypoglycemia unawareness.
    - CGM devices measure glucose level in the interstitial fluid on a continuous basis, providing information about the direction, magnitude, and duration of glycemic fluctuations.
    - CGM devices are now integrated with insulin pumps and provide suspend features for hypoglycemia or hybrid close-loop insulin basal rate adjustments.
    - CGM readings can be shared with family members, or displayed while driving, adding another layer of safety.
    - The use of CGM-directed therapy has been shown to decrease the frequency of hypoglycemia and improve HbA1c.[15,16]

Diet

- Patients should receive medical nutrition therapy (MNT), which is an individualized assessment and instruction on diet and is most effectively provided by a registered dietitian.
- The caloric requirement for people with moderate physical activity is approximately 35 kcal/kg/day, but there is significant variation from person-to-person and day-to-day.[10]
  - Individualized instruction should consider the patient's caloric needs, ethnicity, habits, constraints, and prescribed insulin regimen.
  - The diet for patients with diabetes should aim to achieve an ideal HbA1c, blood pressure, and lipid profile.
  - Attention should be paid to balancing energy intake and expenditure to avoid excess weight gain.
  - Patients on fixed-dose insulin regimens need to have a consistent day-to-day carbohydrate intake.
  - Mastery of either an exchange system or carbohydrate counting allows for flexibility in meal planning, and helps avoid postprandial hypo- or hyperglycemia.
  - Review of dietary principles is a cost-effective way to help the patient achieve treatment targets.

Medications

Insulin Therapy

- Insulin regimens must be individualized to cater to a given patient's lifestyle and comorbidities.
- Insulin types and pharmacokinetics are shown in Table 29-1.
- Flexible insulin regimens with **multiple daily injections (MDI)** or use of an insulin pump can best approximate the physiologic insulin response (Table 29-2).
- Insulin prescriptions consisting of a long-acting basal and rapid-acting preprandial insulin formulations (given based on carbohydrate intake) are best suited for reaching HbA1c goals while minimizing the risk of hypoglycemia.
- **Continuous subcutaneous insulin infusion (CSII)** via an insulin pump has the added benefit of allowing for variable basal rates and flexibility in delivering bolus insulin doses.
- The DCCT and other studies have clearly demonstrated that patients are more likely to achieve glycemic targets using **intensified insulin therapy with basal and bolus components** than with conventional therapy with one or two injections.[11]
  - Decisions about the appropriate insulin regimen should be made with the patient's abilities and scheduling constraints in mind.
  - In general, patients need an **intermediate- or long-acting insulin to cover basal needs** and a **rapid- or short-acting insulin to provide meal coverage**.
  - When initiating or changing an insulin regimen, an estimation of the **total daily dose (TDD)** should be made. Individual requirements vary, but usually range from 0.5 to 0.8 units/kg/day; higher if insulin resistance is present.
- Historically, the most widely prescribed regimen was "split-mixed," which used NPH as the basal insulin and a short- or rapid-acting analog before breakfast and dinner.
  - Use of this regimen presumed that the patient would eat lunch at a standard time, because the morning NPH is likely to peak at about midday. Patient scheduling problems and the erratic pharmacokinetics of NPH have made this regimen less popular.
  - If NPH is used, the dose will be about 0.2 units/kg, twice a day.
- The most commonly prescribed regimens for patients with T1DM by endocrinologists today are **MDI** or **CSII**. These regimens use the concepts of basal and bolus (premeal) dosing.

TABLE 29-1 INSULIN TYPES AND PHARMACOKINETICS/PHARMACODYNAMICS[a]

Insulin	Onset	Peak	Duration
Rapid acting[b]			
Insulin aspart (NovoLog, Fiasp)	10–20 minutes, 3–15 minutes	1–2 hours 60–90 minutes	3–4 hours 3–4 hours
Insulin lispro (Humalog)	10–20 minutes	1–2 hours	3–4 hours
Insulin glulisine (Apidra)	10–20 minutes	1–2 hours	3–4 hours
Technosphere insulin (Afrezza)	10 minutes	30 minutes	2 hours
Short acting			
Regular ("R")	0.5–1.0 hour	2–4 hours	4–8 hours
Regular U-500[c]	1.0 hour	4–6 hours	8–14 hours
Intermediate acting			
NPH ("N")[d]	1.5–3 hours	4–10 hours	10–18 hours
Long acting			
Insulin detemir (Levemir)	1–2 hours	6–8 hours	16–24 hours
Insulin glargine (Lantus, Basaglar, Toujeo)[e]	2–3 hours	None	~24 hours
Insulin degludec (Tresiba)[f]	2–3 hours	None	40 hours

[a]Insulin pharmacokinetics and pharmacodynamics show significant inter- and intra-subject variation. The onset, peak, and duration may be influenced by the dose administered, injection site, skin temperature, and other less well-defined factors.

[b]Rapid-acting insulin should be administered before meals. Injectable rapid-acting insulin is suitable for insulin pump use.

[c]Human regular insulin (Humulin U-500) is 5× concentrated compared to U-100 regular insulin.

[d]Cloudy, suspended formulations require resuspension by rolling and tipping (but not shaking) the vial before administration. Resuspension is a potential source of erratic pharmacokinetics.

[e]Insulin glargine is available in U-100 and U-300 concentrations. Do not mix with any other type of insulin in the same syringe due to incompatible pH. Clear preparation, no resuspension needed.

[f]Insulin degludec is available in U-100 and U-200 concentrations.

Multiple Daily Injections

- The **basal dose** is generally 45% to 55% of the TDD, ~0.4 units/kg/day, and is given in one injection (insulin glargine, insulin degludec) or two injections (human NPH, insulin detemir, insulin glargine).
  - The basal insulin dose is adjusted so that the fasting BG is routinely within the target of 80 to 120 mg/dL, and there is <30 mg/dL variation between evening and morning values.
  - Changes in weight, exercise, persistent hyperglycemia, or frequent hypoglycemia should prompt reconsideration of the basal insulin dose.

TABLE 29-2 MDI OR CSII INSULIN DOSING REGIMEN

Time	Dose	Regimen
Before breakfast, lunch, and dinner	0.15–0.2 × TDD or units determined by carbohydrate counting plus correction factor	Rapid acting insulin
Before bed (can be given in the morning or split into two doses) or continuously in insulin pump	0.4–0.55 × TDD	Insulin glargine, detemir or degludec. If NPH is used, give one-half in the morning and one-half in the evening. Rapid acting insulin is preferred in insulin pumps

- **Bolus doses** are administered to cover carbohydrate intake and to correct high BG readings. Premeal bolus doses are determined by one or more of the following methods:
  - Fixed amount before each meal, ~0.13 U/kg or one-sixth of the TDD.
  - Fixed dose before each meal as above plus a sliding scale "correction factor" (see subsequent text) based on the premeal SMBG.
  - Carbohydrate counting plus "correction factor" uses variable amounts depending on the anticipated carbohydrate intake and the premeal SMBG.
  - Both the patient and the physician need to learn important concepts to succeed in the use of MDI regimens. If fixed amounts of premeal insulin are to be used, the patient should have a clear idea of the prescribed meal plan and be able to follow it precisely.
  - Alternatively, the patient can adjust the premeal dose based on the anticipated carbohydrate content, which allows greater flexibility. To do this, the physician or diabetes educator must determine the **"insulin-to-carbohydrate"** ratio, which can be calculated by dividing 500 by the TDD.
    - A patient who takes 50 U of insulin daily needs 1 U of insulin for every 10 g of carbohydrate intake.
    - The patient needs to learn which foods contain carbohydrate, how to estimate the grams of carbohydrate in the serving provided, and how to calculate the premeal dose.
    - Additional adjustments are sometimes made for high fat meals or for meals that have high fiber content.
    - Timing of bolus dosing is crucial, since even "rapid-acting" insulins do not have an immediate effect. In general, bolus or premeal insulin should be taken before eating, with time to correct higher glucoses if present.
    - Patients may benefit from a more rapid acting insulin such as technosphere insulin (Afrezza), or a newer product in development to keep the postprandial glucose rise to a minimum while avoiding late postprandial hypoglycemia.
- In addition to covering calories, the patient must be able to compensate for high or low BG readings. An individualized sliding scale, known as the **correction factor** is determined, which provides the number of units to be added (or subtracted) to each premeal dose. The correction factor is estimated by dividing 1,800 by the TDD.

Sample Calculations
- Example 1: a modestly overweight patient takes 60 U of insulin daily. His current BG is 178 mg/dL, and he is about to eat a meal with 90 g of carbohydrate. His physician has

told him that his target SMBG is 120 mg/dL. What dose of rapid-acting insulin should he take?

- ○ Insulin-to-carbohydrate ratio = 500/60 = 1 U insulin/8.33 g.
- ○ Correction factor = 1,800/60 = 30 (predicts that 1 U insulin drops the BG 30 mg/dL) 90 g carbohydrates/8.33 g/U insulin = ~10 U insulin to cover carbohydrates.
- ○ SMBG–target BG = 178 mg/dL–120 = 58 mg/dL. He will take 2 U insulin as correction.
- ○ Thus, the patient should take 12 U of rapid-acting insulin.
- Example 2: a thin, insulin-sensitive patient takes 30 U of insulin per day. If this patient has a current BG of 178 mg/dL and is about to eat her usual meal containing 45 grams of carbohydrate, how much insulin should she use?
  - ○ Insulin to carbohydrate ratio = 500/30 = 1 U insulin/16.66 g.
  - ○ Correction factor = 1,800/30 = 60 (predicts that 1 U insulin will drop the BG 60 mg/dL).
  - ○ 45 g carbohydrates/16.66 g/U insulin = ~3 U insulin to cover carbohydrates.
  - ○ SMBG–target BG = 178–120 = 58 mg/dL.
  - ○ She will take 1 U insulin as correction.
  - ○ Thus, this patient should take 4 U of rapid-acting insulin. Using an insulin pen that provides doses in half units, this patient may elect to take 3.5 units.

Continuous Subcutaneous Insulin Infusion

- **Insulin pump therapy** has become a popular alternative to MDI and has both advantages and disadvantages.
- Technologic advances have contributed to smaller pumps with features such as multiple basal rates, dose calculators, and alternate-dosing modalities.
- CSII systems now include continuous glucose monitoring, which assist with dosing adjustments and have suspension features ("closed loop system"). Hybrid systems using both insulin and glucagon may further reduce the risk of hypoglycemia and are in development.
- CSII offers the patient with T1DM the greatest flexibility and is more socially acceptable than needles and syringes for frequent dosing. Insulin pumps are the size of a pager and contain 180 to 300 U of insulin in a specialized syringe that is connected to a subcutaneous (SC) catheter by thin tubing.
- The SC catheter should be changed and repositioned every 3 days. The pump is preprogrammed to infuse the basal rate of insulin, but the patient must activate the pump to deliver bolus doses at the time of the meal or when a correction is needed.
- Only rapid-acting insulin is used. Diabetes education from an educator experienced in CSII is necessary to teach the patient how to use the pump, which requires several hours of instruction.
- **Insulin dose prescribing is conceptually similar to MDI**; however, the TDD is reduced 10% to 20%.
  - ○ The **basal rate** (equal to one-half of the new TDD) is divided by 24 and programmed as an hourly rate. For example, a patient taking 48 U/day with MDI will need ~20 U for basal requirements, or ~0.8 U/hr to start. The basal rate can be adjusted to accommodate nighttime low BG, morning rise, and increased or decreased activity during the day. The basal rate can be temporarily reduced for exercise or the pump can be put in suspended mode for hypoglycemia.
  - ○ **Bolus dosing** is handled similarly to MDI, with a key exception. Today's insulin pumps can administer doses in very small quantities, so the correction factor can be prescribed as a fraction. The opportunity to give smaller doses is helpful for children and insulin-sensitive patients.
- The **major disadvantage** of CSII is the high cost of an insulin pump and supplies. Because only rapid-acting insulin is used, a pump or catheter failure can result in fast-rising BG and DKA within 8 to 12 hours.

- Another potential disadvantage is the risk of catheter-site infection, which is minimized by instruction in semi-sterile techniques.

Adjusting Insulin Doses
- Insulin dose adjustments or changes to the insulin regimen are made after evaluating either SMBG values or a CGM tracing and looking for patterns.
- **The efficacy of a specific rapid-acting insulin dose is monitored by the glucose values that follow the dose in question** (e.g., postprandial or noon glucoses reflect the breakfast dose of rapid-acting insulin).
- Intermediate and long-acting insulin doses are evaluated by scrutinizing the SMBG or CGM tracing after the injection (e.g., morning glucoses to determine adequacy of evening dose) and review of overall frequency of hyper- and hypoglycemia.
- Diabetes educators are skilled at insulin dose adjustments and provide a valuable resource for patients who are experiencing problems keeping their glucose values near the target range.
- Diabetes education is cost-effective and necessary to achieve tight glycemic control while avoiding hypoglycemic episodes.

Adjunct Therapy
- Pramlintide (Symlin), a synthetic analog of the beta-cell secretory product amylin, is approved for use as adjunctive therapy to insulin in patients with T1DM. It is given as a separate injection of 15 to 45 mcg before meals, and helps reduce postprandial glucose excursions by suppressing glucagon and enhancing satiety.
- It has a modest effect on HbA1c of about 0.5%, and may contribute to modest weight loss. Side effects are nausea, vomiting, and increased risk of hypoglycemia. Insulin adjustments are needed when pramlintide is prescribed.[17,18]
- Other adjunct therapy including metformin and SGLT-2 inhibitors are currently under investigation for use in patients with T1DM.

Lifestyle/Risk Modification

Diet
- Patients should receive MNT, which is an **individualized assessment and instruction** on diet and is most effectively provided by a registered dietitian.
- The caloric requirement for people with moderate physical activity is approximately 35 kcal/kg/day, but there is significant variation from person-to-person and day-to-day.[10]
  - Individualized instruction should consider the patient's caloric needs, ethnicity, habits, constraints, and prescribed insulin regimen.
  - The diet for patients with diabetes should aim to achieve an ideal HbA1c, blood pressure, and lipid profile.
  - Attention should be paid to balancing energy intake and expenditure to avoid excess weight gain.
  - Patients on fixed-dose insulin regimens need to have a consistent day-to-day carbohydrate intake.
  - Mastery of either an exchange system or carbohydrate counting allows for flexibility in meal planning, and helps avoid postprandial hypo- or hyperglycemia.
  - Review of dietary principles is a cost-effective way to help the patient achieve treatment targets.

COMPLICATIONS

Diabetic Ketoacidosis
- DKA is the direct result of relative insulin deficiency; dehydration and excess counter-regulatory hormones (glucagon, epinephrine, and cortisol) are accelerating factors.[19]

- Typically, an **exacerbating factor** can be identified: new diagnosis of diabetes, omission of insulin doses, infection, pregnancy, trauma, emotional stress, excessive alcohol ingestion, myocardial infarction, stroke, concurrent illness, hyperthyroidism, Cushing disease, or rarely, pheochromocytoma.
- The major clinical features of DKA are hyperglycemia, dehydration, acidosis, abdominal pain, nausea, vomiting, change in hemodynamic status, and altered mental status.[19]
- **Pathophysiology**
  - The pathophysiology of DKA begins with insulin levels that are insufficient to support peripheral glucose uptake and to suppress hepatic gluconeogenesis.
  - Hyperglycemia is further driven by increases in the counter-regulatory hormones glucagon, catecholamines, cortisol, and growth hormone. Activation of catabolic pathways in muscle and fat produce amino acids and free fatty acids, which fuel hepatic gluconeogenesis and ketone production.
  - The osmotic diuresis imposed by hyperglycemia causes marked fluid and electrolyte losses, further stimulating catecholamine release.
  - Catecholamines are antagonistic to insulin action and contribute to increased lipolysis, which pumps free fatty acids into the circulation that then undergo fatty acid oxidation to ketone bodies.
  - Volume depletion decreases renal blood flow, which contributes to reduced excretion of glucose and ketones and increased serum levels of creatinine and potassium.
  - Acidosis ensues when the levels of acetone, acetoacetate, and β-hydroxybutyrate exceed the buffering capacity of bicarbonate and the respiratory response.
  - Low $PaCO_2$ reflects the respiratory effort and the severity of the metabolic acidosis.
  - The presence of an anion gap and low bicarbonate in the setting of high BG and an ill-appearing patient should prompt immediate treatment for DKA while confirmatory laboratory evaluation is under way.[19,20]
  - Use of point of care ketone meters at triage or in an urgent care setting helps to make the diagnosis of DKA and may prevent delays in treatment.[20,21]
  - The differential diagnosis for anion gap acidosis is outlined in Table 29-3.
- **Symptoms**
  - The symptoms of DKA are nonspecific and include anorexia, nausea, vomiting (coffee-ground emesis in 25%), abdominal pain, and myalgias or weakness.
  - Polyuria and polydipsia are characteristic of high BG, but may become blunted due to vomiting, reduced renal clearance, and altered mental status as the severity of DKA worsens.
  - Hyperpnea is noted with mild acidosis, and the patient may complain of shortness of breath. Kussmaul breathing is a sign of a critically ill patient.
  - The physical examination reveals tachycardia, hypotension, or orthostatic hypotension, dry mucous membranes, poor skin turgor, abdominal tenderness, and other signs of clinical events that may have prompted the DKA episode. Mental status can be normal or severely compromised. Signs of a concurrent illness or event that precipitated the DKA may be present.
- **Laboratory findings**
  - Laboratory findings of DKA include the following: glucose >250 mg/dL, glycosuria, an elevated anion gap (normal gap is ≤12), and the presence of serum or urine ketones or β-hydroxybutyrate.[19–21]
  - The anion gap is calculated as follows: (anion gap = $Na+ - [Cl + HCO3]$). The serum bicarbonate is typically <15 mEq/L, the pCO2 <40 mm Hg, and the arterial pH <7.3, β-hydroxybutyrate >1.5 mmol/L.[19–21]
  - Creatinine and K^+ are generally increased above baseline.
    - If hypokalemia is present at the time of diagnosis, the patient has severe K^+ depletion and requires careful monitoring.

TABLE 29-3	DIFFERENTIAL DIAGNOSIS OF ANION-GAP ACIDOSIS (THE MUDPILES MNEMONIC)

Conditions	Clinical associations
M: Methanol ingestion	Visual impairment/blindness; osmol gap between the calculated and measured osmolality (seen with any alcohol ingestion)
U: Uremia	History of renal failure; increased serum urea and creatinine
D: Diabetic ketoacidosis	History of diabetes, hyperglycemia
P: Paraldehyde	Formaldehyde-like breath odor; increased paraldehyde level
I: Iron; isoniazid	Increased serum iron level; patient may have elevated hepatic transaminases with isoniazid toxicity
L: Lactic acidosis	May be due to hypovolemia/sepsis, infarction, metformin, cyanide, hydrogen sulfide, CO, methemoglobin; lactate levels are elevated
E: EtOH; ethylene glycol	Osmol gap between the calculated and measured osmolality (seen with any alcohol ingestion); increased EtOH level seen with EtOH intoxication; calcium oxalate crystals seen in the urine with ethylene glycol
S: Salicylates	Tinnitus, increased salicylate level, may have a concurrent respiratory alkalosis

EtOH, ethanol.

- Often the initial potassium level is high, and the ECG should be checked for signs of hyperkalemia, which include peaked T waves, shortened QT intervals, widened QRS complexes, and flattened or absent P waves.
- Later in the course of treatment, if hypokalemia occurs, a repeat ECG might show ST-segment depression, flattened or inverted T waves, a prolonged QT interval, and appearance of U waves.
   - Pseudohyponatremia may be present, thus the measured serum sodium should be corrected for the high glucose (add 1.6 to the reported sodium for every 100 mg/dL that the glucose is >100 mg/dL), and may be further depressed by high triglycerides.
   - Amylase and lipase may be elevated via unclear mechanisms, do not necessarily indicate pancreatitis, and resolve with treatment of the DKA.
- **Treatment of DKA**
   - Clinical evaluation and triage
      - Intensive care admission is required for patients with hemodynamic instability or mental status changes, for pediatric patients, or if frequent monitoring is not possible on a medical ward.
      - Hemodynamic monitoring may be required for patients in shock, with possible sepsis, with DKA complicated by myocardial infarction, or in patients with end-stage renal disease or chronic heart failure.
      - Nasogastric tube placement may be needed for patients with hematemesis or for comatose patients.

- ○ **Fluids and electrolytes:** Fluid resuscitation in adults should begin with normal saline at 1 L/hr unless there is a contraindication (chronic heart failure, end-stage renal disease).
  - ▪ The typical total body water deficit is 4 to 6 L, sodium deficit is 7 to 10 mEq/kg, K⁺ deficit is 3 to 5 mEq/kg, and PO4 deficit is 5 to 7 mmol/kg. If the corrected sodium is normal or high on repeat testing, change the intravenous fluids to 0.45% NaCl; continue 0.9% saline if it is low.
  - ▪ When the K^+ drops to <5.0 mEq/L and the patient has adequate urine output, add 20 to 30 mEq K^+ to each liter of intravenous fluid.
  - ▪ Plan to correct the water and salt deficits over 24 hours, slower in children. The starting fluid administration rate for children should be 10 to 20 mL/kg/hr and should not exceed 50 mL/kg over the first 4 hours of therapy.
  - ▪ Patients presenting with DKA have PO4 depletion due to osmotic diuresis, although this may not be apparent on presentation because insulin deficiency and acidosis cause PO4 to shift out of cells. Serum PO4 levels decrease with insulin therapy.
  - ▪ Except in very severe cases of hypophosphatemia (serum PO4 <1.0 mg/dL) or concomitant cardiorespiratory compromise, routine administration of PO4 has not been shown to be beneficial and may, in fact, be harmful because excess replacement can cause hypocalcemia.
  - ▪ Bicarbonate therapy in DKA is controversial and it should not be routinely administered, unless the serum pH is <7.0 or the patient has life-threatening hyperkalemia.
- • **Insulin and glucose**
  - ○ Initial intravenous loading bolus 0.1 to 0.15 units/kg of regular (R) insulin followed by continuous infusion 0.1 units/kg/hr (100 units R insulin/100 mL normal saline solution), though not all guidelines recommend a loading bolus.[19,20] Children should not receive intravenous bolus doses of insulin; infusion should be started.[14]
  - ○ Monitor serum glucose every hour and expect the BG to decline by 50 to 75 mg/dL/hr. A slower response could indicate insulin resistance, inadequate fluid resuscitation, or improper insulin delivery.
    - ▪ As the acidosis clears, the glucose is likely to fall more rapidly. When the serum glucose is <250 mg/dL, add 5% dextrose to the intravenous fluids, and decrease the insulin infusion rate by up to one-half.
    - ▪ If the glucose infusion rate is kept stable, the insulin infusion requirements will be more predictable.
    - ▪ Continue intensive insulin therapy and monitoring until the patient is tolerating oral intake and the anion-gap acidosis has resolved. As the acidosis resolves, the anion gap closes, arterial and venous pH rise, and serum bicarbonate rises.
    - ▪ The ADA position paper regarding the treatment of DKA states that criteria for the resolution of DKA include a glucose <200 mg/dL, a serum bicarbonate ≥18 mEq/L, and a venous pH >7.3.[19,22]
    - ▪ Patients recovering from DKA may develop a transient non–anion-gap hyperchloremic metabolic acidosis that occurs because of urinary loss of "potential bicarbonate" in the form of ketoanions and their replacement by chloride ions from intravenous fluids. This non–anion-gap acidosis is transient and has not been shown to be clinically significant, except in renal failure.
  - ○ **Common error:** the hyperglycemia will respond to treatment faster than the acidosis will resolve. Do not decrease or discontinue the insulin infusion when glucose levels approach the normal range. This can lead to worsening of the ketoacidosis. Instead, continue the intravenous insulin infusion, but adjust the dose and/or add 5% dextrose at a rate of 50 to 75 mL/hr, not at resuscitation rates. If 5% dextrose is infused at excessively rapid rates, the BG will increase, and the transition to SC insulin will be delayed.
- • **Monitoring**
  - ○ Fingerstick BG every hour during insulin infusion.

- Electrolytes, blood urea nitrogen (BUN), and creatinine levels every 2 to 4 hours until the K^+ has stabilized and the anion-gap acidosis is resolved.
- Serum ketones or β-hydroxybutyrate level by fingerstick point-of-care device on admission and in follow-up if available.[20,21]
- Intake and output, weight.

- **Transition to subcutaneous insulin**
  - Continue the intravenous insulin infusion and intravenous fluids until the acidosis has cleared, the glucose is <250 mg/dL, and the patient is able to eat. Note: it is possible for the patient to attempt a small or clear liquid meal while on an insulin drip, but the drip rate may need to be increased for the meal hour and then returned to the usual rate.
  - Make the transition to SC insulin before the insulin drip is discontinued, ideally at a time close to usual insulin administration. Some guidelines recommend continuing the scheduled basal insulin during the initial management of DKA to avoid rebound hyperglycemia when IV insulin is stopped.[20]
  - If the patient has been previously diagnosed, give the usual premeal insulin dose plus any correction factor, and cover basal needs with intermediate- or long-acting insulin. If the patient is newly diagnosed, give basal insulin at ~–0.2 units/kg and bolus doses of ~0.1 units/kg/meal.
    - For example, if the drip can be stopped at noon, give a premeal dose of short-acting insulin according to the patient's usual schedule and add a partial dose of NPH to cover until dinner or bedtime.
    - If basal insulin has not been continued during the acute phase of treatment, start basal insulin (NPH, detemir [Levemir], glargine [Lantus, Basaglar, Toujeo], or deglu-dec [Tresiba]) and short-acting insulin a minimum of 2 hours before stopping the insulin drip.
    - Keep the rate of intravenous dextrose to ≤100 mL/hour or discontinue it if the patient is able to eat.
    - Note that intravenous fluids may need to be continued until the serum creatinine has returned to baseline.

- **Problem solving**
  - Recurring DKA should prompt additional history to search for precipitating causes. Insulin pump malfunction, noncompliance with insulin doses, social distress, medication problems, or concomitant illness should warrant attention of an experienced diabetes care provider.
  - Newly diagnosed patients require additional time in the hospital for the institution of an insulin regimen and diabetes education.
  - DKA is associated with poorer cognitive function, especially in children.[23,24]
  - Recurrent DKA is associated with increased mortality, particularly among young adults with poor glucose control and psychosocial challenges.[25]

Chronic Complications

- Care of the patient with T1DM includes screening for microvascular and macrovascular complications, and the application of proven therapies to reduce morbidity and mortality.
- Tight glycemic control prevents against macrovascular disease, as established by the DCCT and the Epidemiology of Diabetes Interventions and Complications (EDIC) study.[11,12,13]
- Maintaining strict glycemic control in type 1 diabetics has beneficial effects on primary and secondary prevention of microvascular complications; this was demonstrated by the DCCT.[11]
- The best-studied intervention in T1DM is the use of angiotensin-converting enzyme inhibitors (ACEIs) to prevent progression of microalbuminuria to macroalbuminuria and slow the progression of diabetic nephropathy.[26]

- ○ ACEIs should be started if blood pressure increases above the normal range for the patient's age or even at or below goal blood pressure (130/80 mm Hg) when persistent microalbuminuria is identified.[10]
- ○ ACEIs should be avoided in premenopausal women who are not using effective birth control, are planning a pregnancy, or who are pregnant, due to the risk of birth defects.
- Blood pressure control, lipid parameters, and other prevention measures are covered in Chapter 28 and Chapter 30, approaches are similar to patients with T2DM.
- Preconception counseling is mandatory for young women with T1DM, and very tight glucose control with near-normalization of glucoses is recommended before conception and during pregnancy for optimal maternal and fetal outcomes.

REFERENCES

1. Patterson CC, Dahlquist GG, Gyurus E, Green A, Soltész G. Incidence trends for childhood type 1 diabetes in Europe during 1989–2003 and predicted new cases 2005–20: A multicentre prospective registration study. *Lancet* 2009;373(9680):2027–2033.
2. Dabelea D, Mayer-Davis EJ, Saydah S, et al. Prevalence of type 1 and type 2 diabetes among children and adolescents from 2001 to 2009. *JAMA* 2014;311(17):1778–1786.
3. Roep BO, Peakman M. Antigen targets of type 1 diabetes autoimmunity. *Cold Spring Harb Perspect Med* 2012;2(4):a007781.
4. Concannon P, Rich SS, Nepom GT. Genetics of type 1A diabetes. *N Engl J Med* 2009;360(16):1646–1654.
5. Triolo TM, Armstrong TK, McFann K, et al. Additional autoimmune disease found in 33% of patients at type 1 diabetes onset. *Diabetes Care* 2011;34(5):1211–1213.
6. Hughes JW, Riddlesworth TD, DiMeglio LA, Miller KM, Rickels MR, McGill JB. Autoimmune diseases in children and adults with type 1 diabetes from the T1D Exchange Clinic Registry. *J Clin Endocrinol Metab* 2016;101(12):4931–4937.
7. Cooper JD, Smyth DJ, Smiles AM, et al. Meta-analysis of genome-wide association study data identifies additional type 1 diabetes risk loci. *Nat Genet* 2008;40(12):1399–1401.
8. Brownlee M. Biochemistry and molecular cell biology of diabetic complications. *Nature* 2001;414(6865):813–820.
9. Sheetz MJ, King GL. Molecular understanding of hyperglycemia's adverse effects for diabetic complications. *JAMA* 2002;288(20):2579–2588.
10. American Diabetes Association. Classification and diagnosis of diabetes: Standards of medical care in diabetes–2018. *Diabetes Care* 2018;41(Suppl 1):S13–S27.
11. Nathan DM; DCCT/EDIC Research Group. The diabetes control and complications trial/epidemiology of diabetes interventions and complications study at 30 years: Overview. *Diabetes Care* 2014;37(1):9–16.
12. White NH, Sun W, Cleary PA, et al. Prolonged effect of intensive therapy on the risk of retinopathy complications in patients with type 1 diabetes mellitus: 10 years after the Diabetes Control and Complications Trial. *Arch Ophthalmol* 2008;126(12):1707–1715.
13. Writing Team for the Diabetes Control and Complications Trial/Epidemiology of Diabetes Interventions and Complications Research Group. Sustained effect of intensive treatment of type 1 diabetes mellitus on development and progression of diabetic nephropathy: The Epidemiology of Diabetes Interventions and Complications (EDIC) study. *JAMA* 2003;290(16):2159–2167.
14. Albers JW, Herman WH, Pop-Busui R, et al. Effect of prior intensive insulin treatment during the Diabetes Control and Complications Trial (DCCT) on peripheral neuropathy in type 1 diabetes during the Epidemiology of Diabetes Interventions and Complications (EDIC) Study. *Diabetes Care* 2010;33(5):1090–1096.
15. Juvenile Diabetes Research Foundation Continuous Glucose Monitoring Study Group, Bode B, Beck RW, Xing D, et al. Sustained benefit of continuous glucose monitoring on HbA1c, glucose profiles, and hypoglycemia in adults with type 1 diabetes. *Diabetes Care* 2009;32(11):2047–2049.
16. Weisman A, Bai JW, Cardinez M, Kramer CK, Perkins BA. Effect of artificial pancreas systems on glycaemic control in patients with type 1 diabetes: A systematic review and meta-analysis of outpatient randomized controlled trials. *Lancet Diabetes Endocrinol* 2017;5(7):501–512.

17. Edelman S, Garg S, Frias J, et al. A double-blind, placebo-controlled trial assessing pramlintide treatment in the setting of intensive insulin therapy in type 1 diabetes. *Diabetes Care* 2006; 29(10):189–195.
18. Ryan G, Briscoe TA, Jobe L. Review of pramlintide as adjunctive therapy in treatment of type 1 and type 2 diabetes. *Drug Des Devel Ther* 2009;2:203–214.
19. Fayfman M, Pasquel FJ, Umpierrez GE. Management of hyperglycemic crises. *Med Clin North America* 2016;101(3):587–606.
20. Joint British Diabetes Societies Inpatient Care Group. The management of diabetic ketoacidosis in adults. Second edition, update 2013. Retrieved February 6, 2018, from http://www.diabetologists-abcd.org.uk/JBDS/JBDS_IP_DKA_Adults.pdf.
21. Naunheim R, Jang TJ, Banet G, Richmond A, McGill J. Point-of-care test identifies diabetic ketoacidosis at triage. *Acad Emerg Med* 2006;13(6):683–685.
22. Kitabchi AE, Umpierrez GE, Murphy MB, et al; American Diabetes Association. Hyperglycemic crises in diabetes. *Diabetes Care* 2004;27(Suppl 1):S94–S102.
23. Semenkovich K, Bischoff A, Doty T, et al. Clinical presentation and memory function in youth with type 1 diabetes. *Pediatr Diab* 2016;17(7):492–499.
24. Cato MA, Mauras N, Mazaika P, et al. Longitudinal evaluation of cognitive functioning in young children with type 1 diabetes over 18 months. *J Int Neuropsychol Soc* 2016;22(3):293–302.
25. Gibb FW, Teoh WL, Graham J, Lockman KA. Risk of death following admission to UK hospital with diabetic ketoacidosis. *Diabetologia* 2016;59(10):2082–2087.
26. Lewis EJ, Hunsicker LG, Bain RP, Rohde RD. For the Collaborative Study Group. The effect of angiotensin-converting enzyme inhibition on diabetic nephropathy. The Collaborative Study Group. *N Engl J Med* 1993;329(20):1456–1462.

Type 2 Diabetes Mellitus

30

Cynthia J. Herrick and Janet B. McGill

GENERAL PRINCIPLES

Type 2 diabetes is a common metabolic disorder that has acute and chronic manifestations and complications. Type 2 diabetes can be asymptomatic for years prior to diagnosis. In order to reduce the morbidity and mortality associated with diabetes, health care providers need to understand screening guidelines and prevention strategies as well as individualized treatment of the disease.

Definition

- Type 2 diabetes mellitus (T2DM) results from a combination of resistance to insulin action and an inadequate compensatory insulin secretory response.[1]
- T2DM is a metabolic disorder with carbohydrate intolerance as the cardinal feature.
- The diagnosis of diabetes relies on demonstration of hyperglycemia, regardless of underlying etiology, see Table 30-1.

Epidemiology

- Diabetes has an estimated total prevalence of 30.3 million among people ≥18 years of age, or 9.4% of the adult population.[2] T2DM accounts for about 95% of all cases of diabetes in the United States and is a growing public health concern.
- Diabetes is the seventh leading cause of death in the United States and a leading cause of morbidity and mortality.[2]
- Diabetes is the leading cause or contributor of hospitalization, end-stage renal disease, blindness in individuals aged 20 to 74 years, and nontraumatic limb amputation.
- The major cause of mortality in diabetes is cardiovascular, and the diagnosis of diabetes confers a twofold to fourfold increase in cardiovascular risk.

Etiology

- The etiology of T2DM is multifactorial. It is complex and involves the interaction of genetic and environmental factors.
  - Patients often have a family history of T2DM, supporting the role of genetic predisposition in the pathogenesis.
  - Genome-wide association studies have contributed to our understanding of the genetic architecture of T2DM. While many genetic loci have been associated with T2DM, these new discoveries represent but a small proportion of the genetic variation underlying the susceptibility to this disorder.[3]
- A number of environmental factors have been shown to play a critical role in the development of T2DM.
  - Sex, age, and ethnic background are important factors in determining risk of developing T2DM.
  - Excessive caloric intake leading to obesity, especially visceral adiposity, and physical inactivity contribute significantly to insulin resistance and, in epidemiologic studies, are the factors associated with the increasing incidence of T2DM.

278

TABLE 30-1 DIAGNOSIS OF DIABETES

Stage	HbA1c	FPG	OGTT	Random blood glucose
Normal	≤5.6%	<100 mg/dL	2-hour PG <140 mg/dL	—
Prediabetes	5.7–6.4%	<126 mg/dL	2-hour PG <200 mg/dL	—
IFG		≥100 mg/dL and <126 mg/dL	—	—
IGT	—		2-hour PG ≥140 mg/dL and <200 mg/dL	—
Diabetes	≥6.5%	FPG ≥126 mg/dL	2-hour PG ≥200 mg/dL	≥200 mg/dL with symptoms

In the absence of unequivocal hyperglycemia, diagnosis should be confirmed by repeat testing. FPG, fasting plasma glucose; OGTT, oral glucose tolerance test; PG, plasma glucose; IFG, impaired fasting glucose; IGT, impaired glucose tolerance.

○ Lifestyle modification that includes weight loss and exercise improves insulin resistance and prevents diabetes in high-risk cohorts.[4]

Pathophysiology

- **Insulin resistance**, the inability of cells to respond to stimulation by insulin, is present in most individuals with T2DM.[5]
  ○ Insulin resistance precedes the onset of T2DM by years.
  ○ The cellular features of insulin resistance include reduction of nonoxidative glucose storage as glycogen, impaired fatty acid oxidation and reduced ability to switch between fatty acid and glucose oxidation during hyperinsulinemia. Mitochondrial content and oxidative capacity may be reduced in insulin-responsive tissues of persons with insulin resistance.[6]
  ○ Inflammation also plays a role in insulin resistance, and elevated levels of free fatty acids and inflammatory markers are present. Insulin sensitivity declines with age, but this may be due to the changes in body composition that occur with aging.[7]
- **Insulin deficiency**, on the other hand, typically follows a period of hyperinsulinemia, which compensates for insulin resistance.[8]
  ○ The initial defects in insulin secretion are loss of first-phase insulin release and loss of the oscillatory secretion pattern. The clinical correlate of this early defect is postprandial hyperglycemia. Further decline in insulin secretion leads to inadequate suppression of hepatic glucose output and presents clinically as fasting hyperglycemia.
  ○ Hyperglycemia and T2DM develop when insulin secretion by pancreatic β cells is inadequate to meet the metabolic demand.
  ○ Hyperglycemia contributes to impaired β-cell function and worsening insulin deficiency, a phenomenon known as glucose toxicity.[9]
  ○ Chronic elevation of free fatty acids, another characteristic of T2DM, may contribute to reduced insulin secretion and β-cell apoptosis.

- There are no definitive histopathologic findings of insulin resistance; however, increased cellular triglyceride and reduced numbers of mitochondria may be seen. Histopathologic changes in the islets of Langerhans in long-standing T2DM include amyloid accumulation and a reduction in the number of insulin-producing β cells.
- Longitudinal data from the United Kingdom Prospective Diabetes Study (UKPDS) suggest progressive β-cell failure occurs during the lifespan of individuals with T2DM. Early in the course of diabetes, improvement in insulin secretion can be achieved by reducing insulin resistance and improving hyperglycemia, thereby reducing the functional defects imposed by hyperglycemia and elevated free fatty acids.[10]
- The definitive tests for insulin resistance measure insulin-mediated glucose uptake and/or hepatic glucose output and are available in research settings. In the clinical settings, insulin resistance is often inferred when features of the metabolic syndrome are present, with or without a diagnosis of diabetes.

Classification

In addition to type 1 diabetes mellitus (**T1DM**), **T2DM**, and **gestational diabetes mellitus (GDM)**, the American Diabetes Association (ADA) identifies specific types of diabetes due to other causes, including monogenic diabetes, diseases of the exocrine pancreas and drug or chemical-induced diabetes.[1] Screening for diabetes should be considered in patients with the following concomitant illnesses or problems.

- Diabetes can be due to genetic defects of the β-cell and/or insulin action. See Chapter 32 for discussion of **monogenic forms of diabetes**.
- **Pancreatic disease** can result in partial or complete insulin deficiency. Patients with hemochromatosis or cystic fibrosis may present with nonketotic hyperglycemia. Pancreatitis, pancreatectomy, pancreatic neoplasia, or fibrocalculous pancreatopathy may cause insulin deficiency, and insulin therapy may be needed early in the course of the illness.
- **Drugs that increase the risk of diabetes** include glucocorticoids, nicotinic acid, thiazides, β-adrenergic agonists, somatostatin analogs, atypical antipsychotic agents, and some antiretroviral agents. Hyperglycemia can be relatively mild or quite severe with the institution of these therapies. Diabetes can occur with **critical illness** and other endocrine diseases such as **Cushing syndrome** and **acromegaly**, or develop during treatment for these illnesses. Resolution of the diabetes may occur when the hormone excess is corrected.
- **Latent autoimmune diabetes in adults (LADA)** is an insulin-deficient form of diabetes with an autoimmune etiology that develops more slowly than classic T1DM and is associated with other autoimmune diseases.[11] The majority of patients with LADA require exogenous insulin within 5 years of diagnosis. Later in the course of the illness, patients with LADA may become C-peptide negative and are at risk for ketoacidosis. When LADA is suspected, testing for anti-GAD antibodies and C-peptide may help rule in or rule out the diagnosis.

Risk Factors

Individuals at high risk for the development of T2DM can often be identified before the onset of clinical diabetes.[1] Risk factors for the development of T2DM include:

- Older age
- Overweight or obesity (body mass index [BMI] ≥ 25 kg/m^2)
- Physical inactivity
- First-degree relative with diabetes
- Members of high-risk ethnic population (e.g., African American, Latino, Native American, Asian American, Pacific Islander)
- Women who delivered a baby weighing >9 lb or were diagnosed with GDM
- Women with polycystic ovary syndrome

- HbA1c ≥5.7%, impaired glucose tolerance (IGT) or impaired fasting glucose (IFG)
- Other conditions associated with insulin resistance (e.g., metabolic syndrome,[12] defined as three or more of the characteristics listed in Table 30-2)

DIAGNOSIS

Clinical Presentation

- Mild hyperglycemia is asymptomatic. Patients presenting with symptoms of polyuria, nocturia, polydipsia, polyphagia, fatigue, weight changes, or blurred vision are likely to have significant blood glucose elevation and may have been hyperglycemic for some time.
- Patients who present with complaints of extremity pain, sexual dysfunction, or visual changes from diabetic retinopathy are likely to have been hyperglycemic for years before being diagnosed with diabetes.

History

Medical history of a patient with diabetes should include documentation of the following:[13]

- The onset and progression of diabetes, with information about episodes of diabetic ketoacidosis (DKA), prior response to medications, and level of glycemic control.
- Health behaviors, such as frequency of self-monitoring of BG, use of medical nutrition therapy (MNT), and exercise frequency and intensity, should be recorded.
- Usual BG values and problems with both hyperglycemia and hypoglycemia require assessment to plan changes in therapy.
- Symptoms of hyperglycemia and hypoglycemia should be elicited to augment a careful review of glucose records or meter readings.
- The past medical history (PMH) should record history of diabetes-related complications.
  - Macrovascular: coronary heart disease, cerebrovascular disease, peripheral vascular disease.
  - Microvascular: retinopathy, nephropathy, and neuropathy including history of foot ulceration or joint problems.
- Other: psychosocial problems, dental problems.
- The vaccine status should be recorded. Menstrual history, pregnancy history, and use of contraception need to be addressed in the PMH of adolescent and adult women.

Physical Examination

Physical examination may be completely normal or may include hypertension, obesity, or acanthosis nigricans plus evidence of microvascular or macrovascular disease.

TABLE 30-2 METABOLIC SYNDROME

Metabolic syndrome characteristics	Men	Women
Waist circumference	>40 in	>35 in
	>102 cm	>88 cm
Triglycerides	≥150 mg/dL	≥150 mg/dL
High-density lipoprotein	<40 mg/dL	<50 mg/dL
Blood pressure	≥130/85 mm Hg	≥130/85 mm Hg
Fasting glucose	≥100 mg/dL	≥100 mg/dL

- Funduscopic examination may be normal or abnormal (dot hemorrhages, exudates, neovascularization or laser scars).
- The cardiovascular examination for patients with diabetes should include auscultation of the heart and examination of carotid and peripheral pulses.
- Examination of the feet, including skin, nails, joints, and sensation with a 10 g Semmes–Weinstein monofilament, should be done at regular intervals.
- The diagnosis of neuropathy is based on a combination of symptoms and physical findings, with documented decrease in more than one sensory modality (e.g., absent reflexes plus loss of vibratory, temperature, or monofilament sensation).

Diagnostic Criteria

- Classically, the diagnostic criteria for diabetes have been derived from prospective epidemiologic data associating circulating glucose levels with the future development of diabetes retinopathy. The diagnostic criteria for diabetes and prediabetes conditions are listed in Table 30-1.
- **ADA current criteria for the diagnosis of diabetes:**[1]
  - Hemoglobin A1c (HbA1c) ≥6.5%;
  - Fasting plasma glucose (FPG) ≥126 mg/dL, confirmed on a second sample;
  - 2-hour plasma glucose ≥200 mg/dL after a 75-g oral glucose tolerance test (OGTT);
  - Or a random BG ≥200 mg/dL accompanied by classic symptoms of hyperglycemia or hyperglycemic crisis.
  - In the absence of unequivocal hyperglycemia, tests should be confirmed by repeat testing.
- Categories of increased risk for diabetes:
  - This is an intermediate category that includes individuals whose glucose levels do not meet criteria for diabetes, yet are higher than normal.[1]
  - They have been referred to as having **prediabetes**, indicating the relative high risk for the future development of diabetes. They may be at higher risk for cardiovascular events even in the absence of T2DM.
  - Diagnostic criteria for prediabetes includes:
    - IFG (FPG 100 mg/dL to 125 mg/dL) or
    - IGT (2-hour values on the 75-g OGTT of 140 mg/dL to 199 mg/dL) or
    - HbA1c ≥5.7% to ≤6.4%.
- Testing for T2DM in asymptomatic patients
  - Although the effectiveness of early identification of prediabetes and diabetes through mass testing of asymptomatic individuals has not been proven, prediabetes and diabetes meet established criteria for conditions in which early detection is appropriate.
  - ADA recommends testing for diabetes in asymptomatic patients based on their risks.[1]
    - Testing to detect T2DM in asymptomatic people is recommended in adults of any age who are overweight or obese (BMI ≥25 kg/m²) and who have ≥1 risk factors for diabetes. Risk factors include first-degree relative with diabetes, high-risk ethnicity (African American, Native American, Latino, Asian, or Pacific Islander ancestry), history of CVD, history of hypertension, metabolic syndrome, women with polycystic ovary syndrome, physical inactivity.
    - Any woman with history of GDM should be screened with 2-hour OGTT or FPG at 6 to 12 weeks postpartum and every 1 to 3 years thereafter with either of these tests or HbA1c.
    - In those without risk factors, testing should begin at age 45.
    - HbA1c, FPG, or 2-hour 75-g OGTT may be used to test for diabetes.
    - If tests are normal, repeat testing is recommended at least at 3-year intervals.

Diagnostic Testing

- **Routine laboratory testing** of a patient with T2DM should include the following: HbA1c, chemistry panel, fasting lipid profile, urine microalbumin (usually done as microalbumin-to-creatinine ratio on a random spot urine sample), and liver function panel.[13]
  - HbA1c should be done at diagnosis and at least semi-annually. If the HbA1c is significantly above the target of 7% and therapy is being changed, it should be checked every 1 to 3 months.
  - Fasting lipid profile should be done at diagnosis and repeated as needed to adjust therapy to meet lipid goals.
  - Liver function testing should be considered for all patients with obesity and type 2 diabetes due to the increased risk of nonalcoholic fatty liver disease (NAFLD).
  - Kidney function should be monitored with annual checks of urine microalbumin and serum creatinine for calculation of estimated glomerular filtration rate (eGFR). Patients with evidence of kidney damage or reduced kidney function should undergo additional testing to rule out other causes, and more frequent surveillance of kidney function parameters to identify rate of decline of kidney function.
- **A baseline electrocardiogram (ECG)**

TREATMENT

- T2DM is best managed with a multidisciplinary team, including physicians, diabetes educators, pharmacists, dietitians, and support groups.[13]
- Diabetes is a lifelong disease, consequently lifestyle modifications and appropriate self-care behaviors should be carefully taught, encouraged, and monitored. It is critical for the health care professional to understand the social and cultural context in which patients are taking care of their disease, and carefully engage patients in the therapeutic decision making.
- Diabetes therapy should be individually designed to achieve glycemic, blood pressure, lipid, and prevention targets while accommodating the patient's age and socioeconomic and cultural status and presence of complications of diabetes and other medical conditions.
- Glycemic targets are lower (HbA1c <6.5%) in patients requiring less intensive therapy, and who are at low risk for hypoglycemia. The usual glycemic target (HbA1c <7%) is appropriate for most nonpregnant adults. Higher glycemic targets (HbA1c <8%) may be appropriate for patients at risk of severe hypoglycemia, those with shorter life expectancy or persons with significant comorbidities.[14,15]
- Blood pressure and lipid targets are reviewed in Chapter 28. Attainment of these targets is particularly important in patients with T2DM, given the marked increase in risk of CVD.[15]

LIFESTYLE MODIFICATION, NON-PHARMACOLOGIC THERAPY

- Lifestyle modification incorporating both MNT and physical activity is the first-line therapy for the prevention of diabetes and treatment of new-onset T2DM. Also discussed in Chapter 28.
- Weight loss has been shown to reduce insulin resistance. Moderate weight loss (7% body weight) and regular physical activity (150 min/wk) with dietary strategies are effective in reducing the progression from prediabetes to diabetes.[4,15]
- Weight loss is recommended for all overweight or obese individuals who have or are at risk for diabetes.[15,16]
- Individuals who have prediabetes or diabetes should receive individualized MNT instruction to help achieve treatment goals.

- Low-carbohydrate or low-fat calorie-restricted diets are effective for short-term weight loss. Several randomized controlled trials suggested low-carbohydrate diets (<130 g/day) achieved more weight loss than low-fat diets and a greater decrease of HbA1c in T2DM patients.[17]
- Monitoring carbohydrate intake remains a key strategy in achieving glycemic control.
- Structured exercise interventions have been shown to lower HbA1c in T2DM patients.[16] In the absence of contraindications, T2DM patients should be encouraged to perform resistance training three times/week and at least 150 min/wk of moderate-intensity aerobic physical activity, and limit prolonged periods of inactivity.[18,19]
- However, the UKPDS study showed that only 8% of patients treated with dietary therapy alone were able to achieve and maintain glycemic control over a 9-year period.[20]
- All patients with T2DM who smoke or use other forms of tobacco should be counseled to stop such use. Referral to smoking cessation program may be necessary.

Medications

- Treatment of T2DM should be individualized, taking into consideration the patient's age, severity of hyperglycemia, need for weight loss, concomitant conditions such as hypertension, and other comorbidities.[15,21,22] Metformin is generally recognized as the initial therapy if it is tolerated and kidney function is adequate. The choice of second and third line therapies should be based on proven attributes of the drug, especially in cases where cardiovascular risk reduction or delay of progression of diabetic kidney disease (DKD) is an important consideration.[15,21]
- **Oral and non-insulin injectable hypoglycemic agents** are discussed below and listed in Table 30-3, along with dosing considerations for impaired kidney function. Current information about each drug should be obtained by reviewing FDA or other regulatory agency approved prescribing information. Attainment of glucose targets is important to prevent the long-term consequences of hyperglycemia (Chapter 28). Initiating treatment with two or three drugs, or one or more non-insulin drugs plus basal insulin is recommended for patients presenting with higher HbA1c levels.[15,21]
- **Cardiovascular outcome trials (CVOTs),** mandated by the FDA for new drugs approved after 2008, have been completed in a number of the newer anti-diabetes agents. In general, the newer classes of anti-diabetes medications have shown CVD safety or benefit. The sodium–glucose cotransporter type 2 (SGLT2) inhibitors have been shown to reduce progression of DKD, while the glucagon-like peptide 1 receptor agonists (GLP-1 RAs) have a positive effect on proteinuria.[15,21,22]
- **Medication classes** are listed below, with key prescribing considerations. See Table 30-3 for individual medications with usual dosing and renal dosing.
  - **Metformin**
    - Metformin is the only biguanide available in the United States.
    - Metformin decreases hepatic glucose output and lowers fasting glucose.
    - Metformin monotherapy decreases HbA1c by 1% to 2%.
    - Metformin therapy is associated with weight stability or modest weight loss.
    - Metformin does not cause hypoglycemia.
    - The most common adverse effect is gastrointestinal intolerance. Metformin may interfere with vitamin B12 absorption, so measurement of vitamin B12 level is advised in patients taking metformin.
    - Renal dysfunction with eGFR <30 mL/min/1.73m^2 is considered a contraindication to metformin use. Lower doses should be used in patients with eGFR <45 but >30 mL/min/1.73m^2.
    - Limited data suggest the potential for cardiovascular benefit but neutral effects with regard to congestive heart failure (CHF) and progression of DKD.

TABLE 30-3 NONINSULIN ANTIDIABETIC DRUGS

Drug	Doses	Dose adjustment in renal impairment
Biguanide		
Metformin (Glucophage, Riomet)	500, 850, 1,000 mg bid	Reduce dose at eGFR 45 mL/min/1.73 m^2, stop at eGFR ≤30 mL/min/1.73 m^2
Metformin XR (Glucophage XR, Glumetza)	500, 1,000 mg qday or bid	Reduce dose at eGFR 45 mL/min/1.73 m^2, stop at eGFR ≤30 mL/min/1.73 m^2
Sulfonylureas		
Glipizide (Glucotrol)	5, 10 mg qday, bid or tid	No renal dose adjustment
Glipizide XL (Glucotrol XL)	5, 10 mg qday or bid	No renal dose adjustment
Glyburide (Diabeta, Micronase)	1.25, 2.5, 5 mg qday or bid	Renally excreted, lower dose is recommended
Glimepiride (Amaryl)	1, 2, 4 mg qday	Renally excreted, lower dose is recommended
Meglitinides		
Nateglinide (Starlix)	60, 120 mg tid	No renal adjustment
Repaglinide (Prandin)	0.5, 1, 2 mg tid	Use 0.5 mg if CrCl 20–40 mL/min
α-Glucosidase inhibitors		
Acarbose (Precose, Glucobay)	50, 100 mg tid	Contraindicated if CrCl <25 mL/min
Miglitol (Glyset)	25, 50, 100 mg tid	Renal excretion; lower dose if CrCl <60 mL/min; contraindicated if CrCl <25 mL/min
Voglibose (Volicose, others)	0.2, 0.3 mg tid	Not absorbed
Thiazolidinedione		
Pioglitazone (Actos)	15, 30, 45 mg	No renal dose adjustment
Bile acid sequestrant		
Colesevelam (Welchol)	3.75 g/day as 3 tablets, 625 mg, bid or 1 packet, 3.75 mg in water, daily; take with food	No renal dose adjustment
Dopamine receptor agonist		
Bromocriptine mesylate (Cycloset)	0.8 mg, 1–6 tablets daily	No information, use caution

(continued)

TABLE 30-3 NONINSULIN ANTIDIABETIC DRUGS (*Continued*)

Drug	Doses	Dose adjustment in renal impairment
DPPIV inhibitors		
Alogliptin (Nesinia)	6.25, 12.5, 25 mg qday	eGFR 30–60 mL/min/1.73 m², use 12.5 mg; eGFR <30 mL/min/1.73 m², use 6.25 mg
Linagliptin (Tradjenta)	5 mg qday	No dose adjustment for renal function
Saxagliptin (Onglyza)	2.5, 5, 10 mg qday	For eGFR <50 mL/min/1.73 m², use 2.5 mg
Sitagliptin (Januvia)	25, 50, 100 mg qday	If eGFR <50 mL/min/1.73 m², use 50 mg. If eGFR <25 mL/min/1.73 m², use 25 mg
Vildagliptin (Galvus)	50 mg qday or bid	Use 50 mg qday if eGFR <50 mL/min/1.73 m². Insufficient data in ESRD to recommend use
SGLT2 inhibitors		
Dapagliflozin (Farxiga)	5, 10 mg qday	Do not use if eGFR <60 mL/min/1.73 m²
Canagliflozin (Invokana)	100, 300 mg qday	If eGFR <60 mL/min/1.73 m², use 100 mg; stop if eGFR <45 mL/min/1.73 m²
Empagliflozin (Jardiance)	10, 25 mg qday	Do not use if eGFR <45 mL/min/1.73 m²
Ertugliflozin (Steglatro)	5, 15 mg qday	Do not use if eGFR <30 mL/min/1.73 m²; do not initiate if eGFR is <60 mL/min/1.73 m²
GLP1 receptor agonists		
Dulaglutide (Trulicity)	0.75, 1.5 mg qw	No renal dose adjustment
Exenatide (Byetta)	5, 10 mg bid	Do not use if eGFR <30 mL/min/1.73 m²
Exenatide QW (Bydureon Bcise)	2 mg qw	Do not use if eGFR <30 mL/min/1.73 m²
Lixisenatide (Adlyxin)	10, 20 mg qday	Do not use if eGFR is <30 mL/min/1.73 m²
Liraglutide (Victoza)	0.6, 1.2, 1.8 mg	No renal dose adjustment
Semaglutide (Ozempic)	0.5 mg, 1 mg	No renal dose adjustment
Amylin analog		
Pramlintide (Symlin)	30, 60, 120 mcg tid	No renal dose adjustment, not studied in ESRD

Bid, twice daily; qday, daily; tid, three times daily; qw, weekly; eGFR, estimated glomerular filtration rate; CrCl, creatinine clearance.

○ **Sulfonylureas**
  ▪ Sulfonylureas (SFUs) enhance insulin secretion by directly stimulating the β cell.
  ▪ SFUs lower HbA1c by 0.7% to 1.5%.
  ▪ The major adverse effect is hypoglycemia, especially in the elderly. Weight gain is common with sulfonylurea therapy.
  ▪ SFUs carry a warning about increased CV mortality based on a study comparing tolbutamide with insulin. Second-generation SFUs are considered neutral for CV safety and DKD progression.[23]

○ **Glinides**
  ▪ Glinides are short-acting insulin secretagogues. They bind to a different site on the sulfonylurea receptor than SFUs. They have a shorter half-life than the sulfonylureas (SFUs) and must be administered more frequently.
  ▪ Glinides decrease HbA1c by 0.6% to 1.5%
  ▪ The major adverse effect is hypoglycemia, however due to the short half-life hypoglycemia is less frequent and less severe than SFUs.
  ▪ Data about CV and renal safety are limited.

○ **Thiazolidinedione**
  ▪ Thiazolidinedione (TZDs) are peroxisome proliferator-activated receptor γ modulators.
  ▪ TZDs improve the response (sensitivity) of muscle, fat, and liver to insulin.
  ▪ Monotherapy with TZDs has demonstrated a 0.8% to 1.5% decrease in HbA1c.
  ▪ TZDs do not cause hypoglycemia.
  ▪ The most common adverse effects are weight gain, fluid retention, and an increased incidence of fractures in women.
  ▪ Pioglitazone has been shown to reduce the composite MACE endpoint of cardiovascular death, myocardial infarction and stroke, but increase the incidence of heart failure.[24]
  ▪ Pioglitazone may have a slightly increased risk of bladder cancer, though this claim has been disputed.

○ **α-Glucosidase inhibitors**
  ▪ α-Glucosidase inhibitors reduce the rate of digestion of polysaccharide in the proximal small intestine, lowering postprandial glucose without causing hypoglycemia.
  ▪ α-Glucosidase inhibitors decrease HbA1c by 0.6% to 0.9%, and do not cause hypoglycemia.
  ▪ Increased intestinal gas production and gastrointestinal symptoms are the most common side effects.

○ **Bile acid sequestrant (colesevelam hydrochloride)**
  ▪ Colesevelam hydrochloride is a resin originally developed for the treatment of high LDL.
  ▪ Colesevelam hydrochloride lowers HbA1c in patients with T2DM by 0.4% to 0.6%, and does not cause hypoglycemia.[25]
  ▪ Do not use if triglycerides are >500 mg/dL, if the patient has a history of hypertriglyceridemia-induced pancreatitis or history of small bowel obstruction.
  ▪ Colesevelam hydrochloride does not require dose adjustment in patients with renal impairment, and may offer CV benefit due to LDL lowering.

○ **Dopamine agonist (bromocriptine mesylate)**
  ▪ Bromocriptine mesylate lowers HbA1c by 0.4% to 0.6%.
  ▪ The major side effects are orthostatic hypotension and syncope.
  ▪ Bromocriptine mesylate showed a reduction in CV events in a 1-year study.[26]

○ **Dipeptidyl peptidase 4 inhibitors**
  ▪ **Dipeptidyl peptidase 4 inhibitors** (DPP-4 inhibitors) inhibit the enzyme that breaks down endogenous glucagon-like peptide-1 (GLP1) and glucose-dependent

insulinotropic polypeptide (GIP). Therefore, they enhance the effects of GLP1 and GIP, increase glucose-mediated insulin secretion, and suppress glucagon secretion and gastric emptying.

- DPP-4 inhibitors lower HbA1c by 0.6% to 1.2%, are weight neutral and do not cause hypoglycemia.
- Rare side effects include polyarticular arthralgia and other altered immunities.
- Most of the DPP-4 inhibitors need adjustment for reduced renal function except for linagliptin, which is excreted by the liver.
- The CVOTs reported prior to 2018 have been neutral, proving cardiovascular safety.[22,27]
- Saxagliptin and alogliptin CVOTs showed an increase in the rate of hospitalization for heart failure.
- Renal benefit with DPP-4 inhibitors has not been demonstrated.

○ **SGLT2 inhibitors**
- SGLT2 inhibitors lower blood glucose by blocking the glucose reabsorption transporter in the proximal tubule of the kidney, which results in increased glucose excretion in the urine.
- SGLT2 inhibitors lower HbA1c by 0.6% to 1%, and are associated with blood pressure reduction and weight loss.
- The major side effects are increased genital mycotic infections and urinary tract infections. Older patients in particular should be monitored for signs of dehydration. Euglycemic DKA has been reported with use of these drugs.
- Canagliflozin (both doses) and empagliflozin are contraindicated in patients with eGFR <45 mL/min/1.73 m^2; and dapagliflozin and canagliflozin, 300 mg are contraindicated in patients with eGFR <60 mL/min/1.73 m^2. Ertugliflozin is contraindicated if the eGFR is <30 mL/min/1.73 m^2, but should not be started in patients with eGFR <60 mL/min/1.73 m^2.
- Cardiovascular outcome trials have been completed for two of the agents, and show reduced major adverse cardiovascular events (MACE), including cardiovascular death, myocardial infarction, and stroke. The major effect of empagliflozin was to reduce cardiovascular death, while canagliflozin reduced the combined MACE endpoint.[22,28,29]
- SGLT2 inhibitors slow progression of DKD and reduce hospitalization for CHF.[28,29,30]
- Canagliflozin was associated with an increased risk of limb amputation when compared with placebo.[29]

• **Noninsulin injectable hypoglycemic agents**
○ **Glucagon-like-peptide 1 receptor agonists (GLP1 RAs)**
- **Albiglutide, exenatide, dulaglutide, liraglutide, lixisenatide, and semaglutide** are GLP-1 RAs. They bind to the GLP-1 receptors on the pancreatic β cells and augment glucose-mediated insulin secretion. They also suppress glucagon secretion and slow gastric motility.
- GLP-1 RAs decrease HbA1c by 0.5% to 2.5%, and are not generally associated with hypoglycemia; however the risk of hypoglycemia increases when these agents are used with SFUs or insulin.
- GLP-1 RAs have a high incidence of gastrointestinal side effects, but have an ancillary benefit of contributing to weight loss while lowering blood glucose.
- Acute pancreatitis has been a concern, but the incidence was not increased in large clinical trials with GLP-1 RAs. C-cell tumors were identified in animal models, so this class of drugs is contraindicated in patients with C-cell tumors of the thyroid.
- GLP-1 RAs are administered subcutaneously once daily (liraglutide, lixisenatide), twice daily (exenatide) or once weekly (albiglutide, dulaglutide, exenatide XR, semaglutide).

- Albiglutide will no longer be sold in the United States after July 2018.
- CVOTs have shown neutral results for exenatide and lixisenatide, proving cardiovascular safety.[31,32] Liraglutide and semaglutide have been shown to reduce MACE endpoints.[33,34] None of the tested drugs impact hospitalization for CHF.
- Reduction in dose of exenatide is recommended if eGFR <30 mL/min/1.73 m^2, caution is advised when using lixisenatide at that level. No dose restrictions are required for albiglutide, dulaglutide, liraglutide, or semaglutide, however side effects may increase.
- Liraglutide may be beneficial in DKD.[35]
○ **Amylin analog (Pramlintide)**
  - Pramlintide is a synthetic analog of the β-cell hormone amylin. It slows stomach emptying, improves satiety, and inhibits glucose-dependent glucagon production, which is reflected in reduced postprandial glucose and modest weight loss.
  - Pramlintide decreases HbA1c by 0.5% to 0.7%.
  - The major side effects are gastrointestinal, including nausea, vomiting and abdominal discomfort.
  - Pramlintide is administered in doses of 30- to 120-mcg subcutaneously before each meal.
  - Pramlintide is approved for use in patients with T1DM and T2DM patients who are taking insulin.
  - **Insulin** regimens are summarized in Table 30-4 (see Chapter 29 for an overview of insulin types and pharmacokinetics.)
○ When adding insulin for the management of inadequately controlled T2DM, most of the noninsulin oral and injectable antidiabetic agents can be continued. The exceptions are SFUs and glinides, which should be discontinued if prandial insulin is needed.
○ Initially, basal insulin can be added once daily at bedtime. The long-acting insulins glargine (Lantus, Basaglar, Toujeo), detemir (Levemir), and degludec (Tresiba) have been shown to cause less nighttime hypoglycemia when used with oral agents in an evening-dosing regimen.
○ If the patient does not achieve glucose targets, or has hypoglycemia with basal insulin plus noninsulin therapy, a more complex insulin regimen might be required. Multiple daily injection (MDI) regimens have been used to achieve tight glucose control and reduce the risk of hypoglycemia by carefully adjusting the premeal doses according to ambient BG, anticipated carbohydrate intake, and activity level.
○ Patients with diabetes due to pancreatic disease, or who have been shown to be insulin deficient by the presence of a low C-peptide, will require intensive insulin therapy using either MDIs or an insulin pump.
○ Insulin requirements vary with changes in weight, diet, activity, concomitant medication use, acute illnesses, and infections.
○ The regimen should be tailored to the patient's needs and abilities.
○ **Concentrated insulins** are available, and may be useful for patients requiring higher doses of insulin.
  - U500 (500 units/mL) is available only as human regular insulin (Humulin R).
  - U500 human regular insulin is an option for patients who require exceptionally large doses of insulin, generally >200 units daily.
  - U500 human regular insulin can be administered bid or tid with equal efficacy due to the long half-life.[36]
  - An endocrinology consultation should be sought if U500 insulin use is contemplated.
  - U200 (200 units/mL) rapid acting insulin lispro is available by pen injector for patients who require larger doses of premeal insulin. Dosing is the same as with U100 insulin rapid-acting insulins.

TABLE 30-4 INSULIN REGIMENS FOR TYPE 2 DIABETES MELLITUS

Regimen	Oral agents	Insulin types	Glucose monitoring	Starting doses
Oral agents + basal insulin—usual *starting regimen*	Continue all types of oral agents. Use submaximal doses of TZD	Intermediate (NPH) or long-acting (glargine, detemir, degludec)	Fasting and as needed during the day	0.1–0.2 U/kg given at bedtime; increase until FPG is at target. Switch to morning if nocturnal hypoglycemia occurs
Premixed insulin, generally bid—*OK for patients with regular meal schedules*	Stop SFU and meglitinides. Continue metformin and other agents if efficacious and no contraindications. Use submaximal dose of TZD	70/30 NPH/regular; Humalog mix 75/25; NovoLog mix 70/30	2–4 × daily and as needed to avoid hypoglycemia	0.1 U/kg AM and PM; increase doses equally until blood glucose nears the target range; evaluate with qid self-monitored blood glucose
MDI regimens—*helpful for patients with irregular meal schedules; may be necessary to achieve tight control; consider CGM*	Continue metformin, GLP-1 receptor agonists, SGLT2 inhibitors. Reconsider DPP4-inhibitors, other agents. Discontinue secretagogues	Basal insulin: insulin glargine or degludec given morning or evening or detemir/NPH/Lente given qday or bid; premeal insulin: lispro (Humalog), aspart (NovoLog), glulisine (Apidra), faster acting aspart (Fiasp) or human regular insulin. Inhaled insulin is a premeal insulin option	4 × daily is required: before meals and at bedtime	In general, a total dose of 0.5–2 U/kg will be required. Give 50% as basal; divide the remaining 50% into premeal doses. Use adjustable scales ± carbohydrate counting for premeal dosing
Continuous SC insulin infusion—*many attractive features for patients; consider CGM*	See recommendations for MDI patients	Lispro (Humalog), aspart (NovoLog), and glulisine (Apidra), faster-acting insulin aspart (Fiasp)	4 × daily and as needed	Conceptually similar to MDI regimens. Intensive diabetes education is needed

FPG, fasting plasma glucose; MDI, multiple daily injection; TZD, thiazolidinedione.

- U200 (200 units/mL) long-acting degludec is available by insulin pen. Dosing is equivalent to U100 insulin degludec.
- U300 (300 units/mL) insulin glargine is available for use as a basal insulin. Dosing is the same as insulin glargine, but the slightly longer half-life may be beneficial for some patients.
- **Diabetes education** is highly recommended when insulin is started or when the regimen is changed.
  - ○ Instruction in self-monitoring of blood glucose (SMBG) is needed for every patient, but especially in those taking insulin.
  - ○ The frequency of SMBG is based on the need to adjust insulin doses based on glucose values, as with intensive insulin therapy, or the risk of hypoglycemia.
  - ○ Patients on intensive insulin therapy with MDI or insulin pumps may qualify for continuous glucose monitoring (CGM) use, which provides additional information about ambient glucoses and safety. Patients should be instructed in the use of these devices and insulin dosing techniques to maximize the benefit from CGM.
  - ○ Instruction in signs and symptoms of hypoglycemia and in methods of treatment is required.
  - ○ Instruction in the use of glucagon should be provided to the patient's household members.

Surgical Management

- Bariatric surgery is classified as restrictive or malabsorptive (Chapter 34). Sleeve gastrectomy and gastric banding are examples of restrictive approaches, which leave the small intestine absorptive surface area intact. Roux-en-Y bypass surgery typically results in more weight loss, and is the most likely to improve or reverse T2DM. Bariatric surgery is an effective weight loss treatment, particularly for severe obesity.[37]
- Bariatric surgery has been shown to reduce HbA1c, triglyceride levels and use of insulin at 5 years when compared to medical therapy.[38]
- The mechanisms of glycemic improvement, long-term benefits and risks, and cost-effectiveness of bariatric surgery in T2DM need further investigation.
- Bariatric surgery should be considered for T2DM adults with BMI ≥35 kg/m^2, especially if their diabetes is difficult to control with lifestyle modification and medications.
- Currently, there is insufficient evidence to support general recommendation for bariatric surgery in T2DM patients with BMI <35, however some patients may benefit from the procedure.
- Patients who have undergone bariatric surgery need lifelong lifestyle support and medical monitoring.

Prevention

- Randomized controlled trials have shown that lifestyle or medication interventions can significantly decrease the incidence of diabetes in high-risk individuals. The ADA recommends prevention of T2DM, and the CDC currently sponsors lifestyle change programs for diabetes prevention.[4,15,39]
- Weight loss of 5% to 10% of body weight and increase in physical activity to at least 150 minute/wk of moderate activity through a structured support program is recommended for persons with risk factors for diabetes or those with prediabetes.
- In addition to lifestyle counseling, metformin can be considered in those who are at very high risk for developing diabetes (combined IFG and IGT plus other risk factors) and who are <60 years of age. Other medications have shown effectiveness in diabetes prevention and may be considered if metformin is not tolerated (see Chapter 28).
- Follow-up counseling and monitoring for development of diabetes should be performed annually.

SPECIAL CONSIDERATIONS

- **Nonketotic hyperosmolar coma (NKHC)** evolves over a period of time but presents emergently when neurologic deterioration occurs in the setting of high glucose levels and dehydration.
- Elderly or disabled patients with significant hyperglycemia who are unable to compensate for the free water loss with oral intake are predisposed to develop this syndrome.[40]
- Patients with NKHC present with a plasma glucose that is generally >600 mg/dL, normal or slightly elevated anion gap, increased BUN and creatinine, increased serum osmolality, and a free water deficit of 2 to 6 L.
- The initial goal of therapy is to replace volume and correct the free water deficit with the infusion of appropriate intravenous fluids.
  - The nature of the fluids (isotonic vs. hypotonic) administered and the rate of infusion are determined by the clinical circumstances.
  - As in DKA, patients in NKHC also present with total body K^+ deficit.
  - Intravenous insulin should be given as repeated intravenous bolus doses (0.1 U/kg/ every 1 to 2 hours) or via insulin drip (see Chapter 28 for further details).
  - The glucose may decline more rapidly in NKHC than in DKA. Electrolytes and the clinical status of the patient should be checked closely and intravenous fluids adjusted accordingly.
  - Neurologic changes should be evaluated to rule out stroke or other central nervous system (CNS) conditions.
  - Mortality is high in patients who present with NKHC due to age and underlying conditions.

REFERENCES

1. American Diabetes Association. Classification and diagnosis of diabetes: Standards of medical care in diabetes—2018. *Diabetes Care* 2018;41(S1):S13–S27.
2. Center for Disease Control and Prevention. *National Diabetes Statistics Report 2017: Estimates of Diabetes and Its Burden in the United States.* Atlanta, GA: Department of Health and Human Services, Centers for Disease Control and Prevention; 2017. https://www.cdc.gov/diabetes/pdfs/data/statistics/national-diabetes-statistics-report.pdf.
3. Frayling TM. Genome-wide association studies provide new insights into type 2 diabetes aetiology. *Nat Rev Genet* 2007;8(9):657–662.
4. Knowler WC, Barrett-Connor E, Fowler SE, et al; Diabetes Prevention Program Research Group. Reduction in the incidence of type 2 diabetes with lifestyle intervention or metformin. *N Engl J Med* 2002;346(6):393–403.
5. Kitabchi AE, Temprosa M, Knowler WC, et al; Diabetes Prevention Program Research Group. Role of insulin secretion and sensitivity in the evolution of type 2 diabetes in the Diabetes Prevention Program. Effects of lifestyle intervention and metformin. *Diabetes* 2005:54(8);2404–2414.
6. Szendroedi J, Phielix E, Roden M. The role of mitochondria in insulin resistance and type 2 diabetes mellitus. *Nat Rev Endocrinol* 2011;8(2):92–103.
7. Donath MY, Shoelson SE. Type 2 diabetes as an inflammatory disease. *Nat Rev Immunology* 2011:11(2);98–107.
8. Weyer C, Bogardus C, Mott DM, Pratley RE. The natural history of insulin secretory dysfunction and insulin resistance in the pathogenesis of type 2 diabetes mellitus. *J Clin Invest* 1999;104(6):787–794.
9. Leahy JL, Bonner-Weir S, Weir GC. Beta-cell dysfunction induced by chronic hyperglycemia. Current ideas on mechanism of impaired glucose-induced insulin secretion. *Diabetes Care* 1992;15(3):442–455.
10. United Kingdom Prospective Diabetes Study Group. United Kingdom Prospective Diabetes Study 24: A 6-year, randomized, controlled trial comparing sulfonylurea, insulin, and metformin therapy in patients with newly diagnosed type 2 diabetes that could not be controlled with diet therapy. *Ann Int Med* 1998;128(3):165–175.

11. Naik RG, Brooks-Worrell BM, Palmer JP. Latent autoimmune diabetes in adults. *J Clin Endocrinol Metab* 2009;94(12):4635–4644.

12. Park Y, Zhu S, Palaniappan L, Heshka S, Carnethon MR, Heymsfield SB. The metabolic syndrome: Prevalence and associated risk factor findings in the U.S. population from the third national health and nutrition exam survey, 1988–1994. *Arch Intern Med* 2003;163(4):427–436.

13. American Diabetes Association. Comprehensive medical evaluation and assessment of comorbidities: Standards of medical care in diabetes—2018. *Diabetes Care* 2018;41(Suppl 1):S28–S37.

14. American Diabetes Association. Glycemic targets: Standards of medical care in diabetes—2018. *Diabetes Care* 2018;41(Suppl 1):S55–S64.

15. Garber AJ, Abrahamson MJ, Barzilay JI, et al. Consensus statement by the American Association of Clinical Endocrinologists and American College of Endocrinology on the comprehensive type 2 diabetes management algorithm—2018 executive summary. *Endocrine Practice* 2018;24(1): 91–120.

16. American Diabetes Association. Prevention or delay of type 2 diabetes: Standards of medical care in diabetes—2018. *Diabetes Care* 2018;41(Suppl 1):S28–S37.

17. Stern L, Iqbal N, Seshadri P, et al. The effects of low-carbohydrate versus conventional weight loss diets in severely obese adults: One-year follow-up of a randomized trial. *Ann Intern Med* 2004;140(10):778–785.

18. Boulé NG, Haddad E, Kenny GP, Wells GA, Sigal RJ. Effects of exercise on glycemic control and body mass in type 2 diabetes mellitus: A meta-analysis of controlled clinical trials. *JAMA* 2001;286(10):1218–1227.

19. U.S. Department of Health and Human Services. *2008 Physical Activity Guidelines for Americans.* Atlanta, GA: Center for Disease Control and Prevention; 2008.

20. Turner RC, Cull CA, Frighi V, Holman RR. Glycemic control with diet, sulfonylurea, metformin, or insulin in patients with type 2 diabetes mellitus: Progressive requirement for multiple therapies (UKPDS 49). UK Prospective Diabetes Study (UKPDS) Group. *JAMA* 1999;281(21):2005–2012.

21. American Diabetes Association. Pharmacologic approaches to glycemic treatment: Standards of medical care in diabetes-2018. *Diabetes Care* 2018;41(Suppl 1):S73–S85.

22. Cefalu WT, Kaul S, Gerstein HC, et al. Cardiovascular outcomes trials in type 2 diabetes: Where do we go from here? Reflections from a Diabetes Care editors' expert forum. *Diabetes Care* 2018;41(1):14–31.

23. Schwartz TB, Meinert CL. The UGDP controversy: Thirty-four years of contentious ambiguity laid to rest. *Perspect Biol Med* 2004;47(4):564–574.

24. Betteridge J, DeFronzo RA, Chilton RJ. PROactive: Time for a critical appraisal. *Eur Heart J* 2008;29(8):969–983.

25. Handelsman Y, Goldberg RB, Garvey WT, et al. Colesevelam hydrochloride to treat hypercholesterolemia and improve glycemia in prediabetes: A randomized, prospective study. *Endocr Pract* 2010;16(4):617–628.

26. Gaziano JM, Cincotta AH, O'Connor CM, et al. Randomized clinical trial for quick-release bromocriptine among patients with type 2 diabetes on overall safety and cardiovascular outcomes. *Diabetes Care* 2010;33(7):1503–1508.

27. Secrest MH, Udell JA, Filion KB. The cardiovascular safety trials of DPP-4 inhibitors, GLP-1 agonists, and SGLT2 inhibitors. *Trends Cardiovasc Med* 2017;27(3):194–202.

28. Zinman B, Wanner C, Lachin JM, et al. Empagliflozin, cardiovascular outcomes, and mortality in type 2 diabetes. *N Engl J Med* 2015;373(22):2117–2128.

29. Neal B, Perkovic V, Mahaffey KW, et al. Canagliflozin and cardiovascular and renal events in type 2 diabetes. *N Engl J Med* 2017;377(7):644–657.

30. Wanner C, Inzucchi SE, Lachin JM, et al. Empagliflozin and progression of kidney disease in type 2 diabetes. *N Engl J Med* 2016;375(4):323–334.

31. Pfeffer MA, Claggett B, Diaz R, et al. Lixisenatide in patients with type 2 diabetes and acute coronary syndrome. *N Engl J Med* 2015;373(23):2247–2257.

32. Holman RR, Bethel MA, Mentz RJ, et al. Effects of once-weekly exenatide on cardiovascular outcomes in type 2 diabetes. *N Engl J Med* 2017;377(13):1228–1239.

33. Marso SP, Daniels GH, Brown-Frandsen K, et al. Liraglutide and cardiovascular outcomes in type 2 diabetes. *N Engl J Med* 2016;375(4):311–322.

34. Marso SP, Bain SC, Consoli A, et al. Semaglutide and cardiovascular outcomes in patients with type 2 diabetes. *N Engl J Med* 2016;375(19):1834–1844.

35. Mann JFE, Orsted DD, Brown-Frandsen K, et al. Liraglutide and renal outcomes in type 2 diabetes. *N Engl J Med* 2017;377(9):839–848.
36. Hood RC, Arakaki RF, Wysham C, Settles JA, Li YG, Jackson JA. Two treatment approaches for human regular U-500 insulin in patients with type 2 diabetes not achieving adequate glycemic control on high-dose U-100 insulin therapy with or without oral agents: A randomized, titration-to-target clinical trial. *Endocr Pract* 2015;21(7):782–793.
37. Buchwald H, Estok R, Fahrbach K, et al. Weight and type 2 diabetes after bariatric surgery: Systematic review and meta-analysis. *Am J Med* 2009;122(3):248–256.
38. Schauer PR, Bhatt DL, Kirwan JP, et al. Bariatric surgery versus intensive medical therapy for diabetes—5 year outcomes. *N Engl J Med* 2017;376(7):641–651.
39. https://www.cdc.gov/diabetes/prevention/index.html.
40. Ennis ED, Stahl EJVB, Kreisberg RA. The hyperosmolar hyperglycemic syndrome. *Diabetes Rev* 1994;2:115–126.

Inpatient Management of Diabetes

31

Paulina Cruz Bravo and Garry S. Tobin

GENERAL PRINCIPLES

- Hyperglycemia is common in hospitalized patients, and includes those with previously diagnosed diabetes, those with newly diagnosed diabetes, and those with acute illness, stress, or intervention-induced hyperglycemia.
- Guidelines defining appropriate glucose targets are specific to either a critically ill or noncritically ill patient population (Table 31-1).[1]
- Insulin is almost always preferred over oral hypoglycemic therapy in the hospital setting.
- Diabetes care from a multidisciplinary team has been shown to improve glycemic control, reduce length of stay, and improve outcomes.

Epidemiology

- It is estimated that one-third of all inpatient (IP) hospital days are incurred by patients with diabetes.[1]
- Blood glucose (BG) levels greater than 180 mg/dL are found on 46% of all BG readings in intensive care units (ICUs), and 31.7% of all non-ICU readings.[2]

Outcomes

- Hyperglycemia in hospitalized patients increases mortality in both previously diagnosed and newly diagnosed patients.[3] Critically ill patients with newly diagnosed hyperglycemia have higher IP mortality rates than patients with known diabetes or without hyperglycemia.[4]
- Patients who are hyperglycemic at admission and are placed on total parenteral nutrition (TPN) have increased mortality compared to those on TPN who did not have hyperglycemia at admission.[5]
- Patients who have had an episode of hypoglycemia (BG <50 mg/dL) in the hospital have increased in-hospital mortality, longer hospital stays, increased hospital charges, and increased rates of discharge to skilled nursing facilities.[6]
- Intensive insulin therapy administered by a variable dose IV infusion improves many clinical outcomes in ICU settings, including reductions in wound infections and in organ failure after cardiothoracic surgery. However, the risk of hypoglycemia is increased and may contribute to increased mortality in medical ICU settings.[7–9]
- Outcomes with intensive insulin therapy in noncritically ill patients are less well studied.

DIAGNOSIS

- **IP hyperglycemia** can be defined as **any BG value >180 mg/dL**.
- A hemoglobin A1c (HbA1c) should be checked in all hospitalized patients with diabetes or hyperglycemia if none is available within the prior 3 months.[3]
- HbA1c values are affected by hemoglobinopathies, acute blood loss, and blood transfusion.
- For diagnostic criteria for diabetes, see Chapter 28

TABLE 31-1	RECOMMENDED GLUCOSE TARGETS FOR INPATIENTS

Recommended blood glucose targets for inpatients

	Critically ill	Noncritically ill
AACE/ADA	140 mg/dL to 180 mg/dL using IV insulin protocol	Premeal glucose <140 mg/dL Random glucose <180 mg/dL Using basal/prandial regimen with correction dose

AACE, American Association of Clinical Endocrinologists; ADA, American Diabetes Association.

- Glucose Monitoring
  - "Fingerstick" or capillary BG testing using point-of-care (POC) glucose meters is an integral part of diabetes management in hospitalized patients. **The timing of glucose checks should be adjusted to the patient's clinical condition.** Glucose should be checked every hour in patients receiving insulin by IV infusion, every 4 to 6 hours in patients who do not have oral intake of nutrients (NPO) or those receiving enteral or parenteral nutrition, and before every meal and bedtime for patients eating meals.
  - Timing of POC glucose testing and insulin administration within 30 minutes of a meal has been shown to decrease hypoglycemia.[10]
  - The current FDA standard requires that POC glucose meters for IP use have 95% of measured glucose values within ± 15% of a gold standard measurement, and that they should be able to measure accurately BG down to 10 mg/dL and up to 500 mg/dL.
  - Interference with POC BG readings occurs due to low hematocrit, hypoxia, acetaminophen, icodextrin, and high triglycerides.[11]

TREATMENT

Management of the Noncritically Ill

- **Assessment:**
  - A history of diabetes should include the age of onset, duration, **type of diabetes**, complications of diabetes, and history of DKA or other diabetes-related hospitalizations.
  - Self-management skills include ability to perform self-monitoring of blood glucose (SMBG), frequency of SMBG, ability to manage medications including insulin injections.
  - The home regimen should specify doses and frequency of all medications including insulin. Insulin history should reflect the type of insulin(s) and doses taken, and an estimate of the total daily dose (TDD). In general regimens of >1 unit per kilogram (kg) body weight in TDD are considered high risk for hypoglycemia.
  - Ongoing assessment of nutritional intake, including dextrose containing IV fluids, is necessary when prescribing insulin or other diabetes therapies.
- **Oral Hypoglycemic Agents and Injectable Non-insulin Therapies:**
- **Oral and noninsulin injectable hypoglycemic agents are generally discontinued in the hospital setting,** although selected agents may be used in IPs with stable kidney function and nutritional intake (e.g., psychiatric or rehabilitation wards).[1,3,12]
  - Insulin secretagogues (sulfonylureas and glinides) may contribute to hypoglycemia, particularly during periods of poor intake or NPO status.

- Metformin is contraindicated in patients with severe renal impairment or acute kidney injury, and in situations of possible fluctuation in kidney function, such as during IV contrast studies or surgery.
- Dipeptidyl-peptidase IV inhibitors may be an option as monotherapy or with basal insulin and have been shown to be safe and effective in the noncritically ill patients who require less than 0.6 units of insulin per kg body weight.[13]
- The use of thiazolidinediones and GLP-1 analogs is not well studied and discouraged.
- **Therapy Goals:**
  - ADA/AACE guidelines recommend a BG target between 140 and 180 mg/dL for IPs. Less stringent targets are appropriate in patients with severe comorbidities or terminal illness. More stringent targets (<140 mg/dL) are suitable in patients who are successful with tight control in the outpatient setting and are more sophisticated with dosing (e.g., carbohydrate counting).[1,3]
  - Glucose levels <100 mg/dL should prompt a review of insulin doses, and levels below 70 necessitate a dose change (unless the event is easily explained by another factor).[3]
  - DKA and hyperosmolar hyperglycemic nonketotic coma are considered "never events" by CMS and may result in loss of Medicare/Medicaid reimbursement for the hospitalization if the cause is due to inappropriate treatment of patients with diabetes while hospitalized.
- **Starting an Insulin Regimen:**
  - **Patients with diabetes eating meals should generally be started on a basal-bolus regimen consisting of basal, prandial, and correction doses of insulin** (also known as "sliding scale"). American Association of Clinical Endocrinologists (AACE)/American Diabetes Association (ADA) guidelines recommend the use of insulin analogs in the hospital setting.
  - The efficacy and safety of a basal-bolus regimen has been tested against "sliding scale" and has been found superior in achieving glucose targets with no difference in hypoglycemia rates.[14]
  - Basal insulins include insulin glargine, insulin degludec, and insulin detemir, and human NPH. Insulin glargine and detemir have equal efficacy and rate of hypoglycemia, however, insulin detemir often requires twice daily dosing.[15]
  - The starting doses for an IP basal-bolus regimen could be determined in a number of ways:
    - For patients on basal-bolus regimens at home, the TDD should be reduced by 20% to 50%, and divided equally between basal and premeal doses.
    - For "basal only" regimens, the TDD needs to be converted to a basal-bolus regimen, for example, a 80-kg patient with T2DM is taking 50 units of insulin glargine once daily in combination with a SFU or a DPP-4 agent, an IP regimen could be glargine 25 units daily and prandial insulin (lispro, aspart, or glulisine) 8 units with each meal.
    - Patients new to insulin should have weight-based dosing, taking additional patient-specific risk factors into consideration. Please see Table 31-2.
  - Distribution of the TDD can be 50/50 (50% as basal insulin and 50% as prandial insulin divided into 3 meals) or 40/60 (40% basal and 60% prandial).
  - The ADA no longer advocates for a particular type of diet. Some hospitals offer a "diabetic," "carb-consistent," or "carb-restricted" diets. The dose of prandial insulin may need to be reduced if the diet contains <60 g of carbohydrate per meal.[3]
  - The choice of correction dose scale is determined by the patient's sensitivity to insulin. This can be inferred by their TDD of insulin. Those using >100 units/day would require the "insulin resistant" or "high" scale, while those using <40 units/day would apply the "insulin sensitive" or "low" scale on this algorithm.
  - Mixed insulins (such as NPH 70/regular 30 and analog mixes) increase the risk of hypoglycemia in the hospital. Mixed insulin regimens should be converted to basal-bolus regimens during the hospital stay using the same TDD principles.
- **Patients Taking Nothing By Mouth (NPO)**

TABLE 31-2	SUBCUTANEOUS INITIAL INSULIN DOSING ALGORITHM
	TDD (units/kg)
Insulin sensitive:	
Pancreatectomy	0.2 (40% basal and 60% bolus)
AKI/CKD/ ESRD/ESLD	0.3
Malnourished elderly	0.3
T1DM	0.4–0.5
Insulin-naïve T2DM, BMI <30	0.4
Insulin resistant:	
Insulin-naïve T2DM with BMI >30	0.5
Insulin experienced T2DM	0.5–0.6
T2DM on steroids	0.6

- ○ **In general, basal insulin doses should be continued during short periods of NPO status**, such as for tests or surgery. The prandial insulin should be held and correctional doses reconsidered, possibly only administered if the BG is >180 mg/dL.
- ○ During prolonged periods of NPO status, low-dose dextrose (50 to 100 g of dextrose in 24 hours) may be required in addition to basal insulin or an insulin drip for insulin-deficient patients to prevent lipolysis and avoid the development of ketones or iatrogenic diabetic ketoacidosis (DKA).[16,17]
- **Enteral Tube Feeding**
  - ○ Tube feeds with varying amounts of carbohydrate are administered on a continuous, cycled, or bolus schedule. The insulin regimen should match the administration of tube feeds.
  - ○ The carbohydrate content of tube feeds should be calculated, and bolus doses provided every 4 to 6 hours accordingly.[3]
  - ○ To avoid hypoglycemia, orders should include instructions for starting dextrose containing IV fluids if insulin has been administered and the tube feeding has been interrupted.
- **Total Parenteral Nutrition:**
  - ○ Intravenous nutrition containing a mix of macro- and micronutrients has a profound effect on glucose and insulin requirements. Failure to control BG in patients receiving TPN has been associated with increased mortality.[5]
  - ○ Common starting ratios range from 1 unit: 10 g carbohydrate for a known patient with diabetes to 1 unit: 20 g carbohydrate for TPN-induced hyperglycemia. A protocol to titrate insulin in TPN was shown to be superior when compared to ad hoc management.[18]
  - ○ Insulin should be added to the TPN solution. This ensures that when the TPN stops, the insulin also stops, reducing the risk of hypoglycemia. Small doses of basal insulin should be given subcutaneously in patients with T1DM to reduce the risk of DKA during periods between TPN infusions.
  - ○ Cycled TPN carries an additional risk for hypoglycemia once the TPN is stopped. This can be prevented by decreasing the rate of the TPN by 50% in the last 1 to 2 hours of the cycle.

Management of Hyperglycemia in the Critically Ill

- Hyperglycemia is a common finding in patients in the ICU, and is an independent risk factor for morbidity and mortality.[4]

- Table 31-1 lists the most recent recommendations for glucose control in the ICU by the ADA (Position Statement 2016), Society of Critical Care Medicine and the American College of Endocrinology, which includes patients in all ICUs and hospital wards. The authors of the Surviving Sepsis Campaign advocate blood sugar goals of less than 180 mg/dL in critically ill patients in large part to limit hypoglycemia and to simplify management.
- Glucose targets should be individualized, and should consider preillness glucose control.[19]
- Insulin is generally administered by IV infusion, and most ICUs now have standardized glucose algorithms, generally managed by ICU nurses, which have been shown to be valid ways to manage glucose. The most effective glucose algorithms are dynamic and incorporate the rate of glucose change into the insulin dose adjustments (Table 31-3).[20]
- **Measurement of Blood Glucose in ICU, FDA Guidance:**
  - The FDA has issued an off-label designation for POC glucose meters not approved for their use in critically-ill patients. POC glucose meters must automatically correct for hematocrit, hypoxia, and interfering reducing substances to be approved by the FDA for use in critically ill patients.[21]
  - Continuous glucose monitoring in the ICU has shown promise and a number of devices are approved in the European Union. Unfortunately, outcome data showing benefit from their use in critically ill patients remain limited.
- **Insulin Adjustments:**
  - Changes in the insulin-infusion rate are predicated on the current BG, rate of change from past measurements, changes in the clinical condition, and changes in carbohydrate intake.
  - Nutrition, whether enteral or parenteral, should be given as a continuous infusion rather than intermittent boluses to prevent significant fluctuations in BG. Caloric intake should be reassessed every 12 to 24 hours.
  - The **patients most at risk for hypoglycemia are those with kidney or liver failure.** Less aggressive titration of insulin is needed in these patients.
  - Avoidance of hypoglycemia is entirely the responsibility of the physicians and staff managing the insulin and nutrition orders.
  - Computerized calculation of the drip rate has been shown to minimize mistakes and may improve outcomes. Multiple computerized programs are available.
- **Transition from IV to Subcutaneous Insulin**
  - Subcutaneous insulin should overlap with IV insulin to prevent hyperglycemia after discontinuation of an insulin drip. The first dose of long-acting insulin should be given 2 to 4 hours prior to the end of the IV drip.
  - For patients with diabetes, the subcutaneous insulin doses are 75% to 80% of the total insulin received IV in the prior 24 hours.
  - Nondiabetic patients with stress hyperglycemia typically require 60% to 70% of the daily IV dose.
  - The daily insulin requirement may fall as patients recover from stress due to illness or surgery. For example, in patients who are recovering from cardiothoracic surgery, the subcutaneous insulin dose may need to be tapered rapidly, with daily changes in the subcutaneous TDD until a stable regimen is established.

SPECIAL CONSIDERATIONS

- **Corticosteroids:**
  - The use of oral, IV, and IM corticosteroids virtually always exacerbate hyperglycemia in patients with diabetes. The effect is most pronounced in the postprandial state and is dose dependent.
  - We recommend converting the steroid dose to prednisone equivalent. Online calculators are available and utilize this to guide therapy.

TABLE 31-3 IV INSULIN INFUSION PRINCIPLES

Initiating insulin infusion

Standard insulin infusion is 100 units of **regular human insulin** in 100 mL 0.9% normal saline

Preferred administration is via an infusion pump

Give initial bolus if blood glucose (BG) >150 mg/dL;

Divide initial BG by 100 and round to nearest 0.5 U (e.g., BG 255: 255/100 = 2.55, rounded to 2.5, so IV bolus 2.5 U)

After bolus, start infusion at same hourly rate as bolus (2.5 U/hr IV in above example)

If **BG <150 mg/dL**, divide by 100 for initial hourly rate with **NO bolus** (e.g., BG 145 would be 145/100 = 1.45, rounded to 1.5, so start at 1.5 U/hr IV)

Changes to the insulin infusion rate are made hourly, based on: blood glucose, rate of change of glucose, change in nutrition, administration of corticosteroids

Blood glucose monitoring

Check BG q1h until stable (three consecutive values in target range)

Once stable, can change BG monitoring to q2h

If stable q2h for 12–24 hours, can change to q3–4h if no significant change in nutrition or clinical status

Resume q1h BG monitoring for BG >70 md/dL with any of the following:

Change in insulin infusion rate

Initiation or cessation of corticosteroid or vasopressor therapy

Significant change in clinical status

Change in nutritional support (initiation, cessation, or rate change)

Initiation or cessation of hemodialysis or CVVHD

Hypoglycemia (BG ≤70 mg/dL)

If BG <50 mg/dL, *stop infusion* and give 25 g dextrose 50% (1 amp D50) IV

Recheck BG q10–15min

When BG > 100 mg/dL, recheck in 1 hour. If still >100 mg/dL after 1 hour, resume insulin infusion at 50% most recent rate

If BG 50–69 mg/dL, stop infusion

If symptomatic or unable to assess, give 25 g dextrose 50% (1 amp D50) IV

Recheck BG q15min[a]

If asymptomatic, consider 12.5 g dextrose 50% (1/2 amp D50) or 8 oz. fruit juice PO

Recheck q15–30min[a]

---

[a]When, BG >100 mg/dL, recheck in 1 hour. If still >100 mg/dL after 1 hour, resume insulin infusion at 75% most recent rate.

BG, blood glucose; CVVHD, continuous venovenous hemodialysis; IV, intravenous; PO, by mouth.

Data adapted from Goldberg PA, Siegel MD, Sherwin RS, et al. Implementation of a safe and effective insulin-infusion protocol in a medical intensive care unit. *Diabetes Care.* 2004;27:461–467.

○ For **low doses** (10 to 40 mg of prednisone) a dose of NPH at the time of steroid administration can be added. For insulin-naïve patients a starting dose of 10 units with daily titrations is reasonable. In the insulin-experienced patient, higher doses of prandial insulin divided in a 40/60 ratio or higher dosages of NPH can be added with the steroids. Dosages in the range of 0.1 units per kg for each 20 mg of prednisone have been used limiting the initial dosage to 20 units of NPH in insulin-naïve and 40 units in insulin-experienced patients.

○ For **intermediate doses** (40 to 80 mg of prednisone) or insulin resistant patients (TDD >0.6 u/kg), increase their regimen by 30% and titrate daily.

○ For **high doses** (>100 mg of prednisone), the TDD may approach 1.5 to 2 units/kg, with 40% given as basal and 60% as bolus doses. Lunch and dinner doses are higher due to peaking of prednisone. NPH dosed with the steroids can be useful.

○ If the patient has persistent hyperglycemia despite attempts at insulin dose adjustment, consider continuous IV insulin infusion (CII) with titration protocol to achieve glucose targets and to determine daily insulin requirements.

○ Posttransplant patients require special consideration. CII postoperatively can be converted to subcutaneous insulin on day 2 postoperatively.[22]

• **Insulin pump therapy**
  ○ Insulin pumps with patient self-management can be continued in the hospital with appropriate policies and procedures. A patient must show the physical and mental capacity for self-management with the pump, and staff must document the timing and amount of insulin administered in the medical record.

  ○ Obtaining an **endocrinology consultation or assessment by a certified diabetes educator (CDE)** to evaluate the appropriateness of the insulin pump regimen, and to make setting adjustments when hyper- and hypoglycemia occur is recommended.

  ○ Hospitals without policies and procedures in place or experienced staff to ensure safe insulin pump use should disallow pump use and convert patients to an appropriate basal-bolus subcutaneous regimen.

  ○ The use of an insulin pump can increase the risk of DKA due to tube or catheter occlusion or insufficient insulin in the reservoir.

• **U-500 Insulin**
  ○ U-500 insulin contains 500 units of regular insulin per mL, compared to 100 units/mL of U-100. The use of U-500 insulin requires special care and is **generally discouraged in the hospital setting**.

  ○ U-500 insulin is generally prescribed to patients requiring >200 units of insulin daily; and is taken split doses, either twice or three times daily.

  ○ When possible, the U-500 home dose should be converted to a basal/bolus regimen using U-100 insulin in the hospital. Reduce the TDD by 40% and use NPH insulin for basal insulin q12 hours and prandial insulin with each meal.

  ○ If U-500 insulin is needed for control of hyperglycemia, the doses should be written in units of insulin and volume (e.g., 0.1 cc = 50 units) to prevent errors. Errors can be reduced by having the dose predrawn by the pharmacy. Using a U-500 pen device will also reduce errors.

  ○ Lower doses should be given for any missed meal to ensure basal coverage, and to decrease hypoglycemic events while NPO.

  ○ New basal insulin formulations include U-300 glargine, U-100 and U-200 insulin degludec, and insulin/GLP-1 agonist combinations
    ▪ The newer basal insulins have variable half-lives, which must be considered when a patient enters the hospital.
    ▪ Insulin degludec (half-life >24 hours), requires a lower dose of basal insulin in the first 24 hours if the patient will be converted to another basal insulin.
    ▪ U-300 glargine, (half-life 12 hours), has a slightly longer half-life than U-100 glargine. Delaying the first dose and/or reducing the dose of U-100 glargine by 10% to 15% more than the expected reduction may be appropriate.

- Basal insulin/GLP-1 receptor agonist combinations are available. Substituting the insulin portion only with basal insulin is appropriate.

- **Hypoglycemia**
  - IP hypoglycemia is associated with poor outcomes including prolonged length of stay, increased falls, increased mortality, and increased risk of readmissions.
  - **Clinically significant hypoglycemia is defined as a BG ≤54 mg/dL and severe hypoglycemia as a BG ≤40 mg/dL in IPs.**
  - Risk factors for IP hypoglycemia include low weight, advanced age, chronic kidney disease or acute kidney injury, liver dysfunction, autonomic instability, hypoglycemia unawareness, and malnutrition.
  - Strategies to prevent hypoglycemia include standardization of insulin orders and treatment of hypoglycemia; weight-based insulin dosing for the treatment of hyperkalemia; formulary restrictions (e.g., restricted use of secretagogues, U-500 insulin); dosing calculators and computerized dosing algorithms; computerized algorithms to predict and prevent hypoglycemia; and innovative approaches like virtual diabetes care.[23,24]

MONITORING/FOLLOW UP

- **Discharge**
  - Readmission rates are higher in patients with IP hyperglycemia. Clinical inertia at the time of discharge has been identified as a major factor in readmission.[25]
  - Discharge planning should include instruction in basic diabetes management skills, such as SMBG and insulin injections, as appropriate.
  - Outpatient medication regimens should mimic prehospitalization diabetes regimens if the patient's glucoses were at goal on admission, but intensified for patients not at goal.[26]
  - For treatment of type 1 diabetes, see Chapter 29; for treatment of type 2 diabetes, see Chapter 30.
  - For those requiring insulin for corticosteroid-induced hyperglycemia, a plan to taper the insulin dose during steroid taper should be included in the discharge plan.

- **Education and Supplies:**
  - All patients with newly diagnosed diabetes, those with uncontrolled diabetes prior to admission, and those who will require hypoglycemic therapy after discharge would benefit from diabetes education during the hospital stay.[27] Early consultation of a CDE for these services will allow for skill assessment after instruction. Education should include:
    - Assessment of level of understanding related to the diagnosis of diabetes
    - Self-monitoring of BG and explanation of home BG goals
    - Definition, recognition, treatment, and prevention of hyper- and hypoglycemia.
    - Information on consistent eating patterns
    - Insulin administration (if appropriate)
    - Sick day management
  - It is also important to ensure that the patient will have all the needed equipment and supplies at home, and will be able to afford and obtain them. Supplies may include glucose meter, test strips, lancets, needles, syringes, urine ketone strips, and a Glucagon kit.

- **Follow-up Care**
  - Short-term follow up with a health care provider skilled in diabetes management should be scheduled for patients with new or changed diabetes treatment regimens.
  - The discharge summary should include the extent of IP hyperglycemia, the HbA1c on admission, and any medication changes made, and should be communicated in a timely manner to the outpatient provider.

REFERENCES

1. Moghissi ES, Korytkowski MT, DiNardo M, et al. American Association of Clinical Endocrinologists and American Diabetes Association consensus statement on inpatient glycemic control. *Diabetes Care* 2009;32(6):1119–1131.

2. Cook CB, Kongable GL, Potter DJ, Abad VJ, Leija DE, Anderson M. Inpatient glucose control: A glycemic survey of 126 U.S. hospitals. *J Hosp Med* 2009;4(9):E7–E14.

3. American Diabetes Association. Diabetes care in the hospital: standards of medical care in diabetes – 2018. *Diabetes Care* 2018;41(Suppl 1):S144–S151.

4. Umpierrez GE, Isaacs SD, Bazargan N, You X, Thaler LM, Kitabchi AE. Hyperglycemia: An independent marker of in-hospital mortality in patients with undiagnosed diabetes. *J Clin Endocrinol Metab* 2002;87(3):978–982.

5. Olveira G, Tapia MJ, Ocon J, et al. Parenteral nutrition-associated hyperglycemia in non-critically ill inpatients increases the risk of in-hospital mortality (multicenter study). *Diabetes Care* 2013;36(5):1061–1066.

6. Hulkower RD, Pollack RM, Zonszein J. Understanding hypoglycemia in hospitalized patients. *Diabetes Manag (Lond)* 2014;4(2):165–176.

7. van den Berghe G, Wouters P, Weekers F, et al. Intensive insulin therapy in critically ill patients. *N Engl J Med* 2001;345(19):1359–1367.

8. van den Berghe G, Wilmer A, Hermans G, et al. Intensive insulin therapy in the medical ICU. *N Engl J Med* 2006;354(5):449–461.

9. NICE-SUGAR Study Investigators; Finfer S, Chittock DR, et al. Intensive versus conventional glucose control in critically ill patients. *N Engl J Med* 2009;360(13):1283–1297.

10. Engle M, Ferguson A, Fields W. A journey to improved inpatient glycemic control by redesigning meal delivery and insulin administration. *Clin Nurse Spec* 2016;30(2):117–124.

11. Klonoff DC. Point-of-care blood glucose meter accuracy in the hospital setting. *Diabetes Spectr* 2014;27(3):174–179.

12. Umpierrez GE, Pasquel FJ. Management of inpatient hyperglycemia and diabetes in older adults. *Diabetes Care* 2017;40(4):509–517.

13. Pasquel FJ, Gianchandani R, Rubin DJ, et al. Efficacy of sitagliptin for the hospital management of general medicine and surgery patients with type 2 diabetes (Sita-Hospital): A multicentre, prospective, open-label, non-inferiority randomised trial. *Lancet Diabetes Endocrinol* 2017;5(2):125–133.

14. Umpierrez GE, Smiley D, Zisman A, et al. Randomized study of basal-bolus insulin therapy in the inpatient management of patients with type 2 diabetes (RABBIT 2 trial). *Diabetes Care* 2007;30(9):2181–2186.

15. Galindo RJ, Davis GM, Fayfman M, et al. Comparison of efficacy and safety of glargine and detemir insulin in the management of inpatient hyperglycemia and diabetes. *Endocr Pract* 2017;23(9):1059–1066.

16. Modi A, Agrawal A, Morgan F. Euglycemic diabetic ketoacidosis: a review. *Curr Diabetes Rev* 2017;13(3):315–321.

17. John R, Yadav H, John M. Euglycemic ketoacidosis as a cause of a metabolic acidosis in the intensive care unit. *Acute Med* 2012;11(4):219–221.

18. Jakoby MG, Nannapaneni N. An insulin protocol for management of hyperglycemia in patients receiving parenteral nutrition is superior to ad hoc management. *JPEN J Parenter Enteral Nutr* 2012;36(2):183–188.

19. Krinsley JS, Egi M, Kiss A, et al. Diabetic status and the relation of the three domains of glycemic control to mortality in critically ill patients: An international multicenter cohort study. *Crit Care* 2013;17(2):R37.

20. Goldberg PA, Siegel MD, Sherwin RS, et al. Implementation of a safe and effective insulin-infusion protocol in a medical intensive care unit. *Diabetes Care.* 2004;27(2):461–467.

21. Scott MG, Bruns DE, Boyd JC, Sacks DB. Tight glucose control in the intensive care unit: Are glucose meters up to the task? *Clin Chem* 2009;55(1):18–20.

22. Wallia A, Gupta S, Garcia C, et al. Examination of implementation of intravenous and subcutaneous insulin protocols and glycemic control in heart transplant patients. *Endocr Pract* 2014;20(6):527–535.

23. Elliott MB, Schafers SJ, McGill JB, Tobin GS. Prediction and prevention of treatment-related inpatient hypoglycemia. *J Diabetes Sci Technol* 2012;6(2):302–309.

24. Rushakoff RJ, Sullivan MM, MacMaster HW, et al. Association between a virtual glucose management service and glycemic control in hospitalized adult patients: An observational study. *Ann Intern Med* 2017;166(9):621–627.

25. Griffith ML, Boord JB, Eden SK, Matheny ME. Clinical inertia of discharge planning among patients with poorly controlled diabetes mellitus. *J Clin Endocrinol Metab* 2012;97(6):2019–2026.

26. Dungan K, Lyons S, Manu K, et al. An individualized inpatient diabetes education and hospital transition program for poorly controlled hospitalized patients with diabetes. *Endocr Pract* 2014;20(12):1265–1273.

27. Healy SJ, Black D, Harris C, Lorenz A, Dungan KM. Inpatient diabetes education is associated with less frequent hospital readmission among patients with poor glycemic control. *Diabetes Care* 2013;36(10):2960–2967.

Monogenic Diabetes

32

Laura T. Dickens and Louis H. Philipson

GENERAL PRINCIPLES

Definition

- Monogenic diabetes describes a heterogeneous group of inherited forms of diabetes and includes maturity-onset diabetes of the young (MODY), neonatal diabetes, and syndromic forms of diabetes.
- Inherited mutations in genes involved in β-cell development, function, and regulation result in impaired glucose sensing and insulin secretion.[1]
- Diagnosis of monogenic diabetes by genetic testing is important because optimal therapy can differ from type 1 or type 2 diabetes and it can identify at-risk family members to be appropriately screened and diagnosed.

Classification

- Maturity-onset diabetes of the young (MODY) is the most common form of monogenic diabetes and includes the following subtypes:
  - GCK-MODY (previously known as MODY 2)
  - HNF1A-MODY (MODY 3)
  - HNF4A-MODY (MODY 1)
  - HNF1B-MODY (MODY 5)
  - Other: PDX1, NEUROD1, PAX4, KLF11, BLK, INS, CEL
- Neonatal diabetes is defined as diabetes diagnosed within the first 6 months of life and can be transient or permanent.
  - Transient neonatal diabetes typically presents soon after birth and resolves by 12 weeks of age, though type 2 diabetes may develop in early adulthood. It is most commonly caused by overexpression of the imprinted chromosome 6q24 genes *PLAG1* and *HYMAI*.[2]
  - Permanent neonatal diabetes is most commonly caused by mutations in the ATP-sensitive potassium channel including activating mutations in the genes *KCNJ11* and *ABCC8* which cause failure of K_{ATP} channel closure and insufficient β-cell insulin secretion.[3,4] A majority of patients with these mutations can be successfully treated with sulfonylureas, which effectively result in ATP-independent closure of the K_{ATP} channel.[5]
- Syndromic forms of diabetes are rare and include Wolfram syndrome, IPEX syndrome (immune dysregulation, polyendocrinopathy, enteropathy, X-linked), cystic fibrosis transmembrane conductance regulator (CFTR)-related diabetes, and mitochondrial diabetes among others.[6]

Epidemiology

- The prevalence of monogenic diabetes is approximately 1% to 2% of all diabetes cases worldwide.[7]
- Four subtypes account for a majority of MODY cases with a confirmed genetic diagnosis.[8]
  - GCK-MODY accounts for 32% of MODY. GCK-MODY prevalence is approximately 1 in 1,000 in the general population and 1 in 100 in gestational diabetes.[9]
  - HNF1A-MODY accounts for 52% of MODY

- ○ HNF4A-MODY accounts for 10% of MODY
- ○ HNF1B-MODY accounts for 6% of MODY
- Neonatal diabetes occurs in 1:90,000 to 1:260,000 live births.[10]

Etiology

See Table 32-1[6] for description of genetic mutations associated with monogenic diabetes.

Pathophysiology

See Table 32-1[6] for description of pathophysiology associated with each genetic mutation.

Associated Conditions

- Patients with β-cell–specific forms of monogenic diabetes will have less risk of other autoimmune diseases than patients with type 1 diabetes.
- Patients with syndromic forms of monogenic diabetes will have manifestations of the syndrome (optic atrophy, diabetes insipidus, and deafness in Wolfram syndrome, lung disease, and exocrine pancreatic insufficiency in CFTR-related diabetes, immune dysregulation in IPEX, etc).[6]

DIAGNOSIS

Clinical Presentation

- Patients with monogenic diabetes typically present with nonketotic, noninsulin dependent diabetes before the age of 25. A family history of atypical diabetes in 2 to 3 consecutive generations is frequently present.[11]
- A diagnosis of monogenic diabetes should also be considered in patients with a prior diagnosis of type 1 diabetes, type 2 diabetes, or gestational diabetes who lack the typical features of these disorders.[7]
  - ○ Patients with a diagnosis of type 1 diabetes with negative autoantibodies at diagnosis or detectable C-peptide suggesting endogenous insulin secretion outside of the honeymoon period.
  - ○ Patients with a diagnosis of type 2 diabetes or gestational diabetes who are not significantly overweight or lacking signs of insulin resistance or other features of metabolic syndrome.
- See Table 32-1[6] for typical clinical features of the different subtypes of MODY.

History
- Patient history should include birth weight, incidence of neonatal hypoglycemia, age, and body mass index (BMI) at the time of diabetes diagnosis, history of ketoacidosis, prior treatments for diabetes and response to treatment, and any other potentially associated medical diagnoses (glucosuria, renal, or genitourinary abnormalities).
- A thorough multigenerational family history should be taken inquiring about all relatives diagnosed with diabetes and their age at diagnosis, BMI, and diabetes treatment.

Physical Examination
Physical examination should focus on identifying signs of insulin resistance (obesity, acanthosis nigricans) or other indicators of autoimmunity (vitiligo) which may indicate an alternative diagnosis of type 1 or 2 diabetes.

Diagnostic Criteria

- Diabetes is diagnosed by the usual criteria (see Chapter 28, Standards of Care for Diabetes Mellitus).
- The genetic disorder is diagnosed by genetic testing.

TABLE 32-1		GENETIC CAUSES AND CLINICAL FEATURES OF MONOGENIC DIABETES	
Gene	Inheritance	Gene function	Clinical features
GCK	AD	Glucokinase enzyme catalyzes the conversion of glucose to glucose-6-phosphate and functions as the pancreatic β cell's glucose sensor	MODY2: stable, nonprogressive elevated fasting blood glucose; typically does not require treatment; microvascular complications are rare; small rise in 2-hour glucose level on OGTT (<54 mg/dL; <3 mmol/L)
HNF1A	AD	Hepatocyte nuclear factor 1-α is a transcription factor involved in tissue-specific regulator of liver genes and expressed in pancreatic islets[4]	MODY3: progressive insulin secretory defect with presentation in adolescence or early adulthood; lowered renal threshold for glucosuria; large rise in 2-hour glucose level on OGTT (>90 mg/dL; >5 mmol/L); sensitive to sulfonylureas
HNF4A	AD	Hepatocyte nuclear factor 4-α is an upstream regulator of HNF1A transcription factor[5]	MODY1: progressive insulin secretory defect with presentation in adolescence or early adulthood; may have large birth weight and transient neonatal hypoglycemia; sensitive to sulfonylureas
HNF1B	AD	Hepatocyte nuclear factor 1-β is a transcription factor expressed in embryonic development of the kidney, pancreas, liver, and GU tract	MODY5: developmental renal disease (typically cystic); genitourinary abnormalities; atrophy of the pancreas; hyperuricemia; gout

Modified from a previously published version found in: Carmody D, Støy J, Greeley SAW, et al. Chapter 2: A clinical guide to monogenic diabetes. In: Weiss RE, Refetoff S, eds. Genetic Diagnosis of Endocrine Disorders. 2nd ed. Waltham, MA: Academic Press, 2016:21-30.

Differential Diagnosis

The differential diagnosis primarily includes type 1 or type 2 diabetes. See Table 32-2[12] for features distinguishing monogenic diabetes from type 1 and type 2 diabetes.

Diagnostic Testing

Laboratories

- Screening labs can be used to determine patients who are appropriate to undergo genetic testing for monogenic diabetes.
  - **Hemoglobin A1c** that is slightly above normal range from 5.6% to 7.6%, when combined with other clinical data, can identify patients more likely to have GCK-MODY compared to controls without diabetes or patients with type 1 or 2 diabetes.[13]
  - **GAD and IA-2 antibodies** are present in only 1% of patients with MODY and, if positive, strongly suggest a diagnosis of type 1 diabetes.[14]
  - **C-peptide** at the time of diabetes diagnosis can also distinguish MODY from type 1 diabetes. Serum C-peptide <0.2 nmol/L is highly suggestive of type 1 diabetes while C-peptide ≥1.0 nmol/L is associated with a 46% chance of type 2 diabetes or MODY.[15]

TABLE 32-2	COMPARISON OF CLINICAL FEATURES OF MODY, TYPE 1 DIABETES, AND TYPE 2 DIABETES		
	MODY	Type 1 diabetes	Type 2 diabetes
Prevalence	1–5% of diabetes cases	5–10% of diabetes cases	90% of diabetes cases
Age at onset	Typical presentation in adolescence or early adulthood (<35 years)	Typical presentation in childhood	Typical presentation in later adulthood. Pediatric cases occur postpuberty
Family history	Two to three consecutive unilineal generations	Affected parent is rare	Often one or both parents have a history of obesity and/or type 2 diabetes
Obesity or metabolic features	Classically absent, though impact of current obesity epidemic is unclear	Classically absent, though impact of current obesity epidemic is unclear	Frequent
Clinical presentation	Typically without significant ketosis or acidosis	Usually with ketosis and varying degree of acidosis	Insidious onset. Typically without ketosis or acidosis though exceptions occur

- ○ **Urinary C-peptide to creatinine ratio** (UCPCR), a noninvasive alternative to serum C-peptide, also tends to be lower in type 1 diabetes. A cutoff of UCPCR ≥0.2 nmol/mmol can differentiate HNF1A and HNF4A-MODY from type 1 diabetes with 97% sensitivity and 96% specificity.[16]
- ○ **Urinalysis** can demonstrate glucosuria in patients with HNF1A-MODY due to a lower renal threshold for glucose.[17]
- ○ **High-sensitivity CRP** levels tend to be lower in patients with HNF1A-MODY compared to type 1 or 2 diabetes or other MODY subtypes.[18]
- Standard screening tests to identify complications and comorbidities associated with diabetes should also be obtained including serum creatinine and estimated GFR, liver function tests, fasting lipid panel, and urine microalbumin to creatinine ratio. Fundoscopic and comprehensive foot examinations are also indicated.[19]
- A definitive diagnosis of monogenic diabetes can be made by identification of a causative mutation with genetic testing.
  - ○ Genetic testing is covered by some insurances and can be performed by Clinical Laboratory Improvement Amendments (CLIA)-certified laboratories using traditional Sanger sequencing or next-generation sequencing.[20]
  - ○ It is recommended to consult with a specialist in monogenic diabetes when ordering genetic testing and interpreting test results.

Imaging

Imaging is not generally required for a diagnosis of monogenic diabetes. In the case of HNF1B, renal imaging is indicated to identify renal disease which most commonly manifests as renal cysts.[21]

TREATMENT

Medications

- GCK-MODY does not require glucose-lowering therapies because mild hyperglycemia is stable and diabetes-associated complications are rare.[22,23] One potential exception where treatment may be required is during pregnancy with a GCK-unaffected fetus, discussed below.
- HNF1A-MODY should be treated with sulfonylureas as first-line therapy.
  - ○ In patients previously treated with insulin, a majority can be transitioned off insulin to sulfonylureas with equal or improved glucose control.[24] Low doses of sulfonylureas are typically sufficient and starting doses should be one-fourth of typical doses.
  - ○ Sulfonylureas can remain effective for many years. Over time, however, the loss of pancreatic β-cell function can result in deteriorating glucose control and need for additional glucose-lowering therapies.
  - ○ Potential second-line therapies include other insulin secretagogues such as nateglinide and GLP1 receptor agonists, both of which have been shown to effectively lower glucose with lower rates of hypoglycemia compared to sulfonylureas.[25,26]
- HNF4A-MODY may also be effectively treated with sulfonylureas or insulin secretagogues, however since this diagnosis is less common the data supporting these approaches are limited.[27]
- HNF1B-MODY does not typically respond to sulfonylurea therapy and often requires insulin for glycemic control.[28]
- Neonatal diabetes caused by mutations in the ATP-sensitive potassium channel may be effectively treated with sulfonylureas, especially if diagnosed early in infancy or childhood.[5]
- Wolfram syndrome patients and CFTR-related diabetes patients typically require insulin, but are not ketosis prone.[29]
- Patients with IPEX syndrome are managed like type 1 diabetes and are prone to ketosis or ketoacidosis.[30]

Other Nonpharmacologic Therapies

Lifestyle management is particularly important for diabetes related to obesity and metabolic syndrome, which occurs in many inherited syndromes (Down syndrome, Turner syndrome, Klinefelter syndrome, etc).

SPECIAL CONSIDERATIONS

Pregnancy

- GCK-MODY treatment during pregnancy depends upon whether the fetus has inherited the GCK mutation, which can be inferred from abdominal circumference measurements on ultrasound.[31]
  - Beginning at 26 weeks, ultrasound monitoring every 2 weeks can detect accelerated fetal growth based on abdominal circumference >75th percentile.
  - Accelerated fetal growth suggests the fetus has not inherited the GCK mutation and insulin therapy should be initiated and delivery induced at 38 weeks.[31]
  - Normal fetal growth indicates that the fetus has inherited the GCK mutation and senses mild maternal hyperglycemia to be normal, thus no treatment is indicated.
- HNF1A and HNF4A-MODY are optimally treated with sulfonylureas outside of pregnancy, however data regarding management in pregnancy are limited.[32]
  - Studies have shown that sulfonylureas cross the placenta and increase risk of macrosomia and neonatal hypoglycemia.[33]
  - Current recommendations suggest that women with HNF1A or HNF4A-MODY on sulfonylurea treatment prior to pregnancy either switch to insulin before pregnancy or continue sulfonylurea treatment in the first trimester and switch to insulin in the second trimester.[32]
- HNF4A-MODY specifically is associated with risk of macrosomia and neonatal hypoglycemia in affected offspring and monitoring for these complications is recommended.[32] Beginning at 28 weeks, ultrasound monitoring at least every 2 weeks is recommended to identify developing macrosomia and if present, delivery should be considered at 35 to 38 weeks.[32]

COMPLICATIONS

- GCK-MODY patients have low rates of microvascular and macrovascular complications that are not significantly different from control populations. One study demonstrated higher rates of retinopathy in GCK-MODY compared to controls (30% vs. 14%), however this difference was due to an increase in background retinopathy with minimal disease and no patients required laser therapy.[23]
- In HNF1A, microvascular and macrovascular complications occur at similar frequency to patients with insulin-dependent and non-insulin-dependent diabetes and are related to glycemic control.[34]
- In HNF4A, diabetic complications are similarly related to glycemic control.[35]
- HNF1B is a multisystem disorder also known as "renal cysts and diabetes syndrome" owing to the high frequency of renal complications. Affected patients have been seen to have 66% incidence of renal cysts and 86% incidence of renal impairment.[21] Renal dysfunction is thought to be a consequence of developmental renal abnormalities rather than a complication of diabetes.

REFERRAL

Physicians and patients can be referred to the Monogenic Diabetes Registry (http://monogenicdiabetes.uchicago.edu) for advice regarding genetic testing and interpretation.

REFERENCES

1. Fajans SS, Bell GI, Polonsky KS. Molecular mechanisms and clinical pathophysiology of maturity-onset diabetes of the young. *N Engl J Med* 2001;345(13):971–980.

2. Temple IK, Gardner RJ, Mackay DJ, Barber JC, Robinson DO, Shield JP. Transient neonatal diabetes: Widening the understanding of the etiopathogenesis of diabetes. *Diabetes* 2000;49(8):1359–1366.

3. Gloyn AL, Pearson ER, Antcliff JF, et al. Activating mutations in the gene encoding the ATP-sensitive potassium-channel subunit Kir6.2 and permanent neonatal diabetes. *N Engl J Med* 2004;350(18):1838–1849.

4. Babenko AP, Polak M, Cavé H, et al. Activating mutations in the ABCC8 gene in neonatal diabetes mellitus. *N Engl J Med* 2006;355(5):456–466.

5. Pearson ER, Flechtner I, Njølstad PR, et al. Switching from insulin to oral sulfonylureas in patients with diabetes due to Kir6.2 mutations. *N Engl J Med* 2006;355(5):467–477.

6. Carmody D, Støy J, Greeley SAW, et al. Chapter 2: A clinical guide to monogenic diabetes. In: Weiss RE, Refetoff S, eds. *Genetic Diagnosis of Endocrine Disorders.* 2nd ed. Waltham, MA: Academic Press; 2016:21–30.

7. Naylor R, Philipson LH. Who should have genetic testing for maturity-onset diabetes of the young? *Clin Endocrinol (Oxf)* 2011;75(4):422–426.

8. Shields BM, Hicks S, Shepherd MH, Colclough K, Hattersley AT, Ellard S. Maturity-onset diabetes of the young (MODY): How many cases are we missing? *Diabetologia* 2010;53(12):2504–2508.

9. Chakera AJ, Spyer G, Vincent N, Ellard S, Hattersley AT, Dunne FP. The 0.1% of the population with glucokinase monogenic diabetes can be recognized by clinical characteristics in pregnancy: The Atlantic Diabetes in Pregnancy cohort. *Diabetes Care* 2014;37(5):1230–1236.

10. Iafusco D, Massa O, Pasquino B, et al. Minimal incidence of neonatal/infancy onset diabetes in Italy is 1:90,000 live births. *Acta Diabetol* 2012;49(5):405–408.

11. Tattersall RB, Fajans SS. A difference between the inheritance of classical juvenile-onset and maturity-onset type diabetes of young people. *Diabetes* 1975;24(1):44–53.

12. Naylor RN, et al. Monogenic Diabetes: Maturity-Onset Diabetes of the Young (MODY) and Neonatal Diabetes. In: Draznin B, ed. *Atypical Diabetes.* Arlington, VA: American Diabetes Association; 2018:3–36.

13. Steele AM, Wensley KJ, Ellard S, et al. Use of HbA1c in the identification of patients with hyperglycaemia caused by a glucokinase mutation: observational case control studies. *PLoS One.* 2013;8(6):e65326. Available at: https://doi.org/10.1371/journal.pone.0065326. Accessed November 30, 2018.

14. McDonald TJ, Colclough K, Brown R, et al. Islet autoantibodies can discriminate maturity-onset diabetes of the young (MODY) from type 1 diabetes. *Diabet Med* 2011;28(9):1028–1033.

15. Ludvigsson J, Carlsson A, Forsander G, et al. C-peptide in the classification of diabetes in children and adolescents. *Pediatr Diabetes* 2012;13(1):45–50.

16. Besser RE, Shepherd MH, McDonald TJ, et al. Urinary C-peptide creatinine ratio is a practical outpatient tool for identifying hepatocyte nuclear factor 1-alpha/hepatocyte nuclear factor 4-alpha maturity-onset diabetes of the young from long-duration type 1 diabetes. *Diabetes Care* 2011;34(2):286–291.

17. Menzel R, Kaisaki PJ, Rjasanowski I, Heinke P, Kerner W, Menzel S. A low renal threshold for glucose in diabetic patients with a mutation in the hepatocyte nuclear factor-1alpha (HNF-1alpha) gene. *Diabet Med* 1998;15(10):816–820.

18. McDonald TJ, Shields BM, Lawry J, et al. High-sensitivity CRP discriminates HNF1A-MODY from other subtypes of diabetes. *Diabetes Care* 2011;34(8):1860–1862.

19. American Diabetes Association. 3. Comprehensive medical evaluation and assessment of comorbidities: standards of medical care in diabetes-2018. *Diabetes Care.* 2018;41(Suppl 1):S28–S37.

20. Stein SA, Maloney KL, Pollin TI. Genetic counseling for diabetes mellitus. *Curr Genet Med Rep* 2014;2(2):56–67.

21. Bingham C, Hattersley AT. Renal cysts and diabetes syndrome resulting from mutations in hepatocyte nuclear factor-1beta. *Nephrol Dial Transplant* 2004;19(11):2703–2708.

22. Stride A, Shields B, Gill-Carey O, et al. Cross-sectional and longitudinal studies suggest pharmacological treatment used in patients with glucokinase mutations does not alter glycaemia. *Diabetologia* 2014;57(1):54–56.

23. Steele AM, Shields BM, Wensley KJ, Colclough K, Ellard S, Hattersley AT. Prevalence of vascular complications among patients with glucokinase mutations and prolonged, mild hyperglycemia. *JAMA* 2014;311(3):279–286.

24. Shepherd M, Shields B, Ellard S, Rubio-Cabezas O, Hattersley AT. A genetic diagnosis of HNF1A diabetes alters treatment and improves glycaemic control in the majority of insulin-treated patients. *Diabet Med* 2009;26(4):437–441.

25. Østoft SH, Bagger JI, Hansen T, et al. Glucose-lowering effects and low risk of hypoglycemia in patients with maturity-onset diabetes of the young when treated with a GLP-1 receptor agonist: A double-blind, randomized, crossover trial. *Diabetes Care* 2014;37(7):1797–1805.

26. Tuomi T, Honkanen EH, Isomaa B, Sarelin L, Groop LC. Improved prandial glucose control with lower risk of hypoglycemia with nateglinide than with glibenclamide in patients with maturity-onset diabetes of the young type 3. *Diabetes Care* 2006;29(2):189–194.

27. Pearson ER, Pruhova S, Tack CJ, et al. Molecular genetics and phenotypic characteristics of MODY caused by hepatocyte nuclear factor 4alpha mutations in a large European collection. *Diabetologia* 2005;48(5):878–885.

28. Pearson ER, Badman MK, Lockwood CR, et al. Contrasting diabetes phenotypes associated with hepatocyte nuclear factor-1alpha and -1beta mutations. *Diabetes Care* 2004;27(5):1102–1107.

29. Moran A, Doherty L, Wang X, Thomas W. Abnormal glucose metabolism in cystic fibrosis. *J Pediatr* 1998;133(1):10–17.

30. Wildin RS, Smyk-Pearson S, Filipovich AH. Clinical and molecular features of the immunodysregulation, polyendocrinopathy, enteropathy, X linked (IPEX) syndrome. *J Med Genet* 2002;39(8):537–545.

31. Chakera AJ, Steele AM, Gloyn AL, et al. Recognition and management of individuals with hyperglycemia because of a heterozygous glucokinase mutation. *Diabetes Care* 2015;38(7):1383–1392.

32. Shepherd M, Brook AJ, Chakera AJ, Hattersley AT. Management of sulfonylurea-treated monogenic diabetes in pregnancy: Implications of placental glibenclamide transfer. *Diabet Med* 2017;34(10):1332–1339.

33. Balsells M, García-Patterson A, Solà I, Roqué M, Gich I, Corcoy R. Glibenclamide, metformin, and insulin for the treatment of gestational diabetes: A systematic review and meta-analysis. *BMJ* 2015;350:h102.

34. Isomaa B, Henricsson M, Lehto M, et al. Chronic diabetic complications in patients with MODY3 diabetes. *Diabetologia* 1998;41(4):467–473.

35. Colclough K, Bellanne-Chantelot C, Saint-Martin C, Flanagan SE, Ellard S. Mutations in the genes encoding the transcription factors hepatocyte nuclear factor 1 alpha and 4 alpha in maturity-onset diabetes of the young and hyperinsulinemic hypoglycemia. *Hum Mutat* 2013;34(5):669–685.

Hypoglycemia

33

Paulina Cruz Bravo and Philip E. Cryer

GENERAL PRINCIPLES[1]

- Glucose is the sole metabolic fuel for the brain under physiologic conditions. This makes it essential for the body to protect itself against hypoglycemia and for plasma glucose to be maintained in a narrow range.
- This regulation occurs in the postprandial state due to increased insulin secretion from the β cell and increased glucose use and energy storage by target tissues.
- Glucose is derived from three sources: carbohydrate absorption in the intestine, glycogenolysis, and gluconeogenesis. In the postabsorptive (fasting) state, plasma glucose is maintained between approximately 70 and 100 mg/dL(3.9 to 5.5 mmol/L)
- The body has multiple counterregulatory mechanisms to prevent or correct hypoglycemia. These include, in order of occurrence, decreased insulin secretion—followed by increased secretion of counterregulatory hormones (glucagon and epinephrine) that amplify release of glucose from liver stores (glycogenolysis), increase glucose production and release by the liver (gluconeogenesis), and further reduce glucose use by tissues. All of these mechanisms serve to raise plasma glucose levels. Later, other noncritical counter-regulatory hormones (cortisol and growth hormone) assist in defending against hypoglycemia. Finally, symptoms prompt behavioral ingestion of food.

Definition

- In patients without diabetes:
  - Hypoglycemia **is a plasma glucose concentration low enough to cause signs or symptoms.**
  - Hypoglycemia is rare and most convincingly documented by **Whipple triad** of neurogenic and neuroglycopenic symptoms, a low measured plasma glucose concentration, and relief of symptoms or signs on raising the glucose levels.[1]
- In patients with diabetes: Hypoglycemia **is a low plasma glucose concentration with or without symptoms that can result in harm**. The International Hypoglycaemia Study Group defines serious and clinically significant hypoglycemia as a glucose <54 mg/dL (3.0 mmol/L) It is recommended that people with diabetes become concerned when a self-monitored blood glucose (SMBG) or continuous glucose monitoring (CGM) value <70 mg/dL (3.9 mmol/L). At this level, patients should consider actions including repeat measurement, carbohydrate ingestion, and avoiding exercise or driving until the glucose level is raised. This is also the level where neurogenic and neuroglycopenic **symptoms normally begin to occur.**[2]
- Due to shifting thresholds of symptoms with recurrent hypoglycemia (hypoglycemic symptoms occur at lower BG) or poorly controlled diabetes (hypoglycemic symptoms occur at higher BG), it is not possible to identify a single plasma glucose value that defines hypoglycemia.

Pathophysiology

- Hypoglycemia occurs, in general, when disappearance of glucose from the circulation is greater than the appearance of glucose in the circulation.

- Sources of circulating glucose include exogenous glucose from ingested carbohydrates and endogenous processes such as hepatic gluconeogenesis and glycogenolysis and renal gluconeogenesis.[1]

Etiology

- Symptoms of hypoglycemia can be classified as **neurogenic symptoms** that result from activation of the sympathetic nervous system, and **neuroglycopenic symptoms** that result from inadequate delivery of glucose to the brain Table 33-1.
- In patients without diabetes
  - ◦ It is clinically useful to classify hypoglycemia based on patient characteristics: That occurring in those who are ill or on medication or those who are seemingly well.[3]
  - ◦ Reactive hypoglycemia is a term no longer in use that described a functional disorder with postprandial hypoglycemia symptoms without demonstration of Whipple triad.
- In the ill or medicated person without diabetes, there are **four main causes of hypoglycemia** (see Table 33-2):[2]
  - ◦ **Drugs** are the most common cause of hypoglycemia.[4] Insulin, sulfonylureas, and alcohol account for the majority of cases. Although hypoglycemic agents used in the treatment of diabetes are the drugs most often implicated in iatrogenic hypoglycemia, it is important to remember that many other medications—some of which are commonly used—can also lower blood sugar. Included in this list are salicylates, quinine, quinolone antibiotics (especially gatifloxacin), haloperidol, disopyramide, angiotensin-converting enzyme (ACE) inhibitors, β-blockers, pentamidine, trimethoprim-sulfamethoxazole, and propoxyphene. Ingestion of alcohol during prolonged fasting (i.e., an alcohol binge) may lead to hypoglycemia by inhibition of gluconeogenesis Table 33-2.[2]
  - ◦ In **critical illness**, such as end-stage liver disease, renal failure, starvation, and sepsis, glucose utilization may exceed production, thereby causing hypoglycemia.
  - ◦ **Counter-regulatory hormone deficiencies** (adrenal insufficiency, growth hormone deficiency) rarely cause hypoglycemia.
  - ◦ **Nonislet cell tumors** can cause hypoglycemia, albeit rarely. Malignancies such as lymphoma, hepatoma, some sarcomas, and teratomas can cause hypoglycemia by secretion of insulin-like growth factor 2 (IGF-2), which can increase glucose use and suppress production.
- In the seemingly well individual, hypoglycemia generally results from one of two causes:
  - ◦ Hypoglycemia can be accidental, malicious, or surreptitious. (Factitious and hyperinsulinism.)

TABLE 33-1	SYMPTOMS OF HYPOGLYCEMIA
Neurogenic (autonomic)	Neuroglycopenic (brain glucose deprivation)
Palpitations	Confusion
Tremor	Fatigue
Anxiety	Seizure
Sweating	Loss of consciousness
Hunger	Focal neurologic deficit
Paresthesia	

TABLE 33-2 CAUSES OF HYPOGLYCEMIA IN ADULTS

Ill or medicated individual

Drugs
- Insulin or insulin secretagogue
- Alcohol
- Others

Critical illnesses
- Hepatic, renal, or cardiac failure
- Sepsis
- Inanition

Hormone deficiency
- Cortisol
- Glucagon and epinephrine (in insulin deficient diabetes mellitus)

Nonislet cell tumor

Seemingly well individual

Endogenous hyperinsulinism
- Insulinoma
- Functional β-cell disorders (nesidioblastosis)

Noninsulinoma pancreatogenous hypoglycemia

Postgastric bypass hypoglycemia
- Insulin autoimmune hypoglycemia

Antibody to insulin

Antibody to insulin receptor
- Insulin secretagogue
- Other

Accidental, surreptitious, or malicious hypoglycemia

Reprinted from Cryer PE, Axelrod L, Grossman AB, et al. Evaluation and management of adult hypoglycemic disorders. *J Clin Endocrinol Metab* 2009;94(3):709–728.

- Factitious hypoglycemia should be considered in any patient with a history of psychiatric illness, or access to insulin or oral hypoglycemia agents (e.g., health care workers, friends and relatives of people with diabetes).
- Hyperinsulinism may be due to the following:
  - **Insulinoma** is a rare but life-threatening condition characterized by excessive insulin secretion by a pancreatic β-cell tumor, leading to primarily fasting but occasionally postprandial hypoglycemia. The incidence of insulinoma is one to two cases per million patient years. The median age at presentation is 47 with a slight female predominance. Malignant insulinoma, which occurs in 10% of all such tumors, is more common in older patients.[5] In younger patients, insulinoma is more frequently associated with multiple endocrine neoplasia 1 (MEN1). Insulinomas associated with MEN may be multifocal or malignant and may secrete other hormones such as gastrin or adrenocorticotropic hormone (ACTH).
  - **Noninsulinoma pancreatogenous hypoglycemia syndrome** (NIPHS) leads to neuroglycopenic spells typically after a meal. It occurs predominantly in men and is due to diffuse islet hypertrophy and sometimes, hyperplasia.
  - Some patients after Roux-en-Y gastric bypass surgery develop **postprandial endogenous hyperinsulinemic hypoglycemia** through a yet unknown mechanism.

DIAGNOSIS

Clinical Presentation

- A detailed history is essential and should include the following: the circumstances of the episode and its temporal relationship to meals or exercise, associated symptoms, weight changes, recurrence of the episode, drug/alcohol history, medication history, history of gastric surgery, personal or family history of diabetes or of MEN1 or MEN-associated conditions, comorbid conditions, and symptoms of other hormone deficiencies.
- In patients with diabetes:[6]
  - Severe hypoglycemia: An event that requires the assistance of others to administer glucagon or other resuscitative actions
  - Symptomatic hypoglycemia: An event where the typical symptoms of hypoglycemia occur in conjunction with a low plasma glucose measurement
  - Asymptomatic hypoglycemia: Low plasma glucose measurement without the typical symptoms of hypoglycemia
  - Probable hypoglycemia: Typical symptoms of hypoglycemia in the absence of a documented low plasma glucose measurement.
  - Pseudohypoglycemia: An event with symptoms suggestive of hypoglycemia, but the measured plasma glucose is >70 mg/dL (3.9 nmol/L).
- Hypoglycemia in diabetes is usually iatrogenic due to the combination of insulin excess and defective glucose counterregulation and awareness.
- Persons with type 1 diabetes experience innumerable episodes of hypoglycemia each year and most experience at least one severe episode each year.
- Hypoglycemia is less common in type 2 diabetes but carries a bigger burden of morbidity and mortality due to the 20-fold greater prevalence of the disease.[6]
- In both type 1 and long-term type 2 diabetes, glucose counterregulatory mechanisms may be reduced or lost. When hypoglycemia is caused by exogenous insulin or insulin secretagogue, reduction in ambient insulin level is not possible. Both glucagon secretion and epinephrine responses may be attenuated. This cluster of abnormal responses leads to the clinical syndromes of **defective glucose counterregulation** and **hypoglycemia unawareness** which are associated with 25-fold or greater and 6-fold or greater risks of severe hypoglycemia respectively.[7]
- In addition, repeated hypoglycemia shifts glycemic thresholds for epinephrine secretion and awareness of hypoglycemia. This phenomenon is known as **hypoglycemia-associated autonomic failure** (HAAF) and is a common complication of tight glycemic control in people with diabetes. In most cases, avoidance of hypoglycemia for 2 to 3 weeks can restore awareness.[8]

Diagnostic Testing

- In patients with diabetes[9]
  - Minimizing hypoglycemia in diabetes through risk factor reduction is the priority. See Table 33-3.[9]
  - Risk factors can be divided in conventional risk factors in the setting of absolute or relative insulin excess (i.e., decreased insulin clearance in renal failure, excessive doses of insulin or secretagogues, exercise, fasting episodes); and risk factors for HAAF (absolute endogenous insulin deficiency, multiple episodes of severe, hypoglycemia unawareness, antecedent hypoglycemia, and aggressive glycemic therapy per se).
- In patients without diabetes:[3]
  - Confirmation of low blood glucose by a reliable laboratory method rather than with SMBG is essential in the work-up of hypoglycemia in patients without diabetes. If the patient's apparent hypoglycemia was asymptomatic, it is important to consider artifacts caused by improper collection, storage, or error in analytic methods. Measured plasma

TABLE 33-3 MINIMIZING HYPOGLYCEMIA

Acknowledge the problem

Consider each of the risk factors
1. Absolute or relative insulin excess
2. Compromised glucose counterregulation

Apply the relevant principles of intensive glycemic therapy
1. Drug selection. Avoid SUs and glinides. Use more physiologic regimens. Use insulin analogs
2. Technologies. CSII, CGM, CSII + CGM, closed loop CSII

Select an individualized glycemic goal
1. Link HbA1c and risk of hypoglycemia
2. Select the lowest HbA1c that does not cause severe hypoglycemia and preserves awareness of hypoglycemia, preferably with little or no symptomatic or even asymptomatic hypoglycemia

Provide structured patient education
1. Educate patients regarding the risk factors for, symptoms and documentation of, and treatment of hypoglycemia
2. Patients should consider treating all SMBG or CGM values below 70 mg/dL (3.9 mmol/L)

Provide short-term scrupulous avoidance of hypoglycemia in patients with impaired awareness

CSII continuous subcutaneous insulin infusion, CGM continuous glucose monitoring

Adapted from International Hypoglycaemia Study Group. Minimizing hypoglycemia in diabetes. *Diabetes Care* 2015;38(8):1583–1591.

glucose can drop 10 to 20 mg/dL/hr after the blood sample is drawn, so it is important for samples to be processed quickly. In addition, large numbers of blood cells, as in patients with leukemia, can consume plasma glucose, thereby artifactually lowering the measured value, even in the presence of glycolytic inhibitors.[5]

- The focus should then be placed on **documentation of insulin and C-peptide levels during an episode of symptomatic hypoglycemia (plasma glucose <54 mg/dL).**
- When Whipple triad has not been documented or laboratory evaluation has not been done during symptomatic hypoglycemia, it is necessary to recreate the circumstances in which symptoms occur either through a **monitored 72-hour fast for a history of fasting hypoglycemia** or a **mixed meal challenge for a history of postprandial hypoglycemia.**
- If the C-peptide is low in the presence of high measured insulin, exogenous insulin is the probable etiology. With high insulin and high C-peptide, screening for sulfonylurea, and nonsulfonylurea (repaglinide and nateglinide) secretagogues should be performed to rule out surreptitious or inadvertent drug use. Insulin antibodies should also be considered and ordered early in the course of the work-up when there is a suspicion of exogenous insulin administration.
- During a 72-hour fast, the fast is ended once symptomatic hypoglycemia is documented and appropriate samples are collected. Diagnostic values include the following:
  - glucose <54 mg/dL,
  - insulin ≥3 μU/mL,
  - C-peptide ≥0.2 nmol/L,

- proinsulin ≥5.0 pmol/L,
- β-hydroxybutyrate ≤2.7 mmol/L, and
- negative screen for insulin secretagogues.
  - If Whipple triad has been previously documented, the diagnostic fast can be concluded with these measurements at an asymptomatic plasma glucose of <54 mg/dL.
  - If Whipple triad has not been previously documented, the fast should be continued until symptoms occur even if this means a lower blood sugar. Once symptomatic, the patient can be treated with 1-mg intravenous glucagon. An increase in glucose of >25 mg/dL over 30 minutes is consistent with the diagnosis of endogenous hyperinsulinemia.
  - For postprandial hypoglycemia, a mixed meal challenge including foods recognized by the patient to cause hypoglycemia should be performed over 5 hours. An oral glucose tolerance test should never be used to diagnosis postprandial hypoglycemia because of high false positive results. The same laboratories that are obtained in a fasting challenge are obtained in the mixed meal challenge.

Imaging
- Once a diagnosis of endogenous hyperinsulinemia is made clinically and biochemically, insulinoma localization is usually performed first by **dual-phase thin-section multide-tector computed tomography (CT).** Alternative imaging procedures include **MRI** or **transabdominal ultrasonography**. These methods detect 75% of insulinomas.
- **Endoscopic ultrasound** with the possibility of fine needle aspiration allows preoperative localization of the vast majority of insulinomas.

TREATMENT

- In patients with diabetes:
  - Most episodes of symptomatic hypoglycemia or asymptomatic hypoglycemia that are detected by self-monitoring or a CGM can be effectively treated with ingestion of carbohydrates or glucose tablets.
  - An initial dose of 20 g of glucose is reasonable and helps prevent overtreating. With ongoing hyperinsulinemia, the response to oral glucose is limited to about 2 hours and an ingestion of a snack or meal after the glucose has been raised is advisable.
  - Severe episodes of hypoglycemia might require administration of glucagon. A dose of 1 mg can be given subcutaneously or intramuscularly. The effect is quick, but is ineffective in glycogen-depleted individuals. IV glucose is the standard parenteral therapy in the hospital. The response is also transient and should be followed by glucose infusion or feeding. Intranasal glucagon has been recently tested in a randomized clinical trial and proven highly effective in adults with type 1 diabetes when a 3-mg dose was used.[10] A stable liquid, ready-to-use preparation is also available and a dose of 150 mcg appears to be optimal.[11]
  - The duration of hypoglycemia reflects the underlying cause. If secondary to rapid acting insulin or a short-acting secretagogue, the episode will be brief. In contrast, if secondary to long acting insulin or long acting secretagogues, the duration will be more prolonged and event warrant hospitalization.[9]
- In patients without diabetes:
  - Immediate treatment of hypoglycemia is necessary to prevent further decline in blood glucose, neuroglycopenia, and its associated adverse outcomes.
  - To prevent recurrent hypoglycemia, identification and correction of the underlying mechanism are necessary. For insulinoma, surgical resection is preferred.

Medications
- **Immediate treatment of hypoglycemia** is similar to that of patient with diabetes (see above).

- Medical therapy with diazoxide (notable side effects include edema and hirsutism), verapamil, or octreotide is reserved for patients with endogenous hyperinsulinism who are not surgical candidates, who have recurrent disease and refuse reoperation, or who have inoperable disease.
- α-Glucosidase inhibitors, diazoxide, and octreotide may be helpful in NIPHS or post-gastric bypass hypoglycemia.
- Oral formulations of inhibitors of mammalian target of rapamycin (mTOR), such as everolimus, have recently been used with some success for refractory hypoglycemia in malignant insulinoma. Studies have shown improvement in glucose levels with and without tumor regression.

Other Nonpharmacologic Therapies

- If surgical or medical treatments fail, **frequent daytime feedings** and **provision of large amounts of uncooked cornstarch at bedtime** or even overnight gastric glucose infusion may be necessary.
- Patients should be educated about the symptoms of hypoglycemia and the appropriate corrective measures (including when to seek medical attention), and diabetic patients should be provided with a medical alert bracelet and a glucagon emergency kit.

Surgical Management

- The **treatment of choice for insulinoma is surgical resection**, usually via a laparoscpic procedure. For solitary adenomas, surgery is curative.
- Multiple insulinomas associated with MEN1 are treated with an 80% subtotal pancreatectomy, although the recurrence rate is still 21% at 20 years.
- Partial pancreatectomy in NIPHS and postbariatric surgery hyperinsulinemic hypoglycemia is sometimes curative.

REFERENCES

1. Melmed S, Polonsky K, Larsen RP, Kronenberg H. *Williams Textbook of Endocrinology*. Philadelphia, PA: Elsevier; 2015.
2. International Hypoglycaemia Study Group. Glucose concentrations of less than 3.0 mmol/L (54 mg/dL) should be reported in clinical trials: A joint position statement of the American Diabetes Association and the European Association for the Study of Diabetes. *Diabetes Care* 2017;40(1):155–157.
3. Cryer PE, Axelrod L, Grossman AB, et al. Evaluation and management of adult hypoglycemic disorders: An Endocrine Society Clinical Practice Guideline. *J Clin Endocrinol Metab* 2009;94(3):709–728.
4. Murad MH, Coto-Yglesias F, Wang AT, et al. Clinical review: Drug-induced hypoglycemia: A systematic review. *J Clin Endocrinol Metab* 2009;94(3):741–745.
5. Field JB, Williams HE. Artifactual hypoglycemia associated with leukemia. *N Engl J Med* 1961;265:946–948.
6. Spanakis EK, Cryer PE, Davis SN. Hypoglycemia during therapy of diabetes. 2018 Jun 18. In: De Groot LJ, Chrousos G, Dungan K, et al., eds. *Endotext [Internet]*. South Dartmouth, MA: MDText.com, Inc.; 2000. Available from: https://www.ncbi.nlm.nih.gov/books/NBK279100/.
7. Cryer PE. Hypoglycemia, functional brain failure, and brain death. *J Clin Invest* 2007;117(4):868–870.
8. Cryer PE. Hypoglycemia-associated autonomic failure in diabetes: Maladaptive, adaptive, or both? *Diabetes* 2015;64(7):2322–2323.
9. International Hypoglycaemia Study Group. Minimizing hypoglycemia in diabetes. *Diabetes Care* 2015;38(8):1583–1591.
10. Rickels MR, Ruedy KJ, Foster NC, et al. Intranasal glucagon for treatment of insulin-induced hypoglycemia in adults with type 1 diabetes: A randomized crossover noninferiority study. *Diabetes Care* 2016;39(2):264–270.
11. Haymond MW, Redondo MJ, McKay S, et al. Nonaqueous, mini-dose glucagon for treatment of mild hypoglycemia in adults with type 1 diabetes: A dose-seeking study. *Diabetes Care* 2016;39(3):465–468.

Obesity

34

Julia P. Dunn, Susan R. Reeds, and Richard I. Stein

GENERAL PRINCIPLES

Definition

- Obesity is the disease of excessive adiposity.
- Body mass index (BMI; weight in kilograms/square of the height in meters, or kg/m^2) is typically used as a proxy for assessing body fat.

Classification

- Adults:
  - Overweight: BMI 25 to 30 (23 to 26.9 in Asian populations)
  - Obese: BMI ≥30 (≥27 in Asian populations)
    - Class 1: BMI 30 to 34.9
    - Class 2: BMI 35 to 39.9
    - Class 3: BMI ≥40 (extreme)
- Children:
  - Overweight: BMI in 85th to <95th percentile for age/sex (based on normative growth curves).
  - Obese: BMI ≥95th percentile.
    - Normative growth curves are used for youth because of changing BMI distribution over the course of development.
- The term morbid obesity has been used to describe patients with a BMI ≥35, who have a comorbid condition; a BMI ≥40; and with weights >150 kg. This term is now considered derogatory and should be avoided.[1]

Epidemiology

- The National Health and Nutrition Examination Survey (NHANES) has tracked overweight/obesity in the United States since 1960.[2]
  - Prevalence of overweight has remained stable at ~35%.
  - Prevalence of obesity increased significantly from the late 1970s to almost 2000, when the rate of increase began to plateau.
  - Most recent data indicate 36.5% of US adults are obese, nearing three times the prevalence in the 1960s.
  - 6.3% of American adults have extreme obesity, compared to 1% in 1962.
  - Prevalence of obesity is greater in women than men and in middle-aged and older adults compared to younger adults.
  - Non-Hispanic black Americans have the highest prevalence of obesity followed by Hispanic and non-Hispanic white Americans; prevalence in non-Hispanic Asian Americans is significantly lower.[3]
- Health risks associated with obesity may be lower for black than white Americans at the same BMI level.
- NHANES also tracks obesity prevalence in children/adolescents

○ 17% of children aged 2 to 19 had obesity in 2013–2014 (triple the prevalence from 1980; no significant change compared to 2003–2004)
○ Increases with age, but does not vary with sex.
○ Highest among Hispanic boys, followed by Hispanic girls and non-Hispanic black girls
○ Normative growth curves are based on historical data; thus, as the population increases in weight, more than 5% of children may be ≥95th percentile for BMI.

Etiology and Pathophysiology

• Obesity results from interactions among environment, genetic factors, and behavior. Excessive adiposity results from an imbalance between energy intake and energy expenditure, or an imbalance between caloric intake/fat synthesis and fat oxidation.
• **Genetics:**
  ○ Polygenic inheritance plays a large role in susceptibility to obesity.
    ▪ Studies suggest 60% to 90% heritability.
    ▪ Studies have identified at least 97 loci involved in elevated BMI.[4]
    ▪ FTO (fat mass and obesity-related) gene variations are among the most important contributors.[5]
  ○ Identifiable monogenic obesity is very rare.
    ▪ Extreme, early-onset obesity.
    ▪ Mutations of leptin, leptin receptor, prohormone convertase 1 (PC1), pro-opiomelanocortin (POMC), and peroxisome proliferator–activated receptor (PPAR) γ 2 result in syndromic conditions, and are inherited in a recessive pattern.[6]
    ▪ Melanocortin 4-receptor (MC4-R) mutation is nonsyndromic, and autosomal dominant.[7]
    ▪ Prader-Willi syndrome results from a deletion on the long arm of chromosome 15 (q11-13) and is characterized by severe hyperphagia and developmental delay.
    ▪ Bardet–Biedl syndrome
• **Hypothalamic Obesity**
  ○ Results from damage to satiety/hunger signaling regions of the hypothalamus, leading to insatiable appetite and overeating.
  ○ Can occur after any process that significantly disrupts the hypothalamus.
• **Medications that may contribute to obesity**
  ○ Antipsychotics
  ○ Antidepressants
  ○ Neuroleptics
  ○ β-Blockers
  ○ Glucocorticoids
  ○ Some hypoglycemic agents: (insulin, sulfonylureas, thiazolidinediones [TZDs])
  ○ Antiretrovirals
  ○ Oral contraceptives
• **Psychiatric conditions** contributing to obesity or difficulty losing weight include depression and binge eating disorder (BED).

Associated Conditions

• Type 2 diabetes mellitus (T2DM):
  ○ ~75% of people with T2DM have obesity[8]
  ○ Risk for T2DM increases with BMI.
  ○ Weight gain of >5 kg after age 20 increases risk of T2DM[9,10]
• Coronary artery disease (CAD): risk increases with BMI starting within normal range[11]
• Congestive heart failure: risk increases 5% to 7% for every 1 kg/m² increase in BMI above 30[12]
• Cerebrovascular disease

- Hypertension
- Insulin resistance/hyperinsulinemia
- Dyslipidemia (hypertriglyceridemia, low high-density lipoprotein [HDL])
- Obstructive sleep apnea (OSA)
- Obesity hypoventilation syndrome (OHS)
- Venous thromboembolism
- Gastroesophageal reflux disease (GERD), gallstones, nonalcoholic steatohepatitis (NASH)/nonalcoholic fatty liver disease (NAFLD; present in 85% of those with a BMI >40 kg/m²)[13]
- Polycystic ovary syndrome (PCOS)
- Impaired fertility (both male and female)
- Pregnancy complications
- Stress incontinence
- Osteoarthritis (OA), gout
- Vitamin D deficiency; secondary hyperparathyroidism
- Idiopathic intracranial hypertension (IIH)
- Increased risk of colorectal, esophageal, kidney, pancreatic, thyroid, endometrial, gallbladder, and postmenopausal breast cancer. Weaker correlation for leukemia, malignant melanoma, multiple myeloma, non-Hodgkin lymphoma, and premenopausal breast cancer.[14]

Mortality

- Obesity is associated with increased all-cause mortality.
  - In the year 2000, there were 111,909 excess deaths associated with/attributed to obesity, according to conservative interpretation of NHANES data.[15]
  - Mortality rate increases 30% for every 5 kg/m² increase in BMI over 25.[16]
- Disease-specific mortality. Prospective studies show the following mortality hazard ratios[16], with every 5 kg/m² increase in BMI above 25:
  - T2DM (HR 2.16)
  - CAD (HR 1.39)
  - Cancer (HR 1.1)
- The greatest mortality burden of obesity is in adults with BMI ≥30 kg/m², and adults 45 to 64 years of age.[17]

DIAGNOSIS

Clinical Presentation

- Patients often do not present with a complaint about weight, and this can be a delicate issue
  - Be sensitive when raising and addressing the issue; avoid communicating disapproval or blame
  - Preferred language includes weight, unhealthy weight, and overweight.[1]
  - Obesity should be approached as a chronic illness
  - Many patients with overweight and obesity have had negative experiences with medical practitioners; they may be less likely to seek routine healthcare or have recommended screenings.
- Be prepared and welcoming by having bariatric chairs in the waiting room, scales and tables that can accommodate larger weights, appropriately-sized gowns, etc.
- Only rarely, based on specific features in the history and on physical examination, is it necessary to rule out secondary causes of obesity

History

- Medical history—elicit conditions that may contribute to obesity, improve with weight loss and/or guide treatment. Should include cardiovascular disease (CVD)/risk; diabetes,

thyroid disorders and other endocrine conditions; sleep apnea; conditions that limit mobility
- Family history should include overweight/obesity, diabetes, and early-onset CAD
- Weight history:
  - Age/stage of weight gain (for example, pregnancy/menopause in women)
  - Trajectory, high/low adult weights
  - Prior weight-loss attempts and response
  - Outside influences including job, finances
- Modifiable factors
  - Medications
  - Diet
  - Physical activity
  - Stress
  - Sleep history—including evaluation for OSA and sleep schedule
- Dietary history:
  - Meal timing
  - Food preferences, intolerances
  - Cravings
  - Binge eating behavior
  - Hunger versus nonhunger related
  - Cultural/religious influences
  - Who is at home, buys the groceries and does the cooking
- Additional questionnaires, if eating disorder is suspected
  - Questionnaire on eating and weight patterns (QEWP-5)
- Review of systems should include questions to elicit thyroid dysfunction, Cushing's disease, male hypogonadism, menorrhagia, GERD, CVD, then OA, urinary problems, sleep disorders

Physical Examination
- Examination should aim to identify comorbid conditions and secondary causes of weight gain.
- Measure height and weight after removing shoes and heavy clothing. **Do not rely on patient-reported values.**
- Measure waist circumference if BMI<35—the National Cholesterol Education Program recommends measuring at the level of the iliac crest.
  - A waist circumference of >35 in in women or >40 in in men is associated with increased cardiovascular risk (central obesity)
- Blood pressure (BP), measured manually using a size-appropriate cuff (not a thigh cuff)
- Particular attention should be paid to:
  - Features associated with OSA—including neck circumference >17 in
  - Evidence of right-sided heart failure
  - Signs of thyroid dysfunction
  - Skin changes—facial plethora; hirsutism, acne, violaceous abdominal striae, acanthosis nigricans, acrochordon
  - Hepatomegaly
  - Proximal muscle weakness
  - Fat distribution

Diagnostic Testing

Laboratories
- Routine laboratory tests: fasting blood glucose; lipid panel; thyroid-stimulating hormone (TSH); complete metabolic panel, hemoglobin A1c, 25-OH vitamin D, parathyroid hormone

○ Though NAFLD is common in obesity, other causes of liver dysfunction should be considered before ascribing transaminitis to this.
- Additional tests for secondary causes of obesity and comorbidities as suggested by history and physical:
  ○ Cushing syndrome: late-night salivary or 24-hour urinary free cortisol; dexamethasone suppression test
  ○ PCOS: LH, FSH
  ○ OHS: ABG
  ○ Hypogonadism: testosterone level in men
  ○ Routine screening for genetic causes of obesity is not recommended

Electrocardiography
- ECG—look for evidence of structural abnormalities, myocardial damage, and rhythm disturbances as patients will be advised to increase physical activity and may be prone to electrolyte disturbances with dietary interventions.
- Certain ECG abnormalities are more common in patients with obesity—leftward deviation of P/QRS/T axes, low voltages, inferior/lateral T-wave flattening, and changes associated with left ventricular hypertrophy and atrial enlargement.
  ○ May be related to lead placement and body habitus; however, this should not be assumed and significant abnormalities should be evaluated.
  ○ Some changes may improve with weight loss.

Imaging
Imaging only if prompted by abnormalities on examination or laboratory testing—for example, thyroid and hepatic ultrasound.

Diagnostic Procedures
- Referral to a sleep clinic or polysomnography should be obtained if there is evidence of OSA
- Routine evaluation for CAD not indicated in asymptomatic obese patients without diabetes.
  ○ Stress testing, prior to starting exercise or prior to bariatric surgery, should be obtained according to society guidelines.
- **Remember that for tests including cardiac and imaging procedures, the equipment may have size and/or weight limitations; sometimes referral to a tertiary center may be required.**

TREATMENT
- Benefits of weight loss:
  ○ 5% weight loss can improve β-cell function and insulin sensitivity,[18] reduce fasting glucose, and reduce the need for diabetes medications.
  ○ With physical activity, weight loss of as little as 4 kg may prevent progression of pre-diabetes to T2DM.[19]
  ○ Improvement in triglycerides and HDL. Weight loss without changing macronutrients rarely alters LDL cholesterol significantly.[20]
  ○ For every 1-kg loss, systolic and diastolic BP fall 1 mm Hg.[21]
- Weight loss goals
  ○ A reasonable goal is 5% to 10% weight loss, at a rate of ~1 to 2 lb/wk over 6 months followed by efforts toward long-term weight maintenance (as detailed below)
  ○ Note that provider and patient goals may differ (they may want to lose more weight); patients should know that 5% weight loss has significant clinical benefits.

○ Weight loss greater than 2% per week increases the risk of cholelithiasis and should be avoided after the first few weeks, when weight loss is typically more rapid.

○ It should be noted that the recommendations for weight loss in this chapter do not pertain to obese pregnant women. The Institute of Medicine (IOM) recommends that women with a prepregnancy BMI >30 kg/m² gain 11 to 20 lb during pregnancy, and that overweight women (prepregnancy BMI 25.0 to 29.9) gain 15 to 25 lb during pregnancy.[22]

Lifestyle/Risk Modification

Diet

Weight loss requires an energy deficit. This is best achieved by reducing dietary energy intake, which may be accomplished in several ways:[23]

- A general recommendation of a 1,200 to 1,500 kcal/day restriction for women or 1,500 to 1,800 kcal/day for men, adjusted for weight and activity level
- Calculating estimated energy requirements (EER) and prescribing a deficit of 30% or 500 to 750 kcal/day
  ○ Harris–Benedict or Mifflin St. Jeor equations
  ○ A deficit of 500 to 750 kcal/day is estimated to produce a ~1 lb per week weight loss
  ○ NIDDK body weight planner
    ▪ https://www.niddk.nih.gov/health-information/weight-management/body-weight-planner
    ▪ May be used to estimate caloric restriction required to meet a weight loss goal by a target date, or to estimate rate of weight loss over time given a specific caloric intake
- Approaches where reduced caloric intake is produced by elimination of particular foods/food groups in the absence of a set calorie restriction
- With dietary interventions involving moderate calorie restriction, maximal weight loss, averaging 4 to 12 kg, is seen at 6 months, followed by gradual regain resulting in smaller total losses at 1 (4 to 10 kg) and 2 (3 to 4 kg) years.
- Very low-calorie diets (VLCD; <800 kcal/day):
  ○ Can result in more rapid weight loss (20% in 4 months) than low-calorie diets; however, long-term (≥1 year) weight loss is equivalent.
  ○ Include 0.8 to 1.5 g protein/kg ideal body weight per day to preserve lean body mass
  ○ Increased risk of gallstones
  ○ In one study comparing VLCD to LCD, higher percentage fat-free mass lost, but not rate of weight loss, was associated with greater weight regain.[24]
- Specific diets:
  ○ 2013 guidelines for treating obesity from the American Heart Association (AHA), the American College of Cardiology (ACC), and The Obesity Society (TOS)[23] review evidence supporting a wide variety of diets with differing macronutrient compositions and present the conclusion that all are similarly effective if the appropriate calorie deficit is achieved.
    ▪ These included Mediterranean-style, high-protein, low-fat, low-carb, low-glycemic, low-fat vegan-style, and vegetarian diets.
    ▪ In most cases, the comparator diet was calorie-restricted AHA Step 1 or 2 or NHLBI ATP III plan.
    ▪ In all cases, effectiveness was seen only in the setting of an intensive, multidisciplinary program.
  ○ **Low-fat diets:**
    ▪ Contain 20% to 30% of daily calories from fat; very-low–fat plans contain <15% to 20%.

- Compared to low-carbohydrate diets, low-fat diets result in larger reductions in LDL cholesterol, but lesser improvements in HDL cholesterol and triglycerides.
- Very low-fat diets may exacerbate hyperglycemia and hypertriglyceridemia in patients with diabetes
- AHA/ACC guidelines recommend limiting saturated fat intake to 5% to 6% of total calories and reducing trans fats for patients in whom LDL lowering is desired

○ **Low-carbohydrate diets:**
- Contain less than 130 g/day carbohydrate; very-low–carbohydrate diets have less than 60 g/day.
- Compared to low-fat reduced-calorie diets, low-carbohydrate diets produce more weight loss initially, but not long term.
- The Zone® diet limits carbohydrates to 40% of a calorie-restricted diet, but is not ketogenic.
- In ketogenic diets, carbohydrate and protein intake are restricted to the point that glycogen stores are depleted and glucose must be produced through gluconeogenesis.
  □ This begins at an intake of <50 g carbohydrate/day; many diets start with a restriction of ≤20 g/day for the first 1 to 3 months with a gradual increase after initial weight loss
  □ Limited carbohydrate types
  □ Protein typically 25% of total daily calories
  □ Increased satiety with higher-fat foods and limited variety of palatable foods contribute to reduced caloric intake in the absence of a prescribed limit
  □ Ketosis may promote anorexia
  □ Avoid in patients with type 1 diabetes due to risk for diabetic ketoacidosis

○ **High-protein diets 25% daily calories from protein**
- May promote satiety and potentially raise resting energy expenditure[25]
- May have benefit in maintenance of weight loss[26]
- Avoid in patients with chronic kidney disease

○ **Mediterranean-type diet:**
- Features fresh fruits and vegetables, nuts and legumes, whole grains, olive oil, and fish
- One study comparing Mediterranean-type diet and AHA Step 1 diets in individuals newly diagnosed with T2DM showed modest benefits in HbA1c, plasma glucose, triglycerides, HDL-C and BP at 1 year; at 4 years the difference in BP was no longer seen but the other benefits persisted[27]
- May reduce incidence of T2DM and prevent CVD events[28,29]

○ **Low-glycemic diets**
- May moderate insulin response to a meal and promote/prolong satiety
- Often used in the setting of prediabetes or T2DM; however, evidence to support this is lacking

- Given similar efficacy for weight loss (with appropriate energy deficit) of diets of varying macronutrient content, **both the 2013 AHA/ACC/TOS guidelines and the ADA Standards of Care for Diabetes recommend choosing a diet for weight loss based on an individual's dietary preferences and potential effects on other conditions** (e.g., a calorie-restricted DASH-type diet in a patient with hypertension or high CVD risk).
  ○ Note that patients with diabetes may require adjustments in oral or injectable hypoglycemic medications and insulin when starting a reduced-calorie, reduced-carbohydrate diet.

Physical Activity
- An increase in physical activity without caloric restriction, does not result in significant or sustainable weight loss, but regular physical activity may help to maintain weight loss and prevent weight gain during and after successful dieting.[30]

- Considerations prior to starting an exercise program
  - Stress testing or other evaluation for CVD, based on current guidelines[31]
  - ADA guidelines if the patient has neuropathy[32]
  - Physical therapy evaluation for balance problems, fall risk and orthopedic problems or risk for these
  - Ensure the patient has appropriate, well-fitting footwear
- Recommended physical activity to promote weight loss begins with 30 to 45 minutes of moderate-intensity aerobic activity (e.g., brisk walking), 3 to 5 days per week. Frequency and duration may be gradually increased from there. Those who were previously inactive should start with low-intensity activity, 10 minutes/day.
- Patients with BMI >50 kg/m^2 are at high risk for joint strain and stress fracture, and it is recommended to limit weight-bearing activity to no more than 30 minutes.
- To maintain weight loss long term, studies show that 60 to 75 minutes of moderate-intensity activity daily is needed. This kind of exercise can be done in/around the home, and can be divided into several sessions/day to increase compliance.[20]
- Physical activity level and cardiorespiratory fitness are associated with decreased CVD risk factors, independent of obesity. Encourage patients to continue exercise even if weight loss goals are not met.[33]

Lifestyle Change Programs
- Giving a patient a list of goals regarding caloric intake and exercise is unlikely to be effective on its own. It is helpful to:
  - Assess the patient's desire/willingness to make lifestyle changes
  - Set concrete, realistic goals such as limiting fast food to one meal per week, eliminating soda, walking for 30 minutes 3 days/wk
  - Problem solve barriers to achieving goals
  - Use behavior modification techniques to improve lifestyle-change adherence and maintain weight loss
  - Individualize frequency of visits. Monthly visits may be adequate for some patients, while others may benefit from more frequent interactions, which can be through:
    - Ancillary medical staff
    - Referral to a dietitian or comprehensive medical weight management program
    - Commercial (e.g., Weight Watchers) or free (e.g., Take Off Pounds Sensibly [TOPS]) weight-control programs
  - Discuss behavioral topics, including social support for dietary/activity changes, overcoming high-risk situations (e.g., parties, bad weather for exercise), maintaining motivation over time, and emotional eating.[34]
- A common first step is for the patient to keep a food diary, which helps both patient and practitioner get a sense of the patient's current energy intake and eating pattern in order to make recommendations and initiate change
- Food diaries are one of the most useful tools for losing weight, and should be strongly encouraged for awareness of overall dietary intake and for accountability.
  - May be done on paper, with online programs or with phone apps
  - Typically involves recording all foods and drinks for at least 3 days, including at least 1 weekend day
  - Patient self-reporting can be highly inaccurate and unreliable
    - Data indicate that even careful food diaries underestimate energy intake.
    - This should be acknowledged to patients to avoid frustration (e.g., if patients think they are eating a small amount of calories and not losing the expected amount of weight), noting that it is not felt to be intentional.
    - Underestimation may be improved by "real-time" recording, as opposed to recall.

> ○ **To promote honest recording, it is essential for the practitioner to be nonjudgmental when reviewing a patient's food diary.**

Medical Therapy[35]

- Pharmacotherapy should be considered in patients who have a BMI >30 kg/m^2, or >27 kg/m^2 with a significant comorbidity and who have been unable to achieve/maintain weight loss with lifestyle modification alone.
- Medications reinforce behavioral changes, promote adherence to lifestyle, and may increase physical activity potential.
- Lifestyle changes are needed when using a weight-loss medication, and effects appear to be additive.
- When starting medication, evaluate patient monthly for at least 3 months, then quarterly.
  - ○ If inadequate (<5%) weight loss at 3 months on maximum recommended/tolerated dose, discontinue medication
  - ○ If effective and well-tolerated, generally treat long-term (with approved agents)
    - ■ Medications do not permanently affect underlying physiology
- There are limited data on improvements in morbidity, and none on mortality, with drug-induced weight loss.
- See Table 34-1 for information about FDA-approved medications for weight loss.
- **Off-label use** may be considered in the setting of certain comorbidities, when other FDA-approved medications are contraindicated or have failed, or when a desired combination medication is financially prohibitive.
  - ○ Bupropion alone
  - ○ Topiramate alone
  - ○ Zonisamide
  - ○ Metformin
  - ○ Pramlintide
  - ○ SGLT-2 inhibitors
  - ○ Other GLP-1 agonists

Surgical Management

- Also called metabolic surgery, bariatric surgery procedures involve modification of the GI tract for the purpose of weight loss.
- Procedures induce weight loss through restriction, malabsorption, or both.
  - ○ Restrictive procedures physically limit the amount of food that can be eaten in a short amount of time before the patient feels satiated or even nauseated; this reduces caloric intake without inducing hunger.
  - ○ Malabsorptive procedures limit exposure of fully digested food to the small intestinal lumen.
  - ○ Alterations in gut hormones also appear to play a role
- **Appropriate patients.**
  - ○ BMI >40
  - ○ BMI >35 with a significant comorbid condition. T2DM, CAD, OSA, hyperlipidemia, and HTN are generally considered adequate by insurers for coverage of bariatric surgery.
  - ○ There are some proponents of and some evidence to support bariatric surgery in patients with BMI 30 to 35 with significant comorbidities, especially T2DM and metabolic syndrome[36]
  - ○ ADA Standards of Care for Diabetes[37] state that bariatric surgery should be considered for patients with T2DM meeting these criteria:

TABLE 34-1 MEDICATIONS

Name—generic (brand)	Mechanism of action	Dose	Expected weight loss	Contraindications	Adverse effects	Approved for long-term use?	DEA schedule	Additional benefits; other
Phentermine (Adipex-P, Lomaira)	Noradrenergic sympathomimetic; anorexogenic	15–37.5 mg daily in 1–2 doses; 8 mg TID	7.2–8.1 kg in 12 weeks	History of CVD, uncontrolled HTN, glaucoma, MAO-I therapy, pregnancy, breastfeeding	Elevated HR, elevated BP, dry mouth, insomnia, nervousness, constipation	No—≤12 weeks	IV	
Orlistat (OTC—Alli; Rx—Xenical)	Pancreatic lipase inhibitor	60 or 120 mg TID w/meals	5–10 kg; 8–11% TBW	H/O calcium-oxalate stones	Borborygmi, cramps, flatus, fecal incontinence, oily spotting; malabsorption of fat-soluble vitamins; nephrolithiasis; rare reports of severe liver injury	Yes	N/A	↓ total and LDL cholesterol; ↓ HbA1c; ↓ BP
Phentermine and Topiramate (Qsymia)	Exact MOA for topiramate w/r/t weight loss is unknown; anorexogenic	Dose titration from 3.75/ 23 mg to 11.25/69 mg daily; high/ max dose 15/92 mg daily	2 years: For 7.5/46 mg dose—9.6 kg, 9.3% TBW; for 15/92 mg dose 10.9 kg, 10.5% TBW	Same as phentermine	In addition to phentermine alone: HA, paresthesias, increased depression/anxiety, metabolic acidosis, nephrolithiasis, confusion/memory disturbance, acute angle-closure glaucoma	Yes	IV	Teratogenicity— check pregnancy test before starting and monthly while taking; document contraception; certified pharmacy

(continued)

TABLE 34-1 MEDICATIONS *(Continued)*

Name—generic (brand)	Mechanism of action	Dose	Expected weight loss	Contraindications	Adverse effects	Approved for long-term use?	DEA schedule	Additional benefits; other
Lorcaserin (Belviq)	Selective serotonin 2C receptor inhibitor; anorexogenic	10 mg BID	5.8 kg at 1 year	CHF, pregnancy, use of other serotonergic agents, creatinine clearance <30. Caution with mild renal, or mild-moderate hepatic insufficiency	Headache (HA), dizziness, nausea, back pain, upper respiratory symptoms, CBC abnormalities, rarely suicidal ideation	Yes	IV	Slight, but significant reductions in BP, HR, total and LDL cholesterol, CRP, fasting glucose and insulin level CYP 2D6 inhibitor
Bupropion and Naltrexone (Contrave)	NE/DA reuptake inhibitor/opioid antagonist; anorexogenic	8/90 mg tablets—dose titration from 1 qday to 2 bid over 4 weeks	5–6% TBW at 56 weeks	Uncontrolled HTN, seizure d/o or predisposition, eating d/o, chronic opioid use, use of MAO-I w/in 14 days	Nausea, HA, constipation most common; ↑HR, insomnia, vomiting, dizziness, dry mouth; rarely suicidal ideation	Yes	N/A	Some evidence for increased cardiovascular events
Liraglutide (Saxenda, Victoza)	Glucagon-like peptide 1 (GLP-1) analog; anorexogenic; slows gastric emptying and improves insulin action	0.6 mg SC daily; increase by 0.6 mg weekly to maintenance dose of 3 mg daily	8 kg at 56 weeks	Pregnancy, pancreatitis, heart block and medullary thyroid carcinoma, personal or family history of MTC/MEN2	Injection site reaction, N/V, diarrhea, constipation, HA, elevated HR, hypoglycemia, renal insufficiency.	Yes	N/A	↓ CV events in T2DM; may help prevent progression from prediabetes to T2DM

MOA, mechanism of action; TBW, total body weight; MAO-I, monoamine oxidase inhibitor.

- BMI ≥40 (37.5 in Asian Americans) regardless of glycemic control or complexity of treatment regimen
- BMI 35.0 to 39.9 (32.5 to 37.4 in Asian Americans) when glycemia is inadequately controlled with lifestyle and optimal medical therapy.[38]
  - Attempted and failed lifestyle intervention
  - Exclusion criteria:
    - Active substance abuse
    - Mental illness that may prevent safe compliance after the procedure
    - Certain eating disorders
- **Improvement in comorbidities with surgical therapy**
  - T2DM remission, see below
  - Improvement in outcomes in general parallel percent EWL[39]
  - Hypertension: Resolved in 62%. Resolved or improved in 79%
  - OSA: resolved in 86%[40]
  - OHS: resolved in 76%
  - Hypertriglyceridemia, low HDL: 85% remission[41]
  - NAFLD: improvement or resolution in steatosis 92%, steatohepatitis 81%, fibrosis 65%[42]
  - GERD: Roux-en-Y gastric bypass (RYGB)-recommended surgery, 95% resolution/significant improvement almost immediately[43]
  - IHH: 100% resolution papilledema; 90% reduction headache[44]
  - OA: 50% of patients able to decrease pain medication dose.[45] MSK pain improves in spine, upper and lower extremity, and in fibromyalgia syndrome.[46]
  - Mortality: improvements are reported for cohorts of mixed bariatric surgery patients while gastric bypass has the most robust data available.[47,48]
  - 40% decrease in long-term all-cause mortality, 49% decrease CVD and 60% cancer-related deaths
    - Increase in nondisease deaths (e.g., suicides), primarily in younger patients
    - Mortality benefit seen in both sexes and persists into older patient groups
    - In one study of nearly 10,000 patients with >7-year mean follow-up, bariatric surgery prevented 136 deaths per 10,000 surgeries performed.[47]
- **Preoperative Care**[49]
  - Patients with diabetes
    - Optimize glycemic control. A hemoglobin A1c value of ≤6.5% to 7.0%, a fasting blood glucose level of ≤110 mg/dL, and/or a 2-hour postprandial blood glucose concentration of ≤140 mg/dL are appropriate goals and may be associated with improved outcomes. An HbA1c of 7% to 8% may be acceptable in patients with advanced complications, extensive comorbid conditions, or longstanding T2DM which has been difficult to control.
    - A perioperative glycemic control plan typically involves stopping oral hypoglycemic agents and noninsulin injectable agents that may cause hypoglycemia prior to surgery
    - Long-acting insulins may be stopped or reduced
    - Assessment and discussion of likelihood of diabetes remission and postoperative need for medications includes duration of diabetes and presurgical need for insulin. Patients with T2DM requiring insulin prior to surgery, and those who have had T2DM for >10 years are more likely to require medication after surgery.
  - Women:
    - Estrogen-containing therapy should be discontinued 1 month prior to surgery to reduce risk of thromboembolism.
    - Women with PCOS may have rapid improvement in fertility postoperatively and should be counseled appropriately regarding contraception.
  - Smokers should stop smoking at least 8 weeks prior to surgery.

○ Evaluation for deep vein thrombosis in symptomatic or high-risk patients; consideration of preoperative inferior vena cava filter placement
  - Psychological evaluation is mandatory
  - Significant mental illness and eating disorders can result in morbidity/mortality after surgery
  - Assess life stressors, support system and intellectual/mental capability to adhere to postsurgical care
○ Prior to malabsorptive procedures, vitamin and mineral deficiencies including vitamin D, B12, and iron should be assessed and treated.
○ Patients with or at risk for CVD should undergo risk stratification and evaluation according to current guidelines
○ Preoperative weight loss using meal replacements is often done to attempt to reduce liver volume and may improve outcomes.[41] In patients with diabetes, insulin doses will need to be reduced and insulin secretagogues discontinued.
○ All patients should be counseled that obesity is a chronic illness that will require continued vigilance around diet, physical activity, and related factors after surgery and that weight regain is possible, even likely, in the absence of this.

- **Specific procedures**
  ○ RYGB is considered the gold-standard procedure.
  ○ In 2016, the most commonly performed bariatric procedure in the United States was sleeve gastrectomy.
  ○ Use of laparoscopic adjustable gastric band has been declining.
  ○ See Table 34-2[50] for information about specific bariatric surgery procedures.
- **Safety of bariatric surgery**[51,52]
- With increased experience and use of laparoscopic approaches, complication and mortality rates for bariatric surgery approach those of other commonly performed elective operations such as hysterectomy and cholecystectomy
  ○ Mortality rates: 0.1% to 0.5%
  ○ Major complication rates: 2% to 6%
  ○ Minor complication rates: up to 15%
- **Postoperative care**[49]
  ○ Diet
    - Sugar- and caffeine-free clear liquids can usually be started within 24 hours.
    - Staged meal progression:
      □ Critically-ill patients: IV insulin titugar, ≥1.5 L) for 10 to 14 days after hospital discharge
      □ Gradual progression to full liquids and pureed foods, then soft foods, then solid proteins over 3 to 4 weeks
      □ Patients should be instructed to eat protein first, followed by fruits and vegetables
      □ Rice, bread, and pasta should be avoided until the patient is comfortably consuming ≥60 g/day protein along with fruits and vegetables
      □ Avoid drinking until 30 minutes after meals.
      □ By 3 months most patients are able to consume a "normal" diet of balanced meals including adequate protein, fruits, vegetables, and whole grains. Adequate protein is ≥60 g or 1 to 1.5 g/kg ideal body weight per day
      □ Patients should continue to ensure adequate fluid intake of ≥1.5 L/day; avoid concentrated sweets, carbonated beverages, and use of straws
  ○ Diabetes control
    - See Chapter 31 on Inpatient Management of Diabetes.
    - Avoid long-acting insulin in the immediate perioperative period. IV insulin may be used.
    - Oral and noninsulin injectable hypoglycemic agents are avoided during hospitalization.

Procedure	Description	Mechanism	Expected weight loss	Advantages	Disadvantages
Roux-en-Y gastric bypass (RYGB)	• Small pouch divided from top of stomach • Small bowel divided distal to ligament of Treitz • Roux (distal) limb anastomosed to stomach • Proximal limb anastomosed to Roux limb further down	R+M	60–80% EWL with typical maintenance of >50% EWL	• Greater, more rapid weight loss • ↑ PYY, GLP-1, CCK may contribute to reduced appetite • ↓ Ghrelin (but may return to baseline)	• Vitamin/mineral deficiencies—especially Ca, B12, folic acid, iron • Lifelong vitamin/mineral supplementation required • Dumping syndrome
Sleeve gastrectomy (SG)	Gastric antrum divided above pylorus and sleeve created around bougie; ~80% stomach removed	R > M	Similar to RYGB	More/more-rapid early weight loss than LAGB; ↓ ghrelin; ↑GLP-1 and PYY	Potential for vitamin + mineral deficiencies; nonreversible
Laparoscopic adjustable gastric band (LAGB)	Silicone ring placed around upper stomach and connected to subcutaneous access port for introduction or removal of saline	R	40–50% EWL Greater % of patients fail to lose at least 50% EWL	• Least invasive; lowest mortality rate • Adjustable and reversible • Low risk for vitamin/mineral deficiencies	• Less/slower early weight loss • Foreign device • Band slippage, erosion. • Explantation required in 5–6%. • Highest reoperation rate
Biliopancreatic diversion/ duodenal switch (BPD/DS)	• Stomach resected similarly to sleeve • Duodenum separated at pylorus • Ileum divided and distal end anastomosed to stomach • Proximal segment anastomosed to terminal ileum	R+M	≥60–70% EWL	• Greatest weight loss • Most effective against diabetes • Fat absorption reduced by ~70% • May eventually eat near-normal meals • ↓ Ghrelin	• Higher complication rate and mortality risk • Greater potential for vitamin/ mineral deficiencies • Fat-soluble vitamin deficiencies (A, D, E, K) • Protein deficiencies; lifelong vitamin/mineral supplementation required • Strict lifelong follow-up required • Dumping syndrome

EWL data from ASMBS

EWL, excess weight loss; R, restrictive; M, malabsorptive; PYY, peptide YY; GLP-1, glucagon-like peptide 1; CCK, cholecystokinin. American Society for Metabolic and Bariatric Surgery. Bariatric Surgery Procedures. https://www.asmbs.org/patients/bariatric-surgery-procedures.

- Achieving inpatient glucose control should be no different than other postoperative populations.
  - Critically-ill patients: IV insulin titrated per protocol to keep BG in the 140 to 180 mg/dL range.
  - Noncritically ill patients: long-acting insulin analogs (typically started at 50% of the preoperative dose) to achieve fasting glucose <140. A correction dose of rapid-acting insulin is given every 4 to 6 hours for hyperglycemia.
- Basal insulin requirements may fall significantly over several postoperative days as glycogen stores are depleted and insulin resistance wanes. Fixed-dose prandial insulin should not be needed, as the initial diet is carbohydrate free.
- There are no published guidelines regarding outpatient management of hypergly-cemia/T2DM after bariatric surgery. The following represent the authors' recom-mendation:
  - At discharge, some patients may still require basal insulin to maintain a fasting blood glucose <140 mg/dL. Discharge on hospital dose of basal insulin. Check glucose fasting daily. When fasting glucoses fall below 100, basal insulin doses can be reduced by 20%. This process can be repeated until insulin can be discontinued.
  - Discharge on hospital dose of basal insulin. Check fasting glucose daily. When fasting glucoses fall below 100, basal insulin doses can be reduced by 20%. This process can be repeated until insulin can be discontinued.
- Prandial insulin may be used cautiously during the early stages of diet advancement with routine monitoring of postprandial blood glucose and a plan in place to titrate insulin doses down if hypoglycemia occurs.
- Metformin is typically restarted within 1 to 2 days following surgery.
- An HbA1c of ≥7 is generally considered to be consistent with nonremission of dia-betes. There are no published society guidelines for the management of patients with nonremission of T2DM after bariatric surgery, and a detailed discussion of treatment is beyond the scope of this chapter.
  - Metformin is typically used as a first-line agent with use of second-line agents favoring those that promote weight loss.
  - The variable effects of the different bariatric procedures on insulin and incretin effects should be considered.
- **Hyperlipidemia:** statins should not routinely be discontinued postsurgery. Routine monitoring every 6 to 12 months is recommended, with treatment following estab-lished guidelines.[53]
- **Hypertension: hypotension** may develop postoperatively in the setting of poor fluid intake and hypovolemia. Consider holding diuretics until adequate intake is confirmed. BP should be monitored at all follow-up visits and treated according to established standards.
- **Skeletal/mineral homeostasis**
  - Following RYGB, dietary calcium bypasses the duodenum, where vitamin D–depen-dent calcium absorption takes place, resulting in increased risk of hypocalcemia and secondary hyperparathyroidism.[54]
    - Patients with vitamin D deficiency prior to surgery may require higher doses, 50,000 units weekly, after surgery.
    - Secondary hyperparathyroidism may persist.[55]
    - Calcium carbonate preparations should be chewable and taken with food to assist absorption. Calcium citrate will be better absorbed, and can be taken without food.
  - DEXA is recommended 2 years after surgery as, in addition to the above, the decrease in mechanical weight bearing of bones may result in increased bone turnover and a fall in bone density.[56]
  - Endocrine Society guidelines recommend vitamin D, calcium, phosphorus, PTH, and alkaline phosphatase levels be checked semiannually.[53]

- When osteoporosis is present, treatment with IV bisphosphonates is preferred over oral preparations due to concern over absorption and anastomotic ulceration; therapy should be started only after correction of vitamin D deficiency and with adequate calcium supplementation.[41]
  - **Micronutrient Deficiencies**
    - Multivitamin supplementation is recommended after all bariatric procedures (1/day for LAGB; 2/day for other procedures).[49]
    - Iron deficiency is found in 25% to 75% of patients by 5 to 10 years. Levels should be checked biannually. Prophylax in menstruating women after RYGB or BPD/DS—twice-daily 65 mg elemental iron supplementation. Vitamin C coadministration helps iron absorption.
    - B12 deficiency is found in 8% to 40% of RYGB patients by 1 year. Routine supplementation with vitamin B12 >350 µg/day is appropriate. Biannual assessment of levels is recommended in all bariatric surgery patients.
    - Folate deficiency can be prevented with folic acid 400 µg/day.
    - Thiamine deficiency may be seen in patients with recurrent/persistent vomiting needing IV fluids. Consider thiamine supplementation for those patients.
    - Risk for copper deficiency is increased after bariatric surgery. Signs include anemia, leukopenia, and neurologic manifestations similar to B12 deficiency.
    - Zinc levels should be checked if symptoms, including altered taste, hair changes, poor wound healing, or skin changes, are present.
    - Selenium deficiency may be seen after RYGB or BPD/DS and may result in skeletal muscle dysfunction or cardiomyopathy as well as macrocytosis, impaired immune function, and mood disorders
    - Deficiency of other fat-soluble vitamins, A, E, and K (in addition to D) may develop after bariatric procedures, particularly BPD/DS.
  - **Dumping syndrome**
    - Abdominal pain, cramping, nausea, diarrhea, lightheadedness, flushing, and tachycardia occurring shortly after eating in patients who have had RYGB or BPD/DS.
    - Results from consumption of carbohydrate-dense or hypertonic foods/beverages that enter the intestines quickly.
    - Reported in 70% to 76% of RYGB patients
    - May serve an important role in behavior adjustment.
    - Behaviors to prevent or lessen these symptoms include eating small frequent meals, not drinking until 30 minutes after meals, and avoiding simple sugars
  - **Postprandial hyperinsulinemic hypoglycemia**
    - Rare syndrome presenting with neuroglycopenic symptoms after meals
    - Diagnosed by negative 72-hour fast for hypoglycemia, hyperinsulinemia with hypoglycemia after a mixed meal tolerance test, and negative imaging for insulinoma
    - Medical management includes low-carbohydrate meals, acarbose, calcium channel blockers, diazoxide, and octreotide. Refractory patients have been treated with 80% pancreatectomy with improvement, but not absolute resolution. Pathology suggests islet hyperplasia.[57]
  - **Fertility concerns**
    - Pregnancy not recommended for 12 to 18 months following surgery
    - Nonoral contraceptives recommended due to potential for malabsorption.[49]
  - **Other conditions:** prophylaxis for gallstones (with ursodiol) and gout may be considered in at-risk patients.

Endoscopic Bariatric Therapy

Recently, the FDA approved various endoscopically placed devices as adjunct to lifestyle modifications in adults who have not achieved weight loss goals with other nonsurgical interventions. Like bariatric surgery, these modalities should be offered in centers that provide a multidisciplinary weight-loss program. Currently insurance coverage is limited.[58,59]

- **Intragastric balloon (IGB) systems:** IGBs promote satiety by reducing gastric capacity. Devices placed endoscopically are fluid filled; an ingestible option is swallowed as a capsule attached to catheter and inflated after placement is radiographically confirmed.
  - Approved for BMI 30 to 40 kg/m^2 for up to 6 months
  - TBL ~7% to 10% after 3 to 6 months
  - Patients with IGBs must take PPI
  - Adverse events: common early nausea, vomiting, abdominal pain contributing to ~10% early device removal. Other AEs include bowel changes, indigestion, and allergic reaction to device; more serious adverse events include gastric ulcerations, bleeding or perforation, and bowel obstruction.
  - Contraindications include certain GI tract disorders (e.g., large hiatal hernias, motility disorders) or GI surgeries, chronic use of NSAIDs or anticoagulants, pregnancy, eating disorders, alcoholism or drug addiction, or other serious current psychiatric illness. The FDA has issued warnings for fluid-filled IGBs being associated with spontaneous over inflation and acute pancreatitis requiring device removal.[58-60]
- **Gastric Emptying System:** The AspireAssist® system requires endoscopic placement of a percutaneous gastrostomy tube that is connected to a skin port. Patients must chew food longer so particle size is small enough to be removed. Postmeal patients attach an external siphon to the skin port to remove approximately one-third of the ingested meal. This device is for long-term weight loss.
  - Total body loss ~12% after 52 weeks
  - Approved for BMI 35 to 55 kg/m^2
  - Adverse events: common include peristomal granulation tissue, bleeding and irritation, abdominal pain, nausea, vomiting, changes in bowel habits, and electrolyte abnormalities. SAE include tube dislodgement, peritonitis, and severe abdominal pain.
  - Contraindications include increased risks for gastrostomy tube placement, upper GI motility issues, eating disorders, refractory gastric ulcers, advanced pulmonary disease or CVD, coagulation disorders, any reason that would significantly limit adherence to therapy.[58-60]
- Patients should be selected carefully for these recently approved procedures. Authors conclude that future experience will assist in determining the broader role of EBT.

OUTCOME/PROGNOSIS

- National Weight Control Registry—developed to identify and investigate the characteristics of individuals who have succeeded at long-term weight loss:[61]
  - >10,000 individuals who have lost an average of 66 lb and kept it off for an average of 5.5 years
  - Most report maintaining a low-calorie, low-fat diet
  - 78% eat breakfast every day
  - 75% weigh at least weekly
  - 62% watch <10 hours of TV per week
  - 90% exercise; average 1 hr/day
- 8-year follow-up in the Look AHEAD study highlighted similar factors in successful maintenance of weight loss, in addition to noting increased use of meal replacements.[62]

REFERENCES

1. Puhl R, Peterson JL, Luedicke J. Motivating or stigmatizing? Public perceptions of weight-related language used by health providers. *Int J Obes (Lond)*. 2013;37(4):612–619.

2. Ogden CL, Carroll MD, Fryar CD, Flegal KM. *Prevalence of Obesity Among Adults and Youth: United States, 2011–2014. NCHS Data Brief, No. 219.* Hyattsville, MD: National Center for Health Statistics; 2015.

3. Flegal KM, Carroll MD, Ogden CL, Curtin LR. Prevalence and trends in obesity among US adults, 1999–2008. *JAMA* 2010;303(3):235–241.

4. Locke AE, Kahali B, Berndt SI, et al. Genetic studies of body mass index yield new insights for obesity biology. *Nature* 2015;518(7538):197–206.

5. Dina C, Meyre D, Gallina S, et al. Variation in FTO contributes to childhood obesity and severe adult obesity. *Nat Genet* 2007;39(6):724–726.

6. Farooqi IS, Wangensteen T, Collins S, et al. Clinical and molecular genetic spectrum of congenital deficiency of the leptin receptor. *N Engl J Med* 2007;356(3):237–247.

7. Santini F, Maffei M, Pelosini C, Salvetti G, Scartabelli G, Pinchera A. Melanocortin-4 receptor mutations in obesity. *Adv Clin Chem* 2009;48:95–109.

8. Ganz ML, Wintfeld N, Li Q, Alas V, Langer J, Hammer M. The association of body mass index with the risk of type 2 diabetes: A case-control study nested in an electronic health records system in the United States. *Diabetol Metab Syndr* 2014;6(1):50.

9. Colditz GA, Willett WC, Rotnitzky A, Manson JE. Weight gain as a risk factor for clinical diabetes mellitus in women. *Ann Intern Med* 1995;122(7):481–486.

10. Koh-Banerjee P, Wang Y, Hu FB, Spiegelman D, Willett WC, Rimm EB. Changes in body weight and body fat distribution as risk factors for clinical diabetes in US men. *Am J Epidemiol* 2004;159(12):1150–1159.

11. Willett WC, Manson JE, Stampfer MJ, et al. Weight, weight change, and coronary heart disease in women. Risk within the 'normal' weight range. *JAMA* 1995;273(6):461–465.

12. Kenchaiah S, Evans JC, Levy D, et al. Obesity and the risk of heart failure. *N Engl J Med* 2002;347(5):305–313.

13. Klein S, Mittendorfer B, Eagon JC, et al. Gastric bypass surgery improves metabolic and hepatic abnormalities associated with nonalcoholic fatty liver disease. *Gastroenterology* 2006;130(6):1564–1572.

14. Basen-Engquist K, Chang M. Obesity and cancer risk: Recent review and evidence. *Curr Oncol Rep* 2011;13(1):71–76.

15. Flegal KM, Graubard BI, Williamson DF, Gail MH. Excess deaths associated with underweight, overweight, and obesity. *JAMA* 2005;293(15):1861–1867.

16. Whitlock G, Lewington S, Sherliker P, et al. Body-mass index and cause-specific mortality in 900 000 adults: Collaborative analyses of 57 prospective studies. *Lancet* 2009;373(9669):1083–1096.

17. Borrell LN, Samuel L. Body mass index categories and mortality risk in US adults: The effect of overweight and obesity on advancing death. *Am J Public Health* 2014;104(3):512–519.

18. Magkos F, Fraterrigo G, Yoshino J, et al. Effects of moderate and subsequent progressive weight loss on metabolic function and adipose tissue biology in humans with obesity. *Cell metab* 2016;23(4):591–601.

19. Knowler WC, Barrett-Connor E, Fowler SE, et al. Reduction in the incidence of type 2 diabetes with lifestyle intervention or metformin. *N Engl J Med* 2002;346(6):393–403.

20. Klein S, Sheard NF, Pi-Sunyer X, et al. Weight management through lifestyle modification for the prevention and management of type 2 diabetes: Rationale and strategies: A statement of the American Diabetes Association, the North American Association for the Study of Obesity, and the American Society for Clinical Nutrition. *Diabetes Care* 2004;27(8):2067–2073.

21. Neter JE, Stam BE, Kok FJ, Grobbee DE, Geleijnse JM. Influence of weight reduction on blood pressure: A meta-analysis of randomized controlled trials. *Hypertension* 2003;42(5):878–884.

22. Rasmussen KM, Abrams B, Bodnar LM, Butte NF, Catalano PM, Maria Siega-Riz A. Recommendations for weight gain during pregnancy in the context of the obesity epidemic. *Obstet Gynecol* 2010;116(5):1191–1195.

23. Jensen MD, Ryan DH, Apovian CM, et al. 2013 AHA/ACC/TOS guideline for the management of overweight and obesity in adults: A report of the American College of Cardiology/American Heart Association Task Force on Practice Guidelines and The Obesity Society. *Circulation* 2014;129(25 Suppl 2):S102–S138.

24. Vink RG, Roumans NJ, Arkenbosch LA, Mariman EC, van Baak MA. The effect of rate of weight loss on long-term weight regain in adults with overweight and obesity. *Obesity (Silver Spring)* 2016;24(2):321–327.

25. Lejeune MP, Westerterp KR, Adam TC, Luscombe-Marsh ND, Westerterp-Plantenga MS. Ghrelin and glucagon-like peptide 1 concentrations, 24-h satiety, and energy and substrate metabolism during a high-protein diet and measured in a respiration chamber. *Am J Clin Nutr* 2006;83(1):89–94.

26. Claessens M, van Baak MA, Monsheimer S, Saris WH. The effect of a low-fat, high-protein or high-carbohydrate ad libitum diet on weight loss maintenance and metabolic risk factors. *Int J Obes (Lond)*. 2009;33(3):296–304.

27. Esposito K, Maiorino MI, Ciotola M, et al. Effects of a Mediterranean-style diet on the need for antihyperglycemic drug therapy in patients with newly diagnosed type 2 diabetes: A randomized trial. *Ann Intern Med* 2009;151(5):306–314.

28. Estruch R, Ros E, Salas-Salvado J, et al. Primary prevention of cardiovascular disease with a Mediterranean diet. *N Engl J Med* 2013;368(14):1279–1290.

29. Salas-Salvado J, Bullo M, Babio N, et al. Reduction in the incidence of type 2 diabetes with the Mediterranean diet: Results of the PREDIMED-Reus nutrition intervention randomized trial. *Diabetes Care* 2011;34(1):14–19.

30. Catenacci VA, Ogden LG, Stuht J, et al. Physical activity patterns in the National Weight Control Registry. *Obesity (Silver Spring)* 2008;16(1):153–161.

31. Haskell WL, Lee IM, Pate RR, et al. Physical activity and public health: Updated recommendation for adults from the American College of Sports Medicine and the American Heart Association. *Circulation* 2007;116(9):1081–1093.

32. Colberg SR, Sigal RJ, Yardley JE, et al. Physical activity/exercise and diabetes: A position statement of the American Diabetes Association. *Diabetes Care* 2016;39(11):2065–2079.

33. Wing RR, Jakicic J, Neiberg R, et al. Fitness, fatness, and cardiovascular risk factors in type 2 diabetes: Look AHEAD study. *Med Sci Sports Exerc* 2007;39(12):2107–2116.

34. Wadden TA, Foster GD. Behavioral treatment of obesity. *Med Clin North Am* 2000;84(2):441–461, vii.

35. Apovian CM, Aronne LJ, Bessesen DH, et al. Pharmacological management of obesity: An Endocrine Society clinical practice guideline. *J Clin Endocrinol Metab* 2015;100(2):342–362.

36. Choi J, Digiorgi M, Milone L, et al. Outcomes of laparoscopic adjustable gastric banding in patients with low body mass index. *Surg Obes Relat Dis* 2010;6(4):367–371.

37. American Diabetes Association. Standards of Medical Care in Diabetes—2017. *Diabetes Care* 2017;40(Suppl 1):S1–S142.

38. American Diabetes Association. Obesity management for the treatment of type 2 diabetes. *Diabetes Care* 2017;40(Suppl 1):S57–S63.

39. Colquitt JL, Pickett K, Loveman E, Frampton GK. Surgery for weight loss in adults. *Cochrane Database Syst Rev* 2014(8):CD003641.

40. Buchwald H, Avidor Y, Braunwald E, et al. Bariatric surgery: A systematic review and meta-analysis. *JAMA* 2004;292(14):1724–1737.

41. Mechanick JI, Kushner RF, Sugerman HJ, et al. American Association of Clinical Endocrinologists, The Obesity Society, and American Society for Metabolic & Bariatric Surgery Medical guidelines for clinical practice for the perioperative nutritional, metabolic, and nonsurgical support of the bariatric surgery patient. *Endocr Pract* 2008;14 (Suppl 1):1–83.

42. Mummadi RR, Kasturi KS, Chennareddygari S, Sood GK. Effect of bariatric surgery on non-alcoholic fatty liver disease: Systematic review and meta-analysis. *Clin Gastroenterol Hepatol* 2008;6(12):1396–1402.

43. Nelson LG, Gonzalez R, Haines K, Gallagher SF, Murr MM. Amelioration of gastroesophageal reflux symptoms following Roux-en-Y gastric bypass for clinically significant obesity. *Am Surg* 2005;71(11):950–953; discussion 953–954.

44. Manfield JH, Yu KK, Efthimiou E, Darzi A, Athanasiou T, Ashrafian H. Bariatric surgery or non-surgical weight loss for idiopathic intracranial hypertension? A systematic review and comparison of meta-analyses. *Obes Surg* 2017;27(2):513–521.

45. Abu-Abeid S, Wishnitzer N, Szold A, Liebergall M, Manor O. The influence of surgically-induced weight loss on the knee joint. *Obes Surg* 2005;15(10):1437–1442.

46. Hooper MM, Stellato TA, Hallowell PT, Seitz BA, Moskowitz RW. Musculoskeletal findings in obese subjects before and after weight loss following bariatric surgery. *Int J Obes (Lond)* 2007;31(1):114–120.

47. Adams TD, Gress RE, Smith SC, et al. Long-term mortality after gastric bypass surgery. *N Engl J Med* 2007;357(8):753–761.

48. Davidson LE, Adams TD, Kim J, et al. Association of patient age at gastric bypass surgery with long-term all-cause and cause-specific mortality. *JAMA Surg* 2016;151(7):631–637.

49. Mechanick JI, Youdim A, Jones DB, et al. Clinical practice guidelines for the perioperative nutritional, metabolic, and nonsurgical support of the bariatric surgery patient—2013 update: Cosponsored by American Association of Clinical Endocrinologists, The Obesity Society, and American Society for Metabolic & Bariatric Surgery. *Obesity (Silver Spring)* 2013;21 (Suppl 1):S1–S27.

50. American Society for Metabolic and Bariatric Surgery. Bariatric Surgery Procedures. Retrieved June 8, 2018, from https://www.asmbs.org/patients/bariatric-surgery-procedures.

51. Arterburn DE, Courcoulas AP. Bariatric surgery for obesity and metabolic conditions in adults. *BMJ* 2014;349:g3961.

52. National Institute of Diabetes and Digestive and Kidney Diseases (NIDDK). Longitudinal Assessment of Bariatric Surgery (LABS). Retrieved September 12, 2017, from https://www.niddk.nih.gov/health-information/weight-management/longitudinal-assessment-bariatric-surgery.

53. Heber D, Greenway FL, Kaplan LM, Livingston E, Salvador J, Still C. Endocrine and nutritional management of the post-bariatric surgery patient: An Endocrine Society Clinical Practice Guideline. *J Clin Endocrinol Metab* 2010;95(11):4823–4843.

54. Carlin AM, Rao DS, Meslemani AM, et al. Prevalence of vitamin D depletion among morbidly obese patients seeking gastric bypass surgery. *Surg Obes Relat Dis* 2006;2(2):98–103; discussion 104.

55. Carlin AM, Rao DS, Yager KM, Genaw JA, Parikh NJ, Szymanski W. Effect of gastric bypass surgery on vitamin D nutritional status. *Surg Obes Relat Dis* 2006;2(6):638–642.

56. Coates PS, Fernstrom JD, Fernstrom MH, Schauer PR, Greenspan SL. Gastric bypass surgery for morbid obesity leads to an increase in bone turnover and a decrease in bone mass. *J Clin Endocrinol Metab* 2004;89(3):1061–1065.

57. Mathavan VK, Arregui M, Davis C, Singh K, Patel A, Meacham J. Management of postgastric bypass noninsulinoma pancreatogenous hypoglycemia. *Surg Endosc* 2010;24(10):2547–2555.

58. Hurt RT, Frazier TH, Mundi MS. Novel nonsurgical endoscopic approaches for the treatment of obesity. *Nutr Clin Pract* 2017;32(4):493–501.

59. Bennett MC, Badillo R, Sullivan S. Endoscopic management. *Gastroenterol Clin North Am* 2016;45(4):673–688.

60. U.S. Food and Drug Administration. Obesity Treatment Devices. Retrieved June 28, 2017, from https://www.fda.gov/medicaldevices/productsandmedicalprocedures/obesitydevices.

61. Brown Medical School/The Miriam Hospital Weight Control & Diabetes Research Center. The National Weight Control Registry. Retrieved September 10, 2017, from http://www.nwcr.ws.

62. The Look AHEAD Research Group. Eight-year weight losses with an intensive lifestyle intervention: The look AHEAD study. *Obesity (Silver Spring)* 2014;22(1):5–13.

Dyslipidemia

35

Jacqueline L. Cartier and Anne C. Goldberg

GENERAL PRINCIPLES

Definition

- Multiple definitions can be found in guidelines. The following is from the National Lipid Association (NLA) in mg/dL for adults.[1]
  - Low-density lipoprotein cholesterol (LDL-C):
    - <100 desirable
    - 100 to 129 above desirable
    - 130 to 159 borderline high
    - 160 to 189 high
    - ≥190 very high
  - High-density lipoprotein cholesterol (HDL-C):
    - <40 (men) low
    - <50 (women) low
  - Non-HDL-C:
    - <130 desirable
    - 130 to 159 above desirable
    - 160 to 189 borderline high
    - 190 to 219 high
    - ≥220 very high
  - Triglycerides:
    - <150 normal
    - 150 to 199 borderline high
    - 200 to 499 high
    - ≥500 very high
- Dyslipidemia usually fits one of four general patterns:
  - Isolated hypertriglyceridemia
  - Isolated elevation in LDL-C
  - Combined elevation of triglycerides and LDL-C
  - Isolated low HDL-C

Epidemiology

Dyslipidemia is very common in the United States. An estimated 28.5 million adults ≥20 years of age have total cholesterol levels ≥240 mg/dL.[2]

Etiology

- Both genetic and environmental factors play a role in the development of dyslipidemia.
- The underlying pathophysiology of dyslipidemia is often complex. Although specific genetic markers have not been identified for many cases, some have a clear genetic basis with a well-defined underlying mechanism (see Table 35-1).[3,4]
- Differential diagnosis of the major lipid abnormalities is summarized in Table 35-2.

Genetic dyslipidemia	Typical lipid profile	Inheritance pattern	Phenotypic features	Pathophysiology
Isolated LDL elevation				
Familial hypercholesterolemia (FH)	Heterozygous form: LDL >220 mg/dL Homozygous form: LDL >500 mg/dL	Autosomal dominant	• Premature CAD • Tendon xanthomas • Xanthelasma • Premature arcus corneae	Caused by mutations of the LDL receptor that lead to defective uptake and degradation of LDL
Familial defective apo B-100	Similar to familial hypercholesterolemia	Autosomal dominant	• Similar to familial hypercholesterolemia	Caused by a mutation in apo B-100 which impairs the interaction of LDL with the receptor leading to decreased LDL clearance
PCSK9 gain-of-function[3]	Similar to familial hypercholesterolemia	Autosomal dominant	• Similar to familial hypercholesterolemia	Caused by either an increase in PCSK9 levels or formation of a tighter bound between the PCSK9 and LDL receptor. PCSK9 targets LDL receptor for degradation
Isolated triglyceride elevation				
Lipoprotein lipase (LPL) OR apo C-II deficiency	TGs 1,000–25,000 mg/dL	Autosomal recessive	• Diagnosed in childhood • Eruptive xanthomas • Lipemia retinalis • Pancreatitis • Hepatosplenomegaly • Clinical manifestations occur when triglycerides exceed 1,500 mg/dL	Deficiency in LPL or its cofactor apo C-II impairs uptake of triglycerides into peripheral tissues
Familial hypertriglyceridemia	TGs 150–500 mg/dL or higher in the presence of secondary factors (obesity, alcohol use, diabetes)	Autosomal dominant	• Diagnosed in adulthood • Same as for LPL if triglyceride levels are severely elevated	Caused by overproduction of VLDL triglycerides Genetic defects are not established
Combined elevations in LDL and triglycerides				
Familial combined hyperlipidemia (FCH)	Moderately elevated levels of LDL, triglycerides or both	Autosomal dominant	• Premature CAD Tendon and cutaneous xanthomas are absent	Caused by overproduction of VLDL Genetic defects are not established

(continued)

TABLE 35-1 REVIEW OF MAJOR GENETIC DYSLIPOPROTEINEMIAS (Continued)

Genetic dyslipidemia	Typical lipid profile	Inheritance pattern	Phenotypic features	Pathophysiology
Type III hyperlipoproteinemia (familial dysbetalipoproteinemia)	Symmetric elevations of cholesterol and triglycerides (300–500 mg/dL) Emergence of hyperlipidemia often requires a secondary factor	Autosomal recessive	• Premature CAD • Tuberous or tuberoeruptive xanthomas • Planar xanthomas of the palmar creases are essentially pathognomonic	Caused by homozygous mutation in apo E (apo E2/E2) leading to defective clearance of chylomicron and VLDL remnants
Isolated low HDL[4]				
Familial hypoalphalipoproteinemia	HDL levels below the 10th percentile (<30 mg/dL for men and <40 mg/dL for premenopausal women)	Autosomal dominant	• Premature CAD • No characteristic findings on physical examination	Genetic defects are not established
Tangier disease	HDL levels <20 mg/dL	Autosomal recessive	• Peripheral neuropathy • Tonsillar enlargement • Hepatosplenomegaly • Yellow-orange discoloration of the tonsils and rectal mucosa	Mutations of the ABCA1 gene which transports cellular cholesterol to extracellular apoA-I to form HDL
Familial LCAT deficiency	HDL levels <20 mg/dL	Autosomal recessive	• Corneal opacification • Anemia • Progressive renal disease	Essentially complete LCAT deficiency. LCAT catalyzes conversion of free cholesterol to esters that migrate into the core of HDL
Fish-eye disease	HDL levels <20 mg/dL	Autosomal recessive	• Corneal opacification	Milder form of LCAT deficiency

CAD, coronary artery disease; HDL, high-density lipoprotein; LDL, low-density lipoprotein; PCSK9, proprotein convertase subtilisin/kexin type 9; TGs, triglycerides; VLDL, very low-density lipoprotein.

Prevention

Diet, exercise, and weight loss play a large role in the prevention and treatment of dyslipidemia.[5]

Associated Conditions

- Dyslipidemia is a major modifiable risk factor for cardiovascular, cerebrovascular, and peripheral vascular disease. Lower LDL-C levels decrease the incidence of heart attacks, revascularization, and ischemic strokes; it is estimated that for each 1 mmol/L (about 40 mg/dL) reduction, the risk of major vascular events is decreased by about 20%.[6] Elevated triglycerides and low HDL-C may confer additional risk, but the benefit of lowering triglycerides and raising HDL-C is less well established.[4]
- Dyslipidemia is often associated with a constellation of additional metabolic abnormalities including obesity, hypertension, insulin resistance, and fatty liver disease.

Diagnosis

- Screening for dyslipidemia should be performed at least every 5 years beginning at age 20. If non–HDL-C and LDL-C are in the desirable range, repeat in 5 years or sooner based on clinical judgment. Consider earlier rescreening if there is a change in atherosclerotic cardiovascular disease (ASCVD) risk factors, evidence of ASCVD, a premature ASCVD event in a first-degree relative, or a new potential secondary cause of dyslipidemia.[1]
- Certain physical examination findings (see Physical Examination section) can be a clue to a lipid disorder and should prompt a screening lipid panel (see Table 35-1).[3,4]

Clinical Presentation

History

The history should focus on identification of secondary causes of dyslipidemia, family history of premature coronary disease, and evaluation of cardiovascular risk factors. Diet, medications, alcohol consumption, and comorbid conditions can contribute to the expression and severity of dyslipidemia (see Table 35-2). A detailed family history is important because a strong family history of premature coronary disease may suggest a genetic dyslipoproteinemia (see Table 35-1).[1,6] Since cardiovascular risk determines an individual patient's intensity of treatment, assessment of risk factors is necessary (see section Treatment).

Physical Examination

The physical examination should focus on identification of occult vascular disease (bruits) and physical findings that suggest a severe dyslipoproteinemia, such as tendon xanthomas, palmar xanthomas, eruptive xanthomas, tuberous xanthomas, xanthelasma, lipemia retinalis, or premature arcus corneae.

Diagnostic Testing

- The **fasting lipid panel** is the cornerstone of diagnosis.
- Most laboratories directly measure levels of triglycerides, total cholesterol, and HDL-C and calculate LDL-C. If triglycerides are >400 mg/dL, calculated LDL-C measurements are not reliable, and direct LDL-C should be measured.
- New onset of hypertriglyceridemia should prompt screening for diabetes, hypothyroidism, and renal failure.
- Newly elevated LDL-C should prompt screening for hypothyroidism, obstructive liver disease, and nephrotic syndrome.

TREATMENT

Statin benefit groups: The American College of Cardiology/American Heart Association 2013 cholesterol guidelines provide recommendations on the treatment of blood cholesterol

TABLE 35-2	DIFFERENTIAL DIAGNOSIS OF MAJOR LIPID ABNORMALITIES	
Lipid abnormality	Primary disorders	Secondary disorders
Hypercholesterolemia	Polygenic, familial hypercholesterolemia, familial defective apo B-100	Hypothyroidism, nephrotic syndrome, obstructive liver disease, thiazide diuretics
Hypertriglyceridemia	Lipoprotein lipase deficiency, apo C-II deficiency, familial hypertriglyceridemia	Poorly controlled diabetes mellitus, hypothyroidism, renal failure, obesity, high carbohydrate diets, alcohol use, oral estrogen, β blockers, protease inhibitors glucocorticoids, retinoids, bile acid–binding resins, antipsychotics, thiazide diuretics
Combined hyperlipidemia	Familial combined hyperlipidemia, type III hyperlipoproteinemia	Poorly controlled diabetes mellitus, hypothyroidism, glucocorticoids, immuno-suppressants, protease inhibitors, nephrotic syndrome
Low HDL	Familial hypoalphalipo-proteinemia, Tangier's disease, familial HDL deficiency, lecithin: cholesterol acyltrans-ferase deficiency	Anabolic steroids, retinoids, tobacco use

HDL, high-density lipoprotein.

to reduce atherosclerotic cardiovascular risk in adults.[5] The guidelines focus on identifying four statin benefit groups and determining the appropriate intensity of statin therapy (see Table 35-3).[5]

- **Secondary prevention**
  ○ High-intensity statin therapy as first-line therapy in individuals ≤75 years of age who have clinical ASCVD.
  ○ If high-intensity statin therapy is contraindicated, moderate-intensity statin is an option.
  ○ If >75 years of age, evaluate potential ASCVD risk-reduction benefits, adverse effects, drug–drug interactions, and patient preferences. It is reasonable to continue statin therapy in those who are tolerating it.
- **Primary prevention in individuals ≥21 years of age with LDL ≥190 mg/dL**
  ○ Evaluate for secondary causes of hyperlipidemia in individuals with LDL-C ≥190 mg/dL or triglycerides ≥500 mg/dL.
  ○ Adults ≥21 years of age with LDL-C ≥190 mg/dL should be treated with statin therapy (10-year ASCVD risk estimation is not required):
    ▪ Use high-intensity statin therapy unless contraindicated
    ▪ Use the maximum tolerated statin therapy if unable to tolerate high-intensity statin

TABLE 35-3	RECOMMENDATIONS FOR TREATMENT OF BLOOD CHOLESTEROL TO REDUCE ATHEROSCLEROTIC CARDIOVASCULAR RISK IN ADULTS

Prevention type	Treatment group
Secondary	Individuals ≤75 years of age who have clinical ASCVD[a]
Primary	Adults ≥21 years of age with LDL-C of ≥190 mg/dL
Primary	Adults 40 to 75 years of age with diabetes and LDL-C 70–189 mg/dL without clinical ASCVD
Primary	Adults 40 to 75 years of age with LDL-C 70–189 mg/dL without clinical ASCVD[a] or diabetes and with an estimated 10-year ASCVD risk of ≥7.5%

[a]Clinical ASCVD includes acute coronary syndromes, history of MI, stable or unstable angina, coronary or other arterial revascularizations, stroke, TIA, or peripheral arterial disease presumed to be of atherosclerotic origin.

Adapted from Stone NJ, Robinson JG, Lichtenstein AH, et al. 2013 ACC/AHA guideline on the treatment of blood cholesterol to reduce atherosclerotic cardiovascular risk in adults: a report of the American College of Cardiology/American Heart Association Task Force on Practice Guidelines. *J Am Coll Cardiol* 2014;63:2889–2934.

- ○ For individuals ≥21 years of age with an untreated primary LDL-C ≥190 mg/dL:
  - ■ It is reasonable to intensify statin therapy to achieve at least a 50% LDL-C reduction
  - ■ Addition of a nonstatin drug may be considered to further lower LDL-C after the maximum intensity of statin therapy has been achieved
- **Primary prevention in individuals with diabetes and LDL 70 to 189 mg/dL**
  - ○ For adults 40 to 75 years of age with diabetes:
    - ■ Moderate-intensity statin therapy should be initiated/continued.
    - ■ High-intensity statin therapy is reasonable if estimated 10-year ASCVD risk is ≥7.5%.
  - ○ For adults <40 years of age or >75 or LDL <70: It is reasonable to evaluate potential ASCVD risk-reduction benefits, adverse effects, drug–drug interactions, and patient preferences when deciding to initiate, continue, or intensify statin therapy.
- **Primary prevention in individuals without diabetes and with LDL 70 to 189 mg/dL**
  - ○ Use the pooled cohort equations to estimate 10-year ASCVD risk.
  - ○ Adults 40 to 75 years of age with LDL-C 70 to 189 mg/dL without clinical ASCVD or diabetes:
    - ■ If 10-year ASCVD risk ≥7.5%, treat with moderate- to high-intensity statin therapy
    - ■ If 10-year ASCVD risk is 5% to <7.5%, it is reasonable to treat with a moderate-intensity statin
    - ■ If a risk-based treatment decision is uncertain, additional factors may be considered to inform decision-making
    - ■ **A risk discussion between clinician and patient is required before initiation of statin therapy.**

Medications

Statin Therapies

Percent reductions in LDL-C for a specific statin and dose have been calculated from randomized controlled trials (see Table 35-4).[5]

- High-intensity: lowers LDL-C by approximately ≥50%
- Moderate-intensity: lowers LDL-C by approximately 30% to <50%
- Low-intensity: lowers LDL-C by <30%

TABLE 35-4	HIGH-, MODERATE-, AND LOW-INTENSITY STATIN THERAPY
Statin therapy	Drug name and dose
High intensity Daily dose lowers LDL-C, on average, by approximately ≥50%	Atorvastatin 40–80 mg Rosuvastatin 20–40 mg
Moderate intensity Daily dose lowers LDL-C, on average, by approximately 30% to <50%	Atorvastatin 10–20 mg Rosuvastatin 5–10 mg Simvastatin 20–40 mg Pravastatin 40–80 mg Lovastatin 40 mg Fluvastatin XL 80 mg Fluvastatin 40 mg bid, Pitavastatin 2–4 mg
Low intensity Daily dose lowers LDL-C, on average, by <30%	Simvastatin 10 mg Pravastatin 10–20 mg Lovastatin 20 mg Fluvastatin 20–40 mg Pitavastatin 1 mg

LDL-C, low-density lipoprotein cholesterol.
Adapted from Stone NJ, Robinson JG, Lichtenstein AH, et al. 2013 ACC/AHA guideline on the treatment of blood cholesterol to reduce atherosclerotic cardiovascular risk in adults: A report of the American College of Cardiology/American Heart Association Task Force on Practice Guidelines. *J Am Coll Cardiol* 2014;63:2889–2934.

Nonstatin Therapies[7]
- **Please see** Table 35-5[5,8–10]
- **Adults ≥21 years of age with clinical ASCVD, on statin for secondary prevention**
  - **Stable clinical ASCVD without comorbidities:** If a patient has a less-than-anticipated response (<50% reduction in LDL-C)
    - Address statin adherence
    - Increase dose to a high-intensity statin if not on already
    - If unable to tolerate even a moderate-intensity statin, evaluate for statin intolerance
    - Intensify lifestyle modification
    - Consider incorporation of soluble dietary fiber and phytosterols
    - If the patient still has not had <50% reduction in LDL-C, discuss adding a nonstatin:
      - First line: ezetimibe 10 mg daily: lowers LDL and improves cardiovascular outcomes[11]
      - Second line: bile acid sequestrant (BAS) if ezetimibe intolerance and triglycerides <300 mg/dL
      - If patient still has <50% reduction in LDL-C, consider alirocumab or evolocumab (and continue maximally tolerated statin)
  - **Clinical ASCVD with comorbidities**
    - Comorbidities: diabetes, recent (<3 months) ASVD event, ASCVD event while already taking a statin, poorly controlled other major ASCVD risk factors, elevated lipoprotein(a), or CKD not on hemodialysis.
    - Similar approach as outlined above for those without comorbidities but consider a lower LDL-C threshold of <70 mg/dL and non-HDL-C threshold of <100 mg/dL
- **Clinical ASCVD and baseline LDL-C ≥190 mg/dL not due to secondary causes**

TABLE 35-5 CHARACTERISTICS OF THE LIPID-LOWERING DRUGS

Drug class	Agents and daily doses	Lipid/lipoprotein effects	Side effects	Contraindications
HMG CoA reductase inhibitors (statins)	Lovastatin (20–80 mg) Pravastatin (20–40 mg) Simvastatin (20–40 mg) Fluvastatin (20–80 mg) Atorvastatin (10–80 mg) Pitavastatin (1–4 mg) Rosuvastatin (5–40 mg)	LDL-C ↓ 18–55% HDL-C ↑ 5–15% TG ↓ 10–30%	Myopathy Increased liver enzymes	Absolute: active liver disease Relative: concomitant use of certain drugs[a]
Bile acid sequestrants	Cholestyramine (8–16 g) Colestipol (2–16 g) Colesevelam (1.9–3.8 g)	LDL-C ↓ 10–27% HDL ↑ 3–5% TG no change or increase	GI distress Constipation Decreased absorption of other drugs	Absolute: Dysbetalipoproteinemia, TG >400 mg/dL Relative: TG >200 mg/dL
Nicotinic acid[8]	Immediate release (1.5–3 g) Extended release (1–2 g)	LDL-C ↓ 5–20% HDL-C ↑ 10–30% TG ↓ 10–30%	Flushing Hyperglycemia Hyperuricemia GI distress Hepatotoxicity	Absolute: chronic liver disease, severe gout Relative: poorly controlled diabetes, Hyperuricemia, Peptic ulcer disease
Fibric acids[8]	Gemfibrozil (600 mg bid) Fenofibrate (various dose forms 135 to 200 mg)	LDL-C ↓ 5–20%[b] HDL-C ↑ 10–20% TG ↓ 30–50%	Dyspepsia Gallstones Myopathy	Severe renal disease Severe hepatic disease
Cholesterol absorption inhibitor	Ezetimibe (10 mg)	LDL-C ↓ 18% HDL-C No change TG no change	Diarrhea Myalgias	Severe hepatic disease

(continued)

TABLE 35-5 **CHARACTERISTICS OF THE LIPID-LOWERING DRUGS** *(Continued)*

Drug class	Agents and daily doses	Lipid/lipoprotein effects	Side effects	Contraindications
Omega-3 fatty acids[8]	Lovaza (3–4 g) OTC Fish oils (have variable quantities of EPA + DHA: need 3–4 g total)	LDL-C no significant change HDL-C ↑ 5% TG ↑ 20–50%	Eructation Diarrhea Gastrointestinal distress	None
Antisense oligonucleotide inhibitor of apo B[9]	Mipomersen (200 mg SC once weekly)	LDL-C ↓ 25–37% HDL-C no change TG ↓ 9–27%	Injection site reactions Influenza-like symptoms Hepatotoxicity	Moderate or severe hepatic impairment Active liver disease or persistent elevated serum transaminase levels
Microsomal triglyceride transfer protein inhibitor[9]	Lomitapide 5–60 mg	LDL-C ↓ 38–51% HDL-C no change TG ~–30%	GI distress Hepatotoxicity	Concomitant use with strong or moderate CYP3A4 inhibitors Moderate or severe hepatic impairment or active liver disease
PCSK9 Inhibitors[10]	Alirocumab 75 mg or 150 mg every two weeks Evolocumab 140 mg SC every two weeks or 420 mg once per month	LDL-C ↓ 45–71% HDL-C ↑ 5–12% TG ↓ 4–17%	Injection site reactions Nasopharyngitis	None

[a]Cyclosporine, macrolide antibiotics, various antifungal agents, and cytochrome P-450 inhibitors.

[b]May be increased in patients with elevated TG.

LDL-C, low-density lipoprotein cholesterol; HDL-C, high-density lipoprotein cholesterol; TG, triglycerides.

Adapted from Lloyd-Jones DM, Morris PB, Ballantyne CM, et al. 2016 ACC Expert Consensus Decision Pathway on the Role of Non-Statin Therapies for LDL–Cholesterol Lowering in the Management of Atherosclerotic Cardiovascular Disease Risk: A Report of the American College of Cardiology Task Force on Clinical Expert Consensus Documents. *J Am Coll Cardiol* 2016;68(1):92–125.

- More likely to have heterozygous (HeFH) or homozygous (HoFH) familial hyper-cholesterolemia, genetic disorders. If identified, perform cascade screening (systematic assessment of close biologic relatives to identify others with the disease).
- If the patient has not achieved a >50% reduction in LDL-C on statin therapy, it is reasonable to consider a proprotein convertase subtilisin/kexin type 9 (PCSK9) inhibitor as a first step rather than ezetimibe or BAS given PCSK9 inhibitors' greater LDL-C lowering efficacy. Evolocumab reduces risk of cardiovascular events.[12]
- If combination statin and nonstatin therapy with ezetimibe (or a BAS) and a PCSK9 inhibitor have been attempted and the patient still has <50% reduction in LDL-C, refer to a lipid specialist.
  - Mipomersen or lomitapide are only approved for the treatment of HoFH.
  - LDL apheresis: phenotypic HeFH and LDL-C ≥190 mg/dL despite maximally tolerated medical therapy and phenotypic HoFH.
- **Adults ≥21 years of age With LDL-C ≥190 mg/dL (not due to secondary modifiable causes) on statin for primary prevention**
  - Early treatment can substantially reduce the risk of ASCVD
  - Monitor lifestyle modification and maximally tolerated statin therapy
  - Low-saturated fat, low-cholesterol diet should be encouraged and refer to a nutritionist. Even with strict adherence, diet has limited impact on the severity of hypercholesterolemia.
  - Risk markers: family history of premature ASCVD events, tobacco use, diabetes, hypertension, chronic kidney disease, evidence of subclinical atherosclerosis, elevated lipoprotein(a), or elevated high-sensitivity C-reactive protein. Attempt to control to the extent possible
  - If ≤50% reduction in LDL-C (may consider <100 mg/dL or non-HDL-C <130 mg/dL in patients with diabetes) on maximally tolerated statin, consider adding either ezetimibe or a PCSK9 inhibitor (depending on desired additional percentage reduction in LDL-C). BAS may be considered as second line.
- **Adults aged 40 to 75 years without ASCVD, but with diabetes and LDL-C 70 to 189 mg/dL, on statin for primary prevention**
  - If 10-year ASCVD risk <7.5% and without high-risk features:
    - Moderate intensity statin but increase to high-intensity statin if there is failure to achieve a 30% to 50% reduction in LDL-C (or consider if LDL-C ≥100 mg/dL or non-HDL-C ≥130 mg/dL) despite intensification of lifestyle modification.
    - If escalation to high-intensity statin results in <50% reduction in LDL-C, discuss addition of a nonstatin medication:
      - □ Ezetimibe preferred
      - □ BAS second line
      - □ PCSK9 inhibitors are not indicated
  - If 10-year ASCVD risk ≥7.5%:
    - High-intensity statin
    - Consider addition of soluble dietary fiber and phytosterols
    - If <50% reduction in LDL-C
      - □ Ezetimibe preferred
      - □ BAS second line
      - □ PCSK9 inhibitors are not indicated
- **Adults aged 40 to 75 Years without clinical ASCVD or diabetes, With LDL-C 70 to 189 mg/dL and an estimated 10-Year risk for ASCVD of ≥7.5%, on statin for primary prevention**
  - Few patients should be considered for additional therapies beyond a maximally tolerated intensity of statin.
  - May consider nonstatin therapy if there is <30% reduction in LDL-C and ≥1 of the following high-risk markers:

- 10-year ASCVD risk ≥20%
- LDL-C ≥160 mg/dL at baseline
- Poorly controlled ASCVD risk factors
- Family history of premature ASCVD
- Evidence of accelerated subclinical atherosclerosis (e.g., coronary artery calcification)
- Elevated hs-CRP
- Other risk-modifying conditions: CKD, HIV, chronic inflammatory disorders
  ○ Attempt to intensify lifestyle modification and soluble dietary fibers as well as control risk factors. If still <30% reduction in LDL-C, use a high-intensity statin. If this does not result in a >50% reduction in LDL-C and high-risk markers are present, have a discussion with the patient:
    - If treating, ezetimibe (or BAS as a second-line agent) may be considered
    - Do not prescribe a PCSK9 inhibitor

Lifestyle/Risk Modification

For all patient groups, lifestyle modifications including a heart-healthy diet, regular exercise habits, avoidance of tobacco products and maintenance of a healthy weight are critical for ASCVD risk reduction.[5] Referral to a dietician is often helpful.

Diet[13]

Adults who would benefit from LDL-C lowering should make the following changes:

- Consume a diet that emphasizes vegetables, fruits, and whole grains.
- Consume low-fat dairy products, poultry, fish, legumes, nontropical vegetable oils, and nuts.
- Limit sweets, sugar-sweetened beverages, and red meats.
- Reduce percentage of calories from saturated fat and trans fat.
- Aim for a dietary pattern that achieves 5% to 6% of calories from saturated fat.
- Follow plans such as the DASH dietary pattern, the U.S. Department of Agriculture (USDA) Food Pattern, or the AHA Diet.

Activity[13]

- Aerobic physical activity
  ○ Reduces LDL-C by 3 to 6 mg/dL.
  ○ Reduces non-HDL-C by 6 mg/dL.
  ○ May have no consistent effect on triglycerides or HDL-C
- Resistance training reduces LDL-C, triglycerides, and non-HDL-C by 6 to 9 mg/dL and has no effect on HDL-C

SPECIAL CONSIDERATIONS

- Patients with symptomatic heart failure[7]
  ○ It is reasonable to consider use of statins in patients with symptomatic heart failure due to ischemic etiology who are expected to live long enough to achieve benefit from the statin therapy (i.e., 3 to 5 years or more).
  ○ PCSK9 inhibitor is not recommended at this time.
- Maintenance hemodialysis[7]
  ○ Approach should be individualized.
  ○ Decisions about the use of statins and other nonstatin agents is a matter of clinical judgment.
  ○ PCSK9 inhibitor is not recommended at this time.

- Considering pregnancy (or already pregnant)[7]
  - Statins should only be used in premenopausal women who are using effective contraception and are not nursing.
  - Discontinue pharmacologic therapy, with the exception of BAS, at least 1 month (preferably 3 months) before attempted conception. Stop immediately if already pregnant.
    - If patient has clinical ASCVD or baseline LDL-C ≥190 mg/dL, counsel on intensive lifestyle modifications. Referral to a lipid specialist and nutritionist is strongly recommended. If patient is on lipid-lowering therapy in the setting of diabetes or elevated 10-year ASCVD risk, discontinue and monitor for significant elevations in LDL-C during pregnancy. Progressive rise in both LDL-C and triglycerides is physiologic. May be managed with BAS.
    - Statin and ezetimibe can be resumed after completion of breast feeding.
    - Lomitapide not recommended.
    - No available safety/efficacy data for use of mipomersen or PCSK9 inhibitors.
    - Consider LDL apheresis in patients with:
      □ HoFH
      □ Severe HeFH and LDL-C ≥300 mg/dL
      □ ASCVD if LDL-C is ≥190 mg/dL

OTHER DYSLIPIDEMIAS

Elevated Triglycerides[8]

- Base the diagnosis on fasting triglyceride levels.
- Evaluate for secondary causes including obesity, diabetes, hypothyroidism, pregnancy, and medications (diuretics, β-adrenergic blocking agents, oral estrogens, BASs, tamoxifen, steroids, antiretroviral therapy, immunosuppressants, certain second-generation antipsychotics).
- Management
  - Dietary counseling and physical activity to achieve weight reduction.
  - Decreasing alcohol intake.
  - Reducing simple carbohydrate intake and sugar-sweetened beverages.
  - Controlling hyperglycemia in patients with diabetes mellitus.
  - Changing oral estrogen replacement to transdermal estrogen.
  - Fibrate is first-line agent in those at risk for triglyceride-induced pancreatitis. Treatment goal: <1,000 mg/dL.
  - Fibrates, niacin, omega-3 fatty acids alone or in combination with statins to treat moderate (200 to 999 mg/dL) to severe (1,000 to 1,999 mg/dL) triglyceride levels.
    - Fibrates: Do not reduce cardiovascular events when added to simvastatin in the majority of high-risk patients with type 2 diabetes.[14]
    - Niacin: Ingestion after a meal with an uncoated aspirin given prior minimizes flushing. No clinical benefit to adding to a statin in patients with atherosclerotic disease and LDL <70 mg/dL, despite improvements in triglyceride and HDL levels.[15]
  - Do not use heparin infusions to treat very severe (≥2,000 mg/dL) hypertriglyceridemia with pancreatitis.
  - Plasmapheresis for extremely severe hypertriglyceridemia is not generally recommended.

Low HDL-C[4]

- Defined as <40 mg/dL for men or below 50 mg/dL for women.
- Extremely low HDL-C: < 20 mg/dL.
- Eliminate severe hypertriglyceridemia as the cause and then classify as artifactual, primary, or secondary.

- ○ Primary monogenic disorders (apolipoprotein A-I mutations, Tangier disease, lecithin-cholesterol acyltransferase deficiency).
- ○ Secondary causes include androgen use and malignancy.
- Association between low HDL-C and atherosclerosis remains unclear.

SPECIAL CONSIDERATIONS

Statin Intolerance[16]

- Statins can cause myositis: muscle symptoms in association with a substantially elevated serum creatine kinase (CK) concentration. Elevations >10× the upper limit of normal (ULN) occur in 1 per 1,000 to 1 per 10,000 people per year.
- If a patient complains of muscle symptoms
  - ○ Exclude secondary causes such as hypothyroidism, polymyalgia rheumatica, or increased physical activity as well as medications (e.g., glucocorticoids, antipsychotics, immuno-suppressants or antivirals, lipid-modifying drugs, as well as substances of abuse).
  - ○ Withdrawal of statin therapy followed by one or more rechallenges can help determine causality.
    - If symptoms/CK abnormalities resolve after discontinuation, treat with the same statin at a lower dose or switch to an alternative statin.
    - If still not tolerated, treat with alternate day or twice-weekly dosing with lower doses of a high-intensity statin with a long half-life (atorvastatin, rosuvastatin, and pitavastatin)
    - Can reduce LDL-C by 12% to 38%, and are tolerated by ~70% of previously intolerant patients.[16]
    - If CK is >4× the ULN, reassess need for statin. If necessary, continue with monitoring of CK but stop if levels exceed 10× ULN.
    - If LDL-C remains above target despite maximally tolerated statin dosage, consider the use of ezetimibe as first choice, potentially followed by BASs or fibrates in combination with ezetimibe.

Statin Safety and Drug–Drug Interactions[17]

- Gemfibrozil reduces the glucuronidation and elimination of statins. If a fibrate is to be used with a statin, use fenofibrate.
- Grapefruit and sweet orange juice as well as tangerines should be separated from statin administration by 4 hours.
- Avoid St. John's wort and red yeast rice.
- Do not initiate simvastatin at 80 mg daily or increase the dose of simvastatin to 80 mg daily.
- Atorvastatin and fluvastatin are minimally excreted by the kidneys.

Liver Function Test Abnormalities[18]

- Irreversible liver damage resulting from statins is exceptionally rare and likely idiosyncratic in nature.
- Check liver enzyme tests before initiating therapy and as clinically indicated thereafter.
- Decompensated cirrhosis or acute liver failure are contraindications for statin use.
- Statins are safe to use in patients with nonalcoholic fatty liver disease, autoimmune hepatitis, chronic liver diseases, compensated cirrhosis, and liver transplant patients.
- If patient has elevated liver enzymes <3× the ULN:
  - ○ Perform a thorough history and physical examination to possible etiologies.
  - ○ Compare to prior liver tests.
  - ○ Repeat testing to confirm elevation.
  - ○ If total bilirubin is not elevated and CK is normal, decide if the most likely diagnosis is nonalcohol fatty liver disease.

○ If not on a statin, then ok to start.

○ If on a statin, then no clinical reason to stop it.

○ Implement lifestyle changes and then repeat liver blood testing.

○ If total bilirubin is elevated and CK is normal, decide if prior bilirubin levels were elevated, suggesting a benign genetic bilirubin handling disorder. If no other likely cause, the patient is asymptomatic, prior testing indirect bilirubin is elevated but not direct, it suggests Gilberts.

  ▪ If not on a statin, then ok to start.

  ▪ If on a statin, then no clinical reason to stop.

○ If prior total bilirubin was not elevated, especially if direct bilirubin is elevated, then more aggressive diagnostic measures are indicated and would hold/stop statin until etiology is determined.

• If patient has elevated liver enzymes >3× the ULN:

○ Perform a thorough history and physical examination to possible etiologies.

○ Compare to prior liver tests.

○ Repeat testing to confirm elevation.

○ If remains >3× ULN, hold/stop statin until diagnostic clarity is obtained.

REFERRAL

• Patients with hyperlipidemia are often managed very successfully by primary care providers.

• Endocrinology referral should be considered in cases of severe dyslipidemias after exclusion and treatment of secondary causes.

MONITORING/FOLLOW-UP

• Fasting lipid panels can be checked every 6 to 12 weeks during medication titration.

• Once lipid goals are achieved, fasting lipid panels should be assessed every 4 to 6 months.

• Other laboratory studies are assessed to evaluate for side effects as determined by symptoms.

REFERENCES

1. Jacobson TA, Ito MK, Maki KC, et al. National lipid association recommendations for patient-centered management of dyslipidemia: Part 1—full report. *J Clin Lipidol* 2015;9(2): 129–169.

2. Benjamin EJ, Blaha MJ, Chiuve SE, et al. Heart disease and stroke statistics—2017 update: A report from the American Heart Association. *Circulation* 2017;135(10):e146–e603.

3. McKenney JM. Understanding PCSK9 and anti-PCSK9 therapies. *J Clin Lipidol* 2015;9(2): 170–186.

4. Rader DJ, deGoma EM. Approach to the patient with extremely low HDL-cholesterol. *J Clin Endocrinol Metab* 2012;97(10):3399–3407.

5. Stone NJ, Robinson JG, Lichtenstein AH, et al. 2013 ACC/AHA guideline on the treatment of blood cholesterol to reduce atherosclerotic cardiovascular risk in adults: A report of the American College of Cardiology/American Heart Association Task Force on Practice Guidelines. *J Am Coll Cardiol* 2014;63(25 Pt B):2889–2934.

6. Baigent C, Blackwell L, Emberson J, et al. Efficacy and safety of more intensive lowering of LDL cholesterol: A meta-analysis of data from 170,000 participants in 26 randomised trials. *Lancet* 2010;376(9753):1670–1681.

7. Lloyd-Jones DM, Morris PB, Ballantyne CM, et al. 2016 ACC Expert Consensus Decision Pathway on the Role of Non-Statin Therapies for LDL-Cholesterol Lowering in the Management of Atherosclerotic Cardiovascular Disease Risk: A Report of the American College of Cardiology Task Force on Clinical Expert Consensus Documents. *J Am Coll Cardiol* 2016;68(1):92–125.

8. Berglund L, Brunzell JD, Goldberg AC, et al. Evaluation and treatment of hypertriglyceridemia: An Endocrine Society clinical practice guideline. *J Clin Endocrinol Metab* 2012;97(9):2969–2989.

9. Gouni-Berthold I, Berthold HK. Mipomersen and lomitapide: Two new drugs for the treatment of homozygous familial hypercholesterolemia. *Atheroscler Suppl* 2015;18:28–34.

10. Cupido AJ, Reeskamp LF, Kastelein JJP. Novel lipid modifying drugs to lower LDL cholesterol. *Curr Opin Lipidol* 2017;28(4):367–373.

11. Cannon CP, Blazing MA, Giugliano RP, et al. Ezetimibe added to statin therapy after acute coronary syndromes. *N Engl J Med* 2015;372(25):2387–2397.

12. Sabatine MS, Giugliano RP, Keech AC, et al. Evolocumab and clinical outcomes in patients with cardiovascular disease. *N Engl J Med* 2017;376(18):1713–1722.

13. Eckel RH, Jakicic JM, Ard JD, et al. 2013 AHA/ACC guideline on lifestyle management to reduce cardiovascular risk: A report of the American College of Cardiology/American Heart Association Task Force on Practice Guidelines. *Circulation* 2014;129(25 Suppl 2):S76–S99.

14. Ginsberg HN, Elam MB, Lovato LC, et al. Effects of combination lipid therapy in type 2 diabetes mellitus. *N Engl J Med* 2010;362(17):1563–1574.

15. Boden WE, Probstfield JL, Anderson T, et al. Niacin in patients with low HDL cholesterol levels receiving intensive statin therapy. *N Engl J Med* 2011;365(24):2255–2267.

16. Stroes ES, Thompson PD, Corsini A, et al. Statin-associated muscle symptoms: Impact on statin therapy-European Atherosclerosis Society Consensus Panel Statement on Assessment, Aetiology and Management. *Eur Heart J* 2015;36(17):1012–1022.

17. Kellick KA, Bottorff M, Toth PP; The National Lipid Association's Safety Task Force. A clinician's guide to statin drug-drug interactions. *J Clin Lipidol* 2014;8(3 Suppl):S30–S46.

18. Bays H, Cohen DE, Chalasani N, Harrison SA; The National Lipid Association's Statin Safety Task Force. An assessment by the Statin Liver Safety Task Force: 2014 update. *J Clin Lipidol* 2014; 8(3 Suppl):S47–S57.

Lipodystrophy

36

Jacqueline L. Cartier and Anne C. Goldberg

GENERAL PRINCIPLES[1]

- Adipose tissue protects against lipotoxicity and glucotoxicity.
- Fat cells store fuel as lipids and if absent or deficient, lipids accumulate in the muscle, liver, and other areas of the body.
- Metabolic hormones (insulin and steroids) induce the preadipocyte to differentiate into a mature adipocyte
- Lipid droplets (small organelles that store triglycerides) form within adipocytes from circulating fatty acids and triglycerides.
- Adipocytes increase in size (hypertrophy), and number (hyperplasia)
- Peroxisome proliferator–activated receptor γ (PPARγ) is the master regulator of adipogenesis.

Definition

- Lipodystrophies are heterogeneous disorders characterized by selective loss of body fat.
  - Generalized: involves nearly the entire body
  - Partial: only certain body regions
  - Local: smaller, focal areas under skin
- Extent of fat loss determines severity of complications
- Deficiency in adipose →leptin deficiency→hyperphagia and ectopic lipid storage →insulin resistance[2]

Classification

- Congenital generalized lipodystrophy (CGL)
- Familial partial lipodystrophy (FPLD)
- Acquired generalized lipodystrophy (AGL)
- Acquired partial lipodystrophy (APL)

Epidemiology

- More than 1,000 cases have been reported
- Prevalence is <1:1,000,000 (although likely underreported)[2]
- Affected females are recognized more easily

Etiology

Inherited (autosomal recessive and dominant subtypes), acquired (autoimmune mechanisms), or drugs

Associated Conditions

Diabetes mellitus, hypertriglyceridemia, acute pancreatitis, nonalcoholic fatty liver disease, cirrhosis, polycystic ovaries, acanthosis nigricans, premature atherosclerosis, cardiomyopathy, rhythm disturbances

DIAGNOSIS

- Perform a physical examination on patients who appear "lean" and having metabolic complications
  - ○ Evaluate for fat loss and muscular prominence
  - ○ Especially important to examine extremities and hips
- Obtain an in-depth family history to understand mode of inheritance
- Genetic testing is not necessary to make the diagnosis but may help identify at-risk family members
- If genetic testing is negative, the patient may still have lipodystrophy as not all mutations are known
- Lipodystrophy is mainly a clinical diagnosis

Differential Diagnosis

Anorexia nervosa, cachexia, starvation, diencephalic syndrome, Cushing syndrome, truncal obesity, lipomatosis, and rare progeroid syndromes[3]

Diagnostic Testing

Skin-fold thickness measurement

Laboratories

- Laboratory tests provide additional supportive evidence
  - ○ Generalized: extremely low adipocytokines (leptin and adiponectin)[4]
  - ○ Partial: variable amounts of leptin and adiponectin
- Test for glucose intolerance, hyperlipidemia, liver function, and hyperuricemia.
- Measurement of leptin may predict response to metreleptin therapy[3]

Imaging

Fat loss pattern can be better assessed with a whole-body T1-weighted MRI and dual-energy x-ray absorptiometry (DXA)[3]

Diagnostic Procedures

- Skin biopsy can confirm panniculitis or neutrophilic dermatosis
- If cardiomyopathy or coronary artery disease is suspected: EKG, ECHO, stress test, Holter monitoring

DISORDERS

Congenital Generalized Lipodystrophy

- Also known as Berardinelli–Seip syndrome
- Autosomal recessive
- There are four distinct subtypes, please see Table 36-1.[2]
- **Pathophysiology:**[1]
  - ○ CGL type 1 (CGL1): genetic mutation the 1-acylglycerol-3-phosphate-O-acyltransferase 2 (AGPAT2) gene. AGPAT2 catalyzes formation of phosphatidic acid, which is essential in developing young adipocytes.
  - ○ CGL2: genetic mutation of the Berardinelli–Seip congenital lipodystrophy 2 (*BSCL2*) gene. *BSCL2* encodes seipin which promotes adipogenesis in periods of excess energy storage. If altered, adipocyte maturation is severely impeded.
  - ○ CGL3: genetic mutation of caveolin 1 (*CAV1*). *CAV1*: binds and transports fatty acids to lipid droplets.
  - ○ CGL4: genetic mutation of polymerase-I-and-transcriptrelease factor (PTRF). PTRF creates caveolae (involved in signal transduction and transport) and regulates expression of caveolins 1 and 3.

TABLE 36-1	CONGENITAL GENERALIZED (BERARDINELLI–SEIP SYNDROME)	
Variants	Gene mutation	Clinical features
CGL1[2]	AGPAT2	• Most common subtype • ***Absent bone marrow fat*** • Acromegaloid appearance • Hyperhidrosis • Lytic lesions in appendicular bones • Diabetes (median age: 12.5 years)
CGL2[2]	BSCL2	• Second most common subtype • Most severe • ***Lack mechanical adipose tissue (retro-orbital, palm, sole, and periarticular regions)*** • ***Lack bone marrow fat*** • Diabetes (median age: 10 years) • 50% have mild mental retardation
CGL3[2]	CAV1	• Only reported in one patient • Preserved mechanical and bone marrow adipose fat • Short stature • Hypocalcemia • Vitamin D resistance
CGL4[2]	PTRF	• Reported in 30 patients • Preserved mechanical and bone marrow adipose fat • Progress to generalized lipodystrophy during infancy • Congenital myopathy, pyloric stenosis, atlantoaxial instability, distal metaphyseal deformation, cardiac rhythm disturbances that can cause sudden death

- **Diagnosis**
  - Recognizable at birth or within the 1st year of life
  - Infancy: hepatosplenomegaly and umbilical prominence or hernia
  - Childhood: voracious appetite, accelerated growth, advanced bone age, acanthosis nigricans
  - Adolescence: may have diabetes, hypertriglyceridemia, and low HDL in addition to characteristic physical features
  - **History:**
    - May have acute pancreatitis (due to high triglycerides), nonalcoholic fatty liver disease leading to cirrhosis
    - Females may develop hirsutism, clitoromegaly, menstrual irregularity, polycystic ovaries, and infertility[4]
  - **Physical Examination**
    - Near-total lack of body fat
    - Prominent muscularity and subcutaneous veins
- **Diagnostic Testing:**
  - Laboratories: very low leptin, elevated hemoglobin A1c (HbA1c) and triglycerides, low HDL
  - Imaging: skeletal survey can reveal lytic bone lesions

TABLE 36-2	FAMILIAL PARTIAL LIPODYSTROPHY	
Variants	Gene mutation	Clinical features
FPLD1: Koberling[2]	Unknown	• Cushingoid appearance • Prominent ledge of fat above the gluteal area, upper medial thigh, and upper arm • Only in females
FPLD2: Dunnigan[2]	LMNA	• Loss of SC fat from extremities • Gain of fat to face, neck, abdominal viscera, and labia • Acanthosis nigricans, muscle hypertrophy, phlebomegaly, eruptive xanthomata, lipomas, hirsutism • HTN, coronary artery disease, diabetes, hypertriglyceridemia, pancreatitis, hepatic steatosis • Females: PCOS, breast hypoplasia, preeclampsia, miscarriages • Males: less obvious phenotype and milder metabolic abnormalities
FPLD3[2]	PPARG	• No increase in head and neck fat • Typical metabolic complications
FPLD4 FPLD5 FPLD6 AKT2 linked[2]	PLIN1 CIDEC LIPE AKT2	• Onset at puberty • Loss of fat to buttocks and limbs and gain of fat to face, neck, and abdomen • Acanthosis nigricans, phlebomegaly, eruptive xanthomata, hirsutism • Metabolic and cardiovascular complications

Familial Partial Lipodystrophy

• Most are autosomal dominant but also autosomal recessive and X-linked traits
• Several different types (see Table 36-2).[2]
  ○ Dunnigan is the most common variety (prevalence of 1 in 15 million persons)[1]
  ○ Subcutaneous fat loss from upper and lower extremities but variable loss of fat from the trunk[4]
• **Pathophysiology**[1]
  ○ FPLD type 2 (FPLD2): involves the *LMNA* gene. Disruption of lamins A and C alter the structure of the adipocyte nucleus, leading to premature cell death
  ○ FPLD3: involves the PPARγ gene. PPARγ mutations inhibit adipocyte differentiation.
  ○ FPLD4: involves v-AKT murine thymoma oncogene homolog 2 (AKT2). AKT2 mutations inhibit adipocyte differentiation
  ○ FPLD5: involves perilipin 1 (PLIN1). PLIN1 mutations cause development of microadipocytes susceptible to macrophage invasion, yielding fibrotic changes.
• **Diagnosis**
  ○ Infancy and early childhood: normal body fat distribution
  ○ Puberty: fat redistribution
  ○ Adulthood: characteristic lack of fat, metabolic complications[2]

○ Females may have reduced fertility with irregular menses and hirsutism
○ Hypertriglyceridemia is common and severe: high risk of acute pancreatitis
○ **Physical Examination:**
  ▪ Lack of extremity and gluteal subcutaneous fat
  ▪ Preserved adipose tissue in the face, neck, and intra-abdominal areas. The presence of a buffalo hump gives a Cushingoid type of appearance.
  ▪ Acanthosis nigricans is common
  ▪ Muscular hypertrophy
○ Laboratories: elevated HbA1c and triglycerides

Acquired Lipodystrophies

• Several different types, variable etiology (see Table 36-3)[2,3]
• AGL, Lawrence syndrome: female-to-male ratio of 3:1
• APL, Barraquer–Simons syndrome: female-to-male ratio of 4:1

TABLE 36-3	ACQUIRED LIPODYSTROPHIES
Types	Clinical features
AGL: Lawrence syndrome[3]	• Born with normal body fat • Childhood: progressive loss of fat that is usually generalized • Minority have sparing of intra-abdominal and bone marrow fat • Hepatic steatosis and fibrosis, diabetes, hypertriglyceridemia • ~25% have panniculitis prior to loss of fat • ~25% have other autoimmune diseases • Many have low serum levels of complement 4.
APL: Barraquer–Simons syndrome[2,3]	• Craniocaudal direction of fat loss starting in childhood or adolescence • May have excess fat accumulation in the lower body (hips, buttocks, legs) • 20% occurrence of membranoproliferative glomerulonephritis • 80% have low serum levels of complement 3 • Most have complement 3 nephritic factor (a circulating autoantibody) • Rarely patients have drusen on fundus examination • Metabolic complications are **not** usually seen
Lipodystrophy in HIV-infected patients[3]	• Gradually lose fat from arms, legs, and face • Can accumulate excess fat and appear to have a buffalo hump, double chin, and increased weight circumference • Can develop hypertriglyceridemia but only a few develop diabetes
Localized[3]	• Focal loss of fat from small areas of the body • Usually causes one or more dimples • Do **not** develop metabolic abnormalities

- In the United States, over 100,000 HIV-infected patients have lipodystrophy (LD-HIV)[3]
  - Highest incidence among all currently known lipodystophies[1]
  - Usually after receiving protease inhibitors (PI) or nucleoside reverse transcriptase inhibitors (NRTIs) for over 2 years
  - Fat loss worsens with ongoing HAART therapy
  - Does not reverse on discontinuation of PI
  - Predisposed to developing coronary heart disease
- Localized lipodystrophy
  - No metabolic impediments
- Pathophysiology[1]
  - **AGL**
    - 25% triggered by panniculitis
    - 25% autoimmune in origin (stemming from conditions such as RA, SLE, Sjogren syndrome and juvenile dermatomyositis)
    - 50% idiopathic
  - **APL**
    - Precise pathogenesis unknown
    - Possibly complement pathway alterations or variants in the *LMNB2* gene
  - **LD-HIV**
- PI: downregulate PPARγ and C/EBPα which disrupts lipogenesis and adipocyte maturation; also can inhibit zinc metalloprotease which is involved in processing of prelamin A to mature lamin A[4]
- NRTIs: cause mitochondrial dysfunction
  - **Localized lipodystrophy:** Usually occurs due to panniculitis, disproportionate direct pressure, injections of a drug causing injury to the adipose tissue

Rare Genetic Lipodystrophy Disorders

- There are three distinct but overlapping recessive autoinflammatory disorders associated with lipodystrophy (see Table 36-4).[2]

TABLE 36-4	AUTOIMMUNE INFLAMMATORY DISORDERS	
Variants	Gene mutation	Phenotype
JMP[2]	PSMB8	• Joint contractures, muscle atrophy, microcytic anemia • Lipodystrophy begins in childhood • Muscle atrophy, joint contractures, skin lesions, microcytic anemia, hepatosplenomegaly, hypergammaglobulinemia
Nakajo–Nishimura syndrome[2]	PSMB8	• Infancy: rash, periodic fevers, nodular erythematous skin eruptions, myositis • Progressive atrophy of subcutaneous fat and muscles • Joint contractures, hepatosplenomegaly, hypergammaglobulinemia, basal ganglia calcifications
CANDLE syndrome[2]	PSMB8	• First year: recurrent fevers, annular violaceous plaques, arthralgias, anemia, and elevated acute phase reactants • Infancy: loss of subcutaneous fat from face • Childhood: loss of fat from upper limbs

- Lipodystrophy is also a manifestation of many progeroid disorders as well as other rare lipodystrophic disorders (see Table 36-5).[1,2,5–16]
- Pathophysiology
  - Mandibular hypoplasia, deafness, progeroid features (MDP) syndrome: mutations of *POLD1*. *POLD1* is responsible for lagging strand DNA synthesis during DNA replication and has proofreading ability.[10]
  - Neonatal Marfan progeroid syndrome: mutations of *FBN1*. *FBN1* encodes fibrillin-1, components of microfibrils which provide a scaffold for elastin.[11]
  - Short stature, hyperextensibility, ocular depression, Rieger anomaly, and teething delay (SHORT) syndrome: mutations of *PIK3R1*. *PIK3R1* signaling is involved in multiple cellular functions and also plays a role in insulin signaling.[16]
  - Werner syndrome: mutations of the WRN protein. WRN encodes RecQ DNA helicase/exonuclease; and mutations compromise DNA replication, leading to instability and cell death.[1]

TREATMENT

- Challenging as reversal of fat loss is not possible[3]
- Focused on managing metabolic abnormalities and cosmetic appearance[4]

Medications[4]

- Treat severe hypertriglyceridemia with fibrates and fish oil
- Treat diabetes with metformin; insulin may also be required
- Switch PI with other antiretrovirals in LD-HIV
- **Metreleptin**[17]
  - Synthetic analog of the hormone leptin
  - Administered as a daily subcutaneous injection
  - Dose adjustments made every 3 to 6 months based on metabolic parameters and weight change[4]
  - Generalized lipodystrophy
    - Dramatically decreases hypertriglyceridemia and improves glycemic parameters
    - Improves ectopic lipid storage, hyperfiltration and proteinuria, and steatohepatitis
    - Approved for the treatment of CGL by FDA in 2014
  - Partial lipodystrophy
    - Ameliorates hypertriglyceridemia but conflicting effects on hyperglycemia
    - Metreleptin is not approved in this population
  - Only available through a Myalept Risk Evaluation and Mitigation Strategy (REMS) Program
    - Black box warning as there were three cases of T-cell lymphoma and four cases of neutralizing antibodies to leptin in long term uncontrolled studies.[17]
    - Common side effects: hypoglycemia and injection site reactions

Other Nonpharmacologic Therapies

Refer to mental health providers for emotional distress[4]

Surgical Management[4]

- Facial appearance can be improved with autologous adipose tissue transplantation or implantation of dermal fillers
- Liposuction of unwanted excess adipose tissue

Lifestyle/Risk Modification

Diet
- 50% to 60% carbohydrates, 20% to 30% fat, 10% to 20% protein is appropriate for most[4]

TABLE 36-5 OTHER RARE LIPODYSTROPHIC DISORDERS

Disorder	Gene mutation	Clinical features
Mandibuloacral dysplasia (MAD) type A[5]	LMNA	• Skeletal abnormalities: mandibular and clavicular hypoplasia and acroosteolysis • Delayed closure of cranial sutures, crowded teeth, joint stiffness • Partial lipodystrophy • Insulin resistance
Mandibuloacral dysplasia (MAD) type B[6]	ZMPSTE24	• Hypoplasia of the mandible and clavicles, acroosteolysis, cutaneous atrophy • Progeroid appearance • Generalized lipodystrophy
Atypical progeria[7,8]	LMNA	• Partial or generalized loss of fat • Progeroid features
Hutchinson–Gilford progeria syndrome[2,9]	LMNA	• Almost all fat lost but intra-abdominal fat spared • Progeroid features • Cardiovascular complications generally cause death
Mandibular hypoplasia, deafness, progeroid features (MDP)-associated lipodystrophy[10]	POLD1	• Minimal subcutaneous adipose tissue • Increased visceral adipose tissue • Mandibular hypoplasia • Deafness • Progeroid features • Severe insulin resistance • Males: undescended testes and hypogonadism
Neonatal Marfan progeroid syndrome[11,12]	Fibrillin 1	• Generalized lipodystrophy • Progeroid features • Features of Marfan syndrome
Neonatal progeroid syndrome[13]	CAV1	• Generalized loss of body fat and muscle mass • Progeroid appearance at birth
Werner syndrome[1,14,15]	WRN	• Lipoatrophy of the four limbs • Truncal and abdominal fat accumulation • Progeroid appearance occurs after adolescence • Insulin resistance • Hypogonadism • Prone to develop malignancies
Short stature, hyperextensibility, ocular depression, Rieger anomaly, and teething delay (SHORT) syndrome[16]	PIK3R1	• Paucity of fat • Short stature, hyperextentensibility, facial dysmorphism, teething delay, variable ocular anomalies • Insulin resistance and/or diabetes typically presents in adolescence

- Overfeeding can worsen diabetes and hyperlipidemia as well as accelerate hepatic steatosis
- To reduce severe hypertriglyceridemia, give medium-chain triglyceride-based formulas in infants and very low-fat diets in those older[4]

Activity

- Physical activity can lower insulin resistance but avoid strenuous exercise if the patient has cardiomyopathy
- Patients with CGL4, FPLD2, and progeroid syndromes should undergo a cardiac evaluation[4]

Future Directions

Medications to reduce apoC-III levels:

- ApoC-III is a component of VLDL and HDL, is a noncompetitive inhibitor of lipoprotein lipase (hydrolyzes triglycerides to free fatty acids for muscle and adipose tissue uptake), and transforms triglyceride rich lipoproteins to their remnant forms to be cleared by the liver[18]
- Increased apoC-III is associated with insulin resistance and hypertriglyceridemia
- Lowering apoC-III has been shown to reduce triglyceride levels
- Lipodystrophy patients have significantly elevated apoC-III levels[18]
- The BROADEN Study is a randomized, placebo-controlled, double-blind phase 2/3 clinical trial for volanesorsen (an apoC-III antisense oligonucleotide) in the treatment of FPLD that is currently ongoing

REFERENCES

1. Nolis T. Exploring the pathophysiology behind the more common genetic and acquired lipodystrophies. *J Hum Genet* 2014;59(1):16–23.
2. Lightbourne M, Brown RJ. Genetics of lipodystrophy. *Endocrinol Metab Clin North Am* 2017; 46(2):539–554.
3. Garg A. Clinical review#: Lipodystrophies: Genetic and acquired body fat disorders. *J Clin Endocrinol Metab* 2011;96(11):3313–3325.
4. Hussain I, Garg A. Lipodystrophy syndromes. *Endocrinol Metab Clin North Am* 2016;45(4): 783–797.
5. Novelli G, Muchir A, Sangiuolo F, et al. Mandibuloacral dysplasia is caused by a mutation in LMNA-encoding lamin A/C. *Am J Hum Genet* 2002;71(2):426–431.
6. Agarwal AK, Fryns JP, Auchus RJ, Garg A. Zinc metalloproteinase, ZMPSTE24, is mutated in mandibuloacral dysplasia. *Hum Mol Genet* 2003;12(16):1995–2001.
7. Chen L, Lee L, Kudlow BA, et al. LMNA mutations in atypical Werner's syndrome. *Lancet* 2003;362(9382):440–445.
8. Garg A, Subramanyam L, Agarwal AK, et al. Atypical progeroid syndrome due to heterozygous missense LMNA mutations. *J Clin Endocrinol Metab* 2009;94(12):4971–4983.
9. Merideth MA, Gordon LB, Clauss S, et al. Phenotype and course of Hutchinson-Gilford progeria syndrome. *N Engl J Med* 2008;358(6):592–604.
10. Weedon MN, Ellard S, Prindle MJ, et al. An in-frame deletion at the polymerase active site of POLD1 causes a multisystem disorder with lipodystrophy. *Nat Genet* 2013;45(8):947–950.
11. Garg A, Xing C. De novo heterozygous FBN1 mutations in the extreme C-terminal region cause progeroid fibrillinopathy. *Am J Med Genet A* 2014;164A(5):1341–1345.
12. Graul-Neumann LM, Kienitz T, Robinson PN, et al. Marfan syndrome with neonatal progeroid syndrome-like lipodystrophy associated with a novel frameshift mutation at the 3' terminus of the FBN1-gene. *Am J Med Genet A* 2010;152A(11):2749–2755.
13. Garg A, Kircher M, Del Campo M, Amato RS, Agarwal AK; University of Washington Center for Mendelian Genomics. Whole exome sequencing identifies de novo heterozygous CAV1 mutations associated with a novel neonatal onset lipodystrophy syndrome. *Am J Med Genet A* 2015;167A(8): 1796–1806.

14. Donadille B, D'Anella P, Auclair M, et al. Partial lipodystrophy with severe insulin resistance and adult progeria Werner syndrome. *Orphanet J Rare Dis* 2013;8:106.

15. Navarro CL, Cau P, Lévy N. Molecular bases of progeroid syndromes. *Hum Mol Genet* 2006;15 (Spec No 2):R151–R161.

16. Thauvin-Robinet C, Auclair M, Duplomb L, et al. PIK3R1 mutations cause syndromic insulin resistance with lipoatrophy. *Am J Hum Genet* 2013;93(1):141–149.

17. Diker-Cohen T, Cochran E, Gorden P, Brown RJ. Partial and generalized lipodystrophy: Comparison of baseline characteristics and response to metreleptin. *J Clin Endocrinol Metab* 2015;100(5):1802–1810.

18. Kassai A, Muniyappa R, Levenson AE, et al. Effect of leptin administration on circulating apolipoprotein CIII levels in patients with lipodystrophy. *J Clin Endocrinol Metab* 2016;101(4):1790–1797.

37

Multiple Endocrine Neoplasia Syndromes

Cecilia A. Davis, Cynthia J. Herrick, and Thomas J. Baranski

GENERAL PRINCIPLES

- Multiple endocrine neoplasia (MEN) syndromes are sporadic or hereditary neoplastic disorders of more than one endocrine organ. Broadly, there are two distinct syndromes: MEN1 and MEN2 with autosomal dominant inheritance and complete penetrance but variable expression. MEN2 has three main subtypes: MEN2A, familial medullary thyroid cancer (FMTC) and MEN2B.
- MEN1 is caused by loss of function or inactivation of a tumor suppressor gene while MEN2 is caused by gain of function or activation of a proto-oncogene.

Definition

- **MEN1 is defined as presence of at least two of three main MEN1 tumor types: parathyroid, pituitary, and enteropancreatic.** Familial MEN1 is defined as one index case plus one relative with at least one of the three main MEN1 tumor types.
- **MEN2 is subclassified into three syndromes:** MEN2A, FMTC, and MEN2B.
  - **MEN2A:** medullary thyroid cancer (MTC), pheochromocytoma, and parathyroid hyperplasia.
  - **FMTC** is a variant of MEN2A. There is a strong predisposition to MTC but not pheochromocytoma or hyperparathyroidism.
  - **MEN2B:** MTC, pheochromocytoma, and ganglioneuromatosis of the gut and oral mucosa (also marfanoid habitus, medullated corneal nerve fibers)

Epidemiology

- MEN1 is inherited as an autosomal-dominant trait with an incidence of 2 to 20 per 100,000 in the general population (see Table 37-1).[1]
  - 1% to 18% among patients with primary hyperparathyroidism
  - 16% to 38% among patients with gastrinoma
  - <3% among patients with pituitary tumors (see Table 37-2).[1,2]
- MEN2 is a rare autosomal-dominant syndrome with an estimated incidence of 1 to 10 per 100,000 in the general population. It has been identified in 500 to 1,000 kindred worldwide. MEN2A accounts for 80% of cases, FMTC for 15%, and MEN2B for 5%.[3]

Etiology

MEN1

- The mutated gene for MEN1 (see Table 37-1)[1] is a tumor suppressor gene, located on the long arm of chromosome 11 (11q13), and encodes a 610 amino acid nuclear protein called menin. The complete function of menin is not yet fully known, although studies suggest it might have a role in transcriptional regulation. 10% of MEN1 mutations arise *de novo*, and more than 400 different germline mutations have been identified.
- There is no genotype–phenotype correlation in MEN1, making genetic screening and rational therapeutic intervention difficult.

TABLE 37-1	GENERAL FEATURES OF MEN1 AND MEN2 SYNDROMES	
	MEN1	MEN2
Incidence	2–20 per 100,000	1–10 per 100,000
Inheritance	Autosomal dominant	Autosomal dominant
Gene	MEN1 gene	RET gene
Gene product	Menin (nuclear protein)	RET (transmembrane tyrosine kinase–linked protein)
Location	Chromosome 11 (11q13)	Chromosome 10 (10q11-2)
Function	Tumor suppresser gene	Proto-oncogene
Type of mutation in tumors	Inactivation	Activation
Genotype–phenotype correlation	No	Yes
Genetic testing guides intervention to prevent and cure cancer	No	Yes

Adapted from Brandi ML, Gagel RF, Angeli A, et al. Guidelines for diagnosis and therapy of MEN type 1 and type 2. *J Clin Endocrinol Metab* 2001;86:5658–5671.

- More endocrine tumor syndromes are being discovered and new genes implicated including the MEN4 distinction which is clinically like MEN1 but caused by mutation in *CDKN1B*.[4]

MEN2

- **Nearly all patients with the MEN2 syndrome will develop MTC** derived from thyroid C-cells of neural crest origin rather than from thyroid follicular cells. Approximately 25% of patients with MTC have one of the MEN2 variants. **Pheochromocytoma is the second most common tumor in MEN2** and is present in 50% of patients.
- The mutated gene for MEN2 is REarranged during Transfection (RET) proto-oncogene, located on chromosome 10 (10q11-2), containing 21 exons and encoding a membrane-bound tyrosine kinase receptor.
- There is a strong genotype–phenotype correlation in MEN2. 80% to 98% of cases of MEN2A and FMTC involve mutations in exon 10 or exon 11 leading to ligand-independent homodimerization of the receptor with constitutive activation and downstream signaling of the mitogen-activated protein (MAP) kinase pathway.
- In most MEN2A kindreds, one of five cysteine residues (C609, C611, C618, C620, C634) in the RET extracellular domain has been mutated.
- More than 95% of MEN2B cases exhibit a single mutation M918T in exon 16, and 2% to 3% have a mutation at codon 883 in exon 15 that leads to autophosphorylation and alteration of substrate specificity.[3]
- Clinical course in MEN2 is generally predictable based on which mutation is driving the disease process. For example, 50% of individuals with MEN2A and a mutation at C634 will develop both hyperparathyroidism and pheochromocytomas in addition to MTC as compared to only 4% with a C609 mutation.[3] In MEN2B patients, MTC is

TABLE 37-2	CLINICAL MANIFESTATIONS OF MEN1, MEN2A, AND MEN2B	
MEN1	**MEN2A**	**MEN2B**
Hyperparathyroidism (90–95%)	**Medullary thyroid cancer (<100%)**	**Medullary thyroid cancer (<100%)**
Enteropancreatic tumors (30–80%)	**Pheochromocy-toma (~50%)**	**Pheochromocytoma (<50%)**
• Gastrinoma (50%)	**Hyperparathyroidism (<30%)**	**Other**
• Insulinoma (10%)	**Other**	• Mucosal neuroma (95%)
• Glucagonoma	• Cutaneous lichen amyloidosis	• Intestinal ganglioneuromatosis (40%)
• VIPoma	• Hirschsprung disease	
• Nonhormone secreting		• Marfanoid habitus (75%)
Pituitary tumors (15–90%)		
• Prolactinoma (60%)		
• GH secreting (acromegaly) (25%)		
• ACTH secreting (Cushing disease) (2–6%)		
• Nonhormone secreting		
Other tumors		
• Facial angiofibromas and collagenomas (70–88%)		
• Multiple lipomas (30%)		
• Adrenocortical tumors (5–40%)		
• Carcinoid tumors (3%)		

GH, growth hormone; VIP, vasoactive-intestinal polypeptide.
Adapted from Brandi ML, Gagel RF, Angeli A, et al. Guidelines for diagnosis and therapy of MEN type 1 and type 2. *J Clin Endocrinol Metab* 2001;86:5658–5671; Lakhani VT, You YN, Wells SA. The multiple endocrine neoplasia syndromes. *Ann Rev Med* 2007;58:253–265.

less aggressive if they have an A883F mutation compared to the M918T mutation.[3] With the tight genotype–phenotype correlation, both genetic screening and curative therapeutic interventions are feasible.

DIAGNOSIS

Clinical Presentation

MEN1

- Clinically, a patient with primary hyperparathyroidism and either a pituitary adenoma or an islet cell tumor is considered to have MEN1.
- **Primary hyperparathyroidism** is the most common and earliest manifestation (with 95% of patients presenting by age 50). Hyperparathyroidism in MEN1, compared to its sporadic counterpart, typically presents around at age 20 to 25 years (vs. 55 to 60 years), with an equal male-to-female ratio (compared to 1M: 3F ratio), and involves asymmetric four gland hyperplasia (rather than a single adenoma). Although most patients are asymptomatic, they may present with typical symptoms and signs of hypercalcemia (polyuria, myalgias, fatigue, and renal stones). See Table 37-2.[1,2]

- **Enteropancreatic tumors** are the second most common tumors found in (30% to 80% of MEN1-affected individuals). They can be functional or nonfunctional. Symptoms of hormone excess usually occur by age 40, although with biochemical testing and imaging, asymptomatic tumors in carriers can be identified much earlier. Larger tumor size is directly related to aggressive behavior with larger tumors having worse WHO pathologic grade and higher metastatic potential.[5]
- **Gastrinoma** is the most common enteropancreatic tumor (50% of MEN1 patients). MEN1 should be considered in patients initially diagnosed with gastrinoma. The tumor causes hypergastrinemia with increased gastric acid output (Zollinger–Ellison syndrome). Patients may present with peptic ulcer disease, diarrhea, cachexia, and abdominal pain. It is usually multicentric and has malignant potential. More than half of the gastrinomas in MEN1 have already metastasized to lymph nodes before diagnosis. These tumors account for the major morbidity and mortality associated with MEN. They are often located in the duodenum (>85%) and may be associated with nonsecreting pancreatic tumors.[6]
- **Insulinoma** is the second most common enteropancreatic tumor (10% of MEN1 patients). Most insulinomas arise spontaneously because <5% of patients with insulinoma have MEN1 syndrome. Patients typically present with fasting hypoglycemia. Inappropriately elevated plasma levels of insulin, C-peptide, and proinsulin in a hypoglycemic patient are highly suggestive of insulinoma. The tumors are usually too small to be identified by computed tomography (CT) scan or magnetic resonance imaging (MRI), but intraoperative ultrasound usually identifies the tumor within the pancreas. For further details, see Chapter 38.
- **Pituitary tumors.** Anterior pituitary adenomas are the initial presenting tumors in 10% to 25% of cases of MEN1. Two-thirds are microadenomas, which are usually functional and commonly secrete prolactin, resulting in the expected symptoms of prolactin excess (amenorrhea and galactorrhea in women; impotence in men). Nearly one-fourth of these pituitary tumors secrete growth hormone resulting in acromegaly, and a smaller percentage secrete adrenocorticotropic hormone (ACTH) resulting in Cushing disease. The presentation, diagnosis, and management are similar to those of sporadic pituitary adenomas (see Chapter 5).
- **Carcinoid tumors** are present in <3% of MEN1 patients. Nearly all carcinoid tumors in MEN1 originate in tissues arising from the embryologic foregut. Thymic carcinoids are predominantly seen in males, can be asymptomatic until a late stage, and tend to be more aggressive than in sporadic tumors. Bronchial carcinoids, by contrast, tend to occur mainly in females, can secrete ACTH, and may present with Cushing syndrome. Gastric enterochromaffin-like cell carcinoids have been found incidentally during gastric endoscopy for gastrinoma in MEN1. Carcinoid syndrome generally does not occur unless the tumor has metastasized to the liver (see Chapter 38).
- **Other tumors.** Patients with MEN1 syndrome can also present with multiple lipomas, facial angiofibromas, and collagenomas. Adrenocortical tumors, both functional and nonfunctional, occur in 5% to 40% of patients with MEN1.
- **Of note, hypercortisolism** can be ACTH-dependent (pituitary adenoma or ectopic ACTH syndrome) or ACTH-independent (adrenal adenoma). Although statistically most cases are caused by pituitary adenomas, it is important to differentiate between the various causes by biochemical testing (see Chapter 15).

MEN2
- The presenting features of MEN2 are largely dependent on the subtype (see Table 37-2).[1,2] However, the **common underlying feature in virtually all patients with MEN2 is the development of MTC**, which is the most common cause of morbidity and death in patients with the MEN2 syndrome.
- **MTC** is the first clinical manifestation in MEN2 kindreds because of its earlier and higher penetrance. MTC is preceded by C-cell hyperplasia, with resultant secretion of

calcitonin and carcinoembryonic antigen (CEA), which serve as excellent plasma tumor markers. C-cell hyperplasia progresses to microscopic MTC, followed by local disease (usually multicentric), and eventually by metastatic disease (commonly to lymph nodes, lung, liver, and bones).

- MTC usually presents as a thyroid nodule and/or increased serum calcitonin.
- MTC is usually more aggressive in MEN2B, typically presenting before 5 years of age and as early as infancy.[7]
- MTC is the only manifestation of **FMTC** and has an indolent clinical course. FMTC presents later in life, with a peak incidence in the fourth and fifth decades. It tends to be less aggressive than the other subtypes of MEN2. The criteria to characterize kindreds as having FMTC include MTC in more than 10 carriers in the kindred, multiple carriers or affected members older than age 50, and an adequate history to rule out pheochromocytoma or hyperparathyroidism. Some MEN2A patients may manifest only MTC and thus be incorrectly designated as FMTC, with the resulting danger of missing a diagnosis of pheochromocytoma.
- **Pheochromocytoma.** Compared to sporadic cases, pheochromocytoma in MEN2 is almost always benign, bilateral, confined to the adrenal glands, and presents earlier in life. If unrecognized, it can present as hypertensive crisis during surgery for MTC early in childhood. The clinical presentation, diagnosis, and management are similar to that seen in sporadic cases (see Chapter 16).
- **Primary hyperparathyroidism** is seen in about one-third of the patients with MEN2A, but it is absent in MEN2B. It is usually caused by asymmetric four-gland hyperplasia, although it is less aggressive than in MEN1. The clinical presentation, diagnosis, and management are similar to those in MEN1 and that seen in sporadic cases (see Chapter 23). It is important to evaluate the parathyroid glands during thyroidectomy for patients with MEN2A because they may be enlarged even though the preoperative calcium level is normal.
- **Ganglioneuromas** occur in 95% of MEN2B patients, which can present at the lips, eyelids, and tongue, giving these patients a characteristic phenotype that can be apparent at birth. **Intestinal ganglioneuromatosis** can occur as early as infancy with gastrointestinal motility disorders. One study reported 90% of patients had colonic disturbances, typically chronic constipation since birth.[8]
- **Other features in MEN2A/FMTC: Cutaneous lichen amyloidosis** is most often associated with mutations in the RET codon 634. It presents with intensive pruritis, often in the central upper back, and is sometimes difficult to treat.[9] Hirschprung disease has been associated with MEN2A. One series found that 50% of patients with RET mutation in C620 had Hirschprung disease.[10]
- **Other features in MEN2B:** Patients with MEN2B also manifest a characteristic marfanoid habitus, but do not have lens subluxation or aortic disease.[11]

Diagnostic Criteria

- **MEN1** is present if the patient has **two of the three main MEN1-related tumors: parathyroid, pituitary, and enteropancreatic**. Familial MEN1 is diagnosed as at least one case of MEN1 plus a first-degree relative with one of the three tumors.
- **MEN2** is diagnosed in a patient with **personal or family history of MTC and positive germline RET gene mutation.** This is a great example of a disorder in which genetic testing allows for early diagnosis and effective prophylactic surgical intervention. In patients who present with a suspicious thyroid nodule, fine-needle aspiration (FNA) biopsy may establish the diagnosis of MTC.
- **MEN2A** is diagnosed in a patient with **personal or family history of the presence of MTC, pheochromocytoma, and primary hyperparathyroidism associated with a germline RET mutation.** Clinical diagnosis of MEN2A can be made if at least two of the clinical features of MEN2A are present in the index case or two generations, even in

the absence of an autosomal-dominant–familial inheritance pattern or RET mutation. In the presence of a germline RET mutation and in the absence of any clinical features, that individual is at risk for the clinical features of MEN2A, and appropriate medical management should be followed.

- **Familial MTC** is a **clinical variant of MEN2A**. To prove that a kindred has FMTC, it is necessary to demonstrate the absence of a pheochromocytoma or primary hyperthyroidism in two or more generations within a family or to have a RET mutation identified only in kindreds with FMTC.
- **MEN2B** is diagnosed in a patient with **personal or family history of MTC and positive germline RET gene mutation at 918 or 883**. The index patient or family member can have clinical manifestation of MTC, pheochromocytoma, and other **features associated with MEN2B** such as **marfanoid habitus, ganglioneuromas, intestinal ganglioneuromatosis**.

Diagnostic Testing
Laboratories

MEN1
- The diagnostic tests are the same as sporadic counterparts. Laboratory tests are directed to gain evidence for hyperparathyroidism (PTH, total and ionized calcium), pituitary tumors (prolactin, ACTH, IGF-1, alpha subunit, TSH), and enteropancreatic tumors.
- DNA testing in diagnosis or screening MEN1 is still controversial, however current practice guidelines recommend offering MEN1 genetic testing to patients with high clinical suspicion and if positive to their first-degree relatives.[12,13]

MEN2
- **Biochemical tests are not required for diagnosis of MEN2**, but maybe useful for disease follow-up and diagnosis of hyperparathyroidism and pheochromocytoma. Useful tests include calcitonin, CEA, calcium (PTH if hyperparathyroidism is suspected), plasma-free metanephrines and normetanephrines, and 24-hour urine metanephrines and normetanephrines.
- Once an index case is identified (any patient with MTC), the individual should be referred for **genetic counseling**. The counseling should include, but is not limited to, the scope and severity of the disease, potential impact on insurability, survivor guilt, possibility of nonpaternity, responsibility of the competent patient or guardian to inform family members for testing, and the option of prenatal or preimplantation diagnostic testing if the patient is of childbearing age.
- Most laboratories screen for the five most commonly mutated codons in exons 10 (609, 611, 618, 620) and 11 (634) for MEN2A and codons 918 and 883 for MEN2B. If the initial analysis is negative, then the remaining exons can be sequenced.
- **To find a laboratory** that provides specific needs for your patient, go to http://www.ncbi.nlm.nih.gov/gtr. RET molecular genetic analysis should only be extended to the patient's first-degree relatives (parents and children) if the patient tests positive. If either parent tests positive, all the at-risk family members should be tested for that mutation.
- The main indications for molecular genetic testing include:
  ○ Confirmation of diagnosis of MEN2A, FMTC, and MEN2B
  ○ Presymptomatic screening of family members at risk
  ○ Identification of germline mutations to distinguish sporadic from familial MTC
- If an individual tests negative for the RET mutation, he or she is not likely to be at risk for development of the MEN2 syndrome (2% to 5% false negative).
- Less likely is the possibility of a highly unusual or new RET mutation. Although entirely replaced by RET mutation analysis for carrier diagnosis, the calcitonin test can be used in such situations in which the MEN2 carrier ascertainment with DNA testing is not helpful or no RET mutation is detected.

- RET genetic testing does not substitute for biochemical studies needed to detect pheochromocytoma or hyperparathyroidism in MEN2 patients. Also, RET genetic testing before symptoms develop cannot identify spontaneous mutations that have not yet occurred.

Imaging

MEN1

- **Neck ultrasonography** should be done in primary hyperparathyroidism. It has been reported to have a sensitivity of 72% to 89% in detecting solitary adenomas.
- **99mTc-sestamibi scan.** The sensitivity is similar to ultrasound and is reported to be 68% to 95% in detecting single adenomas. An advantage of scintigraphy is that it can detect ectopic glands outside the neck. Therefore, some favor a combined approach to preoperative evaluation, which has been shown to more accurately predict solitary adenomas than either approach alone.
- **Pituitary MRI** should be done if a pituitary tumor is suggested by biochemical testing. MRI is most specific and sensitive for diagnosing pituitary lesions.
- Somatostatin receptor imaging with 111-Indium-penetreotide (**Octreoscan**) and single-photon emission computed tomography (SPECT) has a higher sensitivity than all other imaging modalities in localizing enteropancreatic tumors and is particularly useful in identifying liver and bone metastases. Fluorodeoxyglucose-positron emission tomography (FDG-PET) positive lesions have more aggressive behavior and may influence the decision to operate or monitor a pancreatic neuroendocrine tumor.[14] **Ga Dotatate PET** imaging is a new technology with similar pancreatic neuroendocrine tumor detection rates but with the advantage of detecting lesions in the pituitary, parathyroids, and adrenals.[15]
- **Endoscopic ultrasound** is especially valuable in imaging small pancreatic endocrine tumors.

MEN2

- **Neck ultrasonography** by a skilled neck ultrasonographer is mandatory to visualize superior mediastinum and central and bilateral lateral neck compartments in MEN2 patients or suspecting MTC.
- **Chest CT, neck CT, three-phase contrast-enhanced multidector liver CT, or contrast-enhanced MRI is** indicated if metastatic MTC is suspected.
- Abdominal CT or MRI is required to localize pheochromocytomas, which are typically intra-adrenal in MEN2. Please refer to Chapter 16 for further details.

Diagnostic Procedures

MEN1

- The diagnosis and follow-up of MEN1 components are mainly based on biochemical laboratory tests and imaging.
- Endoscopic biopsy might be useful in diagnosing certain enteropancreatic tumors. Skin biopsy may be helpful in diagnosing cutaneous tumors associated with MEN1, such as angiofibromas and collagenomas.

MEN2

- FNA biopsy is safe for the diagnosis of MTC and suspected lymph node metastasis. Measurement of calcitonin in the FNA washout fluid from suspected local recurrences and lymph node metastases may have higher sensitivity and specificity.
- Skin biopsy may be useful in establishing the diagnosis of **ganglioneuromas** in MEN2B and **cutaneous lichen amyloidosis** in MEN2A.
- Rectal biopsy or endoscopic intestinal biopsy may be useful in establishing the diagnosis of **ganglioneuromatosis**.

TREATMENT

MEN1

- There is no indication for treatment until clinical or biochemical presentation of disease. However, a patient with a known MEN1 mutation should be followed closely for evidence of the tumors that are characteristically associated with this syndrome.
- **Hyperparathyroidism**
  - The principle and modality in treating MEN1-associated hyperparathyroidism is similar to sporadic hyperparathyroidism. For details, please see Chapter 23.
  - Minimally invasive parathyroidectomy is not recommended, as the hyperparathyroidism in MEN1 patients is invariably due to hyperplasia of all four glands so the most common surgical approach is four-gland parathyroidectomy with autotransplantation, or a 3.5-gland parathyroidectomy.[13]
  - A decrease in intraoperative PTH >50% from baseline indicates adequate resection of parathyroid tissue. There is a high incidence of recurrence. One series found that over 20 years of follow-up, patients treated with less than 3 parathyroid gland removal had a high recurrence rate (55%) while total parathyroidectomy with autotransplantation has been associated with high rates of postoperative hypoparathyroidism requiring replacement (50%).[16]
  - Calcimimetics (cinacalcet) have a role in treating persistent or recurrent hypercalcemia following surgery in MEN1 patients.[17]
- **Pancreatic neuroendocrine tumors:** Medical and surgical therapy are discussed individually below. New technologies are offering more treatment modalities to patients. Peptide receptor radionuclide therapy improves progression-free survival and overall survival in functioning and nonfunctioning pancreatic neuroendocrine tumors.[18]
- **Gastrinoma (Zollinger–Ellison syndrome)**
  - Proton pump inhibitors are the treatment of choice to effectively control hypergastrinemia, but they are administered at double the usual dose (e.g., omeprazole 40 mg orally daily; pantoprazole 80 mg orally daily).
  - The role of surgery in management of gastrinoma in MEN1 is still controversial. Both the NANETS and ENETS guidelines suggest conservative approach to MEN1 patients with small tumors where symptoms are controlled.[19,20] Patients with small duodenal or pancreatic gastrinomas (≤2 cm) have a 90% to 100% 15-year survival without surgery.[6] However, in MEN1 patients with advanced metastatic disease, cure rate is almost zero with 10-year survival of 15% to 25% if liver metastases are present.[4] Therefore, surgery is usually reserved for patients who: (a) are refractory to or intolerant of medical therapy; (b) have gastrinomas >2 cm; (c) are at increased risk of metastasis (family history); and (d) are free of liver metastasis.
  - Patients with persistent or recurrent gastrinomas after surgery could undergo repeat surgery or medical therapy with 5-FU, octreotide, or interferon.
  - For patients with hepatic metastases, surgical debulking and/or hepatic artery chemoembolization may be employed. Chemotherapy with streptozotocin and doxorubicin can also be considered for patients with metastatic gastrinomas. However, observation is often preferable due to the indolent behavior of the metastases in many patients and the relative lack of efficacy of these agents.
- **Insulinoma**
  - Surgery is the treatment of choice for insulinoma and is usually curative. For other islet cell tumors, surgery is still a first-line indication, since medical therapy alone is unsatisfactory.
  - Tumor recurrence is treated symptomatically with agents such as octreotide.
- **Other functional tumors, VIPoma, glucagonoma, and somatostatinoma.**
  - These tumors are very rare, but have a high risk of malignancy. When clinically evident, 30% to 50% patients have metastatic lesions.

- First-line medical therapy is typically long acting somatostatin analogs. α-Interferon can be added if additional therapy is required for symptom control.[20]
- Surgical debulking has been done in refractory cases but is controversial as there are no good studies to show that this improves symptoms or survival.[20]
- Patients with liver metastases can be offered radiofrequency ablation, cryoablation, or hepatic artery embolization/chemoembolization.[18–20]
- **Nonfunctioning pancreaticoduodenal tumors**
  - Most experts advocate surgery to cure or to prevent malignant transformation and metastasis if the tumor is >2 cm.[21] Typically enucleation of tumors in the pancreatic head and concomitant distal 80% subtotal pancreatic resection is performed. However, there are limited data on timing of surgical management.
- **Intrathoracic neoplasia**
  - Bronchial carcinoid and thymic carcinoid tumors are rare with estimated prevalence in MEN1 patients of 4.9% and 2.0%, respectively.[22] Thymic carcinoid tumors occur almost exclusively in males and carry a bad prognosis.[22] Transcervical thymectomy at the time of parathyroidectomy has been suggested to decrease morbidity and mortality.[13]
- **Pituitary and other tumors:** treatment is similar to that for patients who develop these tumors sporadically. After medical or surgical treatment, patients should be followed for recurrence or persistent disease.

MEN2

- **Medullary thyroid carcinoma**
  - Total thyroidectomy with regional lymph node dissection is the treatment of choice for MTC. If advanced disease is present at time of diagnosis, more aggressive surgical resections can be appropriate along with consideration for external beam radiation or therapy with tyrosine kinase inhibitors.[9]
  - If the genetic mutation for MTC is known prior to developing the disease, the timing of prophylactic thyroidectomy generally in children is dependent on the RET codon mutation. Many groups have published recommendations. Listed below are the American Thyroid Association revised guidelines from 2016 (see Table 37-3).[9]
  - **For clinically apparent disease,** the preoperative evaluation should include basal calcitonin, CEA, and calcium (albumin corrected or ionized) and RET proto-oncogene

TABLE 37-3	RECOMMENDATIONS FOR WHEN TO PERFORM THYROIDECTOMY		
	Highest risk (ATA-HST)	High risk (ATA-H)	Moderate risk (ATA-MOD)
Surgical recommendation	Thyroidectomy <1 year old possible central LN dissection	Thyroidectomy <5 years old	Thyroidectomy before calcitonin elevated and while thyroid nodules <5 mm
Associated mutations	M918T (MEN2b)	C634, A883F	All other mutations
Initiate pheochromocytoma screening	11 years old	11 years old	16 years old

Adapted from Wells SA Jr, Asa SL, Dralle H, et al. Revised American Thyroid Association guidelines for the management of medullary thyroid carcinoma. *Thyroid* 2015;25:567–610.

TABLE 37-4	SURGICAL APPROACH TO MEDULLARY THYROID CARCINOMA		
	Local disease on imaging	LN metastases on imaging	Distant metastases on imaging
Thyroidectomy Central neck dissection	yes	yes	yes
Ipsilateral neck dissection	no	yes	debulking
Contralateral neck dissection	no	(if calcitonin >200)	debulking
Tyrosine kinase inhibitors	no	(if rapidly progressive)	(if rapidly progressive)

Adapted from Wells SA Jr, Asa SL, Dralle H, et al. Revised American Thyroid Association guidelines for the management of medullary thyroid carcinoma. *Thyroid* 2015;25:567–610.

mutation analysis. The surgical approach and potential chemotherapy depend on the extent of disease on preoperative imaging (please see Table 37-4).[9]

○ If preoperative calcitonin <20, very unlikely to have metastasis to lymph nodes.[9]

○ For patients with local lymph node metastases detected clinically or by ultrasound, or calcitonin >500 pg/dL, further imaging tests such as preoperative contrast–enhanced chest CT, neck CT, and three-phase contrast-enhanced multidetector liver CT or contrast-enhanced MRI can be considered. Axial MRI and bone scintigraphy can be used to detect bone metastases.[23]

○ After thyroidectomy, patients are followed with serial calcitonin measurements, as it is often the first index of persistent or recurrent MTC. Local disease can be surgically resected, whereas widespread metastases are difficult to cure since conventional chemotherapy or radiotherapy is not very effective; however, two tyrosine kinase inhibitors have been approved for locally advanced or metastatic MTC (vandetanib and cabozantanib), with others under study.[9]

• **Pheochromocytoma:** treatment of pheochromocytoma in MEN2 is similar to that in sporadic cases (see Chapter 16). If a pheochromocytoma is detected at the same time as MTC, laparoscopic adrenalectomy should be performed before thyroidectomy with appropriate adrenergic blockade to avoid intraoperative catecholamine crisis.

• **Hyperparathyroidism**

○ Those at risk for hyperparathyroidism (with mutations in codons 609, 611, 618, 620, 630 634, 804, 891) should be screened annually with ionized calcium (or total calcium and albumin) and intact PTH, starting at age 15.

○ Hyperparathyroidism is managed with subtotal parathyroidectomy or total parathyroidectomy with autotransplantation. If parathyroid hyperplasia is found at the time of thyroidectomy, this should be considered as hyperparathyroidism even in the absence of biochemical evidence of disease.[9]

Patient Education

Counseling of patients and family members is an important part of disease management. A genetic counseling referral should be obtained. Useful websites include http://ghr.nlm.nih.gov/condition/multiple-endocrine-neoplasia, and http://www.amend.org.uk/.

MONITORING/FOLLOW-UP

MEN1

- Once an index case of MEN1 is identified, genetic counseling and testing should be considered but not absolutely required for all family members. The age to start screening is still controversial. Direct DNA analysis for mutations in the MEN1 gene identifies patients who have inherited a mutated allele and are destined to develop MEN1.
- Once an individual is identified as high risk for MEN1 (positive gene test or family history), periodic biochemical screening to detect symptoms related to hormone excess associated with the tumors characteristic of MEN1 should be carried out. However, prophylactic treatments have no beneficial role in patients with MEN1. Current consensus guidelines propose screening for tumors in an individual with genetic testing confirming MEN1 mutation or diagnosis of MEN1,[24,25] please see Table 37-5.[13]

MEN2

- **Medullary thyroid carcinoma**
  - **All patients thought to have sporadic MTC should undergo RET mutation analysis as 40% to 50% of putative sporadic cases have been shown to harbor germline RET mutations.**

TABLE 37-5 **PROPOSED SCREENING FOR TUMORS IN MEN1 INDIVIDUALS**

	Biochemical test	Frequency	Imaging	Frequency
Hyperparathyroidism	Alb, Total Ca or iCa, PTH	Q1 year	None	
Enteropancreatic tumors	Fasting gastrin, glucagon, VIP, pancreatic polypeptide, chromogranin A, glucose and insulin	Q1 year	Abdominal CT, MRI, or endoscopic ultrasound	Unclear
Pituitary tumors	Prolactin, IGF-1; further testing if imaging positive	Q1 year	Pituitary protocol MRI	Q3–5 years
Thymic, bronchopulmonary, and gastric tumors	None		Chest CT or MRI Endoscopy and biopsy	Q1–2 years Q3 years
Adrenal tumors	1 mg ONDST, renin: aldosterone for tumors >1 cm		Abdominal CT, MRI	Q3 years

ONDST, overnight 1-mg dexamethasone suppression test; Alb, albumin; Ca, calcium; iCa, ionized calcium; PTH, parathyroid hormone; VIP, vasoactive intestinal peptide; IGF-1, insulin-like growth factor 1; CT, computed tomography; MRI, magnetic resonance imaging.
Adapted from Thakker RV, Newey PJ, Walls GV, et al. Clinical practice guidelines for multiple endocrine neoplasia type 1 (MEN1). *J Clin Endocrinol Metab* 2012; 97:2990–3011.

- ○ For patients with RET mutation who elect to wait for prophylactic thyroidectomy, calcitonin and neck ultrasonography should be obtained every 6 to 12 months.
- ○ For patients who achieve a complete biochemical cure, long-term biochemical monitoring of annual measurement of serum calcitonin is recommended.
- ○ For patients with detectable basal serum calcitonin levels postoperatively, basal calcitonin and CEA levels should be obtained approximately every 6 months to determine their doubling time. Ongoing follow-up of these tumor markers and physical examination should occur at one-fourth the shortest doubling time or annually, whichever is more frequent. The timing of follow-up anatomic imaging may be based on the relative stability of these tests, presence or absence of symptoms, and the location of known or likely sites of metastasis.
- ○ For patients in a family that meets clinical criteria for MEN2A or 2B, or FMTC but no RET gene mutation has been found, periodic screening for MTC (neck ultrasound, calcitonin measurement), associated primary hyperparathyroidism (albumin-corrected calcium or ionized calcium) and pheochromocytoma (plasma-free metanephrines and normetanephrines, or 24-hour urine metanephrines and normetanephrines) should be done as indicated by the family phenotype. Screening should continue at 1- to 3-year intervals at least until age 50 or 20 years beyond the oldest age of initial diagnosis in the family, whichever is latest.
- **Pheochromocytoma**
  - ○ Screening for pheochromocytoma with annual plasma and/or urinary fractionated metanephrine measurements is done in all MEN2 patients. The age at which to begin the screening also depends on specific codon mutations. Screening should start between age 10 and 15 in families with high-risk mutations (codons 918, 634, and 883) and after age 16 in those with mutations in less high-risk codons. An abnormal biochemical test should be followed by CT or MRI to localize tumors.
  - ○ Women with a RET mutation associated with MEN2 who are pregnant or planning to become pregnant should be screened biochemically for pheochromocytoma.
  - ○ After pheochromocytoma resection, biochemical testing should be obtained 4 to 6 weeks after surgery, then yearly if blood pressure is under control. If bilateral adrenalectomy has been done, the screening interval can be lengthened since extraadrenal pheochromocytoma in MEN syndrome is very rare.
- **Hyperparathyroidism:** See MEN1 above.

OUTCOME/PROGNOSIS

MEN1

- The mortality of MEN1 is not well documented. Pancreatic malignancy and malignant thymic carcinoids are the principal causes of disease-related death in MEN1.[26] Our institution reported that nearly half of the patients (46%) died of causes related to MEN1 at a mean age of 50. A report from Mayo Clinic showed 28% patients died of MEN1-related causes, the most common being metastatic islet malignancy (58.8%). The overall 20-year survival of MEN1 patients was 64%, compared to 81% for age- and gender-matched controls.[27]
- Rarely patients die of hyperparathyroidism. Parathyroid malignancy is very rare but is reported.[28] The major problem with hyperparathyroidism is postsurgical recurrence. The recurrence rate for subtotal parathyroidectomy or total parathyroidectomy in MEN1 is as high as 55% in 10 years.[29]

- Malignant insulinoma is the major cause of disease-related death. Malignancy rate is higher with MEN1-associated insulinoma compared to sporadic insulinoma. At diagnosis, more than 50% of patients were found to have metastatic disease.
- Gastrinoma also has higher rate of malignancy in MEN1. The cure rate by surgery is very low (0% to 10%). The majority (50% to 70%) of patients with tumor >2 cm on imaging had lymph node involvement. However, these patients have excellent long-term survival rate without surgery, and even with apparent metastatic disease they have a 15-year survival of 52%.[30]
- Nonfunctioning pancreatic tumor is currently the most common entity requiring surgery.[31] Nonfunctioning tumors account for 35% to 55% of all pancreatic endocrine tumors and most commonly present in the fourth or fifth decade of life. Approximately two-thirds of nonfunctioning pancreatic endocrine tumors are malignant.

MEN2

- Eventually all patients develop medullary thyroid carcinoma, which is the major cause of MEN2-related death. Using a prior TNM classification system, 10-year survival rates for stages I, II, III, and IV are 100%, 93%, 71%, and 21%, respectively.[32] New research suggests that response to initial surgical treatment (persistently elevated calcitonin or evidence of remaining structural disease) may provide additional information to TMN staging in predicting mortality.[33–35]
- Medullary thyroid carcinoma in patients with MEN2B is more aggressive than in MEN2A or FMTC, and surgery is only curative when done early before disease is clinically evident.[9]
- Pheochromocytoma occurs in approximately 40% to 50% of patients with MEN2A and probably a similar percentage in MEN2B. Malignant cases are very rare. The presence of pheochromocytomas does not seem to worsen overall prognosis in patients with MEN2, particularly with C634 mutations.[9]
- Primary hyperparathyroidism occurs in 10% to 25% of patients with MEN2A and is almost always multiglandular. In expert parathyroid surgical centers, the recurrence rate after apparently successful subtotal parathyroidectomy is very low.

REFERENCES

1. Brandi ML, Gagel RF, Angeli A, et al. Guidelines for diagnosis and therapy of MEN type 1 and type 2. *J Clin Endocrinol Metab* 2001;86(12):5658–5671.
2. Lakhani VT, You YN, Wells SA. The multiple endocrine neoplasia syndromes. *Ann Rev Med* 2007;58:253–265.
3. Wells SA, Pacini F, Robinson BG, Santoro M. Multiple endocrine neoplasia type 2 and familial medullary thyroid carcinoma: An update. *J Clin Endocrinol Metab* 2013;98(8):3149–3164.
4. Pellegata NS. MENX and MEN4. *Clinics (Sao Paulo)* 2012;67 (Suppl 1), 13–18.
5. Conemans EB, Brosens LAA, Raicu-Ionita GM, et al. Prognostic value of WHO grade in pancreatic neuro-endocrine tumors in multiple endocrine neoplasia type 1: Results from the Dutch-MEN1 Study Group. *Pancreatology* 2017;17(5):766–772.
6. Ito T, Igarashi H, Jensen RT. Zollinger-Ellison syndrome: Recent advances and controversies. *Curr Opin Gastroenterol* 2013;29(6):650–661.
7. Wohllk N, Schweizer H, Erlic Z, et al. Multiple endocrine neoplasia type 2. *Best Pract Res Clin Endocrinol Metab* 2010;24(3):371–387.
8. American Thyroid Association Guidelines Task Force, Kloos RT, Eng C, et al. Medullary thyroid cancer: Management guidelines of the American Thyroid Association. *Thyroid* 2009;19(6):565–612.
9. Wells SA, Asa SL, Dralle H, et al. Revised American Thyroid Association guidelines for the management of medullary thyroid carcinoma. *Thyroid* 2015;25(6):567–610.

10. Butter A, Gagné J, Al-Jazaeri A, Emran MA, Deal C, St-Vil D. Prophylactic thyroidectomy in pediatric carriers of multiple endocrine neoplasia type 2A or familial medullary thyroid carcinoma: Mutation in C620 is associated with Hirschsprung's disease. *J Pediatr Surg* 2007;42(1):203–206.

11. Eng C, Clayton D, Schuffenecker I, et al. The relationship between specific RET proto-oncogene mutations and disease phenotype in multiple endocrine neoplasia type 2. International RET mutation consortium analysis. *JAMA* 1996;276(19):1575–1579.

12. Newey PJ, Thakker RV. Role of multiple endocrine neoplasia type 1 mutational analysis in clinical practice. *Endocr Pract* 2011;17 (Suppl 3):8–17.

13. Thakker RV, Newey PJ, Walls GV, et al. Clinical practice guidelines for multiple endocrine neoplasia type 1 (MEN1). *J Clin Endocrinol Metab* 2012;97(9):2990–3011.

14. Kornaczewski Jackson ER, Pointon OP, Bohmer R, Burgess JR. Utility of FDG-PET imaging for risk stratification of pancreatic neuroendocrine tumors in MEN1. *J Clin Endocrinol Metab* 2017;102(6):1926–1933.

15. Lastoria S, Marciello F, Faggiano A, et al. Role of (68)Ga-DOTATATE PET/CT in patients with multiple endocrine neoplasia type 1 (MEN1). *Endocrine* 2016;52(3):488–494.

16. Fyrsten E, Norlen O, Hessman O, Stalberg P, Hellman P. Long-term surveillance of treated hyperparathyroidism for multiple endocrine neoplasia type 1: Recurrence or hypoparathyroidism? *World J Surg* 2016;40(3):615–621.

17. Moyes VJ, Monson JP, Chew SL, Akker SA. Clinical use of Cinacalcet in MEN1 hyperparathyroidism. *Int J Endocrinol* 2010;2010:906163.

18. Katona BW, Roccaro GA, Soulen MC, et al. Efficacy of peptide receptor radionuclide therapy in a United States-based cohort of metastatic neuroendocrine tumor patients: Single-institution retrospective analysis. *Pancreas* 2017;46(9):1121–1126.

19. Falconi M, Eriksson B, Kaltsas G, et al. ENETS consensus guidelines update for the management of patients with functional pancreatic neuroendocrine tumors and non-functional pancreatic neuroendocrine tumors. *Neuroendocrinology* 2016;103(2):153–171.

20. Kulke MH, Anthony LB, Bushnell DL, et al. NANETS treatment guidelines: Well-differentiated neuroendocrine tumors of the stomach and pancreas. *Pancreas* 2010;39(6):735–752.

21. Nell S, Verkooijen HM, Pieterman CRC, et al. Management of MEN1 related nonfunctioning pancreatic NETs: A shifting paradigm: Results from the dutchMEN1 study group. *Ann Surg* 2018;267(6):1155–1160.

22. Singh Ospina N, Thompson GB, Nichols F, Cassivi SD, Young, WF. Thymic and bronchial carcinoid tumors in multiple endocrine neoplasia type 1: The Mayo Clinic Experience from 1977 to 2013. *Horm Cancer* 2015;6(5-6):247–253.

23. Machens A, Dralle H. Biomarker-based risk stratification for previously untreated medullary thyroid cancer. *J Clin Endocrinol Metab* 2010;95(6), 2655–2663.

24. Falchetti A. Genetic screening for multiple endocrine neoplasia syndrome type 1 (MEN-1): When and how. *F1000 Med Rep* 2010;2:14.

25. Waldmann J, Fendrich V, Habbe N, et al. Screening of patients with multiple endocrine neoplasia type 1 (MEN-1): A critical analysis of its value. *World J Surg* 2009;33(6):1208–1218.

26. Goudet P, Murat A, Binquet C, et al. Risk factors and causes of death in MEN1 disease. A GTE (Groupe d'Etude des Tumeurs Endocrines) cohort study among 758 patients. *World J Surg* 2010;34(2):249–255.

27. Dean PG, van Heerden JA, Farley DR, et al. Are patients with multiple endocrine neoplasia type I prone to premature death? *World J Surg* 2000;24(11):1437–1441.

28. Shih RY, Fackler S, Maturo S, True MW, Brennan J, Wells D. Parathyroid carcinoma in multiple endocrine neoplasia type 1 with a classic germline mutation. *Endocr Pract* 2009;15(6):567–572.

29. Tonelli F, Marcucci T, Giudici F, Falchetti A, Brandi ML. Surgical approach in hereditary hyperparathyroidism. *Endocr J* 2009;56(7):827–841.

30. Norton JA. Surgical treatment and prognosis of gastrinoma. *Best Pract Res Clin Gastroenterol* 2005;19(5):799–805.

31. Lairmore TC, Chen VY, DeBenedetti MK, Gillanders WE, Norton JA, Doherty GM. Duodenopancreatic resections in patients with multiple endocrine neoplasia type 1. *Ann Surg* 2000;231(6):909–918.

32. Cupisti K, Wolf A, Raffel A, et al. Long-term clinical and biochemical follow-up in medullary thyroid carcinoma: A single institution's experience over 20 years. *Ann Surg* 2007;246(5):815–821.

33. Kwon H, Kim WG, Jeon MJ, et al. Dynamic risk stratification for medullary thyroid cancer according to the response to initial therapy. *Endocrine* 2016;53(1):174–181.
34. Lindsey S, Ganly I, Palmer F, Tuttle RM. Response to initial therapy predicts clinical outcomes in medullary thyroid cancer. *Thyroid* 2015;25(2):242–249.
35. Yang JH, Lindsey SC, Camacho CP, et al. Integration of a postoperative calcitonin measurement into an anatomical staging system improves initial risk stratification in medullary thyroid cancer. *Clin Endocrinol (Oxf)* 2015;83(6):938–942.

Neuroendocrine Tumors

Brian D. Muegge and Thomas J. Baranski

GENERAL PRINCIPLES

- Neuroendocrine tumors (NETs) are a heterogeneous collection of rare neoplasms that arise from the diffuse endocrine epithelium found in most organs in the body. The majority of these tumors are in tissues derived from the embryonic gut, including the pancreas and the digestive tract, but also arise in lung, ovary, and prostate.[1]
- While most well-differentiated NET have histologic features of hormone production, only a minority produce clinically apparent signs of excess hormone secretion.
- **Carcinoid syndrome** refers to the cluster of symptoms mediated by the systemic release of vasoactive compounds and hormones from NET, and is found in fewer than 10% of NET.
- Detection is often delayed and most NET tumors are metastatic at diagnosis. Management is multidisciplinary including surgical removal and medical management of symptoms, if present.

Classification

Historical Aspects

- The term *karzinoide* was first introduced by Oberndorfer in 1907 to describe intestinal tumors that histologically resembled carcinomas but did not behave in their aggressive manner. Recognition of the endocrine-related properties of these tumors occurred several years later, along with recognition of similar tumors outside the intestinal tract.
- It is now well established that these tumors are derived from epithelium but have features of both neural and epithelial cells. Current classification schemes use the term "Neuroendocrine" in place of carcinoid. However, "carcinoid" continues to be used interchangeably in the literature for well-differentiated NETs.

Pathologic Classification of NET

- Pathologic criteria derived from World Health Organization (WHO) recommendations use the framework of other epithelial tumors that emphasizes degree of differentiation and cellular grade.[2] The criteria for gastroenteropancreatic (GEP) NET are presented in (Table 38-1).[2] Slightly different definitions are used for tumors arising from other tissues, for example, lung.
- Well-differentiated NETs have histology similar to the nonneoplastic neuroendocrine tissue, such as small round cells with uniform nuclei and cytoplasm. They characteristically have strong immunostaining for the neuroendocrine markers **chromogranin A (CgA)** and **synaptophysin**. Electron microscopy demonstrates membrane-bound secretory granules which contain a variety of biogenic amines and hormones
- Poorly differentiated NET characteristically has less evidence of secretory granules and diminished or absent immunostaining for neuroendocrine markers. They are more rapidly dividing and generally have greater mortality than well-differentiated forms.

Epidemiology

- According to the Surveillance Epidemiology and End Results (SEER) database, the incidence of NET is about 5 per 100,000 people.[3] These estimates may not fully capture benign or noninvasive lesions, which are not reported to SEER.

TABLE 38-1	WHO GRADING SYSTEM FOR GEP-NET		
Differentiation	Grade	Proliferative rate	Name
Well-differentiated	G1 (low grade)	<2 mitoses/10 HPF and <3% Ki67 index	Neuroendocrine tumor
	G2 (intermediate grade)	2-20 mitoses/10 HPF OR 3–20% Ki67 index	Neuroendocrine tumor
Poorly differentiated	G3 (high grade)	>20 mitoses/10 HPF OR >20% Ki67 index	Neuroendocrine carcinoma (large-cell type OR small-cell type)

HPF, high-power field.
Adapted from Klimstra DS, Modlin IR, Coppola D, Lloyd RV, Suster S. The pathologic classification of neuroendocrine tumors: A review of nomenclature, grading, and staging systems. *Pancreas* 2010;39:707–712.

- Risk factors include inherited tumor syndromes (discussed below), female sex, and African American ancestry.[4,5]
- The incidence of NET has increased in the last 30 years, in the United States and around the world. Multiple studies from Asian countries have documented different distributions of primary tumors compared to Western countries.[6–8]
- The greatest rate of increase in most studies has been measured in rectal tumors, which may reflect incidental discovery during endoscopic screening programs.

Pathophysiology

Molecular Genetics

- Most NETs are sporadic, but about one-third of pancreatic NET arise in patients with germline mutations causing MEN1, von Hipple-Lindau, or tuberous sclerosis syndromes. The diagnosis of a pancreatic NET should prompt an evaluation for these syndromes.
- Whole-exome sequencing has revealed that NET tumors have fewer somatic mutations than most other solid tumors. Recent studies have suggested previously unappreciated germline mutations in in *MUTYH*, *CHEK1*, and *BRCA2* that are overrepresented in pancreatic NET.[9]
- Activating mutations in the mechanistic target of rapamycin (mTOR) pathway are frequently found in NET tumors from all primary sites. Other commonly targeted pathways include apoptosis (DAXX) and chromatin modification (ATRX) in pancreatic NET, and the proto-oncogene SRC and TGF-β signaling pathways in small intestinal NET.[10,11]

Biochemistry

- NETs contain neurosecretory granules that synthesize, store, and release a variety of classic hormones and other substances, such as serotonin, histamine, prostaglandin, kallikrein, bradykinin, substance P, as well as many others.[12]
- The majority of NET are **nonfunctional**, meaning there is no clinical evidence of excessive hormone secretion despite histochemical evidence of mature hormone production.
- **Serotonin** (5-hydroxytryptamine, **5-HT**) is largely responsible for the classic symptoms of carcinoid syndrome, including diarrhea, bronchospasm, and carcinoid heart disease.

The cause of flushing is uncertain, but has been attributed to numerous products including prostaglandins, kinins, substance P, and histamine.

- Key steps in 5-HT metabolism include the conversion of dietary tryptophan to 5-HT by the subsequent actions of **tyrosine hydroxylase (TPH)** and **aromatic L amino acid decarboxylase (AAAD)**, and the breakdown of serum 5-HT to **5-hydroxyindoleacetic acid (5-HIAA)** by monoamine oxidase.

- Some foregut NET tumors do not express AAAD. These tumors do not produce serotonin and thus do not cause classical carcinoid syndrome even when widely metastatic.

- Most NET, including nonfunctional tumors, express somatostatin receptors (SSTRs). Some subtypes, for example, insulinomas and poorly differentiated NET, are less likely to express high levels of SSTR, which diminishes the efficacy of somatostatin analogs (SSAs) for imaging and treatment of these groups.

DIAGNOSIS

Clinical Presentation

- Because most NETs are nonfunctional and slowly growing, they are typically discovered incidentally during surgery, endoscopy, or imaging performed for another indication.

- Abdominal pain is the most frequent presenting complaint, with obstruction or rectal bleeding observed less commonly.[13]

- NET of the small intestine often metastasizes to mesenteric lymph nodes, causing fibrosis and contraction of the mesentery, which can manifest as intermittent bowel obstruction or ischemia.

Carcinoid and Other Hormonal Syndromes

- The **classic carcinoid syndrome (flushing, diarrhea, wheezing, right-sided heart disease) is only seen in 5% to 10% of NET** (Table 38-2).[14–17] The syndrome is more often observed in tumors of the midgut (small bowel) than foregut or hindgut.

- The lungs and liver metabolize many of the substances secreted by NET, thereby preventing their release into the systemic circulation until metastases develop. This may explain why patients who have NET typically have carcinoid syndrome only if they have hepatic metastases. Bronchial and ovarian NET can cause carcinoid syndrome with lower tumor burden and in the absence of hepatic metastasis as they secrete directly into the systemic circulation.

- Symptoms of the carcinoid syndrome vary in intensity and timing and are usually vague, nonspecific, and organ related, causing relatively long delays in diagnosis. The average time from symptom onset to diagnosis is more than 9 years.

- **Carcinoid crisis**—carcinoid crisis is a life-threatening form of carcinoid syndrome that is triggered by specific events such as anesthesia, surgery, or chemotherapy, which presumably stimulates the release of an overwhelming amount of vasoactive compounds.

- Symptoms include flushing with extreme changes in blood pressure, and may also include arrhythmias, bronchospasm, and altered mental status.

- A number of other clinical syndromes can arise more rarely from NETs that secrete excessive amounts of mature endocrine hormones (Table 38-2).[14–17]

Diagnostic Testing

Laboratories

- Functional NETs are very rare, so other more likely causes of symptoms such as diarrhea or flushing should be considered before proceeding to biochemical testing.

- The most useful initial screening test for carcinoid syndrome is a measure of **24-hour urinary excretion of 5-HIAA.**

TABLE 38-2   SYNDROMES OF FUNCTIONAL NET

Syndrome	Symptoms	Incidence	Diagnosis
Carcinoid	*Flushing* • Dry, faint pink to red, face and upper trunk • Provoked by alcohol or tyramine-containing foods (blue cheese, red wine) • Lasts 1 to 5 minutes	Of those with carcinoid syndrome: 85%	Urinary 5-HIAA
	Diarrhea • Secretory, persists with fasting • Usually not temporally related to flushing	30%	
	Bronchospasm • Often with flushing episodes	10–20%	
Carcinoid heart disease[14]	• Tricuspid valve regurgitation and pulmonary valve stenosis most common • Symptoms of right-sided heart failure, including peripheral edema and ascites	4–70%	Echocardiography
Fibrotic disease	Retroperitoneal fibrosis, intestinal/urethral obstruction, Peyronie disease, pulmonary fibrosis	30–60% of those with abdominal symptoms	No specific biochemical test
Pellagra	Glossitis, stomatitis, dermatitis, confusion Hypoalbuminemia Due to shunting of precursor tryptophan toward serotonin synthesis	Up to 20%[15]	Urinary N1-methylnicotinamide
Insulinoma	Reviewed in Chapter 33		

(continued)

TABLE 38-2 SYNDROMES OF FUNCTIONAL NET (*Continued*)

Syndrome	Symptoms	Incidence	Diagnosis
Gastrinoma Glucagonoma[16]	*Common* • Weight loss, diabetes mellitus, necrolytic migratory erythema *Other* • Secretory diarrhea, deep venous thrombosis, neuropsychiatric complaints	~1 to 10 in 10 million	Elevated serum glucagon, typically >500 pg/mL
VIPoma/WDHA syndrome/ Verner–Morrison syndrome[17]	Watery Diarrhea Hypokalemia Achlorhydria or hypochlorhydria	~1 in 10 million	Serum VIP >75 pg/mL on ≥2 occasions Low osmotic gap diarrhea
Somatostatinoma	Paracrine inhibition of hormone release leading to diabetes mellitus, cholelithiasis, diarrhea/steatorrhea	~1 in 40 million	Fasting plasma somatostatin >30 pg/mL

VIP, vasoactive intestinal peptide.

TABLE 38-3 SOURCES OF ERROR IN URINARY 5-HIAA TESTING

False positive	False negative
Foods	**Drugs**
• Avocados, pineapples, bananas, kiwi fruit, plums, eggplant, walnuts, pecans	• Ethanol, aspirin, isoniazid, heparin, monoamine oxidase inhibitors, corticotropin, imipramine, levodopa, methyldopa, phenothiazines
Drugs	
• Nicotine, caffeine, acetaminophen, guafenesin, phenobarbital, reserpine, ephedrine, phentolamine, fluorouracil, melphalan	

- This test has a sensitivity of about 70% and specificity of nearly 90% in patients with *carcinoid syndrome*, and levels are often very elevated (>100 mg/day).[18]
- In patients *without* the clinical carcinoid syndrome, the test is not useful to diagnose NET as levels are normal or only minimally elevated. Elevations in 5-HIAA are also seen with celiac sprue, Whipple disease, or after the ingestion of high tryptophan–containing foods.
- Before ordering the measurement of urinary 5-HIAA, it is critical to note factors that can lead to false-positive test results (see Table 38-3).
- 5-HIAA levels appear to correlate well with tumor mass, and can be used as a marker for the extent of disease and to follow response to treatment among those patients with frank elevation prior to treatment
- Direct measurement of 5-HT in the blood is confounded by diet, medications, and serotonin release from platelets. It is not considered to be a useful diagnostic test at this time.
- Another commonly used biomarker is **CgA**. It is a glycoprotein secreted by NETs along with other hormones. It is a sensitive marker of carcinoid tumors but has poor specificity.[19]
- False-positive results may be seen in renal and liver failure, rheumatoid arthritis, inflammatory bowel disease, physical stress and trauma, hypergastrinemia caused by achlorhydria (e.g., chronic use of proton pump inhibitors, atrophic gastritis, or retained gastric antrum), and multiple myeloma.[20]
- Accordingly, current guidelines do not recommend the use of CgA measurement to diagnose NET.
- Unlike 5-HIAA, plasma CgA testing does not rely on serotonin secretion and can detect nonsecreting tumors. It may be used to monitor tumor progression and treatment response if NET is diagnosed by other means.

Imaging
- Once the biochemical diagnosis of carcinoid syndrome is confirmed, the tumor must be localized.
- **Abdominal CT scanning is the diagnostic procedure of choice for tumor staging**, as it identifies the primary tumor and mesenteric lymph node enlargement.
  - Small tumors of the jejunum, ileum, and appendix are often not detected with conventional CT, due to their small size. CT enterography has been shown to be a sensitive method to detect small bowel tumors when conventional CT is nondiagnostic.[21]
  - Metastatic NETs often have a characteristic CT finding in the mesentery of a speculated, fibrotic mass with stellate projections. Central calcifications may be present.
  - Triphasic CT of the liver should be considered because the liver is the most common site for metastasis.

- **Somatostatin-based imaging**
  - NET typically express SSTRs, which has been useful for therapy and radioimaging.
  - [111]In labelled SSAs have been used for scintigraphy for many years. Sensitivity estimates range from 65% to 100% for the detection of carcinoid tumors. Specificity is limited by tracer uptake in other types of non-NET tumors, granulomas, and autoimmune disease.
  - New PET tracers have been developed which are far more sensitive than scintigraphy or conventional CT. These couple a radionuclide chelator (DOTA) to short peptides derived from octreotide. A large prospective trial of 131 patients with suspected NET showed that ^{68}Ga-DOTATATE–detected lesions in 95% of patients (compared to 45% with conventional CT and 31% with scintigraphy).[22]
- Other modalities like MRI (sensitive for detecting extrahepatic disease) or endoscopic ultrasound/intraoperative ultrasound are usually reserved for those patients with suspected carcinoid tumors that have not been localized by CT or functional imaging.
- Chest CT scan can be used to localize bronchial carcinoid tumors, and echocardiography can help in establishing the severity of carcinoid heart disease.

TREATMENT

The key management issues in patients with carcinoid tumors include symptom control, biochemical control (lowering or normalizing 5-HIAA levels), objective tumor control, and improvement of quality of life.

Medical Management

Hormonal Symptom Control

- SSAs are the mainstay of symptomatic therapy in patients with carcinoid syndrome to control symptoms of hormonal secretion. They may also stabilize the progression of carcinoid heart disease. Short-acting octreotide can be initiated and if tolerated converted to long-acting formulations. Typically doses of depot octreotide LAR are 20 to 30 mg IM qmonth. Lantreotide, another long-acting SSA, has similar clinical efficacy to octreotide LAR (see below).
- Side effects include nausea, abdominal pain, vomiting, and diarrhea but usually resolve within a few days of injection.
- Cholelithiasis and biliary sludge can develop as a long-term complication in up to 50% of patients due to reduced postprandial gallbladder contractility and emptying. Prophylactic treatment with ursodeoxycholic acid may help reduce this complication, and cholecystectomy is sometimes performed at time of primary tumor resection.
- Tachyphylaxis is commonly seen after about 12 months and can be overcome with a higher dose or with the addition of interferon-α.
- **Telotristat ethyl**, a tryptophan hydroxylase inhibitor which blocks the initial conversion of tryptophan to 5-HT, has recently been approved as adjunctive therapy to SSA in patients with inadequate symptomatic relief on SSA alone. Phase III trials demonstrated reduced frequency of bowel movements and urinary 5-HIAA when telotristat ethyl was added to SSA, compared to the addition of placebo.[23]
- Specific treatments for the various symptoms of the carcinoid syndrome in addition to SSA are often helpful. Drugs such as prednisone, phenoxybenzamine, and chlorpromazine have shown efficacy for patients with flushing and severe diarrhea. Histamine blockers are useful for gastric carcinoids that secrete histamine.

Control of Tumor Growth

- For poorly differentiated tumors, cytotoxic chemotherapy is the mainstay, as these tumors are less responsive to targeted therapy. Standard protocols include platinum agents and etoposide.[1]

- For patients with well-differentiated tumors and asymptomatic disease, treatment decision is personalized and observation is possible for small, stable lesions.
- For patients with symptomatic or progressive tumor burden, several options exist.
  - Seminal trials with **octreotide LAR** (PROMID) and **lanreotide** (CLARINET) revealed prolonged progression-free survival (PFS) in well-differentiated metastatic small intestinal and pancreatic NET.[24,25] SSAs are considered first-line therapy for patients with metastatic, symptomatic, or progressive well-differentiated tumors.
  - **Everolimus**, an inhibitor of the mTOR pathway, has been shown in the RADIANT-4 trial to prolong PFS in metastatic NET when used as monotherapy or in addition to SSA.[26] It is approved in the United States for progressive, nonfunctional NET. Grade 3/4 adverse events include stomatitis, diarrhea, infection, anemia, and hyperglycemia.
  - Radiolabelled SSAs, also called peptide receptor radionucleotide therapy (PRRT) are used in Europe and are under review by the FDA for somatostatin receptor–positive NET. The NETTER-1 trial of ^{177}Lu-DOTATATE showed superior PFS and response rate among patients receiving PRRT with low-dose octreotide compared to high-dose octreotide alone.[27] Preliminary analysis indicated superior overall survival with PRRT, but this must be confirmed in planned final analysis. Myelosuppression was observed in about 10% of patients.
  - Numerous small molecule inhibitors, including sunitinib, pazopanib, and bevacizumab have shown modest benefit in phase II and III trials.

Surgical Management

- For the minority of patients who present with locoregional disease and no apparent metastasis, surgical resection with curative intent is first-line treatment.
- In contrast to most kinds of metastatic solid tumor, surgical resection may still be indicated for metastatic NET. Debulking of primary NET or metastasis may improve quality of life and reduce symptomatic burden of hormonal secretion or local mass effect.
- Cytoreductive surgery or targeted ablation of hepatic metastases should be considered in patients with symptomatic NET and hepatic disease burden that is amenable to nearly complete removal. Retrospective series indicate reduced symptom burden and noninferior PFS, though recurrence is nearly universal over 5 to 10 years.[28,29]
- Intraoperative **carcinoid crisis** is a rare but serious potential complication that can be precipitated by surgery or anesthesia. Pre- and intraoperative somatostatin analog administration is required in patients with functional carcinoid syndrome.

MONITORING/FOLLOW-UP

- There is limited evidence to guide follow-up recommendations, so current guidelines are largely the result of expert opinion.[30]
- Very small NET, including NET <2 cm in the appendix and <1 cm in the rectum, are typically cured with surgery and may not need specific follow-up.
- Larger NETs with complete resection should be followed with imaging and possible biochemical testing (if hormone levels were elevated preoperatively) over the first 3 to 12 months after resection, then every 1 to 2 years thereafter.
- Patients with residual or metastatic disease will need more frequent clinical examinations, imagings, and biochemical testings depending on symptom burden, SSA therapy, and evidence of disease progression.
- Routine echocardiography to detect early carcinoid heart disease in patients with carcinoid syndrome might improve prognosis, but has not been tested in randomized control trials.

PROGNOSIS

- Prognosis is based on the location, size, invasiveness, and histology of the primary tumor.
- A review of SEER data indicates that among those patients with well-differentiated NET, median survival with local, regional, or metastatic disease was 223, 111, and 33 months respectively.[3]
- Tumors of the appendix and rectum have an especially good prognosis, with 5-year survival rates exceeding 90% when localized.
- Prognosis for poorly differentiated NET is much worse, with median survival of only 10 months.
- Advanced age is strongly associated with worse outcome. Females had small but significantly improved survival outcomes compared to men.

REFERENCES

1. Kunz PL. Carcinoid and neuroendocrine tumors: Building on success. *J Clin Oncol* 2015;33: 1855–1863.
2. Klimstra DS, Modlin IR, Coppola D, Lloyd RV, Suster S. The pathologic classification of neuroendocrine tumors: A review of nomenclature, grading, and staging systems. *Pancreas* 2010;39:707–712.
3. Yao JC, Hassan M, Phan A, et al. One hundred years after "carcinoid": Epidemiology of and prognostic factors for neuroendocrine tumors in 35,825 cases in the United States. *J Clin Oncol* 2008;26:3063–3072.
4. Broder MS, Cai B, Chang E, Neary MP. Epidemiology of gastrointestinal neuroendocrine tumors in a US commercially insured population. *Endocr Pract* 2017;23:1210–1216.
5. Hauso O, Gustafsson BI, Kidd M, et al. Neuroendocrine tumor epidemiology: Contrasting Norway and North America. *Cancer* 2008;113:2655–2664.
6. Ito T, Igarashi H, Nakamura K, et al. Epidemiological trends of pancreatic and gastrointestinal neuroendocrine tumors in Japan: A nationwide survey analysis. *J Gastroenterol* 2015;50: 58–64.
7. Cho MY, Kim JM, Sohn JH, et al. Current trends in the incidence and pathologic diagnosis of gastroenteropancreatic neuroendocrine tumors (GEP-NETs) in Korea 2000–2009: Multicenter study. *Cancer Res Treat* 2012;44:157–165.
8. Tsai HJ, Wu CC, Tsai CR, Lin SF, Chen LT, Chang JS. The epidemiology of neuroendocrine tumors in Taiwan: A nation-wide cancer registry-based study. *PLoS One* 2013;8:e62487.
9. Scarpa A, Chang DK, Nones K, et al. Whole-genome landscape of pancreatic neuroendocrine tumours. *Nature* 2017;543:65–71.
10. Jiao Y, Shi C, Edil BH, et al. DAXX/ATRX, MEN1, and mTOR pathway genes are frequently altered in pancreatic neuroendocrine tumors. *Science* 2011;331:1199–1203.
11. Banck MS, Kanwar R, Kulkarni AA, et al. The genomic landscape of small intestinal neuroendocrine tumors. *J Clin Invest* 2013;123:2502–2508.
12. Vinik AI, Chaya C. Clinical presentation and diagnosis of neuroendocrine tumors. *Hematol Oncol Clin North Am* 2016;30:21–48.
13. Onaitis MW, Kirshbom PM, Hayward TZ, et al. Gastrointestinal carcinoids: Characterization by site of origin and hormone production. *Ann Surg* 2000;232:549–556.
14. Bhattacharyya S, Davar J, Dreyfus G, Caplin ME. Carcinoid heart disease. *Circulation* 2007; 116:2860–2865.
15. Bell HK, Poston GJ, Vora J, Wilson NJ. Cutaneous manifestations of the malignant carcinoid syndrome. *Br J Dermatol* 2005;152:71–75.
16. Wermers RA, Fatourechi V, Wynne AG, Kvols LK, Lloyd RV. The glucaconoma syndrome. Clinical and pathologic features in 21 patients. *Medicine (Baltimore)* 1996;75:53–63.
17. Ghaferi AA, Chojnacki KA, Long WD, Cameron JL, Yeo CJ. Pancreatic VIPomas: Subject review and one institutional experience. *J Gastrointest Surg* 2008;12:382–393.
18. O'Toole D, Grossman A, Gross D, et al. ENETS consensus guidelines for the standards of care in neuroendocrine tumors: Biochemical markers. *Neuroendocrinology* 2009;90:194–202.
19. Campana D, Nori F, Piscitelli L, et al. Chromogranin A: Is it a useful marker of endocrine tumors?. *J Clin Oncol* 2007;25:1967–1973.

20. Modlin IM, Gustafsson BI, Moss SF, Pavel M, Tsolakis AV, Kidd M. Chromogranin A—biological function and clinical utility in neuroendocrine tumor disease. *Ann Surg Oncol* 2010;17: 2427–2443.

21. Hakim FA, Alexander JA, Huprich JE, Grover M, Enders FT. CT-enterography may identify small bowel tumors not detected by capsule endoscopy: Eight years experience at Mayo Clinic Rochester. *Dig Dis Sci* 2011;56:2914–2919.

22. Sandowski SM, Neychev V, Millo C, et al. Prospective study of 68Ga-DOTATATE positron emission tomography/computed tomography for detecting gastro-entero-pancreatic neuroendocrine tumors and unknown primary sites. *J Clin Oncol* 2016;34:588–596.

23. Kulke MH, Hörsch D, Caplin ME, et al. Telotristat ethyl, a tryptophan hydroxylase inhibitor for the treatment of carcinoid syndrome. *J Clin Oncol* 2017;35:14–23.

24. Rinke A, Müller HH, Schade-Brittinger C, et al. Placebo-controlled, double-blind, prospective, randomized study on the effect of octreotide LAR in the control of tumor growth in patients with metastatic neuroendocrine midgut tumors: A report from the PROMID Study Group. *J Clin Oncol* 2009;27:4656–4663.

25. Caplin ME, Pavel M, Ćwikła JB, et al. Lanreotide in metastatic enteropancreatic neuroendocrine tumors. *N Engl J Med* 2014;371:224–233.

26. Yao JC, Fazio N, Singh S, et al. Everolimus for the treatment of advanced, non-functional neuroendocrine tumours of the lung or gastrointestinal tract (RADIANT-4): A randomised, placebo-controlled, phase 3 study. *Lancet* 2016;387:968–977.

27. Strosberg J, El-Haddad G, Wolin E, et al. Phase 3 trial of ^{177}Lu-Dotatate for midgut neuroendocrine tumors. *N Engl J Med* 2017;376:125–135.

28. Mayo SC, de Jong MC, Pulitano C, et al. Surgical management of hepatic neuroendocrine tumor metastasis: Results from an international multi-institutional analysis. *Ann Surg Oncol* 2010;17:3129–3136.

29. Glazer ES, Tseng JF, Al-Refaie W, et al. Long-term survival after surgical management of neuroendocrine hepatic metastases. *HPB (Oxford)* 2010;12:427–433.

30. Kulke MH, Shah MH, Benson AB 3rd, et al. Neuroendocrine tumors, version 1.2015. *J Natl Compr Canc Netw* 2015;13:78–108.

Polyendocrine Syndromes   39

Jing W. Hughes, Andrea Granados,
and Janet B. McGill

GENERAL PRINCIPLES

- Polyendocrinopathy is a heterogeneous group of disorders leading to destruction or dysfunction of multiple endocrine glands and possibly involving other tissues. The pathogenesis may be immune-mediated, infiltrative, cellular destruction due to various genetic defects, or a combination thereof.
- The autoimmune polyendocrine syndromes (APS) are the most commonly encountered of the polyendocrinopathies, and are characterized by loss of immune tolerance to self-antigens leading to autoimmune destruction of endocrine glands and other tissues.
- Thomas Addison was the first to describe the clinical and pathologic features of adrenocortical failure in patients with pernicious anemia (PA) in 1849.[1] Later, Schmidt described the occurrence of lymphocytic infiltrates of thyroid and adrenal glands in autopsy specimens of two patients dying from addisonian crisis (Schmidt syndrome).[2]
- APS (previously autoimmune polyglandular syndrome) can be classified into APS type 1 (APS1) and APS types 2–4 (APS2, APS3, APS4). Their features are summarized in Table 39-1.

TREATMENT

- At the present time, there are no safe and effective therapies targeting the generalized autoimmunity that underlies the pathogenesis of the APSs. Patients with APS require close monitoring, and the clinician should maintain a high index of suspicion for the development of additional autoimmune diseases in these individuals.
- Therapies for the individual components of the syndromes are discussed in other chapters and the management of each disease is essentially the same for the patient with APS. A few points deserve special consideration:
  - Patients with APS1 and chronic oral candidiasis should be treated aggressively with antifungal medication (fluconazole) and closely monitored given the elevated risk of oral cancers in these individuals. In addition, good oral hygiene and abstinence from smoking and alcohol is helpful to prevent candidiasis.
  - Thyroid hormone replacement in a patient with hypothyroidism may precipitate life-threatening adrenal crisis if concomitant adrenal insufficiency is present. It is wise to evaluate adrenal function by dynamic testing in patients with multiple autoimmune endocrinopathies prior to starting levothyroxine therapy.
  - Hypoglycaemic episodes and a decreasing insulin requirement in a type 1 diabetic can be one of the earliest signs of the development of adrenal failure.
  - PA is treated by oral vitamin B12 in high doses or intramuscular injections of cyanocobalamin.
  - Celiac disease generally responds to a gluten-free diet; however, mineral and vitamin supplementation may be required if significant malabsorption persists.

MONITORING/FOLLOW-UP

- A high index of suspicion is required whenever one autoimmune disease is diagnosed in order to prevent morbidity and mortality from other associated diseases.

TABLE 39-1 AUTOIMMUNE POLYENDOCRINE SYNDROMES

	APS-1	APS-2 (type 2–4)
Prevalence	**Rare**	**Common**
Onset	Infancy/early childhood	Late childhood, adulthood
Genetics	*AIRE* (chromosome21), autosomal recessive	Polygenic, HLA association
Gender	Male = female	Female > male
Common phenotype	Mucocutaneous candidiasis Hypoparathyroidism Adrenal insufficiency Ungual dystrophy Enamel hypoplasia	Adrenal insufficiency Type 1 diabetes Thyroiditis
Associated conditions	Hypogonadism Alopecia Vitiligo Celiac disease Type 1 diabetes Pernicious anemia Thyroiditis Chronic active hepatitis	Hypogonadism Alopecia Vitiligo Pernicious anemia Myasthenia gravis Celiac disease Rheumatoid arthritis Sjögren syndrome

APS, autoimmune polyglandular syndrome; *AIRE*, autoimmune regulator gene, chromosome 21; HLA, human leukocyte antigen.

- Follow-up of children with chronic candidiasis is of particular importance. Children with chronic candidiasis infection should be screened and observed for APS1.
- Follow-up with a specialist, particularly an endocrinologist, is advised.
- Proper psychological and social support is important for these patients.
- Patients should be educated about symptoms of potential new serious components.
- Patients should be provided with appropriate written instructions or should be advised to wear medical alert bracelets in case of emergent situations.

AUTOIMMUNE POLYENDOCRINE SYNDROME 1

General Principles

Definition
- APS1—also called autoimmune polyendocrinopathy-candidiasis-ectodermal dystrophy (APECED)—is a rare monogenic autosomal recessive autoimmune disorder consisting of the **classical triad of chronic mucocutaneous candidiasis, hypoparathyroidism, and adrenal insufficiency (Addison disease)**. APECED develops in childhood and results in tissue-specific autoimmunity, leading to loss of function in multiple organs.
- Apart from the major clinical manifestations, primary hypogonadism, type 1 diabetes mellitus, autoimmune thyroid disease, lymphocytic hypophysitis, chronic atrophic

gastritis with PA, celiac disease, alopecia, vitiligo, and autoimmune hepatitis have also been reported in APS1. Type 1 diabetes mellitus and autoimmune thyroid disease are seen less commonly than in other APS types.

Epidemiology

APS1 is a rare condition, most commonly prevalent in the Sardinians (1:14,000), Finns (1:25,000), and Jewish people of Iranian descent (1:9000).[3]

Etiology

- APS1 is caused by mutations in *AIRE* gene (21.q22.3),[4] which encodes the AIRE protein, a transcription factor exclusively expressed in the medullary thymic epithelial cells. The AIRE protein mediates the expression of peripheral tissue antigens, a function that is required for the deletion of auto reactive T-cells and the establishment of self-tolerance. Mutations in this gene presumably lead to incomplete negative selection and escape to the periphery of self-reactive T-cells, which in turn, initiate the destruction of self-tissues.[5] Approximately 60 types of mutations in *AIRE* gene have been reported thus far.[6]
- The presence of a mutation in the *AIRE* gene leads to proliferation of self-reactive T-cells and formation of autoantibodies with destruction of affected organs.[7,8]

Diagnosis

Clinical Presentation

History

- A complete and thorough history including family history is essential for the proper evaluation and management of patients with the APSs.
- Chronic infection of the skin and mucous membranes with *candida albicans* usually occurs as the first major manifestation of APS1, typically presenting in infancy. It is present in 97% of cases by 30 years of age.[6]
- Clinical symptoms of oral candidiasis include soreness, redness, oral ulceration, and white-gray plaques in the mouth. Esophageal inflammation causes odynophagia and substernal pain. Involvement of intestines causes abdominal pain, flatulence, and diarrhea. Infection of skin manifests with rash, chronic onychomycosis of fingernails and toenails and genital discharge. Transformation to squamous cell carcinoma has been reported when oral and esophageal candidiasis is not strictly controlled.[9]
- Hypoparathyroidism is the second most common major component of APS1 and presents with symptoms of hypocalcaemia including muscle cramps, tetany, circumoral paraesthesia, and seizures, as well as airway obstruction when severe. Hypoparathyroidism usually presents before the 10th birthday.
- Adrenal insufficiency is typically the last major component of the syndrome to develop and presents with symptoms of fatigue, salt craving, weight loss, hyperpigmentation of the skin and mucous membranes, and hypotension. The mean age of diagnosing adrenal insufficiency is 15 years.
- In some cases, these major components may be preceded by symptoms of chronic diarrhea, keratitis, periodic rash with fever, severe constipation, autoimmune hepatitis, alopecia or vitiligo.[9]

Physical Examination

- Evidence of mucocutaneous candidiasis, dental enamel hypoplasia, and nail dystrophy are seen in APS1.
- Presence of Chvostek and Trousseau signs, muscle twitching and cramping suggest hypoparathyroidism.

- Orthostatic hypotension, fatigue, hyponatremia and hyperkalemia are signs of adrenal insufficiency. Adrenal insufficiency that is not diagnosed for a lengthy period of time may lead to Nelson syndrome, characterized by high ACTH and hyperpigmentation with characteristic darkening of the palmar creases.

Diagnostic Criteria

APS1: Classic diagnostic criterion consists of presence of at least two of the major components: chronic mucocutaneous candidiasis, hypoparathyroidism, and primary adrenocortical insufficiency. Confirmation by genetic testing is recommended.

AUTOIMMUNE POLYENDOCRINE SYNDROME 2–4

General Principles

Definition

- **APS2** is characterized by the coexistence of autoimmune adrenal insufficiency with autoimmune thyroid disease and/or type 1 diabetes mellitus. It is more common than APS1. The components may not be diagnosed concurrently; consequently, the entire syndrome may not be manifest until adulthood. The presence of autoimmune adrenal insufficiency and autoimmune thyroiditis was previously termed Schmidt syndrome. The combination of type 1 diabetes mellitus with autoimmune adrenal insufficiency and/or autoimmune thyroiditis and was called the Carpenter syndrome.[10]
- Patients with the more common organ-specific autoimmune disorders such as type 1 diabetes, and autoimmune thyroid disease commonly have coexisting endocrinopathies without the presence of Addison disease. Hence, some experts have proposed to classify them into APS3 and APS4.[11]
- **APS3** presents with the same group of disorders as APS2 but without any defect of adrenal cortex.
- **APS4** includes atypical combinations of two or more organ-specific autoimmune diseases that do not fall into either of the above types, such as the presentation of APS2 with mucocutaneous candidiasis.
- As in APS1, autoimmune involvement of other organs is not uncommon, and may include primary hypogonadism, type 1 diabetes mellitus, chronic thyroiditis, lymphocytic hypophysitis, chronic atrophic gastritis with PA, celiac disease, alopecia, vitiligo, and autoimmune hepatitis.

Epidemiology

- APS2 is has an estimated prevalence in the general population of 1.4 to 2.0 per 100,000.[11] This syndrome occurs in approximately half of the cases of autoimmune Addison disease.[12] It is three times more common in females. Adrenal failure is the initial endocrine abnormality in approximately half the cases.[2]
- APS3 and 4 are the most common, with prevalence of up to 1% of the population.

Etiology

Familial clustering of APS2 and its component disorders suggest a strong genetic component. Pedigree analyses of most APS2 families suggest polygenic inheritance. The association with HLA alleles in chromosome 6p21 has been recognized with autoimmune diseases for several decades. The class II HLA haplotypes DR3 and DR4 are strongly linked with component disorders of this syndrome. The highest risk of development of both Addison disease and type 1 diabetes mellitus is associated with a heterozygous HLA-DR4-DQ8/HLA-DR3-DQ2 genotype.[7] Non-HLA genes including cytotoxic T lymphocyte antigen 4 (CTLA4) and interactions with the environment has also been proposed in pathogenesis of APS2.[8]

Risk Factors

- Apart from genetic factors, environmental factors have been associated with APS2. Administration of interferon-α has been associated with development of 21-hydroxylase autoantibodies, islet autoantibodies, and thyroid autoantibodies along with their respective autoimmune diseases.[7]
- Pregnancy is generally associated with decreased immune function; however, postpartum thyroiditis has been observed in approximately one-third of patients with type 1 diabetes.
- Prolamins, or proteins rich in proline and glutamine that resist intestinal peptidases, are known triggers for celiac disease. Gliadin (from wheat) and related proteins in barley, rye, corn, and some oats are implicated in the pathogenesis of celiac disease.
- The hygiene hypothesis proposes that a decline in communicable diseases, especially helminthic infestation, contributes to an increase in the incidence of allergy, asthma, and autoimmune diseases.[13]

Diagnosis

Clinical Presentation

History

- Family history and knowledge of increased risks for other endocrine disorders is key to the diagnosis of a polyendocrinopathy syndrome.
- Adrenal involvement is the initial manifestation of APS2 in half the cases. Other components may precede the diagnosis of adrenal insufficiency or follow it by years to decades.
- History of polyuria and polydipsia suggests presence of type 1 diabetes mellitus while weight gain/weight loss, heat/cold intolerance, and constipation/hyperdefection suggests autoimmune thyroid disease.
- Amenorrhea and hot flashes in a young woman should prompt a work-up for ovarian failure, whereas decreased libido and sexual function may suggest testicular failure in males. In both cases, gonadotropins LH and FSH will be elevated, while estrogen and testosterone are low. Specific gonadal antibodies have not been identified, so these diagnoses are based on physiologic diagnosis in susceptible individuals.
- Patchy depigmentation of skin, loss of hair, papulovesicular rash, unexplained anemia, chronic diarrhea, or jaundice is typical manifestations of the secondary-associated autoimmune diseases including vitiligo, alopecia areata/totalis, PA, celiac disease, or autoimmune hepatitis.
- Development of additional endocrine disorders may complicate the clinical picture of the pre-existing disease. For example, symptomatic hypotension or hypoglycemia leading to a decrease in insulin dosing in a patient with type 1 diabetes may be manifestations of adrenal insufficiency. In a patient with autoimmune hypothyroidism and APS, an increase in requirement for thyroid hormone replacement to maintain euthyroidism may reflect malabsorption of drug due to the onset of celiac disease.

Physical Examination

- The signs of primary adrenal insufficiency include hypotension, hyponatremia, and hyperpigmentation (see Autoimmune Polyendocrine Syndrome 1 section).
- Patients with type 1 diabetes mellitus will present with hyperglycemia, generally developing more rapidly in younger patients but more slowly in older patients. (See Chapter 29).
- Slow relaxation phases of deep tendon reflexes and periorbital edema are signs of hypothyroidism, while proptosis, presence of lid lag, and fine tremors suggest hyperthyroidism (see Chapter 8 and Chapter 9)

- PA may present with anemia or symptoms of peripheral neuropathy. Undiagnosed, PA can cause profound anemia and neurologic symptoms including cerebellar signs and ataxia.
- Vitiligo and alopecia areata are less common components of all of the autoimmune polyglandular syndromes. Vitiligo associated with these conditions is progressive, with a nonsegmental distribution and often occurs at sites of friction and trauma.[14] Alopecia areata presents as patchy nonscarring alopecia and may progress to total loss of scalp hair (alopecia totalis) or total loss of body hair (alopecia universalis).[15]
- Itchy papulovesicular lesions on extensor surfaces suggest dermatitis herpetiformis, which is associated with celiac disease.

Diagnostic Criteria

- **APS2:** Diagnosis requires presence of autoimmune Addison disease with autoimmune thyroid disorder and/or type 1 diabetes. Autoimmune adrenal insufficiency is the defining component of this syndrome.
- **APS3–4:** The diagnosis rests on the presence of multiple autoimmune diseases in the same individual, diagnosed in any order and at any age.

Differential Diagnosis

- Several genetic and acquired syndromes include multiple endocrine organ failure or dysfunction. These polyendocrinopathy syndromes are listed in Table 39-2.[16–23]
- Other syndromes associated with specific autoimmune glandular dysfunction are noted to occur in conjunction with systemic lupus erythematosus, rheumatoid arthritis, or other collagen vascular diseases. These include type B insulin resistance, immune thrombocytopenia, autoimmune neutropenia, and hemolytic anemia.

Diagnostic Testing

- Many of the autoimmune disorders that make up the APS have long prodromal phases during which time tissue-specific autoantibodies appear in the serum. The repertoire of autoantibodies present in a given individual serves as a guide to diseases that may develop, as the risk for a given disease tends to increase as the number and quantity of autoantibodies targeting that tissue increases. For example, the 5-year risk of developing type 1 diabetes in first-degree relatives of affected individuals is >50% if multiple anti-β cell autoantibodies are present.
- The major laboratory approaches to the diagnosis of the APS are serologic tests for autoantibodies against involved glands and tissues, and evaluation of end-organ function and hormone secretion.
- IgG-neutralizing autoantibodies against type 1 interferons, including interferon-α subtypes and interferon-ω, virtually confirm the diagnosis of APS1 when clinical presentation does not fulfill the classic diagnostic criterion and when thymoma and myasthenia gravis have been excluded. Genetic testing to look for mutations in the *AIRE* gene is now available. A good laboratory can detect mutations in the *AIRE* gene in >95% of cases.[6]
- Evaluation for the presence of adrenal (21-hydroxylase), thyroid (peroxidase and thyroglobulin), islet cell (insulin, glutamic acid decarboxylase, and IA-2A), and parietal cell (H^+/K^+-ATPase) autoantibodies (Table 39-3) may assist in confirming clinical suspicion of tissue autoimmunity or in assessing risk for future endocrine disorders, although serologic testing should not replace careful clinical assessment of organ-specific diseases.
- Endocrine organ function should be evaluated by laboratory measurement of appropriate hormones: adrenal (cosyntropin-stimulation testing, serum electrolytes, aldosterone, and renin), thyroid (thyroid-stimulating hormone and free thyroxine), pancreatic islet (fasting glucose or glucose tolerance testing), parathyroid (ionized serum calcium and intact parathyroid hormone), and gonads (estrogen or testosterone, follicle-stimulating hormone, and luteinizing hormone).

TABLE 39-2   POLYENDOCRINOPATHY SYNDROMES

Polyendocrinopathy syndrome	Etiology	Clinical features
Chromosomal abnormalities (Down syndrome and Turner syndrome)	Unknown	Autoimmune thyroid disease, type 1 diabetes mellitus, celiac disease, autoimmune hepatitis, alopecia areata, vitiligo
DiGeorge syndrome, velocardiofacial syndromes OMIM 188400	Microdeletion of chromosome 22q11.2	Craniofacial, pharyngeal, cardiac dysmorphism, mental retardation. Endocrine: hypoparathyroidism, thyroid agenesis and/ or autoimmune hypo or hyperthyroidism, type 1 diabetes, ITP, GH deficiency
Hereditary hemochromatosis[16]	Mutation in *HFE* gene	Classical triad of hepatomegaly, diabetes mellitus, and hyperpigmented skin along with congestive heart failure Other endocrinopathies: hypopituitarism, hypogonadism, hypothyroidism
Hirata disease, also insulin autoimmune syndrome (IAS)[17]	HLA association with HLA DR4 + drug induction	Spontaneous hyperinsulinemic hypoglycemia. Has been associated with Grave disease, particularly if treated with methimazole
IPEX (immune dysregulation, polyendocrinopathy, enteropathy, X-linked)[18] **OMIM 304930**	Mutation in *FoxP3* gene leads to autoimmunity	Clinical triad of enteropathy (severe diarrhea), endocrinopathy (type 1 diabetes or thyroiditis) and dermatitis. Usually develops in neonates. Others: alopecia universalis, autoimmune hemolytic anemia, thrombocytopenia, neutropenia, interstitial nephritis, autoimmune hepatitis
Kearns–Sayre syndrome[19]	Deletion of mitochondrial DNA	Triad of progressive external ophthalmoplegia, atypical pigmentary retinopathy and cardiac conduction defects. Onset before 20 years of age Endocrinopathy: short stature, hypogonadism, diabetes mellitus, thyroid disease, hyperaldosteronism, hypoparathyroidism

(continued)

TABLE 39-2 POLYENDOCRINOPATHY SYNDROMES *(continued)*

Polyendocrinopathy syndrome	Etiology	Clinical features
McCune–Albright syndrome[20] **OMIM 174800**	Activating mutation in α-subunit of G-protein–coupled receptor	Characterized by triad of café-au-lait spots, polyostotic fibrous dysplasia, and multiple endocrine dysfunction Endocrinopathy: precocious puberty, acromegaly, prolactinoma, hyperthyroidism, Cushing syndrome, hypophosphatemic osteomalacia, testitoxocosis
POEMS syndrome[21]	Unclear; monoclonal gammopathy suggests plasma cell disorder, elevated cytokines, and VEGF are common	Polyneuropathy, organomegaly, endocrinopathy, M protein (monoclonal plasma proliferative disorder), skin changes (POEMS) Others: osteosclerotic bone lesions, Castleman disease, papilledema, edema, pleural effusion/ascites Endocrinopathy: hypogonadism, T2DM, hypothyroidism, adrenal insufficiency, increased PTH
Type B insulin resistance syndrome[22]	Antibody to insulin receptors (not commercially available)	Hyperglycemia, hyperandrogenism, SLE, Hashimoto thyroiditis, primary biliary cirrhosis, hypoglycemia (rarely)
Wolfram syndrome[23] **OMIM 222300**	Mutation of *WFS1* gene	Diabetes insipidus, diabetes mellitus, optic atrophy, and deafness (DIDMOAD) Others: hearing loss, neurogenic bladder, ataxia, dysarthria, dementia, psychiatric disease, other endocrine dysfunctions (hypogonadism, hypothyroidism, and growth retardation) occur in this progressive syndrome

GH, growth hormone; HLA, human leukocyte antigen; ITP, immune thrombocytopenic purpura; OMIM, the GenomeNet classification number; POEMS, polyneuropathy, organomegaly, endocrinopathy, M protein, skin changes; PTH, parathyroid hormone; SLE, systemic lupus erythematosus; T2DM, type 2 diabetes mellitus; VEGF, vascular endothelial growth factor.

TABLE 39-3	ORGAN-SPECIFIC AUTOANTIBODIES	
Autoimmune disease	Antibodies associated	Diagnostic test
Type 1 diabetes mellitus	Antibody to glutamic acid decarboxylase (GAD65), antibody to protein tyrosine phosphatase (IA-2A & IA-2β)[a], insulin autoantibody (IAA), antibody to zinc transporter 8 (ZnT8)	Fasting glucose, oral glucose tolerance test, hemoglobin A1c
Insulin autoimmune syndrome (Hirata disease)	Insulin autoantibodies (IAA), either monoclonal or polyclonal	Fasting and postprandial glucose for evidence of hypoglycemia, insulin and C-peptide levels, antibodies
Thyroiditis	Antithyroid peroxidase antibody (Anti-TPO), TSI (thyroid-stimulating immunoglobulin), antithyroglobulin antibody	TSH, free thyroxine (T4), total triiodothyronine (T3)
Primary adrenal insufficiency	Antibody to 21-hydroxylase (ACA), anti-17α-hydroxylase Ab, anti-P450scc Ab (SCA)	ACTH stimulation test
Autoimmune gastritis Pernicious anemia	Antiparietal cell antibody Anti-intrinsic factor antibody	Vitamin B12, measurement of antibodies, gastrin
Celiac disease	Antibody to tTG, antiendomysial IgA Ab, antigliadin antibody	Measurement of antibodies (in addition to serum IgA), small bowel biopsy
Hypoparathyroidism	Antibody to calcium-sensing receptor	PTH, serum calcium and phosphorus, 24-hour urinary calcium
Autoimmune hepatitis	ANA, antismooth muscle antibody, antimitochondrial antibody, anti-LKM1 antibody, anti-LC1 antibody	Liver function test, measurement of anti-bodies, liver biopsy
Hypogonadism	Antibodies to 17α-hydroxylase, P450 side-chain-cleavage enzyme, 3β hydroxysteroid dehydrogenase, antisperm Ab	FSH, LH, testosterone, estradiol, progesterone
Vitiligo	Antityrosinase antibody	Wood lamp examination

[a]Antibody to transmembrane protein of protein tyrosine phosphatase family is also known as insulinoma-associated antigen (IA-2A & IA-2β), IA-2A is also known as ICA512.

Ab, antibody; ACTH, adrenocorticotrophic hormone; ANA, antinuclear antibody; FSH, follicle-stimulating hormone; LC1, liver cytosol type 1; LH, luteinizing hormone; LKM1, liver kidney microsome type 1; PTH, parathyroid hormone; TSH, thyroid-stimulating hormone; tTG, tissue transglutaminase.

- In a patient with anemia, a low serum vitamin B_{12} level suggests PA which can be further evaluated with antiparietal cell antibodies, anti-intrinsic factor antibodies and fasting serum gastrin level.
- Patients with iron deficiency without a history of blood loss should be evaluated for celiac disease with tissue transglutaminase IgA autoantibodies and total IgA level. Endoscopy with small bowel biopsy is necessary for confirmation of celiac disease.

REFERENCES

1. Addison T. Anemia: Disease of the suprarenal capsules. *Lond Med Gaz* 1849;12:535–546.
2. Schatz DA, Winter WE. Autoimmune polyglandular syndrome. II: Clinical syndrome and treatment. *Endocrinol Metab Clin North Am* 2002;31:339–352.
3. Betterle C, Greggio NA, Volpato M. Clinical review 93: Autoimmune polyglandular syndrome type 1. *J Clin Endocrinol Metab* 1998;83:1049–1055.
4. The Finnish-German APECED Consortium. An autoimmune disease, APECED, caused by mutations in a novel gene featuring two PHD-type zince-finger domains. *Nat Genet* 1997;17:399–403.
5. Waterfield M, Anderson MS. Clues to immune tolerance: The monogenic autoimmune syndromes. *Ann N Y Acad Sci* 2010;1214:138–155.
6. Husebye ES, Perheentupa J, Rautemaa R, Kämpe O. Clinical manifestation and management of patients with autoimmune polyendocrine syndrome type I. *J Intern Med* 2009;265:514–529.
7. Eisenbarth GS, Gottlieb PA. Autoimmune polyendocrine syndromes. *N Engl J Med* 2004; 350:2068–2079.
8. Michels AW, Gottlieb PA. Autoimmune polyglandular syndromes. *Nat Rev Endocrinol* 2010;6:270–277.
9. Perheentupa J. Autoimmune polyendocrinopathy-candidiasis-ectodermal dystrophy. *J Clin Endocrinol Metab* 2006;91:2843–2850.
10. Kriegel MA, Lohmann T, Gabler C, Blank N, Kalden JR, Lorenz HM. Defective suppressor function of human CD4+CD25+regulatory T cells in autoimmune polyglandular syndrome type II. *J Exp Med* 2004;199:1285–1291.
11. Betterle C, Dal Pra C, Mantero F, Zanchetta R. Autoimmune adrenal insufficiency and autoimmune polyendocrine syndromes: Autoantibodies, autoantigens, and their applicability in diagnosis and disease prediction. *Endocr Rev* 2002;23:327–364.
12. Falorni A, Laureti S, Santeusanio F. Autoantibodies in autoimmune polyendocrine syndrome type II. *Endocrinol Metab Clin North Am* 2002;31:369–389.
13. Gale EA. A missing link in the hygiene hypothesis? *Diabetologia* 2002;45:588–594.
14. Taieb A, Picardo M. Vitiligo. *N Engl J Med* 2009;360:160–169.
15. Shapiro J. Hair loss in women. *N Engl J Med* 2007;357:1620–1630.
16. Utzschneider KM, Kowdley KV. Hereditary hemochromatosis and diabetes mellitus: implications for clinical practice. *Nat Rev Endocrinol* 2010;6:26–33.
17. Uchigata Y, Eguchi Y, Takayama-Hasumi S, Omori Y. Insulin autoimmune syndrome (Hirata disease): Clinical features and epidemiology in Japan. *Diabetes Res Clin Pract* 1994;22:89–94.
18. Torgerson TR, Ochs HD. Immune dysregulation, polyendocrinopathy, enteropathy, X-linked: Forkhead box protein 3 mutations and lack of regulatory T cells. *J Allergy Clin Immunol* 2007;120:744–750.
19. Harvey JN, Barnett D. Endocrine dysfunction in Kearns-Sayre syndrome. *Clin Endocrinol (Oxf)* 1992;37:97–103.
20. Dumitrescu CE, Collins MT. McCune-Albright syndrome. *Orphanet J Rare Dis* 2000;3:12.
21. Gandhi GY, Basu R, Dispenzieri A, Basu A, Montori VM, Brennan MD. Endocrinopathy in POEMS syndrome: the Mayo clinic experience. *Mayo Clin Proc* 2007;82:836–842.
22. Arioglu E, Andewelt A, Diabo C, Bell M, Taylor SI, Gorden P. Clinical course of the syndrome of autoantibodies to the insulin receptor (type b insulin resistance): A 28 year perspective. *Medicine (Baltimore)* 2002;81:87–100.
23. Rohayem J, Ehlers C, Wiedemann B, et al. Diabetes and neurodegeneration in Wolfram syndrome: A multicenter study of phenotype and genotype. *Diabetes Care* 2011;34:1503–1510.

Endocrine Effects of Oncology Drugs

Conor J. Best and Karin Hickey

40

GENERAL PRINCIPLES

Hyperglycemia

- Hyperglycemia is common in patients undergoing treatment for cancer both in patients with and without a prior history of diabetes and can be difficult to manage.
- **Glucocorticoids** are used for a variety of reasons in patients with cancer. Dexamethasone remains a mainstay in the prevention of chemotherapy and radiation-induced nausea.
  - Typical doses range from 4 to 20 mg, which may be given as a one-time IV dose with each chemotherapy infusion or as an oral treatment before and after each chemotherapy cycle.[1]
  - Dexamethasone is also given as treatment for cerebral edema in patients with primary central nervous system (CNS) tumor or metastatic disease to the brain.
  - Glucocorticoids have a direct cytotoxic effect on hematologic malignancies and are given in high doses for most forms of lymphoma, leukemia, and multiple myeloma.
  - Topical and systemic steroids are used to control graft versus host disease (GVHD) in patients who have undergone a stem cell transplant.
- **Targeted therapy or tyrosine kinase inhibitors** (TKIs) refer to a broad class of small molecule drugs which mimic ATP and inhibit signaling within cellular growth pathways such as PI3-kinase and Akt. These can induce insulin resistance by partially blocking the signal cascade downstream of the insulin receptor.
  - Many of these agents are still in development. Dabrafenib, a BRAF kinase inhibitor, induced hyperglycemia in 49% of patients.[2]
  - Drugs that inhibit **mTOR** (everolimus, temsirolimus) lead to a similar effect and can also induce hyperlipidemia due to alterations in lipolysis and lipoprotein lipase activity.[3]
  - The degree and duration of hyperglycemia depend on the agent, but are typically manageable with treatment.
- **Immunotherapy,** particularly antibodies targeting programmed cell death protein 1 (PD-1) or programmed death-ligand 1 (PD-L1), has been reported to induce an autoimmune form of diabetes (covered in the immunotherapy-induced endocrine dysfunction section).
- Treatment may need to be adjusted for alterations in food intake or use of **tube feeding** or **total parenteral nutrition (TPN)** in patients with alterations of their GI tract.

Bone Health

- Multiple drugs used for cancer treatment can lead to decrease in bone mineral density (BMD).
- **Glucocorticoids**, used as treatment for GVHD, when given in supraphysiologic doses for prolonged periods of time (prednisone 7.5 mg daily or higher for more than 3 months) can lead to significant loss in bone density. Steroids initially inhibit osteoblast action, resulting in decreased bone formation. With chronic use (more than 6 to 9 months) they can inhibit osteoclast function and bone resorption.[4] Glucocorticoids also lower calcium levels by decreasing its gastrointestinal absorption and increasing its renal excretion.

- **Endocrine therapy** is frequently used in estrogen/progesterone receptor–positive breast cancer and prostate cancer.
  - **Aromatase inhibitors**, such as anastrozole, letrozole, and exemestane, work by inhibiting aromatase, an enzyme that catalyzes the conversion of androgens to estrogens. Aromatase is present in the ovaries, placenta, testis, brain, bone, vasculature, and adipose tissue. In postmenopausal females, AIs are used as first-line adjuvant therapy of hormone receptor (HR)–positive breast cancer. In premenopause, they are used in combination with ovarian ablation. AIs lead to decreased bone density and increased fracture risk by inhibiting the beneficial effects of estrogen on bones.[5]
  - **Selective estrogen receptor modulators** (SERMs), such as tamoxifen and raloxifene, can be used for prevention of HR-positive breast cancer and treatment of HR-positive breast cancer in premenopausal patients with low risk of recurrence. Interestingly, SERMs have opposite effects on bone density depending on menopausal state. During premenopause they act as estrogen-receptor antagonists resulting in decreased bone density. Conversely, in postmenopause, they act as estrogen-receptor agonists, leading to increased bone density.
  - **Androgen deprivation therapy** (ADT) with lowering of serum testosterone levels is the main therapeutic approach in men with metastatic prostate cancer. This is accomplished by using a gonadotropin-releasing hormone (GnRH) agonist or antagonist. GnRH agonists (leuprolide, goserelin, buserelin) and antagonists (degarelix) worsen BMD by increasing bone turnover. They also increase the risk of fractures.[6]
- **Bone marrow transplant** has been found to be an independent risk factor for bone density loss. The decrease in bone density usually occurs within the first 6 to 12 months after transplant and recovery begins after 12 months.[7] Proposed mechanisms include the following:
  - Increase in bone resorption due to:
    - Renal dysfunction: decrease in 1,25 dihydroxyvitamin D3 production and secondary hyperparathyroidism
    - Calcineurin inhibitors (tacrolimus): decrease in renal function and osteoclast activation
    - Chemotherapy: hypogonadism causing decrease in estrogen and testosterone
    - Radiation therapy: hypogonadism
  - Decrease in bone production due to:
    - Malabsorption: decrease in calcium and vitamin D absorption
    - Renal dysfunction: calcium and magnesium wasting
    - Chemotherapy: direct inhibitory effect on osteoblasts
    - Radiation therapy: direct inhibitory effect on osteoblasts and decrease in growth hormone (GH) production

Immunotherapy-Induced Endocrine Dysfunction

- Modern immunotherapy uses antibodies to interrupt signaling between inhibitory antigen–presenting cells (APCs) and T cells, which typically functions to inhibit T-cell activation and prevent autoimmunity.
- By inhibiting these "checkpoints" and lowering the threshold for immune self-tolerance, the immune system can better recognize "neoantigens" produced by mutated cancer cells.
- The adverse effects associated with immunotherapy are typically variants of already recognized autoimmune diseases, although the presentation and the clinical course can be more aggressive and rapid than what is seen naturally. In endocrine organs the damage is often permanent.
- There are two primary classes of immunotherapy antibodies:
  - Antibodies that target cytotoxic T-lymphocyte–associated protein 4 (**CTLA-4**) on T cells interrupting its interaction with CD28 on APCs (ipilimumab)

- ◦ Antibodies that target **PD-1** (pembrolizumab, nivolumab) or **PDL-1** (atezolizumab, avelumab, durvalumab) on T cells and APCs
- ◦ As these events are rare, it is currently unclear if there is a difference in incidence of adverse effects within agents in the same class
- ◦ Use of the two classes in combination is FDA approved for treatment of metastatic melanoma
- CTLA-4 antibodies most commonly induce **hypophysitis** in up to 17% of patients.[8]
  - ◦ In one study, patients presented most commonly with headaches (86%) and fatigue (66%).[9] In 79% of the cases in which MRI was performed, findings consistent with hypophysitis were seen.[9]
  - ◦ Diabetes insipidus is less common but has been reported.
  - ◦ Primary thyroid dysfunction can occur but is less common.
- PD-1/PDL-1 antibodies can induce thyroid dysfunction in up to 19% of patients.[10]
  - ◦ The most common pattern of thyroid abnormalities on these agents is a **transient phase of mild hyperthyroidism followed by a rapid progression to profound hypothyroidism**. Radioactive iodine uptake and ultrasound are consistent with thyroiditis and can confirm the diagnosis if there is any uncertainty. There are rare reports of new-onset Graves disease.
  - ◦ **Type 1 diabetes and primary adrenal insufficiency** have been reported.

Reproductive System

- Anticancer drugs and radiation therapy frequently have been found to cause infertility, usually through **direct toxic effects** on ovaries and testis.
- Common chemotherapeutic agents known to cause gonadal failure include the following:
  - ◦ Alkylating agents: cyclophosphamide, melphalan, dacarbazine
  - ◦ Vinca alkaloids: vinblastine, vincristine
  - ◦ Antimetabolites: cytosine arabinoside (Ara-C), methotrexate, fluorouracil, 6-mercaptopurine
- There is a dose-dependent relationship between radiation therapy and infertility.

Thyroid

- Measurement of thyroid function can be unreliable in patients undergoing treatment for cancer due to illness or suppression of thyroid-stimulating hormone (TSH) by frequent steroid administration. Some therapies for cancer can directly, and sometimes permanently, impact thyroid function.
- Some **TKIs** can impair thyroid function, primarily due to inhibition of thyroid vasculature as demonstrated on ultrasound studies showing a decline in gland size and blood flow.[11]
  - ◦ This has been reported in sunitinib, sorafenib, and others. TKI development continues at a rapid pace, and drug-induced thyroid dysfunction should be considered in any patient on one of these agents.
  - ◦ There is some evidence that TKIs may also act on deiodinases to **inhibit T4 to T3 conversion**, seen clinically in an unexpectedly high levothyroxine requirement or a rise in requirement in patients who have had a thyroidectomy and has been reported with sorafenib, imatinib, and motesanib.[12]
- **Radiation** treatment to the neck, typically given for laryngeal or oropharyngeal cancer or Hodgkin lymphoma, can also induce thyroid damage and hypothyroidism.
- The immune effects of newer CTLA-4 and PD-1/PD-L1 antibodies have been described, but older cancer treatments also termed *immunotherapy* such as aldesleukin (recombinant interleukin-2), interferon-α, and thalidomide/lenalidomide are still used and can induce autoimmune thyroid damage, occasionally with a thyrotoxic phase.[13]

- **Bexarotene**, a retinoid X receptor antagonist now used less commonly for cutaneous T-cell lymphoma, induces central hypothyroidism and increases thyroid hormone clearance in almost all treated patients due to suppression of TSH production.[14]
- Euthyroid sick syndrome is common with cancer and treatment is not typically recommended.

Pituitary Gland

- It is well known that chronic high-dose glucocorticoids suppress the endogenous production of adrenocorticotrophic hormone (ACTH) by the pituitary gland, causing secondary adrenal insufficiency. Similarly, exogenous glucocorticoids frequently suppress gonadotroph hormone production and cause central hypogonadism. TSH secretion can also be decreased but does not result in clinical hypothyroidism. Opioid analgesics have similar effects on the pituitary gland.
- **Radiation treatment** to the hypothalamus and pituitary causes dysfunction in a large percentage of patients, but can occur even in cranial radiation not targeted to the pituitary, depending on the form of radiation, dose, and location.[15]
- Pituitary effects of bexarotene and immunotherapy are discussed in the thyroid and immunotherapy-induced endocrine dysfunction sections, respectively.
- A summary of the most common endocrine effects of anticancer drugs is illustrated in Table 40-1.

DIAGNOSIS

Hyperglycemia

- Serum glucose is typically checked with blood work **before** the administration of chemotherapy. Hyperglycemia induced or exacerbated by steroids can be missed until the patient develops typical symptoms of hyperglycemia or the hyperglycemia persists until the start of the next chemotherapy cycle.
- **Hemoglobin A1C levels are often unreliable** in patients treated for cancer because of alterations in red blood cell turnover due to chemotherapy or blood transfusions.
- Patients on targeted therapies known to induce hyperglycemia often require more frequent blood glucose monitoring, particularly if they are enrolled in a **clinical trial**. If hyperglycemia is induced directly by the chemotherapeutic agent it is classified as an adverse effect. Persistent hyperglycemia can lead to dose reduction or discontinuation of treatment. Adverse effects of chemotherapy are classified by grade by the Common Terminology Criteria for Adverse Events (CTCAE). In most trials, dose reduction or discontinuation is performed for grade 3 (fasting glucose 251 to 500 mg/dL) or grade 4 (fasting glucose >500 mg/dL) hyperglycemia that does not respond to treatment.[3]

Bone Health

Most patients with low bone density are asymptomatic until they develop fractures. Consequently, patients receiving long-term glucocorticoids (more than 7.5 mg of prednisone daily for more than 3 months) need to undergo screening for osteoporosis (see Chapter 26).

Immunotherapy-Induced Endocrine Dysfunction

- Patients on CTLA-4 antibodies should have **screening TSH and free T4 prior to each cycle** to detect early signs of hypophysitis. Findings suggestive of central hypothyroidism, new symptoms concerning for adrenal insufficiency, or new acute headaches should be evaluated by pituitary laboratory studies and MRI.[16]
- Patients on PD-1 and PDL-1 agents should have **thyroid function and serum glucose** monitored prior to each infusion. The onset of diabetes is often so rapid that only mild

TABLE 40-1 ENDOCRINE EFFECTS OF ANTICANCER DRUGS

Drug or drug class	Beta cells		Thyroid		Adrenal		Pituitary	Bone	Reproductive
	Hyperglycemia	Autoimmune DM	Hyperthyroidism	Hypothyroidism	Primary AI	Secondary AI	Hypophysitis	Loss	Hypogonadism
Glucocorticoids	X							X	X
TKIs[d]	X		X[b]	X		X			
PD-1/PD-L1		X	X[b]	X	X	X	X		
CTLA-4				X		X	X		
Aromatase inhibitors								X	
SERMs								X[a]	
ADT								X	
Alkylating agents									X
Vinca alkaloids									X
Antimetabolites									X
Bexarotene				X[c]					

[a]SERMs induce bone loss in premenopausal females and increase bone density in postmenopausal females.

[b]Hyperthyroidism is transient followed by rapid progression to hypothyroidism.

[c]Bexarotene causes central hypothyroidism.

[d]Depends on agent—not a class effect.

ADT, androgen deprivation therapy; AI, adrenal insufficiency; CTLA, cytotoxic T-lymphocyte–associated protein; DM, diabetes mellitus; PD, programmed cell death protein 1; PD-L1, programmed death–ligand 1; SERMs, selective estrogen receptor modulators; TKI, tyrosine kinase inhibitor.

hyperglycemia is typically present before the patient presents with acute hyperglycemia or diabetic ketoacidosis (DKA).

- Patients should be advised on the symptoms of hyperglycemia and asked to present for emergent evaluation with any new-onset polyuria and polydipsia. For a patient with pre-existing diabetes, immunotherapy-induced β-cell damage should be considered if he or she develops acute worsening of hyperglycemia that does not respond to usual therapy or a new insulin requirement with low C-peptide level. GAD-65 antibodies are positive in some, but not all, reported cases.[17]
- Other rare forms of endocrine dysfunction, including isolated primary adrenal insufficiency and hypoparathyroidism, have been reported.

Thyroid

- Thyroid function testing should be performed if the patient is receiving a treatment known to induce thyroid dysfunction or develops suggestive symptoms.
- Bexarotene induces central hypothyroidism reliably within hours of the administration of the first dose and empiric therapy is recommended.
- Patients who receive **radiation** to the neck should have thyroid function monitored long term. Onset of hypothyroidism can occur over 10 years after the radiation treatment.[18]

Reproductive System

- Males with hypogonadism usually complain of low libido, erectile dysfunction, fatigue/low-energy levels. Physical examination findings such as reduced muscle mass, changes in hair growth, or gynecomastia are not always present, as they can take a long time to develop. Laboratory evaluation includes a morning free and total testosterone level (ideally drawn between 8 AM and 10 AM), luteinizing hormone (LH), and follicle-stimulating hormone (FSH) (see Chapter 20).
- Premenopausal females develop amenorrhea, which can reverse after completion of chemotherapy. Laboratory workup includes estradiol, FSH, and LH levels. Anti-mullerian hormone has been used as a biochemical marker of ovarian reserve.
- In general, chemotherapy induces primary hypogonadism, with low testosterone/estradiol and high FSH/LH levels. Glucocorticoids and other drugs that affect the pituitary gland will cause secondary (central) hypogonadism, with low testosterone/estradiol and low FSH/LH levels.

Pituitary Gland

- Hypopituitarism presents with symptoms of hypothyroidism, hypogonadism, or adrenal insufficiency. (See Chapter 6 for details.)
- Patients who receive cranial radiation can have new onset of pituitary dysfunction **years** after therapy and should have appropriate monitoring. In a meta-analysis, GH deficiency was most common, followed by prolactin, gonadotropins, TSH, and ACTH.[15]

TREATMENT

Hyperglycemia

- Management of hyperglycemia during cancer treatment is primarily focused on **reducing acute symptoms and complications**, as the offending agent is usually temporary. However, long-term steroids are occasionally used for patients with chronic myeloma or GVHD. More aggressive treatment is indicated for patients at risk of dehydration or infection or who will undergo surgery in the near future.
- For new-onset steroid-induced hyperglycemia, **metformin** can provide significant improvement, but is often unable to compensate for acute hyperglycemia 1 to 2 days after chemotherapy. An additional agent such as a short-acting sulfonylurea can be helpful if metformin alone is insufficient. Metformin may not be advisable in patients with

fluctuating renal function or hepatic impairment or those who have significant diarrhea with chemotherapy. Many patients, and most of those with pre-existing diabetes, will require a **multiple dose insulin regimen** to achieve adequate control. Insulin may have to be redistributed to 60% to 75% prandial for patients on higher doses of glucocorticoids.

- Hyperglycemia related to targeted therapies can typically be managed similar to type 2 diabetes and is often relatively mild. For patients enrolled in a clinical trial of these agents, more aggressive treatment may be indicated to ensure that any hyperglycemia does not disqualify them from the trial or prompt a dose reduction in what may be an effective medication. If symptomatic, anticancer therapy can be held for 3 to 5 half-lives while treatment is started.[19]

Bone Health

- The fracture risks of patients treated with glucocorticoids as per the American College of Rheumatology are outlined in Table 40-2.[20] These patients should undergo a clinical fracture risk assessment **within 6 months** of the start of steroid treatment. Treatment is recommended for patients with moderate and high risk for fractures and for patients older than 30 years on very high glucocorticoid doses (over 30 mg daily or a cumulative dose of over 5 g in the past year).
  - Lifestyle modifications: balanced diet, smoking cessation, weight-bearing and resistance training exercise and maximum 1 to 2 alcoholic beverages/day
  - Adequate calcium and vitamin D supplementation: 1,000 to 1,200 mg of calcium and 600 to 800 international units of vitamin D daily
  - Medical therapy: oral bisphosphonates, IV bisphosphonates, teriparatide, denosumab, raloxifene (for postmenopausal women)
- Patients receiving therapy with aromatase inhibitors and premenopausal females on SERMs **should be treated** to prevent bone loss.[21]
  - T score >−2.0 and no additional risk factors: lifestyle modifications, calcium and vitamin D, and BMD measurement at 1- to 2-year intervals
  - T score <−2.0 and patients with any two risk factors (age >65, T score <−1.5, smoking, BMI <20, family history of hip fracture, personal history of fragility fracture, glucocorticoid use for <6 months): medical therapy as above and BMD measurement every 2 years

Immunotherapy-Induced Endocrine Dysfunction

- While most autoimmune adverse effects such as rash, colitis, hepatitis, and pneumonitis are treated by holding therapy and giving glucocorticoids, it is **unclear if there is any benefit to steroids** in most endocrine adverse effects. Instead, treatment focuses on identifying deficiencies, replacing the necessary hormones, and monitoring for possible recovery.
- Treatment of hypophysitis with high-dose steroids (1 mg/kg of prednisone daily) is **controversial**. Some experts recommend treatment in all cases, and others reserve treatment for severe headache or visual changes.[9]
- Recovery of some pituitary function is common, but persistent deficiencies can occur, **particularly of ACTH which rarely recovers**. Stimulation tests can be helpful to evaluate for recovery. Enlargement of the pituitary consistently improved on follow-up.[9]
- Immunotherapy-induced diabetes should be treated as **type 1 diabetes** with insulin and intensive care unit admission for DKA if present. Typically, no honeymoon period is present and C-peptide levels rapidly become undetectable. There are rare reports of patients being able to discontinue insulin.
- The thyrotoxic phase of PD-1/PDL-1–induced destructive thyroiditis is typically brief and mild. Propranolol can assist in symptoms, and there is no role for methimazole. **Progression to hypothyroidism is rapid**. TSH should be followed closely and levothyroxine started once it begins to rise.[22]

TABLE 40-2	FRACTURE RISK IN GLUCOCORTICOID-TREATED PATIENTS	
	Adults ≥40 years old	**Adults ≤40 years old**
High-fracture risk	Prior osteoporotic fracture(s) Hip or spine T score ≤−2.5 in men ≥50 years old and post-menopausal females FRAX[a] (CG-adjusted[b]) 10-year risk of major osteoporotic fracture[c] ≥20% FRAX[a] (CG-adjusted[b]) 10-year risk of hip fracture[c] ≥3%	Prior osteoporotic fracture(s)
Moderate-fracture risk	FRAX[a] (CG-adjusted[b]) 10-year risk of major osteoporotic fracture[c] 10–19% FRAX[a] (CG-adjusted[b]) 10-year risk of hip fracture[c] 1–3%	Hip or spine Z score <−3 **or** Rapid bone loss (≥10% at the hip or spine over 1 year) **and** Continuing GC treatment at ≥7.5 mg daily for ≥6 months
Low-fracture risk	FRAX[a] (CG-adjusted[b]) 10-year risk of major osteoporotic fracture[c] <10% FRAX[a] (CG-adjusted[b]) 10-year risk of hip fracture[c] ≤1%	None of above risk factors other than GC treatment

[a]FRAX calculator available at: https://www.sheffield.ac.uk/FRAX/tool.aspx?country=9.
[b]Increase the risk generated with FRAX by 1.15 for major osteoporotic fracture and 1.2 for hip fracture if glucocorticoid (GC) treatment is >7.5 mg daily.
[c]Major osteoporotic fracture includes fractures of the spine (clinical), hip, wrist, or humerus.

- Other rare endocrine autoimmune disorders such as primary adrenal insufficiency and primary hypoparathyroidism have been reported and should be treated as typical endocrine disorders.
- There is little evidence that holding immunotherapy reverses endocrine dysfunction, and if not life-threatening, **immunotherapy treatment should be continued**.

Thyroid

- **Levothyroxine** should be supplemented with a goal to correct TSH into the normal range. The effects of most agents are permanent and levothyroxine should be continued even when the agent is withdrawn, although the dose may be able to be reduced.
- Patients on TKIs may require higher doses of levothyroxine than is typically needed to normalize TSH.
- Central hypothyroidism induced by bexarotene resolves rapidly on discontinuation of treatment, but while treated patients may require 2 to 3 times more thyroid hormone than typically expected.[13]

Reproductive System

Options for fertility preservation in females include ovarian suppression and cryopreservation of embryos and oocytes. Males can use sperm banking as a means of preserving fertility.

Pituitary Gland

- Pituitary deficiencies should be treated by replacement of deficient hormones.
- Recovery from hypophysitis is possible and can be detected by routine monitoring of hormone levels. Replacement glucocorticoids should not be stopped without an ACTH-stimulation test confirming adequate adrenal function.

REFERENCES

1. Basch E, Prestrud AA, Hesketh PJ, et al. Antiemetics: American Society of Clinical Oncology clinical practice guideline update. *J Clin Oncol* 2011;29(31):4189–4198.
2. Welsh SJ, Corrie PG. Management of BRAF and MEK inhibitor toxicities in patients with metastatic melanoma. *Ther Adv Med Oncol* 2015;7(2):122–136.
3. Busaidy NL, Farooki A, Dowlati A, et al. Management of metabolic effects associated with anticancer agents targeting the PI3K-Akt-mTOR pathway. *J Clin Oncol* 2012;30(23): 2919–2928.
4. Canalis E, Mazziotti G, Giustina A, Bilezikian JP. Glucocorticoid-induced osteoporosis: pathophysiology and therapy. *Osteoporos Int* 2007;18(10):1319–1328.
5. Eastell R, Adams JE, Coleman RE, et al. Effect of anastrozole on bone mineral density: 5-year results from the anastrozole, tamoxifen, alone or in combination trial 18233230. *J Clin Oncol* 2008;26(7):1051–1057.
6. Nguyen PL, Alibhai SM, Basaria S, et al. Adverse effects of androgen deprivation therapy and strategies to mitigate them. *Eur Urol* 2015;67(5):825–836.
7. McClune BL, Polgreen LE, Burmeister LA, et al. Screening, prevention and management of osteoporosis and bone loss in adult and pediatric hematopoietic cell transplant recipients. *Bone Marrow Transplant* 2011;46(1):1–9.
8. Corsello SM, Barnabei A, Marchetti P, De Vecchis L, Salvatori R, Torino F. Endocrine side effects induced by immune checkpoint inhibitors. *J Clin Endocrinol Metab* 2013;98(4): 1361–1375.
9. Faje A. Immunotherapy and hypophysitis: clinical presentation, treatment, and biologic insights. *Pituitary* 2016;19(1):82–92.
10. González-Rodríguez E, Rodríguez-Abreu D; Spanish Group for Cancer Immuno-Biotherapy (GETICA). Immune checkpoint inhibitors: review and management of endocrine adverse events. *Oncologist* 2016;21(7):804–816.
11. Makita N, Miyakawa M, Fujita T, Iiri T. Sunitinib induces hypothyroidism with a markedly reduced vascularity. *Thyroid* 2010;20(3):323–326.
12. Abdulrahman RM, Verloop H, Hoftijzer H, et al. Sorafenib-induced hypothyroidism is associated with increased type 3 deiodination. *J Clin Endocrinonl Metab* 2010;95(8):3758–3762.
13. Hamnvik OP, Larsen PR, Marqusee E. Thyroid dysfunction from antineoplastic agents. *J Natl Cancer Inst* 2011;103(21):1572–1587.
14. Sherman SI. Etiology, diagnosis, and treatment recommendations for central hypothyroidism associated with bexarotene therapy for cutaneous T-cell lymphoma. *Clin Lymphoma* 2003;3(4):249–252.
15. Appelman-Dijkstra NM, Kokshoorn NE, Dekkers OM, et al. Pituitary dysfunction in adult patients after cranial radiotherapy: systematic review and meta-analysis. *J Clin Endocrinol Metab* 2011;96(8):2330–2340.
16. Dadu R, Zobniw C, Diab A. Managing adverse events with immune checkpoint agents. *Cancer J* 2016;22(2):121–129.
17. Hughes J, Vudattu N, Sznol M, et al. Precipitation of autoimmune diabetes with anti-PD-1 immunotherapy. *Diabetes Care* 2015;38(4):e55–e57.
18. Kumpulainen EJ, Hirvikoski PP, Virtaniemi JA, et al. Hypothyroidism after radiotherapy for laryngeal cancer. *Radiother Oncol* 2000;57(1):97–101.
19. Goldman JW, Mendenhall MA, Rettinger SR. Hyperglycemia associated with targeted oncologic treatment: mechanisms and management. *Oncologist* 2016;21(11):1326–1336.
20. Buckley L, Guyatt G, Fink HA, et al. 2017 American College of Rheumatology Guidelie for the prevention and treatment of glucocorticoid-induced osteoporosis. *Arthritis Rheumatol* 2017;69(8):1521–1537. Available at: https://www.rheumatology.org/Portals/0/Files/Guideline-for-the-Prevention-and-Treatment-of-GIOP.pdf

21. Hadji P, Aapro MS, Body JJ, et al. Management of aromatase inhibitor-associated bone loss in postmenopausal women with breast cancer: practical guidance for prevention and treatment. *Ann Oncol* 2011;22(12):2546–2555.
22. Morganstein DL, Lai Z, Spain L, et al. Thyroid abnormalities following the use of cytotoxic T-lymphocyte antigen-4 and programmed death receptor protein-1 inhibitors in the treatment of melanoma. *Clin Endocrinol (Oxf)* 2017;86(4):614–620.

Index

Note: Page numbers followed by f refer to figures; page numbers followed by t refer to tables.